MODERN MANAGEMENT OF ACUTE MYOCARDIAL

INFARCTION IN THE COMMUNITY HOSPITAL

MODERN MANAGEMENT OF ACUTE MYOCARDIAL

INFARCTION IN THE COMMUNITY HOSPITAL

Editor

Jeffrey L. Anderson, M.D.
Professor and Chairman
Department of Medicine
Division of Cardiology
University of Utah School of Medicine
Salt Lake City, Utah

MARCEL DEKKER, INC.
New York • Basel • Hong Kong

Library of Congress Cataloging-in-Publication Data

Modern management of acute myocardial infarction in the community
  hospital / editor, Jeffrey L. Anderson.
  p.   cm.
  Includes bibliographical references and index.
  ISBN 0-8247-8432-4
  1. Heart--Infarction--Treatment.   2. Heart--Infarction--Patients--
  Hospital care.   3. Coronary care units.   I. Anderson, Jeffrey L.
  (Jeffrey Lance)
  [DNLM: 1. Emergency Service, Hospital.   2. Hospitals, Community.
  3. Myocardial Infarction--therapy.   WG 300 M6895]
  RC685.I6M574   1991
  616.1'23706--dc20
  DNLM/DLC
  for Library of Congress   91-9917
                                                                        CIP

Marcel Dekker, Inc.
270 Madison Avenue, New York, NY 10016

Acknowledgement: The authors wish to thank the editorial and production
staffs of BioLiterature, Inc., Glenview, IL, USA for their assistance in the
development of this book.

This book was made possible by an educational grant from SmithKline
Beecham, Philadelphia, PA 19486.

Current printing (last digit):
  10   9   8   7   6   5   4   3   2   1

Printed in the United States of America

Editor: Jeffrey Anderson, M.D.
Editorial Support: Susan Rosenthal, M.D.
Editing Supervisor: Brian Green, M.Sc.
Book Design: Kern Kuipers
Production: Kathleen Green

CONTRIBUTORS

Jeffrey L. Anderson, M.D.
Professor and Chairman
Department of Medicine
Division of Cardiology
University of Utah School of Medicine
Salt Lake City, Utah

Michael J. Attubato, M.D.
Department of Medicine
Division of Cardiology
New York University School of Medicine
New York, New York

William R. Bell, Jr., M.D.
Professor of Medicine/Radiology
Department of Medicine
Division of Hematology
The Johns Hopkins University School of Medicine
Baltimore, Maryland

Andrew J. Buda, M.D.
Professor of Internal Medicine
Department of Internal Medicine
Division of Cardiology
University of Michigan Medical School
Ann Arbor, Michigan

Robert M. Califf, M.D.
Associate Professor of Medicine
Director, Cardiac Care Unit
Co-Director, Clinical Biostatistics and Epidemiology
Duke University Medical Center
Durham, North Carolina

Frederick Feit, M.D.
Department of Medicine
Division of Cardiology
New York University School of Medicine
New York, New York

Eduardo D. Flores, M.D.
Department of Internal Medicine
Cardiovascular Division
University of Texas Southwestern Medical Center
Cardiac Catheterization Laboratory
Parkland Memorial Hospital
Dallas, Texas

James S. Forrester, M.D.
Director, Division of Cardiology
George Burns and Gracie Allen Chair
Cedars-Sinai Medical Center
Los Angeles, California

Sidney Goldstein, M.D.
Professor of Clinical Medicine
University of Michigan
Head, Division of Cardiovascular Medicine
Henry Ford Hospital
Detroit, Michigan

Cindy L. Grines, M.D.
Director, Cardiac Catheterization Laboratory
Division of Cardiology
William Beaumont Hospital
Royal Oak, Michigan

Warren Grundfest, M.D.
Department of Surgery
Cedars-Sinai Medical Center
Los Angeles, California

Victor Gurewich, M.D.
Director, Vascular Research Laboratory
New England Deaconess Hospital
Harvard Medical School
Boston, Massachusetts

Richard Helfant, M.D.
Professor of Medicine
University of California
School of Medicine
Los Angeles, California

L. David Hillis, M.D.
Department of Internal Medicine
Cardiovascular Division
University of Texas Southwestern Medical Center
Cardiac Catheterization Laboratory
Parkland Memorial Hospital
Dallas, Texas

Richard A. Lange, M.D
Department of Internal Medicine
Cardiovascular Division
University of Texas Southwestern Medical Center
Cardiac Catheterization Laboratory
Parkland Memorial Hospital
Dallas, Texas

Frank Litvack, M.D.
Co-Director, Cardiac Catheterization Laboratory
Cedars-Sinai Medical Center
Los Angeles, California

Victor J. Marder, M.D.
Professor of Medicine
Chief, Hematology Unit
Department of Medicine
University of Rochester School of Medicine & Dentistry
Rochester, New York

E. Magnus Ohman, M.D.
Coordinator of Clinical Trials
Interventional Cardiovascular Program
Division of Cardiology
Duke University Medical Center
Durham, North Carolina

Joseph P. Ornato, M.D.
Professor of Internal Medicine and Cardiology
Chief, Internal Medicine Section
Emergency Medical Services
Medical College of Virginia
Richmond, Virginia

Jeffrey J. Popma, M.D.
Division of Cardiology
Department of Internal Medicine
University of Michigan Medical Center
Ann Arbor, Michigan

Jacob Segalowitz, M.D.
Surgical Research Fellow
Cedars-Sinai Medical Center
Los Angeles, California

Michael H. Sketch, Jr., M.D.
Associate in Medicine
Interventional Cardiovascular Program
Division of Cardiology
Duke University Medical Center
Durham, North Carolina

Bruce R. Smith, Pharm.D.
Philadelphia Association for Clinical Trials
St. Davids, Pennsylvania

Richard S. Stack, M.D.
Associate Professor of Medicine
Director, Interventional Cardiovascular Program
Division of Cardiology
Duke University Medical Center
Durham, North Carolina

H.J.C. Swan, M.B., Ph.D.
Professor of Medicine
UCLA School of Medicine
Senior Consultant in Cardiology
Cedars-Sinai Medical Center
Los Angeles, California

Eric J. Topol, M.D.
Division of Cardiology
Department of Internal Medicine
University of Michigan Medical Center
Ann Arbor, Michigan

G. Michael Vincent, M.D.
Associate Professor and Vice-Chairman
Department of Medicine
University of Utah School of Medicine
Chairman, Department of Medicine
LDS Hospital
Salt Lake City, Utah

Thomas C. Wall, M.D.
Assistant Professor of Medicine
Department of Medicine
Division of Cardiology
Duke University Medical Center
Durham, North Carolina

W. Douglas Weaver, M.D.
Director, Cardiovascular Critical Care
University of Washington Medical Center
Associate Professor of Medicine
Division of Cardiology
University of Washington
Seattle, Washington

Brian D. Williamson, M.D.
Department of Internal Medicine
Division of Cardiology
University of Michigan Medical School
Ann Arbor, Michigan

D. George Wyse, M.D., Ph.D.
Professor and Chief
Division of Cardiology
Foothills Hospital and University of Calgary
Calgary, Alberta, Canada

Frank G. Yanowitz, M.D.
Associate Professor of Medicine
University of Utah School of Medicine
Division of Cardiology
University of Utah School of Medicine
LDS Hospital
Salt Lake City, Utah

PREFACE

Progress toward understanding the pathophysiology of acute myocardial infarction has occurred in the past decade and has carried with it the basis for dramatic improvements in therapy. The central role of atherosclerotic plaque ulceration or fissuring as the stimulus for coronary thrombosis has been established beyond a reasonable doubt and has led to specific diagnostic and therapeutic maneuvers. The focus of therapy for acute myocardial infarction in the 1990s is coronary reperfusion, and coronary thrombolysis with plasminogen activators forms the standard approach.

The past decade has witnessed enormous growth in knowledge regarding reperfusion therapy with thrombolytic agents for acute myocardial infarction. Keeping abreast of this rapidly changing field represents a major challenge for the cardiologist, cardiovascular surgeon, internist, general practitioner, emergency room physician, and allied health care professionals who regularly see patients with acute myocardial infarction and related coronary artery disease syndromes.

For the 1990s, the critical role of reperfusion therapy has been established, particularly for patients with classic electrocardiographic and clinical findings who present within a few hours of the onset of symptoms and who have no contraindications to thrombolytic therapy. The challenge now is to apply this approach to a broader patient population using a more efficient delivery system. This is particularly important at the level of the community hospital, where the majority of patients with acute myocardial infarction in the U.S. are currently admitted.

The purpose of this book is to provide those who treat patients with acute myocardial infarction with a summary of current information necessary to provide optimal care. The emphasis is on practical application of medical information at the community hospital level. In planning this book, authors with a large experience in specific areas were chosen to summarize our current state of knowledge. In the first section, an introduction to physiologic principles of acute myocardial infarction management and the pathogenesis of the acute ischemic syndromes is provided. In the next section, the general principles of diagnosis and management are discussed. Specific attention is directed to the role of the emergency department in acute myocardial infarction care. Implications for the practicing physician of recent clinical trials of thrombolytic therapy are summarized, followed by a review of the status of other medical therapies during the acute phase of a myocardial infarction.

The thrombolytic agents themselves represent the next area of discussion. A summary of hematologic profiles of all thrombolytic agents is given, followed by specific discussions of the currently available thrombolytic agents anistreplase, streptokinase, tissue plasminogen activator, urokinase, and the experimental agent pro-urokinase.

The use of angioplasty as adjunctive or primary therapy in acute myocardial infarction is discussed next. Management of arrhythmias in the thrombolytic era is then presented, followed by a discussion of convalescent post-infarction management strategies, including medical therapies and dietary and life-style interventions. The use of imaging techniques for diagnosis and prognosis, in both acute and chronic phases, is reviewed. Future directions in the management of acute myocardial infarction comprise the last section of the book, which includes sections on out-of-hospital initiation of thrombolytic therapy and new device therapy in the management of the acute ischemic syndromes.

It is evident that thrombolytic therapy in the community hospital has progressed from experimental novelty to clinical reality and should form the mainstay of therapy in the 1990s. Although refinement and change will no doubt be seen in coming years, basic scientific principles have already been well established. These in turn provide the physician with general management guidelines for the reperfusion era. Substantial benefits have already been achieved in reducing patient morbidity and mortality. Additional benefits are expected as application of these strategies becomes more widespread and more efficient.

It is hoped that this book will provide an interesting and informative resource for the broad group of physicians and other health care professionals involved in the treatment of acute myocardial infarction at the level of the community and tertiary care hospitals.

I am grateful to my co-authors for their excellent contributions and to the many other individuals who have made this book possible. Finally, I would like to thank my wife, Kathleen, for her understanding and patience.

Jeffrey L. Anderson, M.D.
Professor of Medicine
University of Utah School of Medicine
Salt Lake City, Utah

ADDENDUM TO PREFACE

ISIS-3 and Thrombolytic Therapy in the 1990s: As this book goes to press, the preliminary results of the ISIS-3 study in acute myocardial infarction are becoming available (see also chapters on streptokinase and anistreplase). In ISIS-3 the three-way mortality comparison of standard doses of anistreplase (APSAC), streptokinase (SK), and recombinant tissue plasminogen activator (rt-PA, duteplase) yielded virtually identical results for the three agents (five-week mortality of about 10.5%).[1] In these comparisons, the streptokinase regimen had the lowest rate of cerebral hemorrhage; rt-PA had the lowest rate of allergy and hypotension but also the highest rate of cerebral hemorrhage. In the other comparisons, subcutaneous heparin therapy (12,500 u q12 h) added to thrombolysis plus routine aspirin (162 mg/day) yielded a modest additional mortality benefit (5 additional net lives saved and 3 fewer reinfarctions per 1,000 patients treated) at the expense of modestly increased morbidity (2 additional cerebral hemorrhages and 3 major bleeds per 1,000 patients treated).[2]

Why was the streptokinase regimen, known to achieve patency more slowly than rt-PA and APSAC, equivalent in its mortality effects? Three possibilities are suggested: 1) later or "plateau" patency rates (ie, at 3-24 hours or beyond), known to be similar for all three regimens, may predict relative mortality benefits better than very early (ie, 60-90 minute) rates;[3] 2) very early patency is still important, but the subcutaneous heparin regimen was inadequate (too little, too late) to maintain an optimal patency rate, especially after the short-lived rt-PA; or 3) the beneficial effects of thrombolysis are related to factors other than patency. The last possibility seems unlikely, given the wealth of data that show that groups of patients with patent infarct-related arteries, however achieved, have a substantially better prognosis.

The second possibility, that the heparin dosage was inadequate, especially in the rt-PA limb, has been hypothesized by the GUSTO study group (see chapter on rt-PA). GUSTO is testing full-dose heparin with either rt-PA or streptokinase as well as the combination of all three drugs. Five observations, however, make it unlikely that an alteration in heparin dosage and/or more aggressive thrombolysis will lead to *substantial* gains in *net* benefit or differences among agents:

1) Excess reocclusion rates after rt-PA without IV heparin as compared with IV heparin are lower when aspirin in doses of 162-325 mg is given, as used in ISIS-3 and GISSI-2 (ie, about a 10% differential rate), than when very low doses (80 mg) or no aspirin is given (as in the Heparin Aspirin Reinfarction Trial) [ie, about a 30% differential rate].

2) The rate of reinfarction was slightly (but significantly) *lower* for rt-PA versus streptokinase (or APSAC) in ISIS-3 and GISSI-2. Inadequate heparinization leading to excessive reocclusion after rt-PA would have been expected to lead to *higher* rates of reinfarction.

3) APSAC is more effective than streptokinase in achieving early (but not late) patency. When used with or without heparin, APSAC is not prone to the early reocclusion problem of rt-PA due to its long-acting effects. However, no incremental mortality benefit of APSAC over SK was noted.

4) The more aggressive thrombolysis regimens (rt-PA, APSAC) are already associated with an excess of minor bleeding events and more cerebral hemorrhages than streptokinase, even when given *without* full-dose intravenous heparin.

5) Subcutaneous heparin added only a modest increment in survival (0.5%) but at the cost of added bleeding risk. Patients treated out of protocol with intravenous heparin (about 3,000 units) showed similar survival in both the streptokinase and rt-PA groups but experienced about twice the rate of total stroke (2-2.5%). This raises concern that the risk of more aggressive thrombolytic and heparin regimens may outweigh further potential benefits.

Thus, the first hypothesis (plateau patency) appears attractive: achieving patency within the time frame of activity of streptokinase may be adequate to capture most of the mortality benefits of thrombolytic therapy. Faster coronary thrombolysis (as expected for rt-PA and APSAC) is either unable to salvage significantly more myocardium or the beneficial effects of thrombolysis are due to other mechanisms associated with patency, such as better ventricular healing and remodeling and rescue of border-zone myocardium by collateral blood flow.

Because all three regimens achieved an equivalent mortality result, the choice of agent in the 1990s must be based on other factors, including cost, safety, and convenience. Streptokinase plus aspirin and modest doses of heparin may be viewed as a desirable therapeutic option for the present, because of lower costs and lower rates of cerebral hemorrhage. The benefit/risk ratio of other thrombolytic regimens tested in the future should be compared with this standard regimen. Because the rt-PA and APSAC regimens are equivalent in their mortality effects, they may be useful in certain situations. rT-PA, which is non-antigenic, is preferred when readministration of a thrombolytic agent is required after initial use of streptokinase or APSAC, especially within the time window of five days to one year. APSAC, however, is the most conveniently administered of the thrombolytic agents. This may make it particularly well suited for initiation of therapy in the setting of the emergency department, community hospital, clinic, or paramedic van.

Beyond the selection of agents, the use of thrombolytic therapy in a greater proportion of AMI patients should be a continuing goal; only an estimated 20% of AMI patients received thrombolytic therapy in 1988. Despite exclusion criteria that limit the proportion of patients qualifying for therapy, it seems reasonable that about one-half of AMI patients should be receiving reperfusion therapy, based on current knowledge of its benefit/risk profile. Thus, more timely and broader application of reperfusion therapy remain an important challenge for the 1990s.

Jeffrey L. Anderson, M.D.

REFERENCES

1. Sleight P: ISIS-3 Trial: Results of SK versus APSAC versus t-PA. Presentation at the American College of Cardiology Annual Scientific Sessions, Atlanta, March 5, 1991.

2. Collins R: ISIS-3 Trial: Design and results of aspirin versus aspirin and heparin. Presentation at the American College of Cardiology Annual Scientific Sessions, Atlanta, March 5, 1991.

3. Sherry S, Marder V: Streptokinase and recombinant tissue plasminogen activator (rt-PA) are equally effective in treating acute myocardial infarction. Ann Intern Med 1991;114: 417-423.

TABLE OF CONTENTS

Section III
Thrombolytic Agents

Section IV
Mechanical Interventions

Section V
Other Post-Infarction Medical and Diagnostic Care

Section VI
Future Directions in Management of
Myocardial Infarction and the Ischemic Syndrome

This book is dedicated to the memory of
Dr. Jay Curtice, teacher and friend.

B.G.

INTRODUCTION TO PATHOGENESIS AND TREATMENT

Section I

Chapter 1

THROMBOLYSIS IN ACUTE MYOCARDIAL INFARCTION

H. J.C. Swan

CURRENT MANAGEMENT OF ACUTE MYOCARDIAL INFARCTION

Physiological Principles

Coronary atherosclerosis is not synonymous with myocardial ischemia or infarction; however, such disorders are uncommon in its absence. As evidenced by autopsy studies in young soldiers and by demonstration radiographically of early microcalcification, preclinical atherosclerosis is present in the majority of adults, including women, over many years. Adverse consequences can result from slow progression to severe degrees of coronary obstruction, clinically characterized by classical Heberden's angina, a relatively stable disorder. Alternatively, the outcome may be the development of an acute coronary syndrome, the consequences of which may be sudden, unanticipated, and potentially fatal. The acute coronary syndromes are characterized by an abrupt onset of symptoms of myocardial ischemia or infarction or a substantive worsening in severity over a short time.

It is necessary to separate the pathophysiologic matrix of the acute coronary syndromes into those issues which involve the coronary arteries and those related to acute and chronic changes in the subserved myocardium. Coronary artery disease by its nature affects differing branches of the coronary arteries to differing degrees; hence its effects on the myocardium are regional. As a cardinal rule, however, the processes that disturb vascular function are completely different from those pertaining to the myocardium. Each element is dynamic and interactive and requires separate consideration from both physiological and therapeutic standpoints.

THE ROLE OF THROMBOSIS

It has been more than 60 years since Herrick[1] used the term "coronary thrombosis" to describe the entity we now refer to as acute myocardial infarction (AMI). In the ensuing decades, clinicians have recognized the existence of acute coronary syndromes other than acute infarction. The large number of terms used for these entities — "unstable angina, intermediate coronary syndrome, accelerated angina, stuttering infarction" (among others) — indicates the various clinical courses sustained by many patients.

Up until a decade ago the primary role of acute thrombosis was widely questioned. Autopsy studies on patients succumbing from "heart attack" consistently demonstrated atherosclerosis (usually severe) in the culprit vessel, yet acute obstructing thrombus was found with only moderate frequency. In these reports patients with "sudden death" due to primary ventricular tachycardia/fibrillation were included, as were patients who had succumbed from myocardial infarction several days or even weeks after the acute event. However, it is now known that the mechanisms of arrhythmic sudden death do not necessarily include acute persistent coronary obstruction. Also, the now obvious possibility of spontaneous lysis some time after thrombotic obstruction in myocardial infarction was not considered. In 1980 DeWood et al[2] reported the angiographic findings in a series of more than 300 patients admitted for acute surgical revascularization for ongoing clinical myocardial infarction. Complete thrombotic occlusion was demonstrated in 87% of those patients who underwent cardiac catheterization within four hours of symptom onset. Patients studied later had a lesser incidence of complete occlusion, and those entering between 12 and 24 hours after onset showed only a 65% incidence of complete obstructive thrombosis of the culprit artery. This observational study has been confirmed repeatedly, and it is now accepted that acute thrombosis with complete obstruction of an epicardial coronary artery is the precipitating cause of AMI. Exceptions to this general rule are uncommon. Sherman et al[3] have also reported plaque ulceration and thrombus formation in patients with "unstable angina." In contrast, a thrombus is not commonly found in chronic stable angina.

The vascular pathology of atherosclerosis is complex, variable and multifactorial. Coronary atherosclerosis involves from a few millimeters to several centimeters of vessel wall, resulting in moderate luminal alteration with localized areas of severe luminal obstruction. Points of vascular branching may be particularly susceptible. The actual composition of an area of disease may differ markedly within and between individuals. The components of such lesions include cholesterol crystals, fibrous tissue, hyperplastic vascular smooth muscle, calcium deposits, and other elements. Lower levels of blood HDL and higher LDL cholesterol and undoubtedly other lipid factors favor the development of lipid-containing lesions and affect the stability of the surface endothelium. In addition, genetic factors may affect the integrity and other

4

characteristics of the endothelial cells. Mechanical factors, including turbulence and angulation, promote disruption of the endothelial surface and ulceration. Collagen, cholesterol, fibrous tissue and calcium comprise the "lipid gruel" and affect the inter-action between an ulcerated atherosclerotic lesion and the blood components. Activa-tion of platelets at the site of tissue damage is rapid, and the resulting platelet/ulcer surface complex is highly thrombogenic. Also, the absence of normally functioning endothelium may result in a variety of effects, including localized vasoconstriction due in part to the absence of endothelially-derived relaxing factor (EDRF) and to the exposure of smooth muscle to circulating or platelet-derived constrictor substances such as serotonin and thromboxane A2. A balance exists in which naturally occurring lytic substances ordinarily first oppose and then overcome the thrombotic process and pro-thrombotic factors, producing plaque remodeling, final healing and endothelial repair. If the developing thrombus is not spontaneously lysed or mechanically dis-placed, an acute coronary syndrome develops. If the vessel is completely obstructed for a longer duration, a myocardial infarct will result.

While pathologic studies suggest that ulceration and thrombosis occur in severely diseased vessels, it has been proposed that ulcerative lesions in "soft" vessels with more moderate disease but with a high cholesterol content may be in fact more throm-bogenic. The "ulceration-thrombosis" hypothesis[4] is presented in detail in Chapter 2.

DURATION OF OBSTRUCTION — THE TIME DOMAIN

All of the acute coronary syndromes can be modified by the availability of collateral blood flow. Collateral flow may prolong the time of survival in downstream myocar-dium to a greater or lesser degree. However, even the presence of predeveloped collateral vessels does not alone provide protection. Thus, profound hypotension will limit collateral perfusion and fail to prevent the morphologic changes of infarction in the myocardium of the territory at risk. Furthermore, if the culprit vessel is the source of major collaterals, the consequences will involve myocardium remote from the primary distribution of the thrombosed vessel.

The clear demonstration of obstructive thrombi in the coronary arteries in patients with AMI and in patients with unstable angina provides a rational basis for the use of thrombolytic agents. However, it is appropriate to consider the role of spontaneous lysis in the broader concept of the acute coronary syndromes per se. Does the efficacy of natural lytic processes determine the exact outcome and final categorization of an acute coronary syndrome? Is there a temporal hierarchy of the non-infarct states — unstable angina, prolonged myocardial ischemia and "ruled-out" myocardial infarc-tion? From intraoperative angioscopic examination in patients with unstable angina pectoris, non-obstructive thrombi are usual. The clinical syndrome could be explained by an incompletely obstructive thrombus changing in size or with superimposed vaso-

5

motion or vasospasm. Equally possible is a series of occlusive thromboses of short duration, responding to mechanical displacement or undergoing spontaneous lysis.

The extension of this hypothesis[5] to the other acute coronary syndromes suggests a model of complete coronary occlusion persisting for differing intervals, then relieved by a combination of intrinsic thrombolytic mechanisms, vasodilation, and mechanical displacement due to the pressure gradient across the area of disease (Figure 1). Thus, in unstable angina, if thrombotic occlusion is complete, it uncommonly persists for more than a very few minutes. In patients with "prolonged myocardial ischemia" the initial clinical state suggests AMI, and patients are usually transported to an emergency room. On arrival their symptoms have regressed or are absent, and the electrocardiogram shows non-specific ST wave abnormalities. This is consistent with spontaneous reperfusion occurring after 10-20 minutes of ischemia. On observation, T-waves flatten or become upright. A 30-40 minute occlusion followed by spontaneous thrombolysis is consistent with the syndrome of "ruled-out" myocardial infarction. Patients are admitted to an emergency facility and transferred to an observation area or a coronary care unit since important electrocardiographic changes persist. After a determination that cardiac enzyme levels are within normal limits, they are discharged. In actuality, 70 to 80% of such patients have important coronary disease

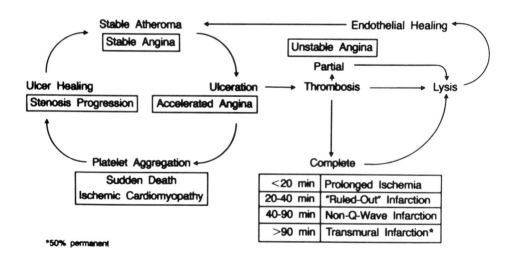

Figure 1. *Ulceration-thrombosis cycle (modified from Forrester et al [4]). Illustrated are the multiple potential clinical outcomes of acute thrombosis superimposed on an ulcerated atherosclerotic plaque. Determining factors include the severity of organic obstruction, the potential for hydrostatic displacement, the completeness and duration of occlusion, and the balance of thrombogenic and thrombolytic forces.*

and deserve a careful cardiac work-up to avoid recurrence of their symptoms or an AMI. Patients with an enzyme rise indicating necrosis include those with non-Q wave and acute transmural myocardial infarctions. Patients with non-Q wave infarction studied at 6 to 8 weeks following their hospitalization demonstrate a low incidence of completely occluded coronary vessels. The incidence of complete occlusion 6 to 8 weeks after transmural myocardial infarction is also less than 50%. Hence, it is likely that thrombosis plays a causative role in the acute coronary syndromes, but in many instances spontaneous thrombolysis takes place. Thus, extensive myocardial necrosis in the clinical syndrome of AMI could be attributed to the failure of timely spontaneous lysis.

Failure of spontaneous lysis may be due to the overwhelming thrombogenicity of the ulcerated intracoronary lesion because of its size, composition, or location. Also, major circadian rhythm fluctuations in plasminogen activator levels have been demonstrated, and PA inhibitor substances are also present in the bloodstream. Conversely, persistent thrombus may be due to a lack of necessary elements in the lytic chain or to an excess of circulating plasminogen activator inhibitors.

CONSEQUENCES OF PERSISTENT OCCLUSION

Myocardial infarction is due to a profound reduction of coronary blood flow to a substantive region of myocardium of a duration sufficient to cause its necrosis. Necrosis may result from deprivation of metabolic substrate, incomplete removal of metabolic product, both processes, or other mechanisms. Jennings et al[6] have elucidated the time course of myocardial necrosis in normothermic animals. Necrosis in the subendocardium commences 20-30 minutes after total occlusion and extends outward towards the epicardium. On average, the final transmural extent of infarction is completed at six hours. Areas of surviving tissue are found in the subendocardium, in the mid-zone of the myocardium, and extensively in the subepicardial myocardium. Since the dog possesses a moderately developed collateral coronary circulation, the time course of extent and completion is relevant to clinical applications. In patients with completed occlusion of the culprit artery, blood flow approaches zero in the most severely affected areas. The relevant time window for survival of this myocardium is dependent on the duration and magnitude of severe ischemia. A temporal sequence of morphologic changes and their therapeutic implications in humans has been proposed[7] and is listed in Table 1.

Limitation of infarct size following a total coronary occlusion may be facilitated by the presence of established collateral vessels perfused with an adequate systemic arterial pressure, spontaneous lysis of the occluding thrombus, or induced lysis. As a general rule, durations of occlusion longer than six hours will result in a completed infarct, the size of which will not be reduced by reflow. Hence, the benefits recently ascribed to antiplatelet agents administered later than 6 and up to 24 hours after

Table 1. *Morphologic subsets following complete coronary occlusion*

Subset	Myocardium	Duration of occlusion
I	Ischemic *	< 20 - 60 mins.
Mixed Pathology *	Ischemic + Necrotic	
II	Necrotic	> 20 mins. - 6 hrs.
III	Absorption of necrotic tissue	hours-days
IV	Healing	weeks-months

* Potential for salvage by thrombolysis
Adapted from Swan et al[7]

occlusion need to be explained by other mechanisms. These include reduction of the incidence of clinical or subclinical reocclusion, optimal remodeling, or a decrease in the incidence of cardiac arrhythmias.

Mechanical Function

Acute coronary artery obstruction causes a profound alteration in the mechanical function of the subtended myocardium.[8] Depression of global function is related to the size of the territory at risk, its compliance, and the presence of other mechanical burdens such as valve regurgitation, septal perforation,and primary or secondary arrhythmias, including heart block. Myocardial contraction ceases within a few seconds of acute coronary obstruction. During short intervals of ischemia, as in patients with angina pectoris, compliance of the affected myocardium decreases. Echocardiographic studies of ventricular wall motion at 4 to 12 hours in patients with large infarcts demonstrate akinesis or dyskinesis of the affected area. The presence of dyskinesis indicates that the contribution of contraction of the perfused myocardium is partially dissipated in distention of the severely ischemic/necrotic segment. Thus, without the protection of the contracting myocytes, the area of injury is subjected to successive distentions during systole which adversely affect not only surviving myocytes, but also the collagen matrix, resulting in less than optimal acute and longer term remodeling of the ventricle, with a higher incidence of aneurysm formation and ventricular hypertrophy, respectively. For relatively large infarcts, the increased compliance of the affected myocardium causes an acute, profound reduction in overall global function, even to levels causing cardiogenic shock.

While clinical trials have stressed the importance of reduction in all-cause mortality as an outcome of thrombolytic therapy — as they certainly should — this alone is an inadequate description of the anticipated clinical benefits. Reduction in morbidity as well as mortality can be expected as a consequence of salvage of ventricular myocardium. The temporal relation of symptom duration, treatment onset and outcome demonstrates that very early treatment causes a statistically significant and clinically important reduction in 30-day mortality. If myocardial function has been preserved to allow for a 50% reduction in short-term mortality, one might anticipate that myocardial function in the surviving patients as a group would be greater than in those who had not received treatment. This evidence has been difficult to obtain because of the heterogeneity of study characteristics, the use of early (< 7 days) angiography during a phase of possible myocardial shunting, and changing physiological status. However, three-week studies have demonstrated remarkable preservation of left ventricular ejection fraction in patients successfully treated with thrombolytic therapy.[9]

SIGNIFICANCE OF THROMBOLYSIS

A reduction in short-term and one-year mortality has been associated with prompt therapy using several of the thrombolytic drugs currently approved for clinical use.[10] Also, in spite of doubt based on studies immediately after lysis, left ventricular function appears to be preserved in treated as compared to untreated patients. Pre-hospital treatment programs may allow for normal levels of performance. But the benefits of effective reperfusion may be far greater.

The natural history of intrinsic "myocardial capacity" as affected by successive episodes of myocardial infarction is shown in Figure 2.[8] In humans, peak capacity is achieved in the late teens or early twenties and declines thereafter. Since necrotic myocytes cannot be replaced, each episode of infarction causes a further reduction in myocardial capacity, with a greater likelihood of cardiac disability. Inappropriate levels of wall stress, even if transient, can cause severe creep deformation of the healing myocardium and adverse late remodeling.

Thus, the overall significance of thrombolytic therapy should be broader than the demonstrated short-term mortality reduction. If myocardial destruction is limited by reperfusion in many patients, this should be reflected in a lower incidence of cardiac enlargement, ventricular hypertrophy, chronic heart failure and perhaps even of cardiac arrhythmias. The stakes involved are high. Thrombolytic therapy offers the potential of accelerating the process of lysis when the natural mechanisms are ineffective or are overcome by intense thrombotic stimuli.

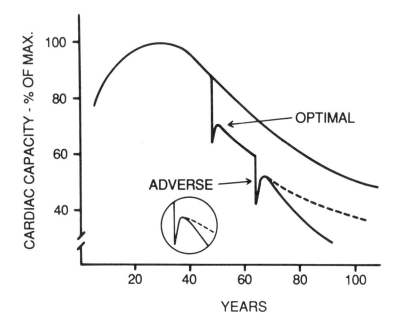

Figure 2. *Relation of intrinsic myocardial capacity to age and its modification by myocardial infarction and adverse remodeling (after Swan et al[8]). Myocardial necrosis reduces the available myocytes (left insert) causing a downward displacement of the age dependent curve. Adverse remodeling (right insert) causes an additional and progressive reduction in myocardial capacity because of chamber dilatation, scar formation, and myocardial hypertrophy and fibrosis due to increased ventricular wall tension.*

Although the ideal lytic agent or combination and/or dosing schedules have yet to be determined, the logic, principles, and efficacy of lysis of an obstructing thrombus in evolving myocardial infarction have been proved beyond any reasonable doubt. Debate must now center on those issues relative to the logistics of application, exclusion criteria, and post-thrombolytic management.

REFERENCES

1. Herrick JB: Clinical features of sudden obstruction of the coronary arteries. JAMA 1912; 59:220-228.

2. DeWood MA, Spores J, Notske RN, et al: Prevalence of total coronary occlusion during the early hours of transmural myocardial infarction. N Engl J Med 1980;303:897-902.

3. Sherman CT, Litvak F, Grundfest W, Lee M, et al: Coronary angioscopy in patients with unstable angina. N Engl J Med 1986;315:913-18.

4. Forrester JS, Litvak F, Grundfest W, Hickey A: A perspective of coronary artery disease seen through the arteries of living man. Circulation 1987;75:505-513.

5. Swan HJC: Acute myocardial infarction: A failure of timely, spontaneous thrombolysis. J Am Coll Cardiol 1989;13:1435-1437.

6. Rymer KA, Lowe JE, Rasmussen MM, Jennings RB: The wave-front phenomenon of ischemic cell death. Myocardial infarct size vs. duration of coronary occlusion in dogs. Circulation 1977;56:786-794.

7. Swan HJC, Shah PK, Rubin S: Role of vasodilators in the changing phases of myocardial infarction. Am Heart J 1982;103:707-711.

8. Swan HJC, Forrester JS, Diamond G, Chatterjee K, Parmley WW: Hemodynamic spectrum of myocardial infarction and cardiogenic shock: A conceptual model. Circulation 1972;45:1097-1110.

9. White HD, Norris RM, Brown MA, et al: Effect of intravenous streptokinase on left ventricular function and early survival after acute myocardial infarction. N Engl J Med 1987;317:850-855.

10. Rapaport E: Thrombolytic agents in acute myocardial infarction. N Engl J Med 1989; 320:861-864.

Chapter 2

UNDERSTANDING THE PATHOGENESIS OF ACUTE MYOCARDIAL INFARCTION
The First Step in Management

James S. Forrester, Frank Litvack,
Warren Grundfest, Jacob Segalowitz,
Richard Helfant

INTRODUCTION

Modern management of myocardial infarction derives from an understanding of the sequences of events on the blood vessel surface that precede and follow the clinical event itself. A clear understanding of these events has finally evolved with the ability to visualize the vessel surface at the time of clinical symptoms, using fiberoptic catheters that are passed directly to the culprit lesion. By comparing these photographic images to histology, it now is apparent that each of the common clinical presentations has a specific, identifiable intimal pathology. This chapter will describe how each syndrome is a stage in a predictable sequence of events at the intimal surface, and focus on how our understanding of these patterns has specific therapeutic implications.

THE STAGES OF ATHEROMA EVOLUTION: AN OVERVIEW

The clinical presentation of coronary syndromes is driven by two unrecognized cycles at the intimal surface which we will call the ulceration and the thrombosis cycles (Figure 1). The ulceration cycle consists of four stages: stable atheroma, endothelial

---

Acknowledgement: The authors are indebted to Dr. Meyer Friedman for retrieving his landmark histologic work from the 1960s and allowing us to republish four of his illustrations.

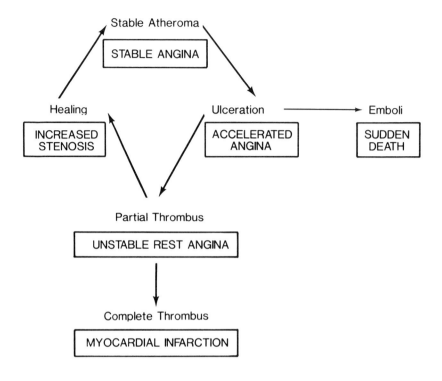

Figure 1. *The evolution of coronary disease in man: new definitions from coronary angioscopy.*

ulceration, platelet adhesion, and ulcer healing.[1] Each stage causes a different clinical syndrome. In stable angina the endothelium is smooth and unbroken and studded with smooth, yellow-white atheroma. When the atheroma ulcerates through the endothelial surface, the patient develops accelerated angina (increased angina frequency without rest pain). Platelet aggregates form on the ulceration.

The thrombosis cycle begins with endothelial ulceration. It also consists of four stages: partial thrombosis, thrombus evolution, thrombus incorporation and stable atheroma. Each stage of the cycle also causes a specific clinical syndrome. The partially occlusive thrombosis causes unstable rest angina. If the thrombosis proceeds to complete occlusion it usually causes acute myocardial infarction (AMI). If the thrombus embolizes, sudden death may result. During ulcer healing there is rapid progression of the coronary stenosis at the site, and a return to chronic stable angina.

THE PERIOD OF CLINICAL STABILITY
BEFORE THE ACUTE SYNDROME

The substrate upon which acute syndromes develop is chronic stable atherosclerotic disease, as illustrated in the following case:

A 65-year-old man presented with a two-year history of stable angina pectoris, 2.5 mm horizontal ST-segment depression during exercise, and a strongly positive thallium test consistent with multivessel disease. At coronary angiography he had greater than 90% stenosis in all three major coronary arteries. Figure 2a shows the typical angioscopic appearances of an atheroma in this patient with stable angina. There is a smooth, crescent shaped yellow-white atheroma protruding into the coronary lumen. The intimal surface is smooth and not disrupted. There is no subintimal hemorrhage.

The histology of stable angina shows a large mature atheroma with an intact intimal surface and a heavy fibrous cap (Figure 2b). At the base of the atheroma is an area of necrosis. Although most of the necrotic core is lost in preparation, macrophages still line its wall.

In patients with stable atherosclerotic disease this atheroma is typical. By angioscopy the smallest lesions are oblong and oriented along the axis of flow. The atheromas are typically eccentric rather than concentric. The atheromas exhibit several stages of histologic development that correspond to angioscopic observations. The small nonocclusive oblong protrusions are fatty streaks, which are composed predominantly of lipid-laden macrophages. Compounds released from macrophages and platelets stimulate smooth muscle cells to migrate from the media into the subintima. These cells lay down the fibrous cap. Thus in stable exercise-induced angina, the normal intimal surface is replaced by a heavy fibrous cap, but the intimal surface itself remains intact. The pathophysiologic basis of pain in stable angina is a transient increase in oxygen demand that exceeds the artery's capacity to deliver flow. Stable angina is, however, the only coronary syndrome in which this mechanism predominates.

THE PRODROME OF ACUTE INFARCTION: UNSTABLE ANGINA

Changes in the intimal surface herald the beginning of acute syndromes. The least severe of the unstable coronary syndromes is a dramatic increase in frequency of angina without rest pain, often called accelerated or progressive angina.

A 66-year-old male presented with a three-week period of accelerated angina, which was only partially responsive to nitrates and β-blockers. At angiography he was found to have severe stenoses in all three major coronary arteries. The electrocardio-

15

gram during pain revealed anterolateral ST-segment depression. Angioscopy shows the intimal surface is irregular and disrupted. There is subintimal hemorrhage, but no thrombus (Figure 3). Serial sections of this type of ulceration show progressive thinning of the fibrous cap at the point of rupture, often with subintimal hemorrhage.

The distinguishing feature between acute and stable coronary disease at angioscopy is intimal disruption. The ulceration is found in the coronary artery identified by electrocardiography as the "offending artery."[2] In our angioscopic experience, all but one of our patients with accelerated angina have had intimal disruption. The cause of this disruption is not established. There are two lines of thought, both of which are probably correct. The first is erosion from within. Atheroma almost always lies beneath the ulceration, and the evolution of ulceration bears a histologic resemblance to rupture-from-within induced by an inflammatory foreign body response.[3] The alternate explanation is a "stress fracture" induced by repetitive bending during cardiac contraction, particularly at points where the intima is made rigid by the atheroma. This theory is supported by the relatively superficial cracks that characterize the histologic appearance of many atheromas. Thus, intimal disruption causes platelet aggregation and subsequent release of vasoconstrictive compounds, leading to unstable angina with rest pain, the beginning of the thrombus cycle. This suggests that a minimal amount of intimal disruption can be tolerated without accelerated symptoms, and a moderate amount can cause an accelerated syndrome that resolves over days as the blood vessel surface heals. The third alternative is that intimal disruption triggers the onset of thrombosis. In this case, a partially occlusive thrombosis can lead to thrombotic occlusion or alternatively to lysis or incorporation with atheroma progression:

A 70-year-old male presented with new onset, unstable rest angina. He had an inadequate in-hospital response to nitrates, β-blockers, calcium channel blockers and heparin. The electrocardiogram showed transient inverted T-waves in the anteroseptal leads, but there was no serum creatine kinase elevation. His coronary angiogram revealed a 95% left anterior descending coronary stenosis. The angioscopic image (Figure 4a) recorded just distal to the stenosis shows a bright red partially occlusive thrombus. The thrombus surface undulated during infusion of the clear viewing solution, but was not dislodged. The histology of this type of lesion is a coronary artery with a partially occlusive intraluminal thrombus (Figure 4b). There is rupture of the fibrous cap that covered an atheroma cavity, and at the point of rupture there is thrombus formation. Beneath the point of rupture lies an atheroma. The thrombus contains cholesterol crystals, suggesting rupture of the contents of the necrotic core into the flowing blood stream.

Hyperacute unstable rest angina is characterized by partially occlusive coronary thrombosis when examined by angioscopy. All but one of our 12 patients in this group have had a thrombus, compared to none in our stable angina group. At autopsy, 90% of coronary thrombi are attached to an intimal ulceration.[4,5] Unstable rest angina, therefore, is usually due to a partially occlusive thrombus. Partially occlusive thrombus is difficult to distinguish from stable plaque by angiography.

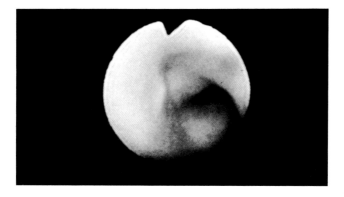

Figure 2a. *A stable atheroma seen in the left descending coronary artery of a patient with stable angina pectoris.*

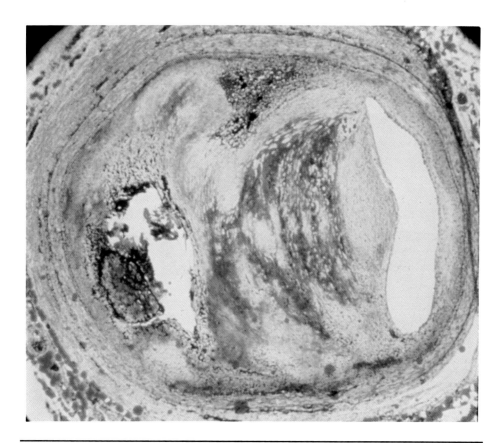

Figure 2b. *An atheroma with a necrotic core covered by a fibrous cap. Reproduced from Am J Pathol 1966;48:19, with permission.*

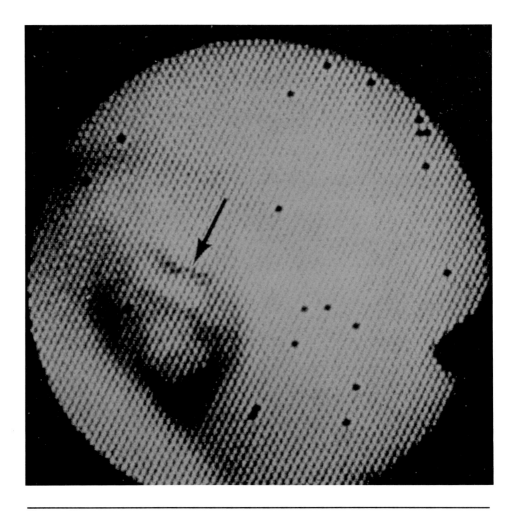

Figure 3. *An intimal disruption in the left descending coronary artery of a patient with accelerated angina.*

Unstable rest angina frequently resolves during supportive medical therapy[6] suggesting that spontaneous lysis is common; ie, that given time, ulceration with thrombosis also heals.

THE ACUTE EVENT: ACUTE MYOCARDIAL INFARCTION

Although unstable angina may precede myocardial infarction, about two thirds of patients with infarction present with a syndrome of sudden onset. In these patients, we assume that the thrombus that forms at the site of intimal disruption is sufficiently

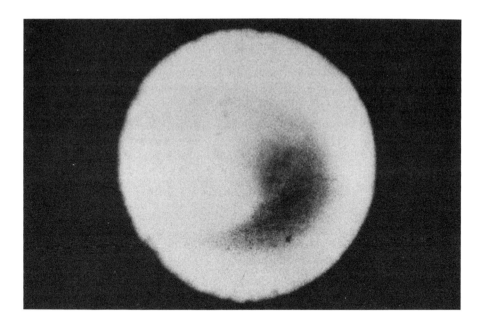

Figure 4a. *A fresh partially occluded thrombosis in a patient with unstable rest angina pectoris (courtesy Dr. Meyer Friedman).*

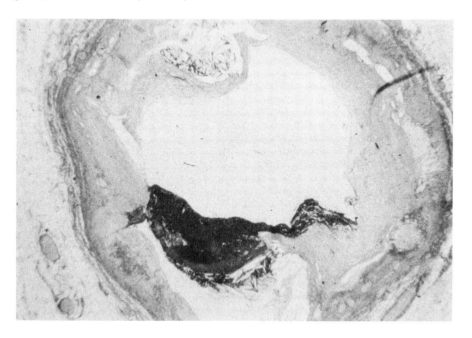

Figure 4b. *A partially occluded coronary thrombosis attached to an endothelial ulceration (courtesy Dr. Meyer Friedman).*

large to rapidly occlude the vessel. The remaining one third of patients probably have a partially occlusive thrombus that progresses to total occlusion over a period of days or weeks. From the world literature collected in the years prior to aggressive therapy we can estimate that 13-40% of unstable angina patients progress to myocardial infarction within the first few days or weeks.[7] Conversely, in patients who have an acute infarction, a prodrome of unstable angina was reported in 30% of patients.[8] This suggests that thrombus progression can be episodic, a concept supported by Falk's autopsy identification of two or more thrombus layers in 81% of the thrombi from unstable angina patients.[9] Thus myocardial infarction can result from a partially occlusive thrombus that progresses slowly and episodically to occlusion, or from an acute coronary occlusion.

Following a one-year history of stable angina, a 66-year-old man presented with the sudden onset of severe chest pain that waxed and waned over several hours. During hospitalization the pain recurred, and an ECG revealed ST-segment elevation in the inferior leads. He immediately received heparin and intravenous tissue plasminogen activator and experienced complete relief of pain within 30 minutes, but soon thereafter symptoms recurred. At angiography he had total left coronary artery occlusion. The angioscopic image shows the left circumflex coronary artery at the site of angiographic occlusion has a coronary thrombus obstructing approximately 90% of the lumen (Figure 5a). The typical histologic appearance of this type of lesion is shown in Figure 5b. It shows a portion of a thrombosed segment of the left anterior descending coronary artery of a patient who died after myocardial infarction. A large atheroma cavity has ruptured into the lumen. The red-staining lipid content of the cavity, containing some cholesterol clefts (arrows), constitutes the upper third of the thrombus which occludes the lumen. The remaining two-thirds of the thrombus consists chiefly of platelets, with an outer fringe composed chiefly of erythrocytes. The atheroma cavity has many cholesterol clefts, similar to the histologic image of the partially occlusive thrombus.

Thus it appears that thrombotic occlusion of a coronary artery is determined by two competing forces. These are the diameter of the blood vessel at the site of atheroma rupture and the efficiency of endogenous thrombolysis. Falk[10] found that complete thrombotic occlusion occurs commonly (79%) when the pre-existing stenosis is greater than 75% of the lumen, but is rare (3%) when the pre-existing stenosis is less than 75%. Furthermore, reocclusion after thrombolysis is also related to the magnitude of pre-existing coronary stenosis. From these data, it seems likely that extensive intimal disruption can heal if the residual stenosis is not severe, and that the most important factor determining the fate of a developing coronary thrombosis is the magnitude of stenosis at the time of intimal disruption.

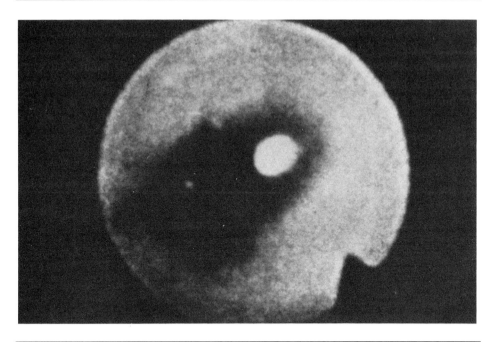

Figure 5a. *A completely occlusive coronary thrombosis in the left anterior descending coronary artery (courtesy Dr. Meyer Friedman).*

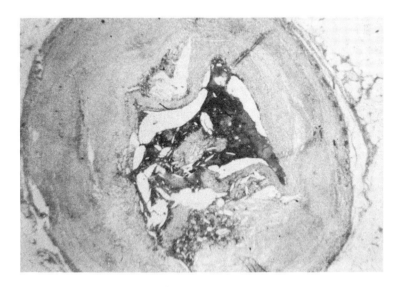

Figure 5b. *A coronary thrombosis containing fragments of the intimal surface and cholesterol clefts in a patient who died soon after the onset of acute myocardial infarction (courtesy Dr. Meyer Friedman).*

21

AFTER MYOCARDIAL INFARCTION:
THE ACUTE HEALING PHASE

The common course after acute thrombotic occlusion is clot lysis, either by therapeutic or by endogenous mechanisms. The angiographic literature suggests that endogenous lysis occurs rapidly. Although the prevalence of complete thrombotic occlusion in the first few hours after acute infarction is 80-90%, it is only 33% after 14 days of conventional therapy including heparin.[11] Figure 6 shows an angioscopic image of the left anterior descending coronary artery in a 64-year-old man two weeks after transmural anterior myocardial infarction. The intimal surface is ulcerated, but there is no thrombosis, suggesting endogenous thrombolysis. Spontaneous lysis is the most common outcome of partially occlusive coronary thrombosis, accounting for the fact that about 15% of patients with unstable angina go on to myocardial infarction.

After myocardial infarction, disrupted intima are observed, which can serve as a nidus for subsequent platelet aggregation. Platelet aggregates and thrombus can embolize. Thus, Davies et al[12] found evidence of microemboli distal to coronary

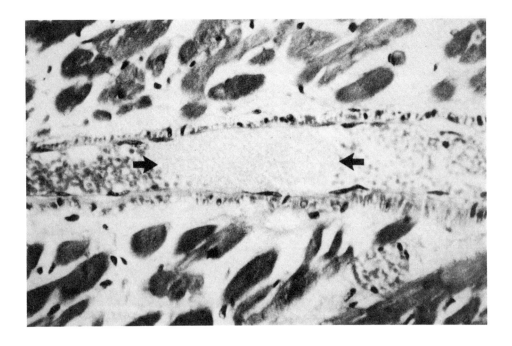

Figure 6. *Embolus to a small intramyocardial vessel distal to an occlusive thrombus in a patient who died post myocardial infarction. (Reproduced with permission of Dr. M. Davies and Circulation 1986;73:418-427.)*

thrombi in 75% of sudden ischemic cardiac deaths, suggesting that microemboli can trigger fatal ventricular arrhythmias.

RAPID PROGRESSION OF CORONARY STENOSIS

When the blood vessels are examined a few weeks to a few months after disruption, healing of the intimal disruption is observed. The vascular healing response has been well defined in the animal laboratory. After vascular injury there is immediate attachment of platelets, and often a fibrin mass forms. The platelets and fibrin are rapidly ingested by macrophages. At about three days, smooth muscle cells begin to migrate into the area. By one week, the damaged intimal surface is covered with a few layers of cells, and the phase of extracellular matrix formation and remodelling begins. By 4-8 weeks, the site of prior intimal damage has healed. This is probably the most common outcome in man.

If the damage has been extensive, however, there is prominent intimal hyperplasia, consisting of a mass of extracellular matrix with many smooth muscle cells. There are factors that increase the probability of this response in the animal. Reintimalization in the presence of hyperlipidemia results in accelerated development of atheroma.[13] It is likely that the same process occurs in man. Thus, in patients with unstable angina who have angiography before and again soon after the acute syndrome, 75% exhibit rapid localized progression of stenosis.[14] Rapid progression typically occurs with the abrupt development of new symptoms and frequently involves previously normal segments.

If endogenous thrombolysis does not occur, the thrombosis cycle may be completed by incorporation of the thrombus into the vessel wall. Figure 7 shows this alternate late fate of a coronary thrombus in a patient who died one month after a myocardial infarction. The thrombus has been covered by a thin layer of intima, and the platelet-fibrin mass is being replaced by macrophages and fibrous tissue. In several more weeks, if the evolution of this thrombus parallels that in the animal, the lesion will be indistinguishable from the chronic stable atheroma. Thus both intimal healing and thrombus incorporation may cause rapid progression of coronary stenosis at the site of intimal disruption.

Therapeutic Implications

From our understanding of the pathogenesis of coronary syndromes, we can speculate that four categories of therapy could interrupt the repeating cycle of ulceration, thrombosis, and healing as the disease progresses. The therapies are those that prevent ulceration, inhibit platelet aggregation, lyse thrombi, or promote healing of the intimal surface.

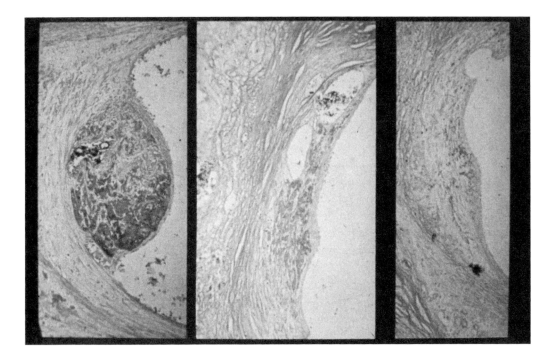

Figure 7. *Incorporation of a coronary thrombosis as seen in three serial sections of the coronary artery.*
(Reproduced from Br J Exp Pathol 1966;47:533, with permission.)

In part because the mechanism of intimal disruption remains largely undefined, there are as yet no preventive therapies. After intimal disruption, platelet inhibitors are effective in preventing further progression of this acute syndrome. Such treatment both reduces platelet emboli and impedes thrombus formation. In the Veterans Administration trial of buffered aspirin, Lewis et al[15] randomized 1266 men with unstable angina to treatment or placebo. There was a 51% lower cardiac event rate at 3 months in the aspirin-treated group. Comparable results have been reported from a Canadian multicenter trial by Cairns et al.[16] Thus we believe that in the absence of contraindication, all unstable angina and acute infarction patients should be placed on a platelet antagonist after hospitalization.

Streptokinase, urokinase and tissue plasminogen activator effectively lyse thrombi. Nevertheless, most data suggest that lytic agents are not as effective as heparin and aspirin in treatment of unstable angina. Two studies serve as exceptions. Gold et al[17] found a sharp reduction in the frequency of persistent angina one week after streptokinase infusion, although lytic therapy alone, without follow-up angioplasty, is probably inadequate. Lawrence et al[18] reported a statistically significant reduction in cardiac event rate at three months in a small group of unstable angina patients who received a 24-hour infusion of streptokinase. At present, we use heparin for systemic anticoagulation in all our patients but do not routinely use lytic agents in unstable rest angina unless the patient is unresponsive to therapy and has an angiographically documented thrombus.[19]

In summary, angioscopy has shown that clinical coronary disease is caused by a cycle of events at the arterial intimal surface. A stable atheroma ulcerates, platelets aggregate, thrombus forms, and the lesion heals. Each stage in this cycle causes a specific clinical syndrome, and each can benefit from specific therapy. Our understanding of the pathogenesis of clinical syndromes described in this chapter provides the basis for our thoughts about management of AMI in the chapters that follow.

REFERENCES

1. Forrester JS, Litvack F, Grundfest W, Fishbein M: New insights into the role of thrombus in the pathogenesis of acute and chronic coronary heart disease. Circulation 1986;75:505-513.

2. Sherman CT, Litvack F, Grundfest WS, Lee M, Hickey A, Chaux A, Kass R, Blanche C, Matloff J, Morgernstern L, Ganz W, Swan HJC, Forrester J: Demonstration of thrombus and complex atheroma by in vivo angioscopy in patients with unstable angina pectoris. N Engl J Med 1986;315:913-919.

3. Friedman M, Van den Bovenkamp GJ: Role of thrombus in plaque formation in the human diseased coronary artery. Br J Exptl Pathol 1966;47:550.

4. Davies MJ, Thomas A: Thrombosis and acute coronary artery lesions in sudden cardiac ischemic death. N Engl J Med 1984;310:1137-1140.

5. Falk E: Plaque rupture with severe pre-existing stenosis precipitating coronary thrombosis: characteristics of coronary atherosclerotic plaques underlying fatal occlusive thrombi. Br Heart J 1983;50:127-134.

6. Mulcahy R, Daly L, Graham I, Hickey N, O'Donoghue S, Owens A, Ruane P, Tobin G: Unstable angina: natural history and determinants of prognosis. Am J Cardiol 1981;48: 525-528.

7. Duncan B, Fulton M, Morrison SL, Lutz W, Donald KW, Kerr F, Kirby BJ, Julian DG, Oliver MF: Prognosis of new and worsening angina pectoris. Br J Med 1976;1:981-985.

8. Solomon HA, Edwards AL, Killip T: Prodromata in acute myocardial infarction. Circulation 1969;40:463-471.

9. Falk E: Unstable angina with fatal outcome: dynamic coronary thrombosis leading to infarction and/or sudden death. Circulation 1985;71:699-708.

10. Falk E: Plaque rupture with severe pre-existing stenosis precipitating coronary thrombosis: characteristics of coronary atherosclerotic plaques underlying fatal occlusive thrombi. Br Heart J 1983;50:127.

11. Rentrop KP, Frederick F, Blanke H, et al: Effects of intracoronary streptokinase and intracoronary nitroglycerin infusion on coronary angiographic patterns and mortality in patients with acute myocardial infarction. N Engl J Med 1984;311:1456-1463.

12. Davies MJ, Thomas AC, Knapman PA, et al: Intramyocardial platelet aggregation in patients with unstable angina suffering sudden ischemic cardiac death. Circulation 1986; 73:418-427.

13. Steele PM, Chesebro JH, Holmes DR, Stanson DW, Badimon L, Fuster V: Balloon angioplasty in pigs. Histologic wall injury as a determinant of platelet deposition and thrombus formation. Circ Res 1985;57:105-112.

14. Stowers M, Short D: Warning symptoms before major myocardial infarction. Br Heart J 1970;32:833-838.

15. Lewis DH, Davis JW, Archibald DG, et al: Protective effects of aspirin against acute myocardial infarction and death in men with unstable angina. N Engl J Med 1983;309: 396-403.

16. Cairns JA, Gent M, Singer J, et al: Aspirin, sulfinpyrazone, or both in unstable angina. Results of a Canadian multicenter trial. N Engl J Med 1985;313:1369-1375.

17. Gold HK, Johns JA, Leinbach RC, Yasuda T, Grossbard E, Zusman R, Collen D: A randomized, blinded, placebo-controlled trial of recombinant human tissue-type plasminogen activator in patients with unstable angina pectoris. Circulation 1987;75:1192-1199.

18. Lawrence JR, Shepard JT, Bone I, Rogen AS, Fulton WFM: Fibrinolytic therapy in unstable angina pectoris. A controlled clinical trial. Thrombosis Res 1980;17:767-777.

19. Theroux P, Quimet H, McCans J, Latour JG, Joly P, Levy G, Pelletier E, Juneau M, Stasiak J, DeGuise P, Pelletier G, Rinzler D, Waters D: Aspirin, heparin, or both to treat acute unstable angina. N Engl J Med 1988;391:1105-1111.

MANAGEMENT PRINCIPLES OF ACUTE MYOCARDIAL INFARCTION

Section II

Chapter 3

DIAGNOSIS AND GENERAL MANAGEMENT PRINCIPLES OF ACUTE MYOCARDIAL INFARCTION

Frank G. Yanowitz

INTRODUCTION

In recent years the availability of aggressive myocardial reperfusion techniques has made the immediate and accurate diagnosis of acute myocardial infarction (AMI) an urgent matter for all primary care and emergency room physicians. Acute interventions including thrombolytic therapy, coronary angioplasty and coronary bypass surgery are not without risk, and since "time is muscle" they must be initiated within hours of the onset of symptoms. Thus the challenge is not only the accurate diagnosis of AMI but establishing the diagnosis in as short a time as possible.

Fortunately, many patients present with easily identifiable symptoms, signs, ECG changes, and laboratory findings which allow the diagnosis of acute coronary syndromes and initiation of the appropriate therapeutic interventions. More difficult, however, are those patients whose presenting symptoms, signs, and ECG findings are atypical for AMI. This chapter considers additional tests and procedures that may be helpful in identifying patients with unusual presentations soon enough to administer appropriate therapeutic interventions.

The final purpose of this chapter is to review routine therapy for AMI including relief of pain and anxiety, diet, and other aspects of general supportive care. Subsequent chapters in this book consider more specific issues of AMI management including thrombolytic therapy, coronary angioplasty, arrhythmia management, and treatment of heart failure and cardiogenic shock.

THE DIAGNOSTIC CHALLENGE

The diagnosis of AMI rests on the triad of classic findings: prolonged chest discomfort typical of AMI, evolution of characteristic ECG changes, and elevations of myocardial specific enzymes. Each of these diagnostic findings is discussed in the following sections. It is generally accepted that any two of the three classic findings are suffi-cient to confirm the diagnosis of AMI.[1]

MEDICAL HISTORY

The importance of a goal-oriented medical history cannot be overemphasized in the initial evaluation of patients suspected of AMI. As many as 80-90% of patients with AMI will give a classic history of cardiac pain, although advancing age and concur-rent illness such as diabetes mellitus or congestive heart failure can alter the presenta-tion considerably. It has been estimated that one-third of elderly patients do not have pain at the onset of AMI but rather present with severe dyspnea, cerebral symptoms or vague complaints of weakness, restlessness and apprehension.[2-4] AMI may also pres-ent with nausea and vomiting, change in mental status, arrhythmias, syncope, or stroke.[5] Interestingly, the mortality in patients with these atypical presentations is much greater than in those presenting with chest pain (50% vs. 18%).[5] Constant vigi-lance is required by admitting physicians to avoid missing the diagnosis of AMI and thus delaying appropriate treatment.

The classic history of AMI is established only after a careful analysis of the presenting symptoms in terms of location, quality, duration, severity, radiation pat-terns, and precipitating and relieving factors, if any. It is also important to determine the time of onset of symptoms in order to establish a therapeutic window for admin-istering thrombolytic agents. Considerable skill is needed by the admitting physician to obtain an unbiased description of chest discomfort in the patient's own words.

The location of chest discomfort is usually substernal and diffuse rather than pin-point. At times, however, the initial location is atypical and involves the right or left chest areas, epigastrium, neck, jaw, teeth, shoulders, arms, or back. Radiation patterns, if any, typically involve the inner aspect of the left arm, although any of the above locations may also be sites of radiating pain. Patients who have had previous ischemic symptoms tend to have recurrent symptoms in the same locations.

The quality of AMI discomfort is often described as crushing, burning, indiges-tion-like, squeezing, pressure, or heaviness. In contrast, complaints such as sharp, stabbing, knife-like, dull, or aching are less likely to be due to myocardial ischemia. Some patients may have trouble describing their symptoms in terms other than a sense of extreme discomfort.

AMI pain is generally minutes to hours in duration rather than seconds or days. The pain duration is categorized as "prolonged" rather than "brief," with 15-20 min-utes being a somewhat arbitrary minimum.[1] Brief ischemic pain lasting 1-15 minutes is more typical of angina pectoris, although if increasing in frequency, severity, or duration, and occurring with less effort or at rest, unstable angina should be considered. Not all unstable angina patients require admission to a coronary care unit, however, if telemetry beds are available on the wards. Prolonged chest discomfort of 20 minutes or longer that is not relieved by rest or nitroglycerine in a middle-aged or older man is the most important warning sign of AMI and deserves urgent evaluation by emergency medical personnel. It is also important that the general public be taught the significance of these symptoms and the procedures for requesting emergency medical services.

Precipitating and relieving factors are helpful in differentiating AMI from other causes of prolonged chest discomfort. Pleuritic chest pain or pain made worse by deep inspiration and various body positions is less likely to be ischemic. Pain aggravated or reproduced by pressing over costochondral junctions or ribs is also unlikely to be due to AMI. Although unusual exertion or emotional excitement are common precipitating events for AMI, it is important to emphasize that AMI symptoms may appear at rest or during usual activities. Also, once symptoms appear patients may be more uncomfortable or anxious at rest and feel the need to move around in order to get relief.

Accompanying symptoms include nausea, vomiting, dyspnea, diaphoresis, palpitations, loss of consciousness, and a sense of impending doom. Although these symptoms are nonspecific, they should be considered as supporting evidence for AMI in patients presenting with prolonged chest discomfort. Table 1 lists the differential diagnosis of conditions whose presentations can mimic AMI and includes entities that can produce ECG changes suggestive of ischemic heart disease.[6]

The past medical history can be quite useful in the differential diagnosis of prolonged chest discomfort. A history of established coronary heart disease such as previous AMI, angina pectoris or coronary artery surgery is most important and generally indicates the need for hospital admission. Manifestations of peripheral vascular diseases such as transient ischemic attacks, strokes, aneurysms, or claudication are indicative of diffuse atherosclerosis and increase the risk for coronary disease. Other cardiac diseases such as valvular heart disease and congestive heart failure are also important to ascertain.

No medical history is complete without a detailed risk factor analysis, since the greater the prior risk for coronary disease the more likely the presenting symptoms represent acute ischemia. This is especially important for men aged 40 and over and women aged 50 and older, since coronary heart disease is the most common cause of morbidity and mortality in these groups. The following risk factors should be assessed in the initial workup: cigarette smoking, hypertension, hypercholesterolemia, hypertriglyceridemia, diabetes mellitus, sedentary life style, and family history of premature coronary heart disease (ie, in first degree relatives under age 55). Although myocardial infarction in younger women is unusual, cigarette smoking and oral contraceptive use are important risk factors in this population.[7]

Table 1. *Differential diagnosis of acute myocardial infarction*

    A. Ischemic heart disease syndromes
       1. Angina pectoris*
       2. Variant (Prinzmetal's) angina*
       3. Unstable angina*
       4. Coronary insufficiency*

    B. Nonischemic cardiac syndromes
       1. Acute pericarditis*
       2. Acute congestive heart failure
          a. Valvular heart disease
          b. Cardiomyopathy
          c. Hypertensive heart disease
          d. Infectious heart disease
       3. Primary arrhythmias

    C. Other cardiovascular or pulmonary syndromes
       1. Acute pulmonary embolus or infarction*
       2. Dissecting aortic aneurysm*
       3. Acute pneumothorax
       4. Asthmatic bronchitis, pneumonitis

Continued

PHYSICAL EXAMINATION

The physical examination is not often helpful in the diagnosis of AMI but is very important in assessing the severity of cardiac dysfunction and in choosing specific therapies. However, in some patients distinctive physical findings suggest an acute coronary event.

The general appearance usually shows a very anxious and restless patient who is diaphoretic and in considerable distress. Before directing attention to cardiac findings an astute clinician may occasionally observe external manifestations of hyperlipidemia including tendinous or tuberous xanthomas, and xanthelasma. Vital signs may be normal or may reveal hypotension, hypertension, bradycardia or tachycardia depending on the patient's hemodynamic status, degree of discomfort and infarct location. Sympathetic excess manifested as hypertension and sinus tachycardia has been observed in over 40% of anterior AMI patients, while parasympathetic overactivity in the form of bradyarrhythmias and hypotension has been noted in 65% of inferior MI patients.[8] Hypotension may also be secondary to volume depletion due to vomiting or

Table 1. *Continued*

---

       5. Mediastinitis, mediastinal tumor,
          mediastinal emphysema
       6. Pleuritis

   D. Gastrointestinal disorders
       1. Esophageal disease (spasm, reflux,
          hiatal hernia)
       2. Stomach and intestinal disease
          (gastritis, ulcer)
       3. Acute pancreatitis*
       4. Acute cholecystitis,*
          choledocholithiasis, etc.

   E. Musculoskeletal disorders
       1. Costochondritis
       2. Arthritis, arthralgias
       3. Myositis, myalgias
       4. Neuritis, neuralgias
       5. Chest wall trauma*

   F. Psychological disorders
       1. Psychogenic causes of chest pain
       2. Hyperventilation

---

* Can present with ECG changes suggestive of ischemia or infarction

diuretic therapy, right ventricular infarction, or left ventricular failure. A persistent sinus tachycardia beyond the first few hours after admission may be a manifestation of heart failure.

The cardiovascular examination should focus on detecting signs of right and left sided cardiac dysfunction. High jugular venous pressure, prominent 'a' and/or 'v' waves, Kussmaul's sign and right-sided gallop rhythms may indicate right ventricular infarction in patients with inferior wall infarcts, although these findings may also occur with severe left-sided failure. Right-sided S3 and S4 gallop sounds are best heard along the left sternal border and increase in intensity during inspiration.

In contrast, left ventricular dysfunction is recognized by an S3 gallop sound at the apex along with inspiratory crackles at the lung bases which progress up the lung fields in proportion to the severity of pulmonary congestion. These findings are associated with a significantly increased risk of mortality when compared to those without them (40% vs. 15%).[9] An atrial or S4 gallop sound at the apex is an expected finding in AMI due to decreased compliance of the infarcted and/or ischemic left ventricle.

The absence of an S4, when properly listened for with the bell of the stethoscope in the left lateral decubitus position, argues against AMI. Signs of peripheral hypoperfusion such as diminished peripheral pulses, cool and clammy skin, altered mental status, and reduced urine output are indicative of low cardiac output states.

A systolic murmur following AMI has an important differential diagnosis including papillary muscle dysfunction or rupture, perforation of the ventricular septum, and acute mitral regurgitation secondary to left ventricular failure.[10] These murmurs may appear within hours of onset of symptoms or at any time during the hospital course. Murmurs due to papillary muscle dysfunction or rupture are more common and are best heard at the apex. Their characteristics vary from typical holosystolic blowing murmurs to atypical harsh, ejection-like murmurs radiating to the base of the heart and mimicking aortic stenosis. A mid-systolic click initiating a late systolic murmur may also indicate papillary muscle dysfunction.

The murmur of ventricular septal defect (VSD) is harsh, holosystolic and usually accompanied by a palpable thrill. Although most often the murmur is best heard along the left sternal border, it may also be well appreciated at the apex. Both VSD and papillary muscle rupture are likely to precipitate profound congestive heart failure and cardiogenic shock and therefore represent serious complications of myocardial infarction. Because the characteristic clinical findings of each overlap, accurate diagnosis usually requires ancillary techniques such as ultrasound or other imaging modalities, or invasive hemodynamic assessment.[10]

ELECTROCARDIOGRAPHIC ABNORMALITIES

The initial ECG in patients presenting with suspected AMI is often the determining factor in the decision to administer thrombolytic therapy. The accuracy of this first ECG in diagnosing AMI was investigated by Rude et al[11] using data from 3,697 patients screened within 18 hours of symptom onset for a multicenter study to limit infarct size (MILIS). ECG criteria used in this study are listed in Table 2. For patients with enzyme documented AMI the sensitivity of these criteria was 81%, and the specificity for non-MI patients was 69%. The overall predictive accuracy for one or more of the ECG criteria was 72% with 28% false positives. When the various ECG criteria were looked at individually, however, the sensitivity of ST-segment elevation alone, a common prerequisite for thrombolytic therapy, was only 46%. In this study over one-half of enzyme-confirmed AMI patients did not have ST-segment elevation on the initial ECG.

The ECG diagnosis of AMI requires an understanding of the temporal sequence of electrocardiographic changes which begin within minutes from the onset of coronary occlusion. The evolution of ECG findings can be divided into three somewhat overlapping phases: 1) the hyperacute phase; 2) the fully evolved acute phase; and

Table 2. *MILIS criteria for the ECG diagnosis of acute myocardial infarction*

Any *one* of the following:

A. New or presumably new Q waves (> 30 ms wide, > 2 mm deep) in at least *two leads* from any of the following:

    1. Leads II, III, aVF, or

    2. Leads V1-V6, or

    3. Leads I and aVL

B. New or presumably new ST segment elevation (> 1 mm at 80 ms after the J point) in *two contiguous leads* of the above lead combinations

C. Complete left bundle branch block

3) the chronic stabilized phase.[12] For Q wave infarctions involving the anterior (V1-V4), lateral (V4-V6, I, aVL), and inferior (II, III, aVF) walls of the left ventricle, the characteristic ECG changes are summarized in Table 3. The ECG leads exhibiting changes of AMI, however, are only crudely reflective of the anatomic sites of necrosis.

The Hyperacute Phase

During this earliest phase of AMI the T waves over the area of injury increase in amplitude and widen as the ST segments change from their usual concave upwards appearance to a straightened or convex upwards appearance (Figure 1). This quickly evolves into manifest ST-segment elevation which, at times, may reach amplitudes of 10-15 mm (1-1.5 mV). The blending of elevated ST segments with the R and T waves results in a "tombstone" appearance to the ECG wave forms (see Figure 4 on page 43). Changes in the QRS complex during this phase include increased R wave amplitude and time to peak R wave reflecting slowed conduction through injured myocardium. The time course of the hyperacute changes is quite variable but is usually measured in hours rather than days. Delay from onset of symptoms to receiving medical attention may result in missing these important indicators of AMI.

    While ST-segment elevation is usually seen in ECG leads facing the injured myocardial surface, depressed ST segments in other leads have traditionally been called "reciprocal changes." Recent evidence, however, suggests that the presence of

Table 3. *ECG changes of myocardial infarction in the inferior, anterior, and lateral wall locations*

Phase I: Hyperacute phase
1. Tall, widened T waves
2. ST segment elevation
3. Increased R wave amplitude

Phase II: Fully evolved acute phase
1. Pathologic Q or QS complexes
2. Elevated, convex upwards ST segments
3. Inverted, arrow-head shaped T waves

Phase III: Chronic, stabilized phase
1. Pathologic Q or QS complexes
2. ST-T changes of chronic coronary insufficiency

these changes especially in leads outside the plane of the myocardial infarction may indicate more extensive myocardial injury and even multivessel coronary artery disease.[13]

Other causes of ST-segment elevation must be considered in the differential diagnosis during this phase of AMI. These include acute pericarditis and normal variant early repolarization. Acute pericarditis is of particular concern since the chest pain presentation may mimic the symptoms of AMI. Unlike AMI where ST-segment elevation is seen only in leads facing the localized area of injury, the ST changes in pericarditis are more diffuse, involving most of the ECG leads except aVR and perhaps V1. Elevated ST segments in pericarditis retain their normal upward concavity, and T waves are low in amplitude. ST-segment elevation in early repolarization is also concave upwards in appearance with normal QRS complexes and T waves. ST-segment elevation in the anterior precordial leads also occurs in left ventricular hypertrophy and left bundle branch block, but these conditions are easily recognized on ECG.

The Fully Evolved Acute Phase

During this phase the ST-segment elevation begins to regress, and the T waves become symmetrically inverted in leads oriented towards the infarcted surface (Table 3).

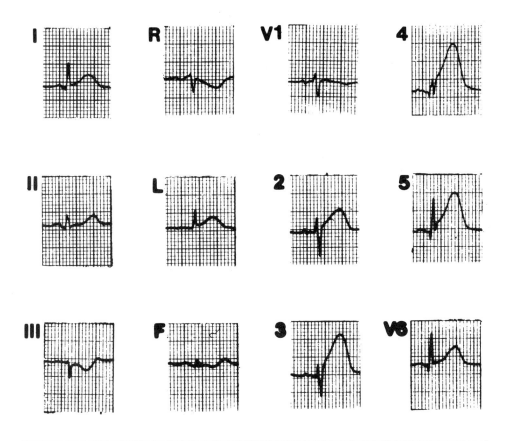

Figure 1. *Hyperacute anterolateral MI with tall, widened T waves in leads V2-6, I, and aVL. Early ST segment elevation is also present in the same leads.*

The ST segments are coved and convex upwards, while the inverted T waves often have an arrow-head appearance (Figure 2). The fully evolved pathologic Q or QS waves, defined as greater than 0.03 seconds in duration and/or more than 30% of the R wave amplitude, are most prominent in this phase.[14] Inverted U waves may also be seen in the precordial leads when the infarction is anterior in location. This finding has not received much attention in the ECG literature.

Resolution of ST-T wave changes is quite variable but is usually complete within two weeks in inferior wall infarct locations. ST-T wave abnormalities rapidly improve after successful reperfusion with thrombolytic therapy.[15] Persistent ST elevation is often seen in anterior locations and is indicative of a large akinetic or dyskinetic myocardial scar.

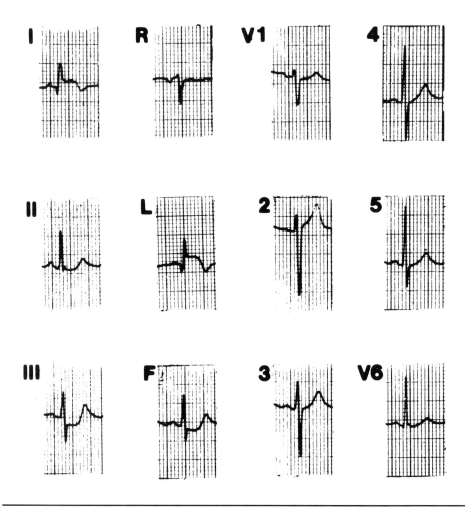

Figure 2. *Fully evolved acute lateral wall MI. Note the pathologic Q waves in leads I and aVL along with ST segment elevation and symmetrically inverted T waves. Reciprocal ST segment depression is present in leads III and aVF.*

The Chronic Phase

Complete resolution of all abnormal ECG findings is very uncommon but may occur in small inferior wall infarctions. More often persistent abnormalities in the form of pathologic Q or QS waves, low amplitude R waves, straightened ST segments and symmetrical T waves are seen for an indefinite period of time.

There is considerable variation in the ECG patterns of myocardial infarction depending on infarct age, size and location, history of previous MI, presence of intraventricular conduction defects and many other confounding variables. The most characteristic changes are more common in patients experiencing their first AMI and in patients with right coronary or left anterior descending coronary occlusions (Table 3). The changes are often more subtle in patients with previous infarcts and in patients with nondominant left circumflex lesions.[16] The rapidity with which the ECG evolves is, in part, determined by whether or not intrinsic recanalization or successful reperfusion following thrombolytic therapy occurs. ST-segment elevation declines more rapidly in patients successfully reperfused, and QRS complex changes tend to be less extensive, although there is much overlap between reperfused and nonreperfused patients.[15]

True Posterior Myocardial Infarction

Table 4 describes the evolution of ECG changes in true posterior wall infarctions which are seen as mirror-image representations in leads V1, V2 and sometimes V3 and V4 (ie, viewed from the opposite anterior leads).[17] ST-segment depression reflects the hyperacute phase in these leads (Figure 3a). Instead of pathologic Q waves, R waves widen and increase in amplitude during the fully evolved phase (Figure 3b). Other causes of prominent anterior forces such as right ventricular hypertrophy, type A WPW, and normal variants must be excluded. In general, however, prominent anterior forces suggest the diagnosis of true posterior wall MI when evolving changes of inferior wall infarction are present in leads II, III, and aVF.

Table 4. *ECG changes in true posterior myocardial infarction*

1. ST segment depression in V1, V2, (V3)

2. R/S > 1.0 in V1 or V2

3. R duration > 0.03 sec in V1 or V2

4. Loss of R waves in V5-6

5. Decreasing ST segment depression with increased T wave amplitude (late change)

6. Associated changes of inferior or infero-lateral wall MI

41

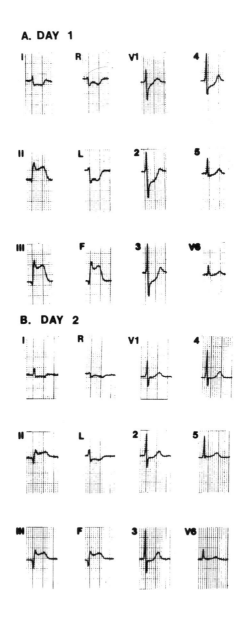

A. DAY 1

B. DAY 2

Figure 3. *(A) Day 1 of an acute inferoposterior MI. Note the ST segment elevation, increased T waves and tall, widened R waves in leads II, III, and aVF (hyperacute inferior wall changes). The corresponding true posterior wall changes include ST segment depression in leads V1-4. (B) By day 2 the fully evolved changes are present including pathologic Q waves with ST segment elevation in leads II, III, and aVF, and pathologic R waves in leads V1 and V2. Reciprocal ST segment depression is present in leads I and aVL.*

Right Ventricular Infarctions

In approximately 30% of inferior wall myocardial infarctions resulting from proximal right coronary artery occlusions there is concomitant infarction of the right ventricular wall. Recognition of RV infarction is important in the hemodynamically compromised inferior wall AMI patient in order to optimize clinical management. ST-segment elevation of 1 mm or greater in one or more of the right sided chest leads V4R to V6R has been found to be both sensitive (90%) and specific (91%) in identifying this infarction location (Figure 4).[18] The presence of a QS or QR complex in both leads V3R and V4R is also a specific marker for RV infarction.[19]

ECG Diagnosis of AMI in Bundle Branch Block

The presence of intraventricular conduction disorders complicates the ECG diagnosis of AMI. This is a particular problem in left bundle branch block (LBBB) where left

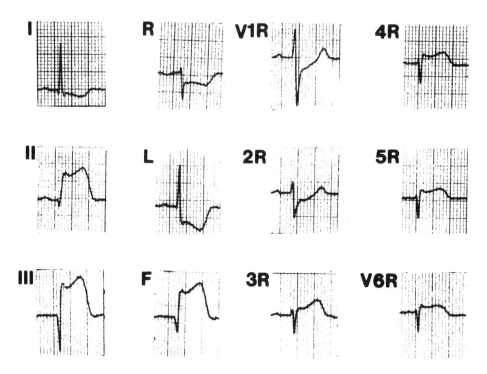

Figure 4. *Acute inferior wall MI with right ventricular infarction. Note the "tombstone" appearance in leads II, III, and aVF of a hyperacute inferior wall MI. Changes of an acute right ventricular infarction consisting of ST segment elevation in the right sided chest leads V3R-V6R are present. Reciprocal ST segment depression is seen in leads I and aVL.*

ventricular activation is delayed and abnormal. Any one of the following ECG criteria have been suggested as evidence for acute or prior myocardial infarction in patients with LBBB: Q waves in at least two of the leads I, aVL, V5, V6; R wave regression from V1 to V4; late notching of S waves in at least two of the leads V3, V4, or V5; and primary ST-T wave abnormalities in two or more adjacent leads.[20] Unfortunately these criteria do not separate acute from old myocardial infarctions.

In right bundle branch block (RBBB) the problem is less difficult, since the usual AMI evolution of ECG findings including hyperacute and fully evolved ST-T wave changes as well as Q wave abnormalities are still seen. True posterior MI, however, may be masked by RBBB because both abnormalities may cause tall R waves and ST depression in the right precordial leads.

Q Wave versus Non-Q Wave Myocardial Infarctions

Although pathologic Q and QS waves have long been considered the most specific ECG markers for transmural myocardial necrosis, there is increasing recognition that the extent of infarction into the left ventricular wall cannot be judged by the presence or absence of Q waves (or pathologic R waves). There are, however, important reasons to consider non-Q wave myocardial infarction (NQMI) as a distinct clinical entity occurring in 25-50% of AMI patients.[21,22] The usual definition of NQMI is the absence of a new abnormal Q wave (> 0.03 sec duration) or the absence of an R wave > 0.03 sec in lead V1 and an R/S ratio > 1 in lead V2 in a patient with enzymatically confirmed AMI (Figure 5).

Opinions differ as to the clinical and prognostic significance of NQMI. To a large extent this is due to the heterogeneous mixture of patients in this group. Some studies have suggested a more favorable short-term outcome in NQMI because of less myocardial damage and smaller infarct size.[21] However, because of the decreased occurrence of total occlusion of the infarct-related coronary artery, residual ischemia and the reinfarction rate are higher than with Q wave MIs.[21]

Spodick has suggested a more comprehensive ECG classification of both Q and non-Q wave infarcts to improve the identification of high-risk and low-risk subsets.[23] When NQMI patients are subdivided into three groups based on the principal ECG abnormality, important prognostic differences can be appreciated.[23] Patients presenting with ST-segment depression as the principal change are older, have more multivessel disease, more hemodynamic complications, and greater in-hospital and long term mortality compared to patients with ST-segment elevation or only T wave inversion. Moreover, the persistence of ST-segment depression until hospital discharge in patients with NQMI is associated with an unusually high (22%) one-year mortality.[24] These data suggest a need for more aggressive management in this high-risk subset of NQMI.

A. DAY 1

B. DAY 4

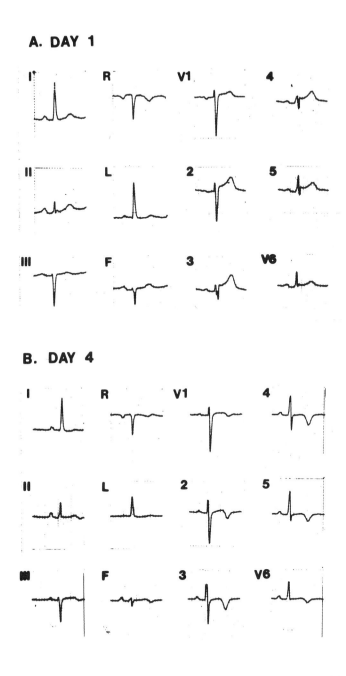

Figure 5. *(A) Day 1 of an acute anterior wall non-Q wave MI shows ST segment elevation with an atypical concave upwards appearance in leads V2-V6. (B) By Day 4 the ST elevation has decreased and symmetrically inverted T waves are present. Note the absence of pathologic Q waves.*

45

Some patients with NQMI present with normal or nearly normal ECG findings. Because these patients have an excellent short term outcome with minimal risk of in-hospital complications, CCU admission may not be necessary if telemetry or intermediate care beds are available.[25,26] Unfortunately the utility of the ECG as a diagnostic test for AMI is lessened when the initial ECG is nearly normal or shows only ST-segment deviation, T wave inversion or minimal nonspecific ST-T wave changes. Under these circumstances the medical history is often the determining factor in the decision to admit or not to admit, and the serum enzymes become the gold standard diagnostic test.

ENZYME ABNORMALITIES

The most sensitive enzyme indicator of AMI is creatine kinase (CK) which begins to rise within 6-8 hours of AMI onset, peaks by 24 hours (earlier if successful reperfusion occurs or in the presence of subtotal occlusion) and returns to normal by 2-4 days. The MB isoenzyme of CK (CK-MB) is very specific for myocardial damage and may increase abnormally in the absence of a significant rise in total CK in approximately 15% of AMI patients with minimal necrosis.[27,28] Because small amounts of CK-MB are also present in the small intestine, tongue, diaphragm, uterus and prostate, injury to these tissues may also elevate this isoenzyme. A two-fold increase in total CK above the normal range for a given laboratory or a CK-MB level greater than 7-8% of the total CK is usually considered diagnostic of myocardial infarction.

The most cost-effective sampling frequency for estimating the peak total CK or CK-MB levels appears to be on admission and every 12 hours for 36 hours.[29,30] Episodes of recurrent chest pain in the hospital might necessitate further sampling to detect infarct extension. If ECG studies for AMI are diagnostic, analysis for CK-MB is not necessary, although aliquots from each blood draw may be frozen and saved for later analysis if uncertainty arises regarding the diagnosis.

In patients whose onset of symptoms is uncertain or begins more than 12-24 hours before admission, analysis of total lactic dehydrogenase (LDH) and the isoenzyme ratio (LDH1/LDH2) is often helpful, since these enzymes rise more slowly, peak at 24-48 hours and remain elevated for up to 10 days after AMI.[30,31] An LDH1/LDH2 isoenzyme ratio greater than 1.0 is indicative of myocardial damage, although injury to kidneys, pancreas, brain, stomach and red blood cells may also give this pattern. It is generally not necessary to order LDH1/LDH2 isoenzyme assays unless CK, CK-MB and ECG studies are inconclusive.

Although serial measurements of CK or CK-MB as often as every 4 hours for up to 72 hours have been used in the past to derive time activity curves for quantifying infarct size or detecting infarct extension, the increasing availability of cardiac imaging modalities to measure infarct size more directly has reduced the need for these enzyme studies. One of the limitations of standard enzyme tests for the diagnosis of AMI is the time required to obtain positive results. For this reason abnormal enzymes are rarely required for hospital admission or administration of thrombolytic therapy. On the horizon, however, are several investigational blood tests that might provide more rapid confirmation of AMI and permit more cost-effective use of critical hospital services.

Recent studies of CK isoenzymes have shown that both CK-MB and CK-MM are converted to subforms when released into plasma.[32] Assays for detecting these subforms and their ratios have been developed which permit earlier detection of myocardial necrosis than conventional CK isoenzymes. The isoenzyme CK-MM, for example, has three subforms — MM1, MM2, and MM3 — of which only MM3 is present in tissue. In healthy individuals the MM3 released into plasma is rapidly converted to MM2 and MM1 and the resulting ratio MM3/MM1 is < 1.0. In AMI, however, large amounts of MM3 are released and the ratio MM3/MM1 is > 1.0 by 6 hours after onset of symptoms when conventional CK levels are still normal.[33] Unfortunately CK-MM is not specific for heart muscle and abnormal ratios are also found after skeletal muscle trauma.

The detection of CK-MB subforms in plasma has been technically more difficult due to the small amounts usually present in normals. A recently developed and validated MB subform assay has identified two subforms, MB1 and MB2, of which only MB2 is present in tissue.[32] Preliminary studies in AMI patients have shown that the ratio MB2/MB1 > 1.5 is highly sensitive (90-100%) and specific (95%) for AMI at 4-6 hours after onset of symptoms.[32]

Elevated serum myoglobin concentrations have been detected as soon as 1-4 hours after onset of AMI symptoms, although current assays do not distinguish cardiac from skeletal muscle myoglobin.[34,35] Elevated myoglobin levels might also be a more sensitive marker for non-Q wave MI than conventional enzyme analyses.[36]

Other studies are investigating the detection of myosin light chains released from the breakdown of cardiac muscle as alternatives to conventional enzyme analyses.[37] Assays specific for cardiac light chains of myosin have been developed, and elevated levels have appeared within 2-3 hours of symptom onset. More work is needed before the role of these new blood assays in the assessment of suspected AMI patients is established.

ADDITIONAL TESTS FOR AMI

Although most patients with AMI satisfy at least two of the three classic diagnostic findings — prolonged chest discomfort, ECG abnormalities, and elevated enzymes — additional tests can be helpful in establishing the diagnosis in some patients. This is particularly important in the emergency room for patients who present with atypical symptoms or nondiagnostic ECG findings, and AMI is still a consideration. In addition, the newer cardiac imaging modalities are being increasingly employed in patients with known or suspected AMI to assess cardiac structure and function, myocardial perfusion and tissue metabolism.

Echocardiography

Recent data have suggested that two-dimensional echocardiography (ECHO) performed in the emergency room can rule in AMI by detecting regional wall motion abnormalities.[38-40] The absence of such findings in patients presenting with chest pain and nondiagnostic ECG findings effectively rules out this diagnosis. The use of the ECHO in this strategy has the potential to reduce hospital admissions for MI rule-out by 38% and overall hospital costs by 31%.[40] It is still too early to assess the utility of this approach since most emergency rooms currently do not have immediate access to an ECHO triage service, and major logistical problems may arise in setting up such a service. In addition some patients with normal ECHO findings may still have unstable angina or non-Q wave MI and require hospitalization on that basis.

ECHO studies are of proven benefit in recently diagnosed AMI to assess the extent of abnormal wall motion, estimate left ventricular ejection fraction, detect the presence of mural thrombus, and differentiate acute mitral regurgitation from ventricular septal rupture as a cause of a new systolic murmur.[41] In patients with recurrent chest pain the detection of regional wall motion abnormalities during an episode of chest pain is evidence for an ischemic origin and may indicate infarct extension.[42] Finally, the ECHO examination may assist in the recognition of right ventricular infarction, a reversible cause of cardiogenic shock in patients with acute inferior wall infarctions.[43,44]

Radionuclide Imaging

Several nuclear imaging techniques can be used in the assessment of patients with equivocal symptoms or ECG or enzyme findings, although their use is generally reserved for patients already admitted to the hospital. Infarcted myocardium may be identified as a "cold spot" from rest thallium-201 images or as a "hot spot" using technetium-99m pyrophosphate scintigraphy. Each technique has advantages and disadvantages.

Cold spot imaging with thallium-201 is dependent on regional myocardial perfusion. Normal functioning myocardial cells extract and concentrate thallium. Cells not perfused, whether ischemic or infarcted, do not. An abnormal perfusion defect, therefore, may be seen in old infarction, acute infarction, or regional ischemia. In acute infarction abnormal thallium scans are seen much earlier than abnormal pyrophosphate (hot spot) scans, although both techniques may miss small or non-Q wave infarcts.[41,45] For prognostic purposes thallium scans permit the assessment of the total extent of myocardial injury including old and new infarctions as well as ischemic tissue. Because of the extremely short shelf life of thallium, this technique is usually not available on short notice.

In hot spot imaging, technetium pyrophosphate is taken up by areas of acute necrosis. Localized patterns of uptake are more specific for transmural MI, whereas diffuse uptake may be seen in unstable angina as well as in normal individuals.[41] Abnormal scans are generally not detected before 24-48 hours after onset of symptoms, and up to 50% of non-Q wave infarcts have negative scans.[46] This technique is most useful in patients who present several days after onset of acute symptoms when enzymes and ECG changes are no longer diagnostic. This study is also useful in detecting right ventricular infarction. Several new radionuclide techniques and imaging agents are being investigated in the AMI population. One of these new methods, positron emission tomography (PET), has the ability to assess myocardial metabolism as well as perfusion.[47] Positron-emitting radioisotopes used in PET studies include rubidium-82 or nitrogen-13 ammonia to measure regional blood flow, 11C-palmitate to measure regional fatty acid metabolism, and 18F-deoxyglucose to measure regional uptake of exogenous glucose. In addition to detection and localization of infarcted myocardium, PET can provide information on tissue viability and discriminate between transmural (Q wave) and nontransmural (non-Q wave) infarcts.[47] PET has also been used to assess the efficacy of thrombolytic therapy in AMI by demonstrating improved regional myocardial metabolism after reperfusion.[48] PET technology is still extremely expensive and only available in large cardiovascular research facilities.

In addition to new imaging techniques, new radiopharmaceuticals are being evaluated which dramatically improve the utility of existing techniques. The most promising new agent is technetium-99m methoxyisobutyl isonitrile (Tc-MIBI) which has better imaging properties and a longer shelf-life than thallium-201.[49] Also, Tc-MIBI does not redistribute when viable myocardium is present, which means that imaging does not have to begin for several hours after injection. As a result this is a better agent to assess reperfusion therapy in AMI. Finally, Tc-MIBI can be used to quantify ejection fractions using first-pass techniques and to detect regional wall motion abnormalities making it a more effective agent for predischarge prognostic assessments.

Other Laboratory Tests

A chest x-ray is routinely ordered in the emergency room or shortly after CCU admission. Although this procedure does not contribute to the diagnosis of AMI, it is often helpful in assessing left ventricular function. Radiographic signs of pulmonary congestion including cephalad redistribution of pulmonary venous flow, perivascular cuffing, air bronchograms, Kerley B lines, alveolar edema and pleural effusions have important prognostic and therapeutic implications. It should be recognized, however, that time-lag discrepancies occur between the observed x-ray findings and the pulmonary vascular pressures. Diagnostic lags of several hours and post-therapeutic lags of several days may occur. The presence of cardiomegaly may indicate existing heart disease such as previous myocardial infarctions with left ventricular enlargement. The chest X-ray may also provide clues to the differential diagnosis of acute chest pain by revealing pneumothorax, rib fractures, aortic aneurysm, subdiaphragmatic air from a ruptured viscus, and abdominal ileus.

Other laboratory tests that are routinely ordered include a complete blood count with differential and a multichannel biochemistry panel to assess chemistries, liver and renal function. Fasting glucose and a lipid screen are also useful soon after admission to the CCU.

TRIAGE DECISIONS/RULES

Although the definitive diagnosis of AMI is usually made after CCU admission on the basis of enzyme and ECG criteria, in many patients who present with chest pain or other symptoms, the diagnosis of acute ischemic heart disease is uncertain. The decision to admit these patients and to what type of hospital bed is a most difficult problem with serious medical and financial implications. The challenge is to minimize false negative errors (ie, sending patients with acute ischemia home) while, at the same time, avoiding unnecessary admissions to expensive and limited intensive care beds. Currently about half of the 1.5 million patients admitted annually to CCUs for suspected AMI are ruled out, and about 5% of AMI patients are mistakenly sent home.[50]

The decision to admit a particular patient is usually based on one or more of the following clinical features: 1) the characteristics of the chest pain and other presenting complaints; 2) a history of previous coronary heart disease events; 3) coronary risk factors; 4) the initial ECG findings; and 5) the presence of life-threatening complications or unstable co-morbidity requiring CCU admission. Often the decision is an easy one if symptoms and ECG findings are typical for AMI or unstable angina. At other times, however, there is considerable uncertainty as to the nature of the patient's complaints. Under these circumstances the decision is generally based on the admitting physician's clinical judgement and the perceived benefit of intensive care treatment over intermediate care, ward care or home care.

Recent studies have now shown that some patients admitted to rule out AMI can be safely managed outside of the CCU if they meet certain low-risk criteria.[51-53] In particular, the initial ECG in conjunction with clinical findings has been found to be a useful triage tool for separating patients into low and high risk subgroups for AMI and its complications.[25,51] Table 5 lists the "positive" and "negative" ECG criteria proposed by Slater et al[51] for classifying suspected AMI patients. In their study of almost

Table 5. *ECG criteria for triage of suspected acute myocardial infarction patients*

Positive ECG

1. Infarction: Any Q of 0.03 sec or more (excluding lead III) or > 25% of R amplitude (15% of R amplitude in I, V4-6), or R duration of > 0.03 sec in V1 or V2 with R/S ratio > 1.0 (in absence of RVH), or decrease in R amplitude in V1-V4 in absence of RVH.

2. Injury: ST elevation of > 0.1 mV (0.2 mV in V1-V3) measured 0.08 sec from the J-point.

3. Ischemia: ST depression of > 0.1 mV (0.2 mV in V1-V3) measured 0.08 sec from the J-point, or inverted T waves of > 0.3 mV.

4. QRS duration of > 0.11 sec, or LVH, RVH, or bundle branch block.

5. 2nd or 3rd degree AV block.

6. Any sustained rhythm disturbance other than sinus tachycardia.

Negative ECG

1. Normal ECG.

2. Nonspecific ST-T changes: inverted T waves < 0.03 mV in a lead with predominantly positive QRS, all T waves < 0.05 mV in limb leads and < 0.15 mV in precordial leads, or any ST deviation > 0.05 mV but not meeting criteria for ischemia or injury.

800 patients admitted with suspected AMI only 10% of patients with normal initial ECGs and 8% of those with nonspecific ST-T wave changes developed AMI. In contrast, 41% of those with "positive" ECG findings (Table 5) were diagnosed to have AMI. Furthermore, only 1% of patients with normal initial ECGs and 6% of those with nonspecific ST-T changes had complications requiring intensive care. This study also reinforces the importance of the medical history and presenting symptoms in the decision to admit a suspected AMI patient to the hospital, since a normal or minimally abnormal initial ECG was found in almost 10% of proven AMI admissions.

Clinical algorithms for assisting in the triage of patients from the emergency room have been successful in improving CCU bed utilization.[50,54] In one study involving six New England hospitals and over 5000 patients, the proportion of nonischemic patients admitted to CCUs (ie, false positives) dropped from 44 to 33% without an increase in missed diagnoses of acute ischemia (ie, false negatives) as a result of using a predictive instrument to compute the probability of acute ischemia.[50] This decision tool requires only a "yes" or "no" answer to 7 questions (Table 6) and can be implemented on a hand-held programmable calculator or a personal computer.

Decision rules for early transfer of hospitalized patients from CCU or intermediate care beds to general ward beds have the potential to shorten length of stay and improve bed availability for incoming patients.[55,56] Weingarten et al[56] considered patients eligible for transfer to a non-monitored bed 24 hours after admission if none of the following criteria were present: 1) ECG or enzyme evidence for AMI; 2) recurrent ischemic-like chest pain; 3) presence of serious cardiac complications; 4) ongoing intervention requiring CCU care; 5) major therapeutic intervention such as angioplasty or surgery planned; and 6) unstable co-morbidity such as a gastrointestinal bleed. In their observational study 57% of low-risk patients would have been transferred by these guidelines earlier than by clinical judgement. It remains to be seen, however, whether or not these triage rules for early transfer actually work in practice, since a prospective study of these rules has yet to be carried out.

EVALUATION OF INITIAL CLINICAL STATUS

Patients admitted to the CCU represent a wide range of clinical conditions with varying medical requirements. The purpose of the CCU is not only to treat existing symptoms and abnormalities in critically ill patients but also to prevent serious com-

Table 6. *Prediction of acute ischemia from emergency room data*

Clinical Variable	Coefficient*
Pain in the chest or left arm?	0.9988
Pressure, pain or discomfort in the chest as most important symptom?	0.7145
History of heart attack?	0.4187
History of nitroglycerine use for chest pain?	0.5091
ST segment elevation or depression of >1.0 mm?	0.7682
ST segment straightening, elevation or depression of >1.0 mm?	0.8321
T wave peaking or inversion of >1.0 mm?	1.1278

* Probability of acute ischemia: $P = [1 + \exp(b_o + \Sigma\, b_i\, X_i\,)]^{-1}$ where X is 1 if variable is present and 2 if variable is absent; $b_o = -7.5698$

plications from developing in clinically stable individuals who are there for observation only. The two major issues in CCU monitoring are the detection of electrical abnormalities in the form of arrhythmias and conduction disorders and the early recognition of cardiac mechanical problems. Both of these are common in the AMI population, and short-term prognosis is largely determined by how well these problems are managed.

Arrhythmia monitoring has always been a major CCU function in the care of patients admitted with known or suspected AMI. Since the risk of death from electrical instability in AMI is greatest during the acute phase of illness, continuous monitoring of ECG rhythm is essential from the moment the patient presents to the emergency room until CCU discharge.

A great deal of controversy still exists concerning the necessity of administering prophylactic lidocaine to monitored patients who do not have any rhythm abnormalities. Although prophylactic lidocaine clearly reduces the incidence of ventricular fibrillation in AMI, a recently published meta-analysis of 14 randomized controlled trials involving over 9000 patients failed to demonstrate a reduction in mortality in the lidocaine-treated patients.[57] In fact, the analysis suggested that lidocaine prophylaxis actually increased mortality in hospitalized patients with uncomplicated AMI.

In addition to ECG rhythm monitoring, CCU patients should be carefully followed to detect the onset of mechanical abnormalities involving the right or left ventricle. Although hemodynamic monitoring is often necessary to manage left ventricular failure and cardiogenic shock, repeated clinical observations at the bedside will usually suffice to classify most patients into different hemodynamic subsets requiring different therapies.

Forrester et al[58] have defined 4 clinical subsets of AMI patients on the basis of bedside and radiographic findings:

Class 1: No evidence for pulmonary congestion or peripheral hypoperfusion
Class 2: Pulmonary congestion without peripheral hypoperfusion
Class 3: Peripheral hypoperfusion without pulmonary congestion
Class 4: Both pulmonary congestion and peripheral hypoperfusion

Recognition of pulmonary congestion requires bilateral rales over the posterobasal lung fields as well as radiographic evidence of pulmonary congestion. Peripheral hypoperfusion is defined by the presence of reduced skin temperature, confusion, oliguria, and hypotension (systolic BP < 100 mm Hg) or sinus tachycardia (> 125 beats/min).

When correlated with invasively determined cardiac index (CI) and pulmonary wedge pressures (PC), these clinical subsets accurately predicted the patients' hemodynamics in 83% of cases.[58] In this study pulmonary congestion was defined hemodynamically as PC > 18 mm Hg, and peripheral hypoperfusion was defined as CI < 2.2

L/min/square meter. Mortality rates in the four subsets of patients when verified by hemodynamic measurements were 3%, 9%, 23% and 51% for classes 1, 2, 3, and 4 respectively.

Most class 2 patients have mild-to-moderate left ventricular failure which responds to diuretic therapy. Invasive hemodynamic monitoring is generally not indicated unless severe pulmonary edema refractory to conventional therapy is present. Class 3 patients with peripheral hypoperfusion are a heterogeneous group, since several possible causes exist for low cardiac output states in AMI. In cases of inferior wall AMI, particularly when the proximal right coronary artery is occluded, right ventricular infarction should be excluded before using inotropic drugs or more invasive therapies. Fluid administration may be all that is necessary to correct low cardiac output when right ventricular infarction is present. However, invasive measurements of central venous and pulmonary wedge pressures may be necessary to confirm this diagnosis. Class 4 patients are in cardiogenic shock and require invasive monitoring and intensive management strategies to reverse this severe hemodynamic complication. Treatment of these conditions is beyond the scope of this chapter.

GENERAL THERAPEUTIC MEASURES

The treatment of AMI is directed towards accomplishing three major objectives: to relieve pain and anxiety, to minimize infarct size, and to detect and manage AMI complications. Specific therapeutic measures for minimizing infarct size and AMI complications are considered in other chapters of this book. This section discusses aspects of general AMI care that are appropriate for the CCU and post-CCU phases of hospitalization.

In the modern era of interventional cardiology, in which there is a major focus on aggressive early management of the AMI patient, it is important not to lose sight of the need to maintain patient comfort. For many patients, the acute event is their first clinical experience with coronary heart disease; it often occurs unexpectedly and has a major negative impact on their lives. For others with preexisting coronary heart disease the AMI represents one more indication that their disease is progressing and their long term outlook is poor. It is essential, therefore, to assess each patient's psychological needs as well as their specific medical needs in order to develop a comprehensive treatment plan that will minimize both functional and mental disability.

RELIEF OF PAIN AND ANXIETY

For optimal management of discomfort and anxiety, it is important to begin and maintain a dialogue with the patient as soon as possible after admission. The information content of this doctor-patient or nurse-patient interaction will vary depending upon the particular needs of each patient but should be informative as well as reassuring. Patients are generally better able to cope with their illness and respond to therapy when they understand what is going on and become active participants in their care.

The initial approach to pain relief may include one or more of the following: nitrates, narcotics, or β-blockers. The decision is generally made on the basis of pain severity, vital signs, hemodynamic status, and infarct location. Although once contraindicated in AMI, nitroglycerine is now often the initial therapy for chest pain. The dose of sublingual nitroglycerine is 0.3-0.4 mg repeated two or three times as needed, provided that the systolic blood pressure is adequate (> 100 mm Hg). This therapy has the potential to increase coronary blood flow across high grade lesions, relieve coronary spasm, improve collateral flow, and decrease ventricular preload and afterload. Resolution of chest pain may also be accompanied by reversal of ECG abnormalities.

Response to sublingual nitroglycerine should be followed by long acting nitrate preparations such as nitroglycerine ointment (1/2 to 2 inches every 4-6 hours) or intravenous nitroglycerine. The initial IV dose is 5 µg/min administered by an infusion pump with close monitoring of blood pressures and symptoms. The dose can be increased slowly to 50-200 µg/min until pain relief is complete, or until a 10 mm Hg or 10% fall in systolic blood pressure occurs (whichever is greater), or a 10% or greater increase in heart rate occurs. The usual duration of treatment is 24-48 hours, and this may be followed with long acting oral or topical nitroglycerine therapy. Intravenous nitroglycerine is also useful in the management of left ventricular failure; the dose is usually titrated upwards until a desired fall in left ventricular filling pressures is observed (pulmonary wedge pressures < 18 mm Hg).

For patients who do not respond adequately to sublingual nitroglycerine or who cannot tolerate the intravenous preparations, narcotic analgesia is recommended. Morphine sulfate, 2-4 mg IV every 10 minutes to 20 mg, has both effective analgesic properties as well as useful anxiolytic and sedative effects. Some patients, particularly those with inferior wall infarcts complicated with bradyarrhythmias, respond better to meperidine (25-50 mg IV) because of its vagolytic properties in contrast to morphine's vagotonic properties. The use of nitrates and IV β-blockers can substantially reduce the need for narcotic analgesia.[56] Diazepam (2-5 mg tid or qid) also provides sedation and anxiety relief with fewer side effects than the narcotic agents.

The need for oxygen in the AMI patient is controversial except in those patients who are clearly hypoxemic. Studies have shown little effect of routine oxygen therapy on survival, arrhythmias or cardiac function when compared to patients on room air.[59,60] On the other hand, routine arterial blood gas determinations to determine the need for oxygen therapy may not be appropriate either. An approach viewed as prudent by most authorities is to administer supplemental oxygen therapy by nasal prongs or face mask at 2-4 L/min for 1-3 days in uncomplicated patients. Patients with heart failure and other AMI complications may need longer and more aggressive oxygen and respiratory therapy. In patients with chronic obstructive lung disease, the dose of oxygen must be carefully titrated by blood gas determinations in order to avoid respiratory depression.

DIETARY MANAGEMENT

The diet in the CCU should be individualized according to the patient's clinical status. For the first 24 hours most patients are restricted to clear liquids with 1 gram or less of sodium. Total fluid intake should be limited to 1500-2000 ml to maintain a urine output of 800-1000 ml. Patients seriously ill with congestive heart failure or shock may require longer periods of fluid restrictions. If nausea or vomiting is present, oral intake should be limited and IV fluids administered (eg, 1500 ml glucose in half-normal saline).

Uncomplicated patients can advance to a soft, low cholesterol, low fat diet on day 2. This is an excellent time to begin education on dietary management of coronary heart disease. Patients will never be more motivated to consider life-style changes that might prevent progression of atherosclerosis than they are in the CCU. If the patient's lipid profile is not known, this should be done soon after admission, if possible, since it has been shown that these data accurately reflect the profile obtained 3 months post-MI.[61] Subsequent dietary recommendations can be based on these laboratory results. By day 4, patients with uncomplicated AMI can tolerate a regular diet with sodium, cholesterol, saturated fat, and caloric restrictions according to individual needs.

Bowel and Bladder Care

A bedside commode is recommended for most patients from the time of admission to the CCU. Constipation is a common problem associated with bed rest, narcotic analgesia, and reduced dietary bulk. A standing order for stool softeners such as dioctyl sodium sulfosuccinate (100 mg once or twice daily) or bulking agents such as methylcellulose (1 teaspoon twice daily) is useful for minimizing the distress and discomfort of constipation. Although once contraindicated, rectal examinations have been found to be safe in stable AMI patients, and the utility of this procedure in detecting abnormalities merits its inclusion in the physical examination.[62]

Urinary retention is also a complication of narcotic analgesia or atropine use in AMI, especially in elderly men with clinical or subclinical prostatic hypertrophy. A one-time urinary straight catheterization is recommended for the initial episode of urinary retention. An indwelling catheter can be used for recurrent urinary retention or in more critically ill patients with cardiogenic shock in whom careful monitoring of outputs is necessary.

REST AND PHYSICAL ACTIVITY

Although the initial treatment for AMI involves bed rest, uncomplicated patients may begin limited activities as soon as they are stable (ie, within 12-24 hours after admission). This includes use of a bedside commode and self-care activities such as eating, washing, teethbrushing, and hair-combing. Seriously ill patients may require more prolonged restriction of activities, at least until they are hemodynamically and electrically stable. While in the CCU patients are encouraged to exercise their feet against the footboard ten times per waking hour and to practice deep-breathing and coughing exercises.

Figure 6 illustrates a seven-step progressive ambulation schedule for a 7-10 day average hospital stay. This Phase I cardiac rehabilitation program is designed to minimize problems associated with prolonged bed rest, to reassure patients that they are not likely to become permanently disabled, and to prepare them to return to a more active lifestyle after hospital discharge. Levels 1 and 2 are carried out while still in the CCU, and the remaining levels on the hospital wards or in a cardiac rehabilitation center. Each level includes self care and bedside activities as well as light calisthenics and breathing exercises. More advanced levels may also include supervised treadmill, bicycle and stair exercises. As seen in Figure 6 the schedule can also be modified for post-op cardiac surgery patients.

The rate of advancement through these levels is determined by the patient's clinical condition and the response to the current level's activities. Older and sicker patients should progress more slowly than younger, uncomplicated patients. Contraindications to physical activities include persistent chest pain, uncontrolled arrhythmias or conduction disorders, heart failure or shock, severe hypertension (systolic blood pressure > 200 mm Hg, diastolic blood pressure > 100 mm Hg), uncontrolled diabetes, recent embolism, and active pericarditis. Careful monitoring of blood pressure, heart rate, ECG rhythm, and symptoms is required during the early phases of this program to insure that there are no hemodynamic or arrhythmic complications associated with physical activities.

The attending physician is ultimately responsible for advancing the patient through each level, although, in practice, the nursing or rehabilitation staff follow a standard routine based on the patient's daily progress. The actual supervision of activities is done by nurses, physical therapists or cardiac rehabilitation specialists. The supervising staff should review each patient's progress in order to provide appropriate feedback to the patient and physician.

CARDIOVASCULAR CENTER AT LDS HOSPITAL

Daily Activity Levels for Patients

During your hospital stay, your activity will gradually increase with the supervision of the medical staff. This is to facilitate your recovery and subsequent discharge from this hospital. Self care and activity levels, along with suggested exercises, are listed here so that you know exactly what you may do. Help us with your progress by doing only what your physician, nurses, and exercise therapists feel is allowable for your individual condition. To monitor your exercise after you leave the ICU, a wristwatch would be helpful.

	SELF CARE	BEDSIDE ACTIVITIES	CALISTHENICS/BREATHING *See Additional Notes on Supervised Exercise on the other side of this sheet.	WALKING/BICYCLING/STAIRS *See Additional Notes on Supervised Exercise on the other side of this sheet. MI	SURGERY
1	•Feed self •Use bedside commode •Wash hands/face •Brush teeth	•Sit in bed with firm back support	•Passive ROM, all extremities •Active plantar/dorsiflexion •Ankle circles •Diaphragmatic breathing	none	none
2	•Bathe self at bedside •Wash hands, face, upper body and personal areas (nurse assist with back and legs) •Comb hair •Shave self	•Dangle legs on side of bed •Sit up in chair for 20 minutes (NOT at mealtime or immediately before or after another activity such as bathing) •Light reading	Same as above, plus: •Active assisted ROM, all extremities •Shoulder shrugs	MET level: -- Walk in halls: --	1.5 100-200 ft. (2-5 min)
3	•Bathe self at bedside or sitting in chair in front of sink (nurse assist with back and legs)	•Walk to bathroom in room with assistance •Sit up in chair as tolerated •Sit in bedside chair for meals	Same as above plus: •In supine position flex knees to 75°	MET level: -- Walk in halls: --	1.5 200-360 ft (2-5 min)
4	•Take warm shower if appropriate	•Sit in bedside chair as tolerated •Sit in bedside chair for meals •Walk to bathroom with assistance as needed.	Same as above, plus 1 minute each of the following: •In supine position flex knees to 75° •Sitting knee extension •Sitting push and pull	MET level: 1.5-2.0 Walk in halls: 100-200 ft (2-5 min) Treadmill/Bike: --	1.5-2.0 400-600 ft (5-7 min) 5-7 min
5	•Take warm shower if desired	•Increased beside chair sitting time as tolerated	Same as above, plus 1.25 min. each, 3x a day of the following •Sitting knee extension •Sitting with lateral trunk bender •Sitting push and pull	MET level: 1.5-2.0 Walk in halls: ≤500 ft (5-7 min) Treadmill/Bike: 5 min Stairs: 3-6	1.2-2.5 ≤ 1000 ft (5-10 min) 5-10 min 3-6
6	•Continue as above plus standing self care	•Continue with bedside chair and bathroom priveleges	Same as above, 1.5 min each, 3x a day	MET level: 1.5-2.5 Walk in halls: ≤ 1000 ft (5-10 min) Treadmill/Bike: 5-10 min Stairs: 6-12	1.2-2.5 ≤ 2000 ft (10-15 min) 10-15 min 6-12
7	•Up ad lib	•Up ad lib	Same as above plus add the following: •Standing one arm overhead •Standing lateral bend°	MET level: 1.5-2.5 Walk in halls: ≤2000 ft (10-15 min) Treadmill/Bike: 10-15 min Stairs: up to 14	2.0-3.0 ≤ 3300 ft (15-20 min) 15-20 min up to 14

Additional Notes on Supervised Exercise

•Blood pressure is recorded before and immediately after each exercise session.
•Heart rate is recorded before, during, and one minute after each exercise session.
•Exercise therapists will supervise calisthenics, treadmill, bicycling, and stairs two times a day; and nursing staff will assist patients once a day.

Specific Learning Objectives

•Patients will be encouraged to attend all scheduled cardiac classes.
•Exercise therapists and nursing staff will review concepts taught in cardiac classes and during exercise sessions and will help patients learn pulse monitoring during each exercise session.
•Home program preparation will begin on level 6.

Figure 6. *Seven-step progressive ambulation schedule used in the Phase I cardiac rehabilitation program at LDS Hospital in Salt Lake City, Utah.*

In addition to the various physical activities listed in Figure 6, some hospital programs offer group classes for patients and their spouses dealing with such topics as psychosocial adjustments to coronary heart disease, cardiac risk factors, nutrition, exercise, and sexual activities. The purpose is to enhance the recovery process by providing information and emotional support to patients and their families. These classes can be administered by nursing, dietary, social work and rehabilitation personnel.

REFERENCES

1. Gillum RF, Fortmann SP, Prineas RJ, et al: International diagnostic criteria for acute myocardial infarction and stroke. Am Heart J 1984;87:577-583.

2. Solomon CG, Lee TH, Cook EF, et al: Comparison of clinical presentation of acute myocardial infarction in patients older than 65 years of age to younger patients. Am J Cardiol 1989;63:772-776.

3. Bayer AJ, Chadha JS, Farag RR, et al: Changing presentation of myocardial infarction with increasing old age. J Am Geriatr Soc 1986;34:263-266.

4. Librach G, Schadel M, Seltzer M, et al: The initial manifestations of acute myocardial infarction. Geriatrics 1976;31:41-46.

5. Uretsky BF, Farquhar DS, Berezin AF, et al: Symptomatic myocardial infarction without chest pain: Prevalence and clinical course. Am J Cardiol 1977;40:498-503.

6. Clark JA, Anderson JL: Assessing the patient with possible acute myocardial infarction, in Anderson JL (ed): *Acute Myocardial Infarction: New Management Strategies.* Rockville, Aspen Publishers Inc. 1987, p 57.

7. Jalowiec DA, Hill JA: Myocardial infarction in the young and in women. Cardiovasc Clinic 1989;20:197-206.

8. Hancock EW: Ischemic heart disease: Acute myocardial infarction, in Rubenstein E, Federman DD (eds): *Scientific American Medicine.* New York, Scientific American Inc. 1989, chapter 10, p 5.

9. Riley CP, Russell RO, Rackley CE: Left ventricular gallop sound and acute myocardial infarction. Am Heart J 1973;86:598-602.

10. Dugall JC, Pryor R, Blount SG: Systolic murmur following acute myocardial infarction. Am Heart J 1974;87:577-583.

11. Rude RE, Poole K, Muller JE, et al: Electrocardiographic and clinical criteria for recognition of acute myocardial infarction based on analysis of 3697 patients. Am J Cardiol 1983;52:936-942.

12. Schamroth L: *The 12-Lead Electrocardiogram, Book 1.* Oxford, Blackwell Scientific Publications, 1989, p 145.

13. Pichler M, Shah PK, Peter T, et al: Wall motion abnormalities and electrocardiographic changes in acute transmural myocardial infarction: Implications of reciprocal ST-segment depression. Am Heart J 1983;106:1003-1009.

14. Marriott HJL: *Principles of Electrocardiography.* Baltimore, Williams & Wilkins, 1983, Chapter 26.

15. Bren GB, Wasserman AG, Ross AM: The electrocardiogram in patients undergoing thrombolysis for myocardial infarction. Circulation 1987;76(II):II18-II24.

16. Huey BL, Beller GA, Kaiser DL, et al: A comprehensive analysis of myocardial infarction due to left circumflex artery occlusion: Comparison with infarction due to right coronary artery and left anterior descending artery occlusion. J Am Coll Cardiol 1988;12:1156-66.

17. Segal MS, Swiryn S: True posterior myocardial infarction. Arch Intern Med 1983;143:983-985.

18. Croft CH, Nicod P, Corbett JR, et al: Detection of acute right ventricular infarction by right precordial electrocardiography. Am J Cardiol 1982;50:421-427.

19. Morgera T, Alberti E, Silvestri F, et al: Right precordial ST and QRS changes in the diagnosis of right ventricular infarction. Am Heart J 1984;108:13-18.

20. Hands ME, Cook EF, Stone PH, et al: Electrocardiographic diagnosis of myocardial infarction in presence of complete left bundle branch block. Am Heart J 1988;116:23-31.

21. Andre-Fouet X, Pillot M, Leizorovicz A, et al: "Non-Q wave," alias "nontransmural," myocardial infarction: A specific entity. Am Heart J 1989;117:892-902.

22. Krone RJ, Friedman E, Thanavaro S, et al: Long-term prognosis after first Q-wave (transmural) or non-Q-wave (nontransmural) myocardial infarction: Analysis of 593 patients. Am J Cardiol 1983;52:234-239.

23. Spodick DH: Comprehensive electrocardiographic analysis of acute myocardial infarction by individual and combined waveforms. Am J Cardiol 1988;62:465-467.

24. Schectman KB, Capone RS, Kleiger RE, et al: Risk stratification of patients with non-Q wave myocardial infarction: The critical role of ST segment depression. Circulation 1989;80:1148-1158.

25. Brush JE, Brand DA, Acampora D, et al: Use of the initial electrocardiogram to predict in-hospital complications of acute myocardial infarction. N Engl J Med 1985;312:1137-1141.

26. Stark ME, Vacek JL: The initial electrocardiogram during admission for myocardial infarction. Use as a predictor of clinical course and facility utilization. Arch Intern Med 1987;147:843-846.

27. Dillon MC, Calbreath DF, Dixon AM, et al: Diagnostic problem in acute myocardial infarction: CK-MB in the absence of abnormally elevated total creatine kinase levels. Arch Intern Med 1982;142:33-38.

28. Yusuf S, Collins R, Lin L, et al: Significance of elevated MB isoenzyme with normal creatine kinase in acute myocardial infarction. Am J Cardiol 1987;59:245-250.

29. Fisher ML, Carliner NH, Becker LC, et al: Serum creatine kinase in the diagnosis of acute myocardial infarction: Optimal sampling frequency. JAMA 1983;249:393-395.

30. Lee TH, Goldman L: Serum enzyme assays in the diagnosis of acute myocardial infarction. Recommendations based on a quantitative analysis. Ann Intern Med 1986;105:221-233.

31. Sobel BE, Shell WE: Serum enzyme determinations in the diagnosis and assessment of myocardial infarction. Circulation 1972;45:471-482.

32. Puleo PR, Roberts R: An update on cardiac enzymes. Cardiol Clin 1988;6:97-109.

33. Muller-Hansen S, Mathey DG, Bleifeld W, et al: Isoelectric focusing of creatine kinase MM isoforms and its application for diagnosis of acute myocardial infarction. Clin Biochem 1989;22:125-130.

34. McComb JM, McMaster EA, Mackenzie G, et al: Myoglobin and creatine kinase in acute myocardial infarction. Br Heart J 1984;51:189-194.

35. Gibler WB, Gibler CD, Weinshenken E, et al: Myoglobin as an early indicator of acute myocardial infarction. Ann Emerg Med 1987;16:851-856.

36. Carpeggiani C, L'Abbate A, Marzullo P, et al: Multiparametric approach to diagnosis of non-Q wave acute myocardial infarction. Am J Cardiol 1989;63:404-408.

37. Katus HA, Yasuda T, Gold HK, et al: Diagnosis of acute myocardial infarction by detection of circulating cardiac myosin light chains. Am J Cardiol 1984;54:964-970.

38. Sasaki H, Charuzi Y, Beeder C, et al: Utility of echocardiography for the early assessment of patients with nondiagnostic chest pain. Am Heart J 1986;112:494-497.

39. Oh JK, Miller FA, Shub C, et al: Evaluation of acute chest pain syndromes by two-dimensional echocardiography: Its potential application in the selection of patients for acute reperfusion therapy. Mayo Clin Proc 1987;62:59-66.

40. Sabia P, Atrookteh A, Touchstone D, et al: Two-dimensional echocardiography can reduce hospital admissions for acute myocardial infarction by more than one-third: Results of a prospective study performed in the emergency room. J Am Coll Cardiol 1989;13:159A.

41. Buda AJ: Diagnosis of myocardial infarction: Traditional methods and new approaches with cardiac imaging, in Anderson JL (ed): *Acute Myocardial Infarction: New Management Strategies.* Rockville, Aspen Publishers Inc. 1987, p 67.

42. Isaacsohn JL, Earle MG, Kemper AJ, et al: Post myocardial infarction pain and infarct extension in the coronary care unit: Role of two-dimensional echocardiography. J Am Coll Cardiol 1988;11:246-251.

43. Jugdutt BI, Sussex BA, Sivaram CA, et al: Right ventricular infarction: Two-dimensional echocardiographic evaluation. Am Heart J 1984;107:505-518.

44. Cecci F, Zuppioli A, Favilli S, et al: Echocardiographic findings in right ventricular infarction. Clin Cardiol 1984;7:405-412.

45. Iskandrian AS, Hakki AH: Thallium-201 myocardial scintigraphy. Am Heart J 1985;109:113-128.

46. Massie BM, Botvinick EH, Werner JA, et al: Myocardial scintigraphy with technetium-99m stannous pyrophosphate: An insensitive test of nontransmural myocardial infarction. Am J Cardiol 1979;43:186-192.

47. Geltman EM: Cardiac positron emission tomography. West J Med 1985;143:764-772

48. Sobel BE, Geltman EM, Trifenbrunn AJ, et al: Improvement of regional myocardial metabolism after coronary thrombolysis induced with tissue-type plasminogen activator or streptokinase. Circulation 1984;69:983-990.

49. Berman DS, Kiat H, Maddahi J, et al: Radionuclide imaging of myocardial perfusion and viability in assessment of acute myocardial infarction. Am J Cardiol 1989;64:9B-16B.

50. Bzen MW, D'Agostino RB, Selker HP, et al: A predictive instrument to improve coronary care unit admission practices in acute ischemic heart disease. N Engl J Med 1984;310:1273-1278.

51. Slater DK, Hlatky MA, Mark DB, et al: Outcome in suspected acute myocardial infarction with normal or minimally abnormal admission electrocardiographic findings. Am J Cardiol 1987;60:766-770.

52. Fineberg HV, Scadden D, Goldman L: Care of patients with a low probability of acute myocardial infarction: Cost effectiveness of alternatives to coronary care unit admission. N Engl J Med 1985;310:1301-1307.

53. Dubois C, Pierard LA, Albert A, et al: Short-term risk stratification at admission based on simple clinical data in acute myocardial infarction. Am J Cardiol 1988;61:216-219.

54. Goldman L, Weinberg M, Weisberg M, et al: A computer-derived protocol to aid in the diagnosis of emergency room patients with acute chest pain. N Engl J Med 1982;309:588-596.

55. Mulley AG, Thibault GE, Hughes RA, et al: The course of patients with suspected myocardial infarction. N Engl J Med 1980;302:943-948.

56. Weingarten SR, Ermann B, Riedinger MS, et al: Selecting the best triage rule for patients hospitalized with chest pain. Am J Med 1989;87:494-500.

57. Hine LK, Laird N, Hewitt P, et al: Meta-analytic evidence against prophylactic use of lidocaine in acute myocardial infarction. Arch Intern Med 1989;149:2694-2698.

58. Forrester JS, Diamond GA, Swan HJC: Correlative classification of clinical and hemo-dynamic function after acute myocardial infarction. Am J Cardiol 1977;39:137-145.

59. Rawles J, Kenmore ACF: Controlled trial of oxygen in uncomplicated myocardial infarction. Brit Med J 1976;1:1121-1123.

60. Loeb HS, Chuquimia R, Sinno MZ, et al: Effects of low-flow oxygen on the hemodynamic and left ventricular function in patients with uncomplicated acute myocardial infarction. Chest 1971;60:352-358.

61. Fyfe T, Baxter RH, Cochran KM, et al: Plasma lipid changes after myocardial infarction. Lancet 1971;2:997-999.

62. Earnest DL, Fletcher GF: Danger of rectal examination in patients with acute myocardial infarction - fact or fiction? N Engl J Med 1969;281-238-241.

Chapter 4

TRIAGE AND MANAGEMENT STRATEGIES FOR ACUTE MYOCARDIAL INFARCTION
Roles of the Community and Referral Hospitals

Eduardo D. Flores
Richard A. Lange
L. David Hillis

INTRODUCTION

Ischemic heart disease is the leading cause of death in industrialized societies. Each year in the United States alone, more than 1,500,000 adults sustain a myocardial infarction. About 25% of all deaths occur as a consequence of myocardial infarction.[1] It is estimated that more than half the deaths due to coronary artery disease occur outside the hospital.[2] Of those with myocardial infarction who survive long enough to reach the hospital, many are taken to community hospitals of small or moderate size. In fact, over half of all patients with myocardial infarction are treated in hospitals with less than 300 beds.[3] Therefore, if morbidity and mortality due to myocardial infarction are to be reduced substantially, management strategies *in the community* will be necessary to encourage early hospitalization and interventions to limit the extent of myocardial ischemic injury.[4]

Over the past decade a remarkable evolution in the management of myocardial infarction has occurred,[5] based largely on observations concerning the pathogenesis and course of infarction. First, pathologic and angiographic studies demonstrated that total thrombotic occlusion of a coronary artery was present in about 90% of patients in the early hours of acute transmural infarction.[6,7] Second, studies in experimental animals showed that total coronary occlusion led to progressive myocardial necrosis over several hours; if coronary perfusion was reestablished quickly, myocardium was salvaged and infarct size limited.[8,9] Third, it became clear that left ventricular function after infarction was an important predictor of quality of life and survival.[10-12] As a result, aggressive therapeutic strategies designed to reestablish antegrade coronary flow in patients with evolving myocardial infarction were developed, including direct balloon angioplasty, emergent coronary artery bypass surgery, and intracoronary or intravenous thrombolytic therapy.[13] At present, a great deal of new information is available concerning the therapy of myocardial infarction, but several questions remain for the practicing physician in the community. This chapter will address the following questions: (a) Which strategy for reperfusion should be adopted in the community hospital for patients with acute myocardial infarction (AMI)? (b) What are the indications for transfer to a referral center, catheterization, and subsequent revascularization (balloon angioplasty or bypass surgery)? (c) What is the role of the referral center in this management scheme?

REPERFUSION STRATEGIES IN THE COMMUNITY HOSPITAL

Direct Balloon Angioplasty

Only about 20% of acute care hospitals in the United States have catheterization facilities, and angioplasty is available in only some of them.[14] Furthermore, in those centers where the facilities are available, the widespread application of angioplasty to patients with evolving myocardial infarction requires that a team of physicians, nurses, and support personnel be available at all times. Since coronary reperfusion should be accomplished within 4 to 6 hours, direct balloon angioplasty without antecedent thrombolytic therapy is impractical for patients who present to most community hospitals. However, for the patient with rapid access to a center experienced with this technique, good results have been reported.[15,16] In a series of 500 patients with evolving myocardial infarction treated with direct balloon angioplasty, O'Keefe et al[15] accomplished reperfusion in 94%, with subsequent reocclusion in only 15%. Global left ventricular function improved significantly, and the hospital mortality was only 7.2%. Survival at one year was excellent. Although similar favorable results with direct balloon angioplasty have been reported from a community hospital,[17] logistic, geographic, and economic limitations preclude its widespread use.

Thrombolytic Therapy

Of the available methods to achieve reperfusion in patients with evolving myocardial infarction, intravenous thrombolytic therapy is the most appropriate for use in the community hospital. Several randomized trials have shown that early intravenous administration of a thrombolytic agent limits infarct size, improves left ventricular function,[18-27] decreases the incidence of late fatal arrhythmias,[28,29] and improves early[30-36] and long-term[31,33,35,37,38] survival. In addition, patients given thrombolytic therapy have a reduced incidence of congestive heart failure,[22] cardiogenic shock, ventricular fibrillation, and pericarditis[25] in the weeks to months after infarction.

Since intravenous thrombolytic therapy, unlike direct angioplasty, does not require immediate access to catheterization facilities, it can be administered to many patients with evolving infarction in the community hospital setting. Several studies have documented the feasibility, efficacy, safety, and improved timing of thrombolytic therapy in the community hospital.[14,39-46] McNamara et al[40] gave intravenous streptokinase to patients with evolving infarction in eight rural hospitals where most of the physicians were not cardiologists and did not have experience with thrombolytic therapy. In comparison to patients treated at a referral center, there was no difference in the incidence of clot lysis, bleeding complications, or death, and the time from onset of chest pain to infusion of drug was similar. Topol et al[14] compared the efficacy and safety of t-PA administration at a community hospital to that by a helicopter transport team before or after transfer to a referral center. In those treated at the community hospital, therapy was initiated earlier (2.1 versus 3.8 hours, p < 0.001), and left ventricular ejection fraction was better (54% versus 50%, p < 0.01). Although interhospital helicopter transport was feasible and safe, the subset of patients in which this modality should be used was undefined. In addition, the cost of a helicopter transfer averaged about $2,000.

Despite its established benefits, thrombolytic therapy has several limitations. First, a thrombolytic agent must be given soon (ie, within 4 to 6 hours) after the onset of chest pain to exert a substantial effect on morbidity and mortality. Unfortunately, many patients with evolving infarction do not seek medical attention within this time frame. For example, over half the patients not randomized in the GISSI trial were excluded because they arrived at the hospital more than 12 hours after the onset of chest pain.[32] Likewise, about 75% of those excluded from the ASSET trial were ineligible because they arrived at the hospital more than 5 hours after symptom onset.[34] If, in addition to arrival at the hospital within 4 to 6 hours of the onset of chest pain, other standard inclusion criteria are utilized (aged < 75 years, electrocardiographic ST-segment elevation, and the absence of contraindications to thrombolytic therapy), it is estimated that only about 15 to 25% of patients with myocardial infarction are eligible for thrombolytic therapy.[47,48]

Second, with conventional doses of currently available thrombolytic agents, early *reperfusion* (within 60-90 minutes), defined as angiographic reopening of closed vessels, is achieved in only about 40-70% of patients[49-57] and early *patency* (90 minutes), defined angiographically after therapy, is achieved in about 50-80%. Streptokinase has the lowest efficacy in establishing early *reperfusion* (average, 39%), whereas t-PA and APSAC have higher rates. The early data for anisoylated plasminogen streptokinase activator complex (APSAC) are intermediate (Table 1). Patency rates at later time points (within 24 hours), however, have been similar for all three agents, provided that full-dose heparin is given after t-PA. "Front-loaded" regimens of t-PA (eg, 100 mg given in 90 rather than 180 minutes, with a substantial percentage of

Table 1. *Reperfusion rates with intravenous thrombolytic therapy*

Author	Time from pain to drug (hours)	Reperfusion*	
		n	%
Streptokinase			
Neuhaus et al[51]	3.4	24/40	60
Spann et al[52]	3.5	21/43	49
Chesebro et al[49]	4.7	37/119	31
Hillis et al[53]	4.5	11/34	32
TOTAL		93/236	39
Tissue Plasminogen Activator			
Collen et al[54]	4.7	25/33	76
Williams et al[55]	4.8	25/37	68
Gold et al[56]	3.0	24/29	83
Chesebro et al[49]	4.5	70/113	62
TOTAL		144/212	68
APSAC			
Bonnier et al[57]	2.5	23/36	64
Anderson et al[50]	3.4	47/79	59[†]
TOTAL		82/151	54

* Reperfusion denotes angiographic confirmation of reestablished flow in a previously totally occluded vessel.
† For patients who were treated within four hours of pain onset.

the total dose given in the first 15 to 30 minutes) are currently being tested, because of a higher early *patency* rate (91%) in one study.[58]

Third, most patients successfully treated with thrombolytic therapy have a significant residual stenosis in the infarct artery,[59] and reocclusion with new thrombus may occur. Such reocclusion often results in early recurrent ischemic events,[49,55,59,60] such as recurrent angina, infarct extension, and occasionally, death. Although a number of studies have demonstrated that the severity of the residual stenosis after successful thrombolysis is related to the propensity for reocclusion,[61-63] the pooled data from TAMI-I and TAMI-III (in which t-PA was administered) failed to relate recurrent ischemic events with angiographic evidence of a severe residual stenosis of the infarct artery.[59]

Although most authors agree that thrombolytic therapy can and should be administered in the community hospital, patient management after its administration is controversial. Some community physicians advocate a strategy of immediate[41] or early (within 12 to 72 hours) transfer to a referral center[42-45] for angiography and possible revascularization, whereas others[40] advocate a more conservative approach, with transfer and catheterization reserved for specific patients. Those who advocate an aggressive strategy argue that: 1) currently used clinical markers of reperfusion fail to identify reliably the 30% or so of patients in whom early patency is not achieved[64] and in whom "salvage" angioplasty might be beneficial,[65] particularly those with cardiogenic shock;[66] 2) the high incidence of severe residual coronary stenoses after successful thrombolysis may promote recurrent thrombosis and reinfarction, and this course of events may be favorably influenced by angioplasty; and 3) early catheterization allows identification of high-risk patients, such as those with left main or severe three vessel coronary artery disease, who would likely benefit from early surgical intervention, or low-risk patients who may be discharged early (ie, at 3 to 5 days).[67]

Again, logistic and economic constraints do not favor approaches mandating interhospital transfer, cardiac catheterization, and angioplasty for all patients with myocardial infarction. Fortunately, several recent randomized trials utilizing "aggressive" and "conservative" management strategies after either t-PA or APSAC administration suggest that no additional benefit is achieved with early emergent catheterization and angioplasty.

MANAGEMENT AFTER THROMBOLYTIC THERAPY

Role of Immediate Catheterization and Angioplasty

Advocates of immediate catheterization and angioplasty after thrombolytic therapy hoped that such a strategy would open vessels in patients in whom thrombolytic therapy had been unsuccessful (ie, those whose infarct arteries were still occluded) and reduce the residual stenosis in patients in whom thrombolytic therapy had been successful. In turn, this management strategy might improve coronary perfusion, limit infarct size, preserve left ventricular function, and reduce the incidence of recurrent ischemic events. In practice, however, the results of such an aggressive strategy have been disappointing. Three large randomized trials have compared the efficacy and safety of immediate catheterization and angioplasty to those of delayed catheterization and angioplasty performed routinely[68,69] or for a recurrence of symptoms[70] (Table 2). In all three studies, t-PA was given. As the data in Table 2 indicate, immediate catheterization and angioplasty following thrombolytic therapy offered no improvement in left ventricular function and short-term mortality when compared to delayed catheterization and angioplasty[68,69] or a completely noninvasive management strategy.[70] Furthermore, immediate catheterization and angioplasty were associated with an increased incidence of hemorrhagic complications, emergent coronary artery bypass surgery, and death. Although all three trials used t-PA, similar data have been reported

Table 2. *Trials assessing immediate catheterization and angioplasty after thrombolytic therapy*

	TAMI[68]		ECSG[70]		TIMI IIA[69]	
	Immediate	7-10 d	Immediate	None	Immediate	18-48 h
Predischarge LVEF (%)	53	56	51	51	50	49
In-hospital mortality (%)	4	1	7	3*	7	6
Success rate of PTCA (%)	85	94	90	—	84	93
Recurrent infarction (%)	—	—	4	7	7	4
Emergent surgery (%)	7	2	—	—	4	2
Transfusion (%)	22	18†	10	4	20	7*
Complications (%)	—	—	—	—	12	4*

* p < 0.05 in comparison to immediate
† Transfusion rates of 22% and 18% were obtained from the data of Topol et al.[16]
LVEF = left ventricular ejection fraction
PTCA = percutaneous transluminal coronary angioplasty

when immediate catheterization and angioplasty were utilized following intravenous streptokinase.[71]

Role of Routine Revascularization Before Discharge

The question of whether routine catheterization and angioplasty prior to hospital discharge are beneficial in patients who have received thrombolytic therapy has been addressed by 2 large randomized trials. In the TIMI IIB trial,[72] 3262 patients were treated with intravenous t-PA and then randomly assigned to an invasive management strategy (catheterization and angioplasty, if coronary anatomy was suitable, 18 to 48 hours after t-PA) or a conservative one (catheterization and angioplasty only for those with recurrent angina or a positive exercise test). In comparison to the conservative management strategy, the invasive strategy did not improve left ventricular function or reduce the incidence of reinfarction or death (Table 3). In fact, adverse clinical events (emergent coronary artery bypass surgery, intracranial hemorrhage, non-fatal reinfarction, or death) occurred more frequently in those treated aggressively (13.0%

Table 3. *Trials assessing delayed catheterization and angioplasty after thrombolytic therapy**

	TIMI IIB[72]		SWIFT[73]	
	Conserv n = 1626	Invasive n = 1636	Conserv n = 403	Invasive n = 397
Lytic agent	t-PA		APSAC	
Duration of follow-up	42 days		90 days	
Reinfarction	5.8%	6.4%	9.7%	13.9%
Mortality	4.7%	5.2%	3.2%	4.8%
Mortality at 1 year	7.6%	7.0%	—	—

* In both trials, conservative and invasive management strategies were statistically similar for all variables.

versus 10.6%, p = 0.04). The SWIFT (**S**hould **W**e **I**ntervene **F**ollowing **T**hrombolysis) study[73] reached similar conclusions. In this trial, 800 patients were treated with APSAC and then randomly assigned to routine delayed catheterization and revascularization or careful observation, with catheterization and angioplasty only for those with recurrent angina. Left ventricular function (measured at hospital discharge or at six weeks after infarction) and survival were similar for the two groups.

Both of these trials provide support for a conservative management strategy for patients with myocardial infarction who have received thrombolytic therapy. According to this strategy, the patient who has received thrombolytic therapy should undergo catheterization and angioplasty for recurrent angina or a positive pre-discharge exercise test. In the absence of either of these events, the patient may be discharged from the hospital on low-dose aspirin and observed closely during rehabilitation.

ROLE OF THE COMMUNITY HOSPITAL IN THE MANAGEMENT OF MYOCARDIAL INFARCTION

Minimizing Delay from Onset of Symptoms to Initiation of Appropriate Therapy

If the patient with AMI is to obtain maximal benefit from thrombolytic therapy, treatment must be instituted as soon as possible after the onset of ischemic injury.[4,32,33] The time from the onset of chest pain to the initiation of effective therapy consists of the time in which the patient decides to seek medical assistance, the time required for travel to the site of assistance, and the time required for medical personnel to evaluate the patient, arrive at a diagnosis, and begin therapy.

In most studies the time in which the patient decides to seek medical assistance accounts for most of the delay.[74,75] When symptoms first appear, many patients minimize their severity and significance (denial); others misinterpret them; and still others cannot expeditiously decide on a proper plan of action.[76] Surprisingly, patients with known ischemic heart disease often take longer to seek medical assistance than those without a history of heart disease.[74,77] As demonstrated in studies from Canada and Sweden,[78,79] the time in which the patient decides to seek medical assistance can be favorably influenced by public education through the mass media. In Göteborg, Sweden, early presentation to hospital for chest pain of >15 minutes duration was encouraged through the mass media, after which the elapsed time from onset of symptoms to hospitalization fell from 3 to 2 hours.[79] The community hospital should play a role in educating its patient population to the symptoms and signs of myocardial infarction as well as the importance of prompt medical assistance.

In urban areas the time required for travel to the site of medical assistance is usually the shortest of the three reasons for delay from onset of symptoms to initiation of therapy. However, for the patient in a remote location, the time required for transport may be substantial.[75] Previous studies have shown that patient transport is made safer by mobile coronary care systems.[80,81] Unfortunately, only about half the patients with myocardial infarction who have access to such facilities utilize them. Interestingly, such sophisticated transport facilities are used least often by patients with the greatest amount of formal education.[82]

In addition to transporting patients to a medical facility quickly and safely, mobile coronary care systems may be beneficial in other ways. The trained paramedical personnel who staff these units can identify the patient with evolving myocardial infarction and notify the receiving medical institution in advance, minimizing the delay from arrival at the facility to the initiation of appropriate therapy.[83,84] Preliminary studies have shown that these paramedical personnel may begin thrombolytic therapy *during transport,* drastically reducing the delay from onset of symptoms to initiation of therapy.[85-87] However, the efficacy and safety of "pre-hospital" thrombolytic therapy are as yet undetermined.

Finally, the time required for medical personnel to evaluate the patient, arrive at a diagnosis, and begin therapy may contribute substantially to the overall delay from onset of symptoms to initiation of appropriate therapy. To minimize this in-hospital delay: 1) an electrocardiogram should be obtained immediately on any patient presenting to the emergency room with chest pain; and 2) once a diagnosis of myocardial infarction is made and the contraindications for thrombolytic therapy excluded, such therapy should be initiated immediately in the emergency room and should not be deferred until the patient is moved to an inpatient setting.

ADMINISTRATION OF THROMBOLYTIC THERAPY

In the community hospital intravenous thrombolytic therapy should be considered for the following patients, regardless of whether catheterization facilities are immediately available:

Patients with Evolving Transmural (Q wave) Infarction

Thrombolytic therapy should be administered to patients with ST-segment elevation in two or more contiguous leads, since previous studies have demonstrated that totally occlusive coronary thrombi are present in 85-90% of these patients.[6] In contrast, totally occlusive coronary thrombi are infrequently observed during evolving non-Q wave infarction,[88] and the efficacy of thrombolytic therapy in these patients is unproven. The GISSI[32] and ISIS-2[33] trials included patients with ST-segment elevation (evolving Q wave infarction) or depression (evolving non-Q wave infarction), but neither showed that streptokinase improved survival in the latter group. Similarly, several small studies have assessed the efficacy of t-PA,[89-92] streptokinase,[93] or urokinase[94] in patients with unstable angina at rest or non-Q wave infarction, but the results have been disparate and inconclusive. Several large trials of thrombolytic therapy in patients with unstable angina or non-Q wave infarction are currently ongoing. Until their results are available, the administration of thrombolytic agents should be restricted to patients with electrocardiographic evidence of evolving Q wave infarction.

Patients Who Can be Treated Within Six Hours of the Onset of Chest Pain

As previously emphasized, the efficacy of thrombolytic therapy is related to the elapsed time from onset of chest pain to initiation of drug treatment. In the GISSI trial,[32] patients given streptokinase within 1 hour of symptom onset had a 47% reduction in mortality; in contrast, those given streptokinase more than six hours after symptom onset derived no benefit in survival in comparison to those treated without thrombolytic therapy. Although the ISIS-2 trial[33] showed a diminished mortality even in patients given streptokinase 13 to 24 hours after the onset of chest pain, the reduction in mortality was most marked in those treated early.

The finding in ISIS-2 that survival was improved in patients given streptokinase as late as 13 to 24 hours after the onset of symptoms has stirred considerable interest, particularly since most studies fail to demonstrate that such late therapy influences left ventricular function. This apparent dissociation between the effects of coronary reperfusion on left ventricular function and survival has been reported by others.[36,95,96] A patent infarct artery, even if accomplished late after the onset of infarction, may exert a beneficial effect by limiting infarct expansion and improving left ventricular

73

remodeling,[97-100] interrupting a "stuttering" infarction, restoring collateral perfusion supplied by the infarct artery,[101] and/or diminishing the propensity for arrhythmic events.[28,29,102,103] However, until the results of ongoing trials assessing the effects of late reperfusion are available, thrombolytic therapy should be given only to patients who can be treated within six hours of the onset of chest pain, unless persistent ischemic pain is present.

Patients Without a Contraindication to Thrombolytic Therapy or Subsequent Anticoagulation

Many of the large randomized trials of thrombolytic therapy have limited enrollment to patients less than 65 to 70 years of age because of a concern for an increased incidence of bleeding complications in elderly individuals.[104] In the TIMI study,[105] patients aged 65 or older had an increased incidence of bleeding complications in comparison to those below 65. However, half these patients received 150 mg of t-PA, and urgent catheterization was performed in all of them. In the GISSI trial,[32] streptokinase did not exert a beneficial effect in patients older than 65 years, but in the ISIS-2 trial,[33] streptokinase induced a 50% reduction in mortality in octogenarians. At present, advanced age should be considered only a relative contraindication to thrombolytic therapy. Table 4 lists the absolute and relative contraindications to thrombolytic therapy.

Complications Following Administration of Thrombolytic Therapy

During and immediately after the administration of a thrombolytic agent, several complications may arise, including:

Hypotension

About 5-10% of patients given intravenous streptokinase or APSAC develop hypotension during the infusion, which for the former is related in part to the rate of infusion.[19-21,32,33,106-109] The hypotension is usually transient and almost always responsive to intravenous fluids or pressor agents. Hypotension occurs less frequently during the intravenous infusion of urokinase or t-PA.

Allergic reactions

Allergic reactions occur in 2 to 10% of patients who are given a thrombolytic agent derived from bacterial proteins (eg, streptokinase, APSAC).[20,21,27,32,33,35,49,107-109] These allergic reactions are rarely life-threatening and include pyrexia, rigors, pur-

Table 4. *Contraindications to thrombolytic therapy*

ABSOLUTE

Active internal bleeding

Recent (< 2 months) cerebrovascular accident

Recent (< 10 days) major surgery

Recent (< 10 days) serious GI bleeding

Recent (< 10 days) serious trauma

Uncontrolled severe arterial hypertension

Intracranial neoplasm

RELATIVE

Age > 75 years

Hemostatic abnormality

Severe hepatic or renal disease

Diabetic hemorrhagic retinopathy

Cerebrovascular disease

pura, or rash; vasculitis, bronchoconstriction, and anaphylaxis occur rarely. Therapy with antihistamines and corticosteroids is effective for milder allergic reactions; more aggressive measures may be needed for the more severe ones. Thrombolytic agents consisting of human proteins (t-PA and urokinase) do not usually induce an antigenic response or an allergic reaction.

Arrhythmias

Coronary thrombolysis may induce arrhythmias associated with reperfusion including ventricular premature beats, ventricular tachycardia, and accelerated idioventricular rhythm. Reperfusion of the right coronary artery may cause bradycardia and hypotension due to the Bezold-Jarisch reflex.[110,111] Conversely, bundle branch block and complete heart block may resolve with reperfusion, even when accomplished relatively late after infarction.[112] Standard antiarrhythmic measures should be employed for ventricular arrhythmias and bradycardia, but accelerated idioventricular rhythm usually requires no treatment.[113]

Hemorrhagic complications

Major hemorrhagic events occur frequently when thrombolytic therapy is given in close temporal proximity to invasive procedures.[49] Major hemorrhagic complications are uncommon when invasive procedures are avoided.[32,72,73] The incidence of major hemorrhagic events appears to be similar for each of the thrombolytic agents.

Recurrent ischemia

During the days immediately after administration of thrombolytic therapy, some patients develop recurrent ischemia. In the TIMI-II trial,[72] about 25% of those treated conservatively had a recurrence of chest pain or evidence of painless ischemia during hospitalization. Therefore, after thrombolytic therapy is given, the patient should be monitored closely for evidence of recurrent ischemia, including chest pain, arrhythmias, hypotension, or electrocardiographic alterations. Recurrent ischemia is often an indication for catheterization and subsequent angioplasty or bypass surgery.

INDICATIONS FOR TRANSFER TO A REFERRAL CENTER

Once the patient with evolving myocardial infarction receives intravenous thrombolytic therapy in the community hospital, he or she should be transferred to a referral center for catheterization and consideration for revascularization for any of the following:

Cardiogenic Shock or Mechanical Complications of Infarction

Patients with cardiogenic shock or mechanical complications of infarction have a short-term mortality of 80 to 90% when treated conventionally. Therefore, they are best managed at a referral center with access to facilities for catheterization, angioplasty, intraaortic balloon counterpulsation, and cardiothoracic surgery. Survival is substantially improved with emergent surgery in patients with mechanical complications of infarction such as rupture of the ventricular septum, left ventricular free wall, or papillary muscle.

In anecdotal reports an occasional patient with cardiogenic shock has benefitted from thrombolytic therapy,[114] but the GISSI trial[32] failed to demonstrate that streptokinase exerted a beneficial effect in patients classified as Killip class 3 or 4. Recent reports have suggested that immediate balloon angioplasty may reduce mortality in patients with cardiogenic shock,[15,66,115] even when it is performed relatively late after the onset of ischemic injury. In the study of Lee et al,[66] mortality was reduced in patients who underwent angioplasty an average of 20 hours after the onset of cardiogenic shock. Therefore, the patient who presents to a community hospital with AMI and cardiogenic shock should receive thrombolytic therapy in the emergency room, and arrangements should be made for immediate transfer to a referral center for catheterization and possible PTCA.

Recurrent Myocardial Ischemia

After the patient with myocardial infarction receives thrombolytic therapy, he or she may have recurrent chest pain. These patients should be transferred to a referral center for catheterization and subsequent revascularization. In the TIMI IIB and SWIFT trials,[72,73] patients managed conservatively after thrombolytic therapy were referred for catheterization and revascularization if spontaneous or inducible ischemia occurred. With such a management strategy, their short and long-term outlook was excellent.

Several noninvasive techniques — exercise testing (with or without radionuclide imaging), ambulatory electrocardiographic monitoring, and echocardiography — may identify patients at high risk of early mortality if treated conservatively. These individuals may have improved survival with transfer to a referral center, catheterization, and subsequent revascularization.[116,117]

Complex Ventricular Tachyarrhythmia Requiring Electrophysiologic Evaluation

Patients with sustained ventricular tachycardia or ventricular fibrillation occurring more than 48 hours following myocardial infarction should be transferred immediately to a referral center for catheterization and electrophysiologic assessment. Such a management strategy allows identification of severe coronary artery disease and/or left ventricular aneurysm, which may be amenable to surgical correction.[118]

INTERHOSPITAL TRANSPORT OF THE PATIENT

There is considerable experience with the emergency interhospital transport of acutely ill cardiac patients,[119-122] including those with an intraaortic balloon counterpulsation device in place.[119] Such interhospital transfer, by helicopter, fixed wing aircraft, or ground ambulance, has been shown to be feasible and safe. Rubenstein et al[122] transferred 755 consecutive patients who received intravenous streptokinase and had recurrent chest pain or evidence of myocardium at risk. Only 1 — a patient with an unexpected ruptured aortic aneurysm — died during transport.[122]

ROLE OF THE REFERRAL CENTER

Many patients with AMI can receive effective treatment, including thrombolytic therapy in the community hospital. The referral center should provide telephone consultation for physicians in the community, helping them to decide which patients should be transferred and when such transfers should be accomplished. The referral center should have facilities and experienced personnel for catheterization, balloon angioplasty, and cardiothoracic surgery. In addition, the physicians at the referral center should keep those at the community hospital updated on the latest advances in the management of patients with evolving myocardial infarction.

CONCLUSION

The patient with evolving Q wave myocardial infarction who presents to a community hospital within 4 to 6 hours of the onset of chest pain should receive intravenous thrombolytic therapy, provided that there is no contraindication to it. Such therapy should be initiated as soon as possible, preferably while the patient is still in the emergency room. Subsequently, the patient can be managed conservatively, with progressive ambulation and discharge 7 to 10 days after admission, provided that complications do not occur. However, if the patient has recurrent chest pain, ventricular tachyarrhythmia, mechanical complications, cardiogenic shock, or evidence by noninvasive testing of inducible myocardial ischemia, he or she should be transferred to a referral center for catheterization and consideration of angioplasty or surgery.

REFERENCES

1. American Heart Association: 1989 Heart Facts. American Heart Association National Center, Dallas, TX; 1988.

2. Wennerblom B: Early mortality from ischemic heart disease and the effect of a mobile coronary care. Acta Med Scand 1982(suppl);667:1-58.

3. Graves EJ: National Hospital Discharge Survey: Annual summary, 1987. National Center for Health Statistics. Vital Health Stat 1989;13(99):38-39.

4. Rude RE, Muller JE, Braunwald E: Efforts to limit the size of myocardial infarcts. Ann Intern Med 1981;95:736-761.

5. Lange RA, Hillis LD: Evolving concepts in the treatment of acute myocardial infarction. Am J Med Sci 1988;296:143-152.

6. DeWood MA, Spores J, Notske R, et al: Prevalence of total coronary occlusion during the early hours of transmural myocardial infarction. N Engl J Med 1980;303:897-902.

7. Buja LM, Willerson JT: Clinicopathologic correlates of acute ischemic heart disease syndromes. Am J Cardiol 1981;47:343-356.

8. Reimer KA, Lowe JE, Rasmussen MM, et al: The wavefront phenomenon of ischemic cell death: 1. Myocardial infarct size vs duration of coronary occlusion in dogs. Circulation 1977;56:786-794.

9. Ellis SG, Henschke CI, Sandor T, et al: Time course of functional and biochemical recovery of myocardium salvaged by reperfusion. J Am Coll Cardiol 1983;1:1047-1055.

10. Sanz G, Castaner A, Betriu A, et al: Determinants of prognosis in survivors of myocardial infarction: A prospective clinical angiographic study. N Engl J Med 1982;306:1065-1070.

11. De Feyter PJ, van Eenige MJ, Dighton DH, et al: Prognostic value of exercise testing, coronary angiography and left ventriculography 6-8 weeks after myocardial infarction. Circulation 1982;66:527-536.

12. White HD, Norris RM, Brown MA, et al: Left ventricular end-systolic volume as the major determinant of survival after recovery from myocardial infarction. Circulation 1987;76:44-51.

13. Braunwald E: The aggressive treatment of acute myocardial infarction. Circulation 1985;71:1087-1092.

14. Topol EJ, Bates ER, Walton JA Jr, et al: Community hospital administration of intravenous tissue plasminogen activator in acute myocardial infarction: Improved timing, thrombolytic efficacy and ventricular function. J Am Coll Cardiol 1987;10:1173-1177.

15. O'Keefe JH Jr, Rutherford BD, McConahay DR, et al: Early and late results of coronary angioplasty without antecedent thrombolytic therapy for acute myocardial infarction. Am J Cardiol 1989;64:1221-1230.

16. Topol EJ: Coronary angioplasty for acute myocardial infarction. Ann Intern Med 1988;109:970-980.

17. Miller PF, Brodie BR, Weintraub RA, et al: Emergency coronary angioplasty for acute myocardial infarction: Results from a community hospital. Arch Intern Med 1987;147:1565-1570.

18. Serruys PW, Simoons ML, Suryapranata H, et al: Preservation of global and regional left ventricular function after early thrombolysis in acute myocardial infarction. J Am Coll Cardiol 1986;7:729-742.

19. The I.S.A.M. Study Group: A prospective trial of intravenous streptokinase in acute myocardial infarction (I.S.A.M.): Mortality, morbidity, and infarct size at 21 days. N Engl J Med 1986;314:1465-1471.

20. Kennedy JW, Martin GV, Davis KB, et al: The Western Washington intravenous streptokinase in acute myocardial infarction randomized trial. Circulation 1988;77:345-352.

21. White HD, Norris RM, Brown MA, et al: Effect of intravenous streptokinase on left ventricular function and early survival after acute myocardial infarction. N Engl J Med 1987;317:850-855.

22. Guerci AD, Gerstenblith G, Brinker JA, et al: A randomized trial of intravenous tissue plasminogen activator for acute myocardial infarction with subsequent randomization to elective coronary angioplasty. N Engl J Med 1987;317:1613-1618.

23. National Heart Foundation of Australia Coronary Thrombolysis Group: Coronary thrombolysis and myocardial salvage by tissue plasminogen activator given up to 4 hours after onset of myocardial infarction. Lancet 1988;1:203-208.

24. O'Rourke M, Baron D, Keogh A, et al: Limitation of myocardial infarction by early infusion of recombinant tissue-type plasminogen activator. Circulation 1988;77:1311-1315.

25. Van de Werf F, Arnold AER, for the European Cooperative Study Group for recombinant tissue type plasminogen activator: Intravenous tissue plasminogen activator and size of infarct, left ventricular function, and survival in acute myocardial infarction. Br Med J 1988;297:1374-1379.

26. Armstrong PW, Baigrie RS, Daly PA, et al: Tissue plasminogen activator: Toronto (TPAT) placebo-controlled randomized trial in acute myocardial infarction. J Am Coll Cardiol 1989;13:1469-1476.

27. Bassand JP, Machecourt J, Cassagnes J, et al: Multicenter trial of intravenous anisoylated plasminogen streptokinase activator complex (APSAC) in acute myocardial infarction: Effects on infarct size and left ventricular function. J Am Coll Cardiol 1989;13:988-997.

28. Vermeer F, Simoons ML, Lubsen J: Reduced frequency of ventricular fibrillation after early thrombolysis in myocardial infarction. Lancet 1986;1:1147-1148.

29. Sager PT, Perlmutter RA, Rosenfeld LE, et al: Electrophysiologic effects of thrombolytic therapy in patients with a transmural anterior myocardial infarction complicated by left ventricular aneurysm formation. J Am Coll Cardiol 1988;12:19-24.

30. Kennedy JW, Ritchie JL, Davis KB, et al: Western Washington randomized trial of intracoronary streptokinase in acute myocardial infarction. N Engl J Med 1983;309:1477-1482.

31. Simoons ML, Serruys PW, van den Brand M, et al: Improved survival after early thrombolysis in acute myocardial infarction: A randomised trial by the Interuniversity Cardiology Institute in the Netherlands. Lancet 1985;2:578-582.

32. Gruppo Italiano per lo Studio della Streptochinasi nell'Infarto Miocardico (GISSI): Effectiveness of intravenous thrombolytic treatment in acute myocardial infarction. Lancet 1986;1:397-402.

33. ISIS-2 (Second International Study of Infarct Survival) Collaborative Group: Random-ised trial of intravenous streptokinase, oral aspirin, both, or neither among 17,187 cases of suspected acute myocardial infarction: ISIS-2. Lancet 1988;2:349-360.

34. Wilcox RG, von der Lippe G, Olsson CG, et al: Trial of tissue plasminogen activator for mortality reduction in acute myocardial infarction: Anglo-Scandinavian Study of Early Thrombolysis. Lancet 1988;2:525-530.

35. AIMS Trial Study Group: Effect of intravenous APSAC on mortality after acute myo-cardial infarction: Preliminary report of a placebo-controlled clinical trial. Lancet 1988; 1:545-549.

36. Meinertz T, Kasper W, Schumacher M, et al: The German multicenter trial of anisoy-lated plasminogen streptokinase activator complex versus heparin for acute myocardial infarction. Am J Cardiol 1988;62:347-351.

37. Gruppo Italiano per lo Studio della Streptochinasi nell'Infarto miocardico: Long-term effects of intravenous thrombolysis in acute myocardial infarction: Final report of the GISSI-study. Lancet 1987;2:871-874.

38. Simoons ML, Vos J, Tijssen JGP, et al: Long-term benefit of early thrombolytic therapy in patients with acute myocardial infarction: 5 year follow-up of a trial conducted by the Interuniversity Cardiology Institute of the Netherlands. J Am Coll Cardiol 1989;14: 1609-1615.

39. Taylor GJ, Mikell FL, Moses HW, et al: Intravenous versus intracoronary streptokinase therapy for acute myocardial infarction in community hospitals. Am J Cardiol 1984; 54:256-260.

40. McNamara CA, Burket MW, Brewster PS, et al: Comparison of thrombolytic therapy for acute myocardial infarction in rural and urban settings. Am J Med 1987;82:1095-1101.

41. Leimbach WN, Hagan AD, Vaughan HL, et al: Cost and efficacy of intravenous strepto-kinase plus PTCA for acute myocardial infarction when therapy is initiated in commu-nity hospitals. Clin Cardiol 1988;11:731-738.

42. Morse HG, Epperson WJ, Kovaz JM, et al: Coronary thrombolysis in a community hospital: Experience with an intravenous streptokinase protocol. South Med J 1988;81: 691-694.

43. Hartmann J, McKeever L, Bufalino V, et al: A system approach to intravenous throm-bolysis in acute myocardial infarction in community hospitals: The influence of para-medics. Clin Cardiol 1988;11:812-816.

44. Vogel JHK, Setty RK, Coughlin BJ, et al: Intravenous streptokinase in acute myocardial infarction at the community hospital: A six-year experience. Am J Cardiol 1988;62:25-27K.

45. Rowe WW, Simpson RJ Jr, Tate DA, et al: Nonemergent cardiac catheterization and risk-stratified revascularization following thrombolytic therapy for acute myocardial infarction: A critical analysis of therapy in the community setting. Arch Intern Med 1989;149:1611-1617.

46. Mark DB, Hlatky MA, O'Connor CM, et al: Administration of thrombolytic therapy in the community hospital: Established principles and unresolved issues. J Am Coll Car-diol 1988;12:32-43A.

47. Lee TH, Weisberg MC, Brand DA, et al: Candidates for thrombolysis among emergency room patients with acute chest pain: Potential true- and false-positive rates. Ann Intern Med 1989;110:957-962.

48. Eisenberg MS, Ho MT, Schaeffer S, et al: A community survey of the potential use of thrombolytic agents for acute myocardial infarction. Ann Emerg Med 1989;18:838-841.

49. Chesebro JH, Knatterud G, Roberts R, et al: Thrombolysis In Myocardial Infarction (TIMI) Trial, Phase I: A comparison between intravenous tissue plasminogen activator and intravenous streptokinase. Clinical findings through hospital discharge. Circulation 1987;76:142-154.

50. Anderson JL, Rothbard RL, Hackworthy RA, et al: Multicenter reperfusion trial of intravenous anisoylated plasminogen streptokinase activator complex (APSAC) in acute myocardial infarction: Controlled comparison with intracoronary streptokinase. J Am Coll Cardiol 1988;11:1153-1163.

51. Neuhaus KL, Tebbe U, Sauer G, et al: High dose intravenous streptokinase in acute myocardial infarction. Clin Cardiol 1983;6:426-430.

52. Spann JF, Sherry S, Carabello BA, et al: Coronary thrombolysis by intravenous strepto-kinase in acute myocardial infarction: Acute and follow-up studies. Am J Cardiol 1984; 53:655-661.

53. Hillis LD, Borer J, Braunwald E, et al: High-dose intravenous streptokinase for acute myocardial infarction: Preliminary results of a multicenter trial. J Am Coll Cardiol 1985;6:957-962.

54. Collen D, Topol EJ, Tiefenbrunn AJ, et al: Coronary thrombolysis with recombinant human tissue-type plasminogen activator: A prospective, randomized, placebo-controlled trial. Circulation 1984;70:1012-1017.

55. Williams DO, Borer J, Braunwald E, et al: Intravenous recombinant tissue-type plas-minogen activator in patients with acute myocardial infarction: A report from the NHLBI Thrombolysis In Myocardial Infarction trial. Circulation 1986;73:338-346.

56. Gold HK, Leinbach RC, Garabedian HD, et al: Acute coronary reocclusion after throm-bolysis with recombinant human tissue-type plasminogen activator: Prevention by a maintenance infusion. Circulation 1986;73:347-352.

57. Bonnier HJRM, Visser RF, Klomps HC, et al: Comparison of intravenous anisoylated plasminogen streptokinase activator complex and intracoronary streptokinase in acute myocardial infarction. Am J Cardiol 1988;62:25-30.

58. Neuhaus KL, Feuerer W, Jeep-Tebbe S, et al: Improved thrombolysis with a modified dose regimen of recombinant tissue-type plasminogen activator. J Am Coll Cardiol 1989;14:1566-1569.

59. Ellis SG, Topol EJ, George BS, et al: Recurrent ischemia without warning: Analysis of risk factors for in-hospital ischemic events following successful thrombolysis with in-travenous tissue plasminogen activator. Circulation 1989;80:1159-1165.

60. Schaer DH, Ross AM, Wasserman AG: Reinfarction, recurrent angina, and reocclusion after thrombolytic therapy. Circulation 1987;76(suppl II):II-57-62.

61. Serruys PW, Wijns W, van den Brand M, et al: Is transluminal coronary angioplasty mandatory after successful thrombolysis? Quantitative coronary angiographic study. Br Heart J 1983;50:257-265.

62. Harrison DG, Ferguson DW, Collins SM, et al: Rethrombosis after reperfusion with streptokinase: Importance of geometry of residual lesions. Circulation 1984;69:991-999.

63. Badger RS, Brown BG, Kennedy JW, et al: Usefulness of recanalization to luminal diameter of 0.6 mm or more with intracoronary streptokinase during acute myocardial infarction in predicting "normal" perfusion status, continued arterial patency and survival at one year. Am J Cardiol 1987;59:519-522.

64. Califf RM, O'Neill W, Stack RS, et al: Failure of simple clinical measurements to predict perfusion status after intravenous thrombolysis. Ann Intern Med 1988;108:658-662.

65. Califf RM, Topol EJ, George BS, et al: Characteristics and outcome of patients in whom reperfusion with intravenous tissue-type plasminogen activator fails: Results of the Thrombolysis and Angioplasty in Myocardial Infarction (TAMI) I trial. Circulation 1988;77:1090-1099.

66. Lee L, Bates ER, Pitt B, et al: Percutaneous transluminal coronary angioplasty improves survival in acute myocardial infarction complicated by cardiogenic shock. Circulation 1988;78:1345-1351.

67. Topol EJ, Burek K, O'Neill WW, et al: A randomized controlled trial of hospital discharge three days after myocardial infarction in the era of reperfusion. N Engl J Med 1988;318:1083-1088.

68. Topol EJ, Califf RM, George BS, et al: A randomized trial of immediate versus delayed elective angioplasty after intravenous tissue plasminogen activator in acute myocardial infarction. N Engl J Med 1987;317:581-588.

69. The TIMI Research Group: Immediate vs delayed catheterization and angioplasty following thrombolytic therapy for acute myocardial infarction: TIMI IIA results. JAMA 1988;260:2849-2858.

70. Simoons ML, Arnold AER, Betriu A, et al: Thrombolysis with tissue plasminogen activator in acute myocardial infarction: No additional benefit from immediate percutaneous coronary angioplasty. Lancet 1988;1:197-203.

71. Stack RS, O'Connor CM, Mark DB, et al: Coronary perfusion during acute myocardial infarction with a combined therapy of coronary angioplasty and high-dose intravenous streptokinase. Circulation 1988;77:151-161.

72. The TIMI Study Group: Comparison of invasive and conservative strategies after treatment with intravenous tissue plasminogen activator in acute myocardial infarction: Results of the Thrombolysis in Myocardial Infarction (TIMI) Phase II trial. N Engl J Med 1989;320:618-627.

73. de Bono DP, Pocock SJ, for the SWIFT Investigators Group: The SWIFT study of intervention versus conservative management after anistreplase thrombolysis. Circulation 1989;80(suppl II):II-418 (abstract).

74. Moss AJ, Wynar B, Goldstein S: Delay in hospitalization during the acute coronary period. Am J Cardiol 1969;24:659-665.

75. Herlitz J, Blohm M, Hartford M, et al: Delay time in suspected acute myocardial infarction and the importance of its modification. Clin Cardiol 1989;12:370-374.

76. Hacket TP, Cassem NH: Factors contributing to delay in responding to the signs and symptoms of acute myocardial infarction. Am J Cardiol 1969;24:651-658.

77. Turi ZG, Stone PH, Muller JE, et al: Implications for acute intervention related to time of hospital arrival in acute myocardial infarction. Am J Cardiol 1986;58:203-209.

78. Mitic WR, Perkins RRT: The effect of a media campaign on heart attack delay and decision times. Can J Public Health 1984;75:414-418.

79. Herlitz J, Hartford M, Blohm M, et al: Effect of a media campaign on delay times and ambulance use in suspected acute myocardial infarction. Am J Cardiol 1989;64:90-93.

80. Crampton RS, Aldrich RF, Gascho JA, et al: Reduction of prehospital, ambulance and community coronary death rates by the community-wide emergency cardiac care system. Am J Med 1975;58:151-165.

81. Lewis RP, Stang JM, Fulkerson PK, et al: Effectiveness of advanced paramedics in a mobile coronary care system. JAMA 1979;241:1092-1094.

82. Schaeffer SM, Eisenberg MS, Ho MT, et al: The relationship of education to use of 911 for symptoms of myocardial infarction. Circulation 1989;80(suppl II):II-637 (abstract).

83. Karagounis L, Ipsen SK, Jessop MR, et al: Impact of field-transmitted electrocardiography on time to in-hospital thrombolytic therapy in acute myocardial infarction. Circulation 1989;80(suppl II):II-352 (abstract).

84. Sharkey SW, Brunette DD, Ruiz E, et al: An analysis of time delays preceding thrombolysis for acute myocardial infarction. JAMA 1989;262:3171-3174.

85. Koren G, Weiss AT, Hasin Y, et al: Prevention of myocardial damage in acute myocardial ischemia by early treatment with intravenous streptokinase. N Engl J Med 1985;313:1384-1389.

86. Weaver WD, Martin J, Litwin P, et al: Prehospital thrombolytic therapy - MITI project report on phase I: Feasibility, characteristics of patients. J Am Coll Cardiol 1989;13:152A (abstract).

87. Castaigne AD, Herve C, Duval-Moulin AM, et al: Prehospital use of APSAC: Results of a placebo-controlled study. Am J Cardiol 1989;64:30-33A.

88. DeWood MA, Stifter WF, Simpson CS, et al: Coronary arteriographic findings soon after non-Q-wave myocardial infarction. N Engl J Med 1986;315:417-423.

89. Gold HK, Johns JA, Leinbach RC, et al: A randomized, blinded, placebo-controlled trial of recombinant human tissue-type plasminogen activator in patients with unstable angina pectoris. Circulation 1987;75:1192-1199.

90. Topol EJ, Kleiman NS, Joelson JM, et al: Tissue plasminogen activator for unstable angina pectoris: A multicenter, randomized, double-blind, placebo-controlled trial. J Am Coll Cardiol 1989;13:191A (abstract).

91. Nicklas JM, Topol EJ, Kander N, et al: Randomized, double-blind, placebo-controlled trial of tissue plasminogen activator in unstable angina. J Am Coll Cardiol 1989;13:434-441.

92. Van den Brand M, van Zijl A, de Feyter PJ, et al: Intravenous rt-PA does not improve the severity of coronary artery stenosis, or the clinical course in patients with refractory unstable angina. Circulation 1989;80(suppl II):II-344 (abstract).

93. Mont L, Betriu A, Sanz G, et al: Thrombolysis in unstable angina. A prospective randomized trial. Circulation 1989;80(suppl II):II-344 (abstract).

94. Schreiber TL, Macina G, Bunnell P, et al: Thrombolytic therapy in unstable angina and non Q-wave myocardial infarction: A randomized trial of urokinase versus aspirin. J Am Coll Cardiol 1989;13:15A (abstract).

95. Van de Werf F: Discrepancies between the effects of coronary reperfusion on survival and left ventricular function. Lancet 1989;1:1367-1369.

96. Cigarroa RG, Lange RA, Hillis LD: Prognosis after acute myocardial infarction in patients with and without residual anterograde coronary blood flow. Am J Cardiol 1989;64:155-160.

97. Braunwald E: Myocardial reperfusion, limitation of infarct size, reduction of left ventricular dysfunction, and improved survival: Should the paradigm be expanded? Circulation 1989;79:441-444.

98. Hochman JS, Choo H: Limitation of myocardial infarct expansion by reperfusion independent of myocardial salvage. Circulation 1987;75:299-306.

99. Schroder R, Neuhaus KL, Linderer T, et al: Impact of late coronary artery reperfusion on left ventricular function one month after acute myocardial infarction (results from the ISAM study). Am J Cardiol 1989;64:878-884.

100. Fedele FA, Thomas ES, Drew TM, et al: Late improvement in left ventricular function after t-PA and PTCA in acute myocardial infarction: Importance of stenosis free patency of the infarct artery. Circulation 1989;80(suppl II):II-352 (abstract).

101. Rentrop KP, Feit F, Sherman W, et al: Late thrombolytic therapy preserves left ventricular function in patients with collateralized total coronary occlusion: Primary end point findings of the Second Mount Sinai-New York University Reperfusion Trial. J Am Coll Cardiol 1989;14:58-64.

102. Kersschot IE, Brugada P, Ramentol M, et al: Effects of early reperfusion in acute myocardial infarction on arrhythmias induced by programmed stimulation: A prospective, randomized study. J Am Coll Cardiol 1986;7:1234-1242.

103. Gang ES, Lew AS, Hong M, et al: Decreased incidence of ventricular late potentials after successful thrombolytic therapy for acute myocardial infarction. N Engl J Med 1989;321:712-716.

104. Lew AS, Hod H, Cercek B, et al: Mortality and morbidity rates of patients older and younger than 75 years with acute myocardial infarction treated with intravenous streptokinase. Am J Cardiol 1987;59:1-5.

105. Chaitman BR, Thompson B, Wittry MD, et al: The use of tissue-type plasminogen activator for acute myocardial infarction in the elderly: Results from Thrombolysis in Myocardial Infarction Phase I, open label studies and the Thrombolysis in Myocardial Infarction Phase II pilot study. J Am Coll Cardiol 1989;14:1159-1165.

106. Lew AS, Laramee P, Cercek B, et al: The hypotensive effect of intravenous streptokinase in patients with acute myocardial infarction. Circulation 1985;72:1321-1326.

107. White HD, Rivers JT, Maslowski AH, et al: Effect of intravenous streptokinase as compared with that of tissue plasminogen activator on left ventricular function after first myocardial infarction. N Engl J Med 1989;320:817-821.

108. Magnani B, for the PAIMS investigators: Plasminogen Activator Italian Multicenter Study (PAIMS): Comparison of intravenous recombinant single-chain human tissue-type plasminogen activator (rt-PA) with intravenous streptokinase in acute myocardial infarction. J Am Coll Cardiol 1989;13:19-26.

109. Gruppo Italiano per lo Studio della Sopravvivenza nell'Infarto Miocardico: GISSI-2: A factorial randomised trial of alteplase versus streptokinase and heparin versus no heparin among 12,490 patients with acute myocardial infarction. Lancet 1990;336:65-71.

110. Wei JY, Markis JE, Malagold M, et al: Cardiovascular reflexes stimulated by reperfusion of ischemic myocardium in acute myocardial infarction. Circulation 1983;67:796-801.

111. Gacioch GM, Topol EJ: Paradoxical, sudden clinical deterioration after reperfusion of the right coronary artery: A hazard of primary or rescue coronary angioplasty for myocardial infarction. Circulation 1988;78(suppl II):II-111 (abstract).

112. Wilber D, Walton J, O'Neill W, et al: Effects of reperfusion on complete heart block complicating anterior myocardial infarction. J Am Coll Cardiol 1984;4:1315-1321.

113. Norris RM, Mercer CJ: Significance of idioventricular rhythms in acute myocardial infarction. Prog Cardiovasc Dis 1974;16:455-468.

114. Lew AS, Weiss AT, Shah PK, Fishbein MC, et al: Extensive myocardial salvage and reversal of cardiogenic shock after reperfusion of the left main coronary artery by intravenous streptokinase. Am J Cardiol 1984;54:450-452.

115. Ellis SG, O'Neill WW, Bates ER, et al: Implications for patient triage from survival and left ventricular functional recovery analyses in 500 patients treated with coronary angioplasty for acute myocardial infarction. J Am Coll Cardiol 1989;13:1251-1259.

116. Cheitlin MD: Finding the high-risk patient with coronary artery disease. JAMA 1988;259:2271-2277.

117. DeBusk RF: Specialized testing after recent acute myocardial infarction. Ann Intern Med 1989;110:470-481.

118. Kleiman RB, Miller JM, Buxton AE, et al: Prognosis following sustained ventricular tachycardia occurring early after myocardial infarction. Am J Cardiol 1988;62:528-533.

119. LoCicero J III, Hartz RS, Sanders JH Jr, et al: Interhospital transport of patients with ongoing intraaortic balloon pumping. Am J Cardiol 1985;56:59-61.

120. Kaplan L, Walsh D, Burney RE: Emergency aeromedical transport of patients with acute myocardial infarction. Ann Emerg Med 1987;16:55-57.

121. Bellinger RL, Califf RM, Mark DB, et al: Helicopter transport of patients during acute myocardial infarction. Am J Cardiol 1988;61:718-722.

122. Rubenstein DG, Treister NW, Kapoor AS, et al: Transfer of acutely ill cardiac patients for definitive care: Demonstrated safety in 755 cases. JAMA 1988;259:1695-1698.

Chapter 5

THE ROLE OF THE EMERGENCY DEPARTMENT IN REDUCING THE TIME TO THROMBOLYTIC THERAPY IN PATIENTS WITH AMI

Joseph P. Ornato

INTRODUCTION

Thrombolytic therapy can reduce mortality and morbidity due to acute myocardial infarction (AMI), but its effectiveness is inversely related to time.[1-3] The goals of this chapter are to identify the emergency department (ED) as an important, rate-limiting site affecting the timing of thrombolytic administration in the majority of AMI patients and to outline steps that can be taken to minimize time delay in the ED.

THE CHAIN OF EVENTS LEADING TO THROMBOLYSIS

Like sequential links in a chain, several factors can contribute to delay from the onset of AMI symptoms to initiation of thrombolytic therapy. Failure of the patient to recognize early symptoms of AMI and procrastination in seeking medical assistance (**patient factors**) have been recognized since the 1960s as major reasons for delayed hospital presentation.[4-15] Prior to the advent of thrombolytic therapy, treatment soon after onset of symptoms by paramedics or medical personnel in the hospital or coronary intensive care unit (CICU) was primarily directed at the relief of symptoms and the prevention of life-threatening AMI complications (eg, ventricular fibrillation, congestive heart failure, shock). Now, early entry into the medical system is even more important because thrombolysis can reduce AMI mortality by 25-50% or more, and the earlier the treatment, the greater the effect.[1-3]

Early entry into the medical care system is no longer the appropriate endpoint with which to judge success; what really matters most is the interval from symptom onset to thrombolytic administration and subsequent reperfusion. **Medical system**

factors (both in- and out-of-hospital) include the time that it takes for medical personnel to evaluate the patient's symptoms and to initiate thrombolytic therapy.

Patient Factors — The Limited Value of Public Education

Although many factors are associated with patient delay in seeking medical care for AMI symptoms (Table 1),[4-15] little is known about whether the average patient's response to AMI symptoms can be altered and at what economic cost. Preliminary efforts to improve patient response to AMI symptoms have met with limited success. In Seattle, a four and one-half month, $139,272 public education campaign using multiple media techniques resulted in no statistically significant difference in the number of AMI patients who presented to the medical system for early treatment (Table 2).[16] In Göteborg, Sweden, a similar public education program reduced the median time delay from symptom onset to CICU admission in patients with con-

Table 1. *Factors commonly associated with patient delay in seeking medical care for AMI*

1. Patient denial
2. Mistaking symptoms for a more benign medical condition
3. Being alone (or at home) at the time of symptom onset
4. Having prodromal symptoms
5. Previous myocardial infarction or angina
6. Attempting to contact personal physician

Table 2. *Effect of a 4.5 month ($139,272), multi-media public education program on the delay in seeking medical care for AMI in Seattle*

	Before	After	Significance
Transport to hospital by paramedic ambulance	42%	44%	ns
> 4 h delay in seeking medical help	37%	41%	ns
Median delay in seeking medical help (hrs)	2.6	2.3	ns

Adapted from Ho et al[16]

firmed AMI from 3 hours to 2 hours 20 minutes.[17,18] There was a significant increase (56%) in the number of "false negative" ED visits (patients with chest pain but no evidence of AMI) during the campaign, while the number of AMI patients presenting to the ED increased by only 9%. Thus, attempts to persuade the public to seek help for AMI symptoms more rapidly have been relatively unsuccessful. Indiscriminate campaigns have the *potential* to significantly increase the volume of chest pain patients in the ED, further congesting already overloaded units and delaying the prompt evaluation of true AMI patients. More research is needed to develop strategies of public education that can target AMI patients or bystanders who may be taught to (1) recognize early signs or symptoms of AMI; (2) deal with patient denial; and (3) summon emergency medical assistance quickly.

Medical System Factors — Limitations of Prehospital Treatment

Much more is known about the rate-limiting steps influencing the administration of thrombolytic therapy once the patient presents to the medical care system. In U.S. hospitals, thrombolytic therapy is usually started in the ED or the CICU. Throughout the world, prehospital thrombolytic administration by physicians[19-23] or paramedics[24,25] has been proposed and implemented to shorten the time between AMI symptom onset and definitive therapy.

Regardless of how effective these prehospital approaches prove to be, they have the potential to shorten the time to thrombolytic therapy in only a minority of the affected U.S. population because many AMI patients are not transported by the EMS system. For example, in Seattle where there has been intense public education regarding emergency medical services (EMS), more than half of all AMI patients still proceed directly to the hospital without activating the EMS system.[16,19]

Experience in other countries has been similar. In one report from Australia,[15] only a third of patients who were admitted to the CICU came to the hospital by ambulance. Another third were transported to the hospital by private automobile. The remainder contacted their doctor directly, resulting in a CICU arrival delay that was more than 2.5 times greater (212 vs. 83-88 minutes) than that of the previous two subgroups. In another study in Ottawa, Canada, only half of the patients hospitalized for suspected AMI were transported by ambulance.[12] In Göteborg, Sweden, a public media campaign failed to increase the number of AMI patients transported to the hospital by ambulance (58% before vs. 57% after the campaign).[17,18]

Even if it is proven that prehospital thrombolytic therapy can be administered by paramedics appropriately and that a measurable improvement in outcome results, it will likely be feasible only in relatively large urban and suburban areas, where the number of calls will suffice to maintain paramedic skills and to justify the expense of prehospital ECG equipment and convenient cellular telephone communication. Cellular telephone coverage is currently adequate only in urban and suburban areas where EMS transport times to the hospital are relatively short. Paramedics in more rural areas (where transport times are often long) could transmit a patient's ECG to the hospital by patching into a standard telephone line, if available. However, maintenance of advanced life support skills (eg, starting an IV) is a problem in many rural systems, which are staffed by volunteers who run very few EMS calls.

Other potential problems relating to prehospital thrombolytic administration include the high cost of maintaining a field stock of drugs, special requirements (eg, refrigeration or daily rotation of the field drug stock into the hospital environment), and overhead expense for breakage. Litigation expenses and damages from an inappropriate thrombolytic use that results in significant patient injury or death could dramatically halt enthusiasm for this type of administration in the U.S.

Medical System Factors — The ED Role in Thrombolytic Therapy

As the hospital entry point for both ambulance patients and walk-ins, the ED is a strategic location that can substantially affect the timing of thrombolytic therapy. The delay from ED arrival until initiation of thrombolytic therapy averages between 45 and 90 minutes in most U.S. studies.[26-29] An ideal average time of 15-20 minutes to complete the initial ED evaluation and to begin treatment has been suggested[30] but has not been achieved in any study reported to date.

There has been an obvious trend towards a shorter treatment delay in more recent studies,[26,28] particularly when patients are brought in by paramedics (107 minutes) rather than when they walk in to the ED (182 minutes).[26] The recent improvement in ED treatment time likely represents increased experience with thrombolytic therapy and use of a team or protocol approach. Field transmission of an ECG by cellular telephone can shorten the time from ED arrival to thrombolytic therapy by at least 20 minutes by allowing ED staff to prepare for arrival of the patient.[26,31]

Decreasing the ED Delay to Thrombolytic Therapy

Several factors can delay the start of thrombolytic therapy in the ED (Table 3). Necessary equipment and personnel are not always available immediately since, unlike the paramedic team in the field, the ED staff is responsible for treating many patients simultaneously. A precipitous increase in the number and acuity of patients (due to changes in the health care reimbursement system, the acquired immune deficiency syndrome, and drug-related violence) and a relative deficiency of intensive care beds has forced most urban EDs to hold admitted patients for long periods of time. This results in frequent ED overcrowding, stretching limited resources to the breaking point and making it difficult to provide timely triage and intervention for

Table 3. *Steps that can contribute to a delay in the ED administration of thrombolytic therapy to an AMI patient*

1. Administrative

    a. Triage

    b. Registration

    c. Patient overcrowding in the ED due to increased volume and acuity, acuity, and a relative deficiency of intensive care unit beds

2. Diagnostic

    a. Nurse and ED physician evaluation

    b. Laboratory procedures (eg, electrocardiogram, drawing bloods, x-rays)

3. Therapeutic (eg, starting IV lines)

4. Political (eg, consultation with the patient's private physician, a cardiologist, cardiologist, or internist)

5. Pharmacy

    a. Time to obtain the drug from the pharmacy

    b. Mixing and preparation

patients who may present with AMI symptoms. Steps that can be taken to minimize the ED delay to treatment are listed in Table 4.

Who Should Make the Decision to Use a Thrombolytic Agent in the ED?

For "political" or perceived medicolegal reasons, the ED physicians in many hospitals are required to involve other physicians (eg, family physician, internist, or cardiologist) in the decision to use thrombolytic therapy. At times, such consultation can be extremely valuable; often, it only delays the administration of thrombolytic therapy that is obviously indicated. Understandable reasons for ED physicians to consult with other physicians prior to initiating thrombolytic therapy include: 1) calling the patient's personal physician to verify the past medical history or prior ECG findings; 2) requesting a cardiologist's help in interpreting a complex or subtle ECG [cardiologists correctly diagnose the presence of AMI from the ECG more often than ED physicians in difficult cases[32]]; 3) asking assistance from an internist or cardiologist in estimating the time of onset of infarction in a "stagger-start" presentation; or 4) seeking help from the patient's personal physician, internist, or cardiologist in diffi-

Table 4. *Steps that can be taken to minimize the ED delay to thrombolytic therapy for AMI patients*

1. Paramedic identification of high risk patients
   a. Checklist
   b. Prehospital ECG
2. Bypass triage based on radio information
3. Team approach to initial evaluation
   a. Nurse and physician simultaneously
   b. Protocol and checklist
   c. ED physician makes decision to treat
4. Drug available in ED at all times

cult cases when there is a relative contraindication to thrombolytic therapy and when other therapy (eg, primary percutaneous transluminal angioplasty) might be a wiser option. However, it is important to emphasize that the majority of AMI cases do *not* require consultation prior to treatment by the ED physician. The internist and cardiologist can play a more important role by helping the ED physician to develop protocols and procedures for rapid institution of thrombolytic therapy, including guidelines for consultation.[33-35]

Use of ED Protocols for Thrombolytic Therapy

Establishment of protocols, procedures, and special training for ED personnel can significantly shorten the time to thrombolytic treatment.[33-35] The time between ED arrival and initiation of thrombolytic therapy averaged 91 minutes (range 80-144 minutes) in the Western Washington IV streptokinase trial.[36-37] In a more recent trial by the same investigators and clinical centers,[38] a conscious effort was made to reduce the time to treatment to less than one hour by establishing a program of in-service training for ED and CICU staff. The result was an average delay of only 52 minutes (range 43-72 minutes) from ED arrival to initiation of IV t-PA. The use of streamlined screening procedures and simplified thrombolytic regimens (eg, bolus dosing with anistreplase) may help to further reduce this time delay.

Early notification of the ED staff by the paramedic team shortens the delay to ED treatment. The shortest ED delays reported in the U.S. have occurred when paramedics transmit a diagnostic electrocardiogram (ECG) by cellular telephone to the ED.[26,31,39] In Seattle, only 4% of prehospital patients with chest pain are potential candidates for prehospital thrombolytic therapy.[26] Thus, if thrombolytic therapy is not started in the field, only about 1 out of every 20 chest pain patients brought in by paramedics will require ED thrombolytic therapy. When paramedics use a checklist to identify potential AMI patients and transmit a diagnostic ECG from the field to the hospital, the ED team can prepare more effectively for the patient who really has an AMI. When Seattle paramedics transmitted an ECG from the field to the ED as part of a pilot study prior to the use of thrombolytic therapy in the field, the time to from ED arrival to the initiation of thrombolytic therapy was reduced from 76 to 56 minutes (p < 0.01).[25]

Standing order flowsheets and checklists can also be used in the ED. This approach streamlines the initial patient screening process, sets appropriate priorities, and provides a high-quality record for medical, medico-legal, and quality assurance audit purposes. An example of an ED screening protocol relating to the use of thrombolytic therapy for AMI is shown in Figure 1.

Problems in the Identification of AMI Patients in the ED

The leading cause of malpractice loss in the ED setting is missed AMI.[40] From 1982-1986 the average cost per claim was $98,054. Undiagnosed AMI patients as a group tend to be younger, present more atypically, and are less likely to have an initial ECG that is typical of AMI.[40] In addition, undiagnosed AMI patients were evaluated by physicians who documented less detailed histories, misread more ECGs, had less ED experience, and admitted fewer patients to the hospital than concurrent controls.[40]

A careful history is of paramount importance in evaluating the patient with chest pain. The history supplies 65-92% of the best discriminators between cardiac and non-cardiac causes of chest pain.[41] One of the most significant discriminators is the quality or character of the pain.[41] The clinical challenge is to obtain consistent information from the patient, since the story may change with repeated questioning.[42,43]

Patients with acute myocardial ischemia due to AMI can have typical, atypical, or no clinical symptoms. "Textbook" symptoms of myocardial ischemia include pressure-like substernal heaviness often with radiation down the ulnar distribution of the left arm, diaphoresis, nausea, shortness of breath, and a sense of impending doom.[44] Prodromal symptoms, often resembling classical angina pectoris but beginning at rest or with less activity than usual (unstable angina), occur in 10-50% of patients.[45] These classic textbook symptoms, however, are found in only about 50% of AMI patients.[46] Approximately 25% of all AMI patients present atypically (eg, they have acute indigestion or other atypical pain location, syncope, shock, pulmonary edema, profound weakness, or peripheral embolization). The remaining 25% are asymptomatic or cannot give a history (because of stroke, aphasia, coma, etc.). Painless infarction or

Date: _____ / _____ / _____   Time: _____ : _____   AM PM (circle)

Patient's name: _____ , _____ _____ .

Hospital Registration #: _____ .   Sex: Male / Female.

Patient's age: _____ yrs.   Patient's weight: _____ Kg

Duration of chest pain: _____ hrs.

Inclusion Criteria: (X = meets criterion)

_____ Cardiac chest pain < 6 hours in duration, and unresponsive to nitroglycerin.

_____ ECG evidence of acute transmural MI with or without Q waves (0.1 mV ST segment elevation 0.08 secs after the J point in 2 inferior leads, 2 contiguous precordial leads, or leads I and aVl). Other considerations include ST segment depression with signs of true posterior MI.

Potential Exclusion Criteria: (X = meets criterion)

May be superceded in specific circumstances based on risk:benefit assessment.

_____ Age > 76 years
_____ Active internal bleeding
_____ Pregnancy, suspected pregnancy, menstruation
_____ Cerebrovascular accident, seizures within 2 months
_____ CNS surgery within 6 months
_____ Surgery, trauma, or organ biopsy within 6 weeks
_____ Known bleeding diathesis
_____ Hemorrhagic retinopathy (Kimmelstiel-Wilson nephropathy III or IV)
_____ Terminal cancer, severe diabetes, liver or kidney disease
_____ Gastrointestinal bleed within 2-6 months
_____ Intracranial mass, neoplasm, arteriovenous malformation, or aneurysm
_____ Acute hypertension (initial BP >180/110 mm Hg)
_____ Puncture of a noncompressible vessel or traumatic CPR
_____ Concurrent therapy with oral anticoagulants
_____ Heme-positive rectal exam
_____ Evidence of aortic dissection (R to L arm SBP difference >15 mm Hg)

_____ , M.D.

Figure 1. *Thrombolytic ED screening protocol*

atypical symptoms are significantly more likely to occur in women,[47] older men,[47] and diabetics.[48]

The ED ECG has a positive predictive value of only 76% in patients who are proven to have AMI.[32] In a recent multicenter chest pain study,[32] cardiologists performing the official interpretation of the ED ECG were slightly better at detecting AMI than the ED physician (cardiologists read the ED ECG as probable AMI in 51% of patients later proven to have an infarction compared to 46% of the ECGs interpreted as probable AMI by the ED physicians). Similarly, cardiologists interpreted only 1% of ECGs as probable AMI in patients later shown *not* to have AMI as opposed to a 2% misinterpretation by ED physicians. When the cardiologists and the ED physicians disagreed on the ECG interpretation, the cardiologists were correct 71% of the time, while the ED physicians were correct in only 29% of these difficult cases.

Common errors in ECG interpretation in the ED include both failing to recognize the ECG signs of acute infarction and mistaking the changes of a benign ECG variant or non-ischemic disease for those of infarction.[49] "Hyperacute" MI changes (tall, peaked, symmetrical T-waves) may be easily overlooked. If there is any doubt about whether borderline peaked T-waves are of significance in a patient with a vague clinical presentation, a repeat ECG within 30-60 minutes will often answer the question. The peaked T-waves of hyperkalemia resemble the "hyperacute" changes of infarction except that hyperkalemia does not cause ST-segment elevation. Serum potassium determination may be of help in a questionable case.

True posterior AMI (causing an increase in the R-wave amplitude in V1-V2 with an upright T-wave) or high lateral AMI (causing ST elevation in I, aVL, or V6) can be easily missed. Conversely, AMI can be mistakenly diagnosed in young healthy patients with "early repolarization," which results in elevation of the ST-segment primarily in the mid-anterior leads (V2-V5).[50] The lack of reciprocal ST-segment depression in any leads should always suggest the possibility of this benign variant. It is most common in young, healthy (especially black) males. Another condition commonly mistaken for AMI on ECG is acute pericarditis. ECG features of pericarditis that help to distinguish it from AMI are listed in Table 5.[51-53]

It is often difficult to distinguish the ECG changes of pericarditis from those of early repolarization. ST elevation in both limb and precordial leads with an ST axis to the left of the T wave axis and ST depression in V1 favor pericarditis.[54] A vertical ST axis to the right of the T wave axis and an isoelectric ST-segment in V6 are more likely due to early repolarization.

Stat cardiac enzymes are of limited value in the ED decision process.[55-57] The MB isoenzyme of creatine phosphokinase (CPK-MB) is the most valuable confirmatory test in patients hospitalized within 24 hours of the onset of symptoms. This test has an eventual positive predictive value of 0.98 and a negative predictive value of 0.99 in serial testing.[57] However, since CPK-MB does not rise until 4-8 hours after the onset of symptoms and does not peak until 14 hours after infarction,[58] it is of no use diag-

Table 5. *ECG features of pericarditis that help distinguish it from AMI*

1. ST segment elevation (usually < 5 mV) with a concave upward ST segment in all leads except aVR and V1;

2. lack of reciprocal ST-segment changes (ST depression only in aVR and V1);

3. depression of the P-R segment due to atrial current of injury;

4. ST segment changes usually resolve before the T-waves invert;

5. lack of pathologic Q waves.

nostically in the majority of patients who present early enough in their clinical course to be considered prime candidates for thrombolytic therapy.

Determination of CPK or CPK-MB in the ED is thus unnecessary and may be misleading. Eisenberg et al[55] found that the availability of stat cardiac enzymes (CPK, aspartate transaminase, alanine transaminase, LDH, and α-hydroxybutyrate dehydrogenase) in the ED could have prevented the inappropriate ED discharge of only one of 80 patients presenting to the ED with chest pain. False positive results led to the inappropriate admission of 11 patients and false negative results led to the discharge of 5 patients. Isolated elevation of cardiac enzymes with a non-diagnostic history and negative ECG is particularly misleading. Seager[56] found that two of 221 patients admitted to the coronary care unit to rule out an AMI were hospitalized solely on the basis of an isolated enzyme elevation. Neither patient was subsequently shown to have had an AMI.

Increasing the Appropriate Use of Thrombolytics in the ED

Because of problems in accurately diagnosing AMI early, the Multicenter Chest Pain Study (which involved 7734 chest pain patients who presented to 3 university and 4 community hospital EDs) found that only 23-25% (based on whether a 4- or 6-hour time limit is chosen as the upper limit for treatment) of the 1118 patients subsequently shown to have AMI were eligible for thrombolytic therapy based on ECG and clinical signs of infarction.[32] When standard contraindications for thrombolytic therapy were considered, only 12-17% of AMI patients were candidates for such treatment in the ED.[32]

A recent editorial[59] discussing the Multicenter Chest Pain Study[32] addressed the question of why most AMI patients are not being treated with thrombolytic therapy. Untreated patients fall into three groups: 1) those with legitimate contraindications to treatment, where the risk:benefit ratio is clearly unfavorable; 2) those in whom the risk:benefit ratio is controversial (inferior infarction, previous infarction, advanced age, late presentation, or equivocal ECG); and 3) underutilization of thrombolytic therapy by practitioners who are still uncomfortable with its use. The editorial points out that physician use of thrombolytics to treat AMI patients is directly proportional to the number of such patients treated by the physician per year.[60] Physicians in solo or small group practices, general internists, and family practitioners were less likely than cardiologists to use thrombolytic therapy to treat their AMI patients.[60] Formation of a consortium or collaborative arrangement between physicians in smaller community hospitals and those in larger facilities can help the former to develop and use thrombolytic protocols in an appropriate and timely fashion.[60-62]

In many settings, innovative technology may help to bridge the gap between ED physicians and their cardiology consultants. Facsimile technology is now widely available, relatively inexpensive, and portable.[63] A small briefcase unit linked to any standard or cellular telephone could transmit the ED ECG to a cardiologist in minutes. This strategy would encourage prompt input from the cardiologist on difficult ECGs and direct discussion between the ED physician and consultant in a timely fashion. In addition, further enhancement of computer ECG algorithms that can accurately diagnose early AMI could benefit the ED physician. In a recent report,[64] cardiologists were more sensitive (69% vs. 51%, p = 0.009) but less specific (96% vs. 99%, p = 0.02) than a computer in detecting AMI in 460 patients who had ECGs taken by paramedics in the field.

CONCLUSION

Until more is known about how to influence patient behavior, the ED should be targeted as the most practical location for decreasing the time to thrombolytic administration in AMI patients. Current evidence suggests that ED thrombolytic treatment plans and protocols can lessen the delay for many patients who present with AMI, especially if paramedics can transmit diagnostic quality ECGs to the hospital in advance of patient arrival. Although not as accurate as cardiologists in detecting AMI on the initial ECG, emergency physicians can make the correct diagnosis in the majority of cases that have an ECG indicating acute transmural infarction. Cardiologists and internists must work together closely with their hospital emergency physicians to develop prospective protocols and guidelines for the timely use of thrombolytic therapy in the ED setting.

REFERENCES

1. Gruppo Italiano per lo studio dells streptochinasi nell'infarto miocardico (GISSI): Effectiveness of intravenous thrombolytic treatment in acute myocardial infarction. Lancet 1986;1:397-401.

2. ISIS-2 (Second International Study of Infarct Survival) Collaborative Group: Randomized trial of intravenous streptokinase, oral aspirin, both or neither among 17,187 cases of suspected acute myocardial infarction: ISIS-2. Lancet 1988;2:349-360.

3. Long-term effects of intravenous anistreplase in acute myocardial infarction: final report of the AIMS study. AIMS Trial Study Group. Lancet 1990;335:427-431.

4. Hackett TP, Cassem NH: Factors contributing to delay in responding to the signs and symptoms of acute myocardial infarction. Am J Cardiol 1969;24:651-658.

5. Moss AJ, Wynar B, Goldstein S: Delay in hospitalization during the acute coronary period. Am J Cardiol 1969;24:659-665.

6. Simon AB, Feinleib M, Thompson HK: Components of delay in the pre-hospital phase of acute myocardial infarction. Am J Cardiol 1972;30:476-482.

7. Kamaryt P, Minarik J, Miklis P: Total delay between first appearance of symptoms in and hospitalization of patients with acute myocardial infarction. Cor Vasa 1972;14:1-8.

8. Goldstein S, Moss AJ, Green W: Sudden death in acute myocardial infarction: Relationship to factors affecting delay in hospitalization. Arch Intern Med 1972;129:720-724.

9. Schroeder JS, Lamb IH, Hu M: The prehospital course of patients with chest pain: Analysis of the prodromal, symptomatic, decision-making, transportation, and emergency room periods. Am J Med 1978;64:742-748.

10. Sjogren A, Erhardt LR, Theorell T: Circumstances around the onset of a myocardial infarction: A study of factors relevant to the perception of symptoms and to the delay in arriving at a coronary care unit. Acta Med Scand 1979;205:287-292.

11. Gudmundsson S, Hardarson T: The determinants of the duration of admission delay in acute myocardial infarction. Danish Med Bull 1980;27:51-55.

12. Wielgosz ATJ, Nolan RP, Earp JA, et al: Reasons for patients' delay in response to symptoms of acute myocardial infarction. Canad Med Assoc J 1988;139:853-857.

13. Hofgren K, Bondestam E, Johansson FG, et al: Initial pain course and delay to hospital admission in relation to myocardial infarct size. Heart Lung 1988;17:274-280.

14. Rawles JM, Haites NE: Patient and general practitioner delays in acute myocardial infarction. Brit Med J 1988;296:882-884.

15. Leitch JW, Birbara T, Freedman B, et al: Factors influencing the time from onset of chest pain to arrival at hospital. Med J Aust 1989;150:6-10.

16. Ho MT, Eisenberg MS, Litwin PE, et al: Delay between onset of chest pain and seeking medical care: The effect of public education. Ann Emerg Med 1989;18:727-731.

17. Herlitz J, Hartford M, Blohm M, et al: Effect of a media campaign on delay times and ambulance use in suspected acute myocardial infarction. Am J Cardiol 1989;64:90-93.

18. Herlitz J, Blohm M, Hartford M, et al: Heart-pain-90,000. Effect of a media campaign on delay times and ambulance use in acute chest pain. Circulation 1989;80(suppl II):353.

19. Weaver WD, Litwin PE, Martin JS, et al: A call for more aggressive management of acute myocardial infarction. Circulation 1989;80(suppl II):353.

20. Applebaum D, Weiss AT, Koren G, et al: Feasibility of pre-hospital fibrinolytic therapy in acute myocardial infarction. Am J Emerg Med 1986;4:201-204.

21. Weiss AT, Fine DG, Applebaum D, et al: Prehospital coronary thrombolysis: A new strategy in acute myocardial infarction. Chest 1987;92:124-128.

22. Castaigne AD, Duval AM, Dubois-Rande JL, et al: Prehospital administration of an-isoylated plasminogen streptokinase activator complex in acute myocardial infarction. Drugs 1987;33(suppl 3):231-234.

23. European Myocardial Infarction Project (E.M.I.P.) Sub-committee: Potential time saving with pre-hospital intervention in acute myocardial infarction. Eur Heart J 1988;9:118-124.

24. Castaigne AD, Herve C, Duval-Moulin A, et al: Pre-hospital use of APSAC: Results of a placebo-controlled study. Am J Cardiol 1989;64:30A-33A.

25. Kennedy JW, Weaver WD: Potential use of thrombolytic therapy before hospitalization. Am J Cardiol 1989;64:8A-11A.

26. Weaver WD, Martin J, Litwin P, et al: Prehospital thrombolytic therapy - MITI project report on Phase I: Feasibility, characteristics of patients. J Am Coll Cardiol 1989;13:152A.

27. Hartmann J, McKeever L, Bufalino V, et al: A system approach to intravenous thrombolysis in acute myocardial infarction in community hospitals: The influence of paramedics. Clin Cardiol 1988;11:812-816.

28. Passamani E, Hodges M, Herman M, et al: The thrombolysis in myocardial infarction (TIMI) phase II pilot study: Tissue plasminogen activator followed by percutaneous transluminal coronary angioplasty. J Am Coll Cardiol 1987;10:51B-64B.

29. Alderman EL, Jutzy KR, Berte LE, et al: Randomized comparison of intravenous versus intracoronary streptokinase for myocardial infarction. Am J Cardiol 1984;54:14-19.

30. Kennedy JW, Atkins JM, Goldstein S, et al: Recent changes in management of acute myocardial infarction: Implications for emergency care physicians. J Amer Coll Cardiol 1988;11:446-449.

31. Karagounis L, Ipsen SK, Jessop MR, et al: Impact of field-transmitted electrocardiography on time to in-hospital thrombolytic therapy in acute myocardial infarction. Circulation 1989;80(suppl II):352.

32. Lee TH, Weisberg MC, Brand DA, et al: Candidates for thrombolysis among emergency room patients with acute chest pain: Potential true- and false-positive rates. Ann Intern Med 1989;110:957-962.

33. Smith M, Eisenberg MS: Thrombolytic therapy for myocardial infarction: Pivotal role for emergency medicine. Ann Emerg Med 1987;16:592-593.

34. Eisenberg MS, Smith M: The farmer and the cowman should be friends: Emergency physicians and cardiologists must work together to ensure rapid initiation of thrombolytic therapy. Ann Emerg Med 1988;17:653-654.

35. Martin LH: Implementation of a thrombolytic protocol in the emergency department. J Emerg Nursing 1989;15:182-187.

36. Maynard C, Althouse R, Olsufka M, et al: Early versus late hospital arrival for acute myocardial infarction in the western Washington thrombolytic therapy trials. Am J Cardiol 1989;63:1296-1300.

37. Kennedy JW, Martin GV, Davis KB, et al: The western Washington trial of intravenous streptokinase in acute myocardial infarction. Circulation 1988;77:345-352.

38. Althouse R, Maynard C, Olsufka M, et al: The Western Washington tissue plasminogen activator emergency room study. J Am Coll Cardiol 1989;13:94A.

39. Grim P, Feldman T, Martin M, et al: Cellular telephone transmission of 12-lead electrocardiograms from ambulance to hospital. Am J Cardiol 1987;60:715-720.

40. Rusnak RA, Stair TO, Hansen K, et al: Litigation against the emergency physician: Common features in cases of missed myocardial infarction. Ann Emerg Med 1989;18:1029-1034.

41. Pipberger HV, Klingeman JD, Cosma J: Computer evaluation of statistical properties of clinical information in the differential diagnosis of chestpain. Method Inform Med 1968;7:79-92.

42. Rose GA: The diagnosis of ischaemic heart pain and intermittent claudication in field surveys. Bull WHO 1962;27:645-658.

43. Myers G, Freeman R, Scharf D, et al: Cervicoprecordial angina: Diagnosis and management. Am J Cardiol 1977;39:287 (abstract).

44. Alpert JS, Braunwald E: Pathological and clinical manifestations of acute myocardial infarction. In: Braunwald E (ed), *Heart Disease: A Textbook of Cardiovascular Medicine*. Philadelphia, WB Saunders Co. 1980, pp 1327-1328.

45. Alonzo AM, Simon AB, Feinleib M: Prodromata of myocardial infarction and sudden death. Circulation 1975;52:1056.

46. Zarling EJ, Sexton H, Milnor P: Failure to diagnose acute myocardial infarction. JAMA 1983;250:1177-1181.

47. Kannel WB, Abbott RD: Incidence and prognosis of unrecognized myocardial infarction: An update on the Framingham Study. N Engl J Med 1984;311:1144-1147.

48. Soler NG, Bennett MA, Pentecost BL, Fitzgerald MG, Malins JM: Myocardial infarction in diabetics. Quart J Med 1975;44:125.

49. Ornato JP: Computer-assisted diagnosis of chest pain. In: Ornato JP (ed), *Cardiovascular Emergencies*. New York, Churchill Livingstone, 1986, pp 1-22.

50. Kambara H, Phillips J: Long-term evaluation of early repolarization syndrome (normal variant RS-T segment elevation). Am J Cardiol 1976;38:157.

51. Surawicz B, Lasseter KC: Electrocardiogram in pericarditis. Am J Cardiol 1970;25:471.

52. Bruce MA, Spodick DH: Atypical electrocardiogram in acute pericarditis; characteristics and prevalence. J Electrocardiol 1980;13:61.

53. Spodick DH: Electrocardiogram in acute pericarditis. Distributions of morphologic and axial changes by stages. Am J Cardiol 1974;33:470.

54. Spodick DH: Differential characteristics of the electrocardiogram in early repolarization and acute pericarditis. N Engl J Med 1976;295:523.

55. Eisenberg JM, Horowitz LN, Busch R, et al: Diagnosis of acute myocardial infarction in the emergency room: A prospective assessment of clinical decision making and the usefulness of immediate cardiac enzyme determination. J Commun Health 1979;4:191-196.

56. Seager SB: Cardiac enzymes in the evaluation of chest pain. Ann Emerg Med 1980;9:346-340.

57. Grande P, Christiansen C, Pedersen A, et al: Optimal diagnosis in acute myocardial infarction: A cost-effectiveness study. Circulation 1980;61:723-728.

58. Turi ZG, Rutherford JD, Roberts R, et al: Electrocardiographic, enzymatic and scintigraphic criteria of acute myocardial infarction as determined from study of 726 patients (a MILIS study). Am J Cardiol 1985;55:1463-1468.

59. Tate DA, Dehmer GJ: New challenges for thrombolytic therapy. Ann Int Med 1989; 110:953-954.

60. Hlatky MA, Cotugno H, O'Connor C, et al: Adoption of thrombolytic therapy in the management of acute myocardial infarction. Am J Cardiol 1988;61:510-514.

61. Rowe WW, Simpson RJ Jr, Tate DA, et al: Non-emergent cardiac catheterization and risk-stratified revascularization following thrombolytic therapy for acute myocardial infarction: A critical analysis of therapy in the community setting. Arch Intern Med 1989; 149:1611-1617.

62. Topol EJ, Bates ER, Walton JA Jr, et al: Community hospital administration of intravenous tissue plasminogen activator in acute myocardial infarction: Improved timing, thrombolytic efficacy and ventricular function. J Am Coll Cardiol 1987;10:1173-1177.

63. Yamamoto LG, Wiebe RA: Improving medical communication with facsimile (fax) transmission. Am J Emerg Med 1989;7:203-208.

64. Kudenchuk PJ, Ho MT, Litwin PE, et al: Accuracy of cardiologist vs. computerized ECG analysis in selecting patients for out-of-hospital thrombolytic therapy. Circulation 1989; 80(suppl II):354.

Chapter 6

REPERFUSION THERAPY
Significance of Recent Trials to the Practicing Cardiologist

Thomas C. Wall
E. Magnus Ohman
Robert M. Califf

INTRODUCTION

Over the last decade, a dramatic change has occurred in the management of patients with acute myocardial infarction (AMI). Standard care in the late 1960s and early 1970s consisted of bed rest, analgesia, and cardiac rhythm surveillance. In the late 1970s, treatment of cardiac dysrhythmias made a substantial impact on the clinical outcome of patients, yet mortality remained substantial. Acute and long-term mortality was still largely unaffected because a means of minimizing left ventricular dysfunction was not available. In the 1980s, strategies directed at restoring infarct related artery patency during AMI by either thrombolytic therapy or coronary angioplasty were initiated. The improvement in survival in treated patients compared with placebo or conservatively treated controls has been a most important observation over the last decade.

Although many details remain to be resolved, several general principles about thrombolytic therapy have become apparent. First, the overwhelming evidence in favor of general benefit is indisputable, given the fact that over 50,000 patients have enrolled in randomized clinical trials. Second, a confluence of information from experimental and clinical studies has stressed the importance of early treatment. Third, therapy is applicable to a much wider variety of patients than envisioned initially, so that the "window" of treatment needs to be broadened. Fourth, the overall environment including the medical care setting and specific ancillary, pharmacologic and mechanical therapies have an important bearing on the outcome of reperfusion therapy. Finally, the individual nature of each patient mandates a careful assessment by the practitioner, with integration of large amounts of data about that patient before a course of action is taken. Each decision must be made only after carefully weighing the potential benefits and risks to the individual.

IMPACT OF THERAPY

Now that over 50,000 patients have been randomized into trials of reperfusion therapy, the general benefit cannot be disputed. In fact, the direction of the treatment effect has been on the side of mortality reduction in every subgroup investigated in clinical trials except for patients with ST-segment depression. Meta-analyses have convincingly demonstrated that when the therapeutic benefit has been "statistically insignificant," the most likely explanation has been inadequate sample size. The data have now been evaluated in many subgroups (inferior MI, elderly, late patients), and it now appears that all available agents (rt-PA, streptokinase, anistreplase/APSAC) have benefits. Thus, the clinician now must search for reasons not to use reperfusion therapy in the individual patient, rather than agonizing over the decision to treat.

EARLY DIAGNOSIS AND TREATMENT

Early identification of AMI has become increasingly important, since earlier administration of thrombolytic therapy is associated with lower mortality rates[1], less myocardial necrosis, and better left ventricular function (Table 1).[2] Accordingly, the clinician must stay abreast of methods to rapidly identify and expeditiously treat patients who are candidates for reperfusion therapy.[3] For instance, phase I of the Myocardial Infarction Triage and Intervention (MITI) trial demonstrated that treatment could be

Table 1. *Mortality in the ISIS-2 study*

Hours from pain onset	Vascular deaths		Reduction in mortality (%)
	SK & Aspirin	Placebo	
0-1	11/178	25/179	56
2	31/476	62/480	50
3	41/617	84/617	51
4	36/590	74/590	51
5-12	179/1823	252/1820	29

SK = Streptokinase. ISIS-2 study data from reference 1. Patients were randomized in a factorial design to streptokinase (1.5 million IU), aspirin (162.5 mg), both or neither. Data displayed are from patients randomized to both streptokinase and aspirin versus neither (placebo).

initiated 56 minutes earlier by paramedics in the field as compared to conventional therapy in the hospital emergency room.[4]

The time to diagnosis and treatment ("door to needle time") can be shortened substantially through a systematic evaluation of structural components of the local medical care setting. Inordinate delays in patient transport and processing remain in many communities. One of the most common problems is a prolonged delay in obtaining a 12-lead electrocardiogram. Another common delay results from obtaining unnecessary subspecialty consultation. Given the substantial evidence for the benefit of early treatment, every medical facility responsible for emergency care should scrutinize its structural components of health care delivery.

The majority of patients with AMI present with typical symptoms of chest discomfort and associated electrocardiographic abnormalities. However, many patients have atypical symptoms and nonspecific changes on the electrocardiogram. Therefore, additional diagnostic studies that can rapidly and accurately identify patients with myocardial infarction are needed. Until new methods are available, a high level of clinical suspicion should be maintained in the emergency department.

Cardiac enzymes are both a sensitive and specific test in the early phase of infarction. Serum tests are now available with assay times of 10-15 minutes for creatine kinase MB, its MB-2 subunit and myoglobin.[5] The utility and accuracy of the MB-2 assay and the serum myoglobin assay in rapidly identifying patients with AMI are currently under investigation. There is little doubt that concerted use of both the electrocardiogram and serum studies will enhance diagnostic capabilities in the early phases of AMI.

CRITERIA FOR USING THROMBOLYTIC THERAPY

Currently, all patients less than 75 years of age, with symptoms consistent with myocardial infarction less than six hours in duration, and associated ST-segment elevations should be considered candidates for reperfusion therapy. Standard contraindications and guidelines for the use of thrombolytic therapy are listed in Table 2. There is general agreement on the specific contraindications, although the interval between events such as stroke and the administration of therapy remains controversial.

The benefit of thrombolytic therapy in patients older than 75 years of age has been documented in the ISIS-2 trial.[1] Data from other clinical trials in which older patients were included have also suggested substantial reduction in mortality rates when reperfusion therapy has been given[1,6-9] (Table 3). However, the potential increase in bleeding, especially intracranial, mandates a more careful assessment of risks in these elderly patients. The use of thrombolytic therapy in elderly patients must be individualized and guided by clinical judgement, with emphasis placed on physiological rather than chronological age. At present, age should not be an absolute contraindication to reperfusion therapy.

Table 2. *Contraindications to thrombolytic therapy*

Contraindication	Time interval
Suspected aortic dissection	
Pregnancy	
Bleeding diathesis/current anticoagulants	
History of active bleeding	4 weeks
Recent surgery or trauma	4 weeks
Prolonged cardiopulmonary resuscitation	> 10 minutes
Stroke	
Intracranial hemorrhage	life-time
Embolic stroke	6 months
Intracranial vascular malformation/neoplasm	life-time
Poorly controlled hypertension (≥ 200/120 mm Hg)	at admission to hospital

Experimental studies in the canine model which demonstrated completed transmural infarction within four to six hours of coronary occlusion led to the concept of "a window of opportunity" for the initiation of thrombolytic therapy and restoring coronary blood flow.[10] However, the ISIS-2 study demonstrated a 25% reduction in mortality in patients enrolled 6-24 hours after symptom onset.[1,7,11] Previous experience with late administration of thrombolytic therapy is summarized in Table 4. The benefit from late administration of thrombolytic therapy suggests that several other mechanisms independent of myocardial salvage may be important for survival. Indeed, sustained patency of the infarct related vessel has been associated with decreased long term mortality, better infarct healing, less aneurysm formation, and a more stable electrophysiologic state.[12] Three large studies (EMERA with SK, LATE with rt-PA, and ISIS-3) and one pilot study are currently examining patients treated after six hours of symptom onset. Until results of these large studies confirm the findings of the ISIS-2 study, a definitive recommendation for treating patients with symptoms greater than six hours in duration cannot be given.

MANAGEMENT OF PATIENTS WITH CONTRAINDICATIONS TO THROMBOLYTIC THERAPY

The standard care of patients in whom thrombolytic therapy is contraindicated includes intravenous heparin, nitroglycerin, aspirin, and β-blockers.[13] Of these agents,

Table 3. *Thrombolytic therapy during myocardial infarction in elderly patients*

Study	Age (years)	Mortality rate Active (%)	Mortality rate Placebo (%)	Reduction in mortality (%)	P value
ISAM[6]	< 70	5.1	6.6	23	0.21
	70-75	13.0	9.6	(+ 35)	0.37
GISSI[7]	< 75	8.7	10.6	18	0.001
	≥ 75	28.9	33.1	13	0.11
ISIS-2[1]	< 70	7.0	9.6	27	0.0001
	≥ 70	18.2	21.6	16	0.01
ASSET[8]	< 66	5.4	6.3	14	0.24
	66-75	10.8	16.4	34	0.001
AIMS[9]	< 65	5.2	8.5	39	0.06
	65-70	12.2	30.2	60	0.003

ISAM – Intravenous Streptokinase in Acute Myocardial Infarction; GISSI – Group Italiano per lo Studio della Streptochinasi; ISIS-2 – Second International Study of Infarct Survival Collaborative Group; ASSET – Anglo-Scandinavian Study Evaluating rt-PA; AIMS – APSAC in Myocardial Infarction Study

intravenous heparin and aspirin have been shown to decrease recurrent ischemia and reinfarction in the acute setting. An overview of trials comparing β-blockers with placebo demonstrated a reduction in death, reinfarction, recurrent ischemia, and serious arrhythmias.[13, 14]

In selected patients, direct angioplasty of the infarct related vessel has been used as primary therapy. The majority of hospitals in the United States are not capable of performing acute cardiac catheterization or coronary angioplasty. In hospitals where facilities are available, this approach appears to have many advantages. Direct angioplasty is successful in restoring acute coronary patency in > 90% of patients and is associated with a significant improvement in left ventricular function.[15] In addition, direct angioplasty even in the setting of anticoagulation has not led to significant complications including bleeding. No intracranial hemorrhage has been reported in any of the carefully collected series. Data from series of direct angioplasty in AMI have shown similar improvements in clinical outcomes when compared to intravenous thrombolytic therapy. Therefore, patients unable to receive intravenous throm-

Table 4. *Mortality rates following late administration of thrombolytic therapy*

Time	Mortality rate Active (%)	Placebo (%)	Reduction in mortality (%)	P value
6-12 hours				
* 33 studies pooled[11]	18.0	21.0	14	0.42
GISSI[7]	13.5	13.9	3	0.77
ISIS-2[1]	10.4	12.1	14	0.02
12-24 hour				
* 33 studies pooled[11]	12.0	22.0	45	0.0007
ISIS-2[1]	8.7	10.8	19	0.08

GISSI – Gruppo Italiano per lo Studio della Streptochinasi; ISIS-2 – Second International Study of Infarct Survival Collaborative Group
*   Data from Yusuf et al[11]

bolytic therapy who are otherwise considered candidates for reperfusion should have direct angioplasty if prompt access to cardiac catheterization facilities can be arranged. Several multicenter studies (**P**rimary **A**ngioplasty **R**egistry–PAR; **D**irect **A**ngioplasty in **M**yocardial **I**nfarction Trial–DAMI) are currently evaluating this approach.

CHOICE OF THROMBOLYTIC AGENT

At present, recombinant tissue plasminogen activator, (rt-PA), streptokinase and anisoylated plasminogen streptokinase activator complex/anistreplase (APSAC) are approved for intravenous reperfusion therapy in AMI. Intravenous urokinase in this setting has received considerable investigation but is not currently approved.[16,17,18] The early patency and recanalization rates of the various agents are shown in Table 5. It can be seen that APSAC and rt-PA have been associated with higher patency rates followed by urokinase and streptokinase. Tissue plasminogen activator is very effective in achieving rapid reperfusion, but its short half-life and fibrin specificity have resulted in a higher reocclusion rate.[19] On the other hand, longer-acting agents such as APSAC, urokinase, and streptokinase, are associated with less reocclusion and a sustained reperfusion state.

Table 5. *Overview of reperfusion rates*

Agent	n	Recanalization rate*		n	Patency rate*	
		Mean	95% ci[†]		Mean	95% ci[†]
Streptokinase	222	38	32-44	793	55	52-58
Urokinase				265	62	56-68
APSAC	182	55	48-62	255	77	72-82
rt-PA	212	68	62-74	1597	73	70-75

* At 90 minutes after dosing
† ci = confidence interval
APSAC – Anisoylated plasminogen streptokinase activator complex
rt-PA – Recombinant tissue plasminogen activator

Currently, there is ongoing debate concerning which thrombolytic agent leads to the best overall clinical outcome. The high cost of rt-PA and APSAC, as opposed to streptokinase, have made this an issue the health care budget. The GISSI 2/International study, which was recently completed,[20,21] was the first large trial to compare rt-PA and streptokinase head to head in a randomized controlled fashion. No significant difference in hospital mortality was found between the two agents. However, heparin was given only to half the patients on a randomized basis. When heparin was given, it was administered subcutaneously 12 hours after the rt-PA infusion. This approach leads to subtherapeutic partial thromboplastin times for up to 18-24 hours. Furthermore, data from two recent studies evaluating rt-PA suggested that concomitant heparin given intravenously is necessary for sustained patency of the infarct vessel.[22,23] As a consequence, another study is soon to be launched, comparing these two agents while administering heparin intravenously starting during thrombolytic infusion. The Global Utilization of Streptokinase and rt-PA for Occluded Coronary Arteries (GUSTO) trial will compare standard streptokinase therapy with rapid rt-PA infusion (weight-adjusted dose over 90 minutes) and a combination of streptokinase and rt-PA (Figure 1).

Studies employing combination therapy with rt-PA and streptokinase or urokinase have demonstrated improved clinical outcomes including less recurrent ischemia, reocclusion and better regional infarct zone function. These studies are shown in Table 6.[24-28] Also, salvage or rescue angioplasty for thrombolytic therapy was better tolerated with fewer complications including abrupt closure and reocclusion, without an increase in bleeding. Therefore, the combination of agents is effective in not only maximizing acute reperfusion but also in sustaining coronary patency. As a result, in the TAMI 5 study overall hospital charges to the patient were no higher with combination therapy than with monotherapy.

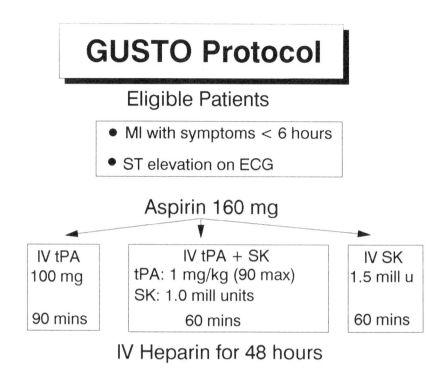

Figure 1. *Therapeutic algorithm for Global Utilization of Streptokinase and rt-PA for Occluded Coronary Arteries.*

The outcome of the GUSTO and ISIS-3 trials should have a substantial impact on the choice of thrombolytic therapy in myocardial infarction. Until these studies are completed, a definitive statement concerning which agent or agents to use cannot be made. Patients who have previously received either streptokinase or APSAC should probably not receive these agents within one year of drug administration for the management of AMI because of a possible concern that neutralizing antibodies may inhibit the fibrinolytic activity of these agents.[29]

NOVEL DOSING REGIMENS FOR THROMBOLYTIC THERAPY

A major shortcoming of intravenous thrombolytic therapy has been the limitation imposed by a "ceiling" rate of reperfusion. The maximum rate of acute patency has been in the mid 70% range. Clinically, this means that 1 out of every 4 patients who are treated will fail to obtain the maximum benefit of early reperfusion. As a conse-

Table 6. *Combination thrombolytic therapy*

Study	n	Dose rt-PA	Dose UK or SK	Patency 90 min (%)	Reocclusion (%)
rt-PA & UK					
TAMI 2	112	1 mg/kg over 60 min	0.5-2.0 million IU over 60 min	73	9
TAMI 5	191	1 mg/kg over 60 min	1.5 million IU over 60 min	78	2
TAMI 7	42	1 mg/kg over 30 min	1.5 million IU over 60 min	74	6
URALMI	129	20 mg-1 mg/kg over 60 min	1.0-2.0 million IU over 60 min	81	9
rt-PA & SK					
KAMIT - PILOT	40	50 mg over 60 min	1.5 million IU over 60 min	75	8
KAMIT	208	50 mg over 60 min	1.5 million IU over 60 min	79	3

rt-PA – Recombinant tissue plasminogen activator; UK – Urokinase; SK – Streptokinase; TAMI – Thrombolysis and Angioplasty in Myocardial Infarction Study Group; URALMI – Urokinase and Alteplase in Myocardial Infarction (personal communication); KAMIT – Kentucky Acute Myocardial Infarction Trial
Adapted from references 24-28

quence, new dosing strategies for thrombolysis have been recently investigated, particularly with intravenous rt-PA. These regimens have employed a rapid infusion of rt-PA in the hope of improving the rate of reperfusion. Of all the studies thus far,[25,30-36] only two have demonstrated an acute coronary patency rate greater than 90% in this setting, while the majority have demonstrated reperfusion rates similar or slightly superior to the approved dosing (Table 7). Thus, at present, it appears that the impact of frontloading the dose of intravenous rt-PA will be modest. The risk of intracranial hemorrhage following rapid infusion of rt-PA has not been fully explored and will need to be evaluated in large numbers of patients. Based upon our experience and that of others, a weight-adjusted dose of rt-PA over 90 minutes appears to be optimal.

Accumulated data from thrombolytic trials with all of the available agents have clarified the risks and side effects associated with this therapy. The major risk is intracranial hemorrhage, which occurs in 0.3-0.7% of patients, even when a carefully

Table 7. *Rapid rt-PA dosing strategies*

Study	n	Dose	rt-PA Max dose (mg)	Patency (%) 60 min	Patency (%) 90 min	Reocclusion (%)
Smalling et al[30]	84	2.0 mg/kg (1.2 mg/kg first hour)	150	65	84	11
Neuhaus et al[31]	80	15 mg bolus 50 mg 30 min 35 mg 60 min	100	74	91	11
Tebbe et al[32]	20	50 mg/2 min	50	75		22
Tranchesi et al[33]	25	70 mg/1-3 min	70	72		25
Lew et al[34]	42	10 mg bolus 90 mg first hour 50 mg second hour	150	86*		11
McKendall et al[35]	36	20 mg bolus wait 30 min 80 mg over 2 hours	100	82	94	
Khan et al[36]	14	10 cL mu x 4 at 20 mins interval	40 cL mu		79	

* At a mean of 41 minutes following the start of therapy
cL mu = clot lysis megaunits

selected population is evaluated.[37,38] Interestingly, the risk is counterbalanced by an apparent decrease in the risk of embolic stroke, so that the total stroke rate is similar in patients treated with thrombolytic therapy compared with controls. Nevertheless, the clinician evaluating the patient in the emergency department must be prepared to deal with a 1/150 to 1/300 chance of creating a clinically obvious deleterious or even lethal effect of the drug within hours after its administration. This fact reinforces the need for careful explanation to the patient and family of the risks and benefits of reperfusion.

DETECTION OF EARLY REPERFUSION

The ability of the clinician to predict infarct vessel reperfusion after thrombolytic therapy has been disappointing. Indeed, only about 25% of patients will obtain complete chest pain resolution within 90 minutes of the infusion despite successful thrombolysis. In addition, complete normalization of ST-segment changes occurs in less than 10% of patients within the first 90 minutes. "Reperfusion arrhythmias" occur in as many patients who remain occluded as in those who successfully open.[39]

Recently, two innovative technologies for noninvasive detection of reperfusion have been investigated. The first of these is a 12-lead electrocardiographic ischemia monitor.[40] This device can be placed on the patient at the time of acute presentation and can be programmed to obtain a 12-lead EKG tracing every 30 seconds. The entire period of monitoring can then be down loaded into a personal computer to give a graphic display of ST-segment changes over time. The device is also capable of sounding an alarm if significant ST-segment shifts indicative of either ischemia or infarction are detected. Preliminary analysis of the data acquired with this device has demonstrated considerable promise in its ability to differentiate patients who reperfuse or remain closed after thrombolytic therapy.

The second technology is a novel enzyme kit for expeditiously measuring creatine kinase levels in the emergency room setting.[41] Enzyme levels measured 30 and 60 minutes after thrombolytic therapy have demonstrated a significant change over time and are capable of predicting early reperfusion.[41] Therefore, with a combination of bedside clinical skills, noninvasive ischemia monitoring and serial CK-MB enzyme changes, the possibility of accurately identifying patients who fail to reperfuse in the emergency setting may soon be available. This would allow clinicians to effectively triage patients in need of acute catheterization.

ADJUNCTIVE PHARMACOLOGICAL STRATEGIES

The "ceiling" rate of reperfusion and early reocclusion remain significant limitations of reperfusion therapy. Current thrombolytic agents are fibrinolytic and are less effective in opening vessels which have platelet rich, fibrin poor thrombus. Furthermore, ongoing thrombin formation continues as the clot lyses. Platelets and thrombin appear to be responsible for not only decreasing the efficacy of reperfusion therapy but also for creating an environment favorable for producing recurrent ischemia and reocclusion.[42,43] The ISIS-2 trial was instrumental in demonstrating a 21% reduction in mortality due to the effect of aspirin, and several studies have now documented the importance of the use of heparin in conjunction with rt-PA.[1, 22,23]

New agents are currently being investigated to more effectively inhibit platelet interaction and function. One such agent, called 7E3, is a monoclonal antibody directed against the IIB, IIIA receptor on the platelet membrane.[44] These receptors are believed to be responsible for platelet aggregation with its subsequent effects on the initiation of thrombin formation, vasoconstriction and elaboration of growth factors responsible for smooth muscle cell proliferation. In preliminary studies, this agent has been shown to eliminate platelet aggregation to a variety of stimuli in a matter of minutes after administration. It is hoped that this agent, along with intravenous thrombolytic therapy, may enhance thrombolysis and decrease recurrent ischemia and reocclusion.

Because the impact of reperfusion on systolic left ventricular function has been less than anticipated, adjunctive therapy to decrease myocardial reperfusion injury is currently an active area of interest. In the canine model, reperfusion of infarcted myocardial tissue with whole blood creates an extensive amount of inflammation and necrosis, which is termed reperfusion injury. White blood cells, particularly neutrophils, are believed to be largely responsible through production of toxic metabolites and plugging of the microcirculation. Initial studies with superoxide dismutase have been disappointing, but new agents are now available. Fluosol, a commercially available perfluorochemical, has been shown to reduce canine infarct size by 40-50% in the setting of reperfusion.[45,46] This agent is not only capable of binding a large amount of oxygen but can deliver it through poorly developed collaterals to the infarct zone at the time of infarction. By creating an aerobic environment, it can theoretically inhibit neutrophil activation and wash out any toxic metabolites. This agent, in conjunction with intravenous rt-PA is currently being investigated in a randomized trial for its possible clinical benefit.

THE ROLE OF CARDIAC CATHETERIZATION

The role of cardiac catheterization in the setting of an AMI has been an area of considerable debate. Some investigators have advocated a "watchful waiting" strategy where cardiac catheterization is only performed when evidence of residual ischemia exists after the administration of thrombolytic therapy.[47] However, early reperfusion and sustained patency of the infarct related vessel appear to be two major factors for improving acute and long term mortality in patients with AMI. The TAMI studies have suggested a better overall clinical outcome in patients who had acute cardiac catheterization compared with a deferred strategy.[24] Presumably the improved outcome was due to knowledge of the coronary anatomy and the ability to perform rescue angioplasty in this setting. In a logistic regression model, a closed infarct related artery at the time of acute catheterization was equivalent to 23 fewer years of life, the loss of 25 ejection fraction points, and 1.6 more diseased vessels.[48] Without catheterization, the status of the infarct related vessel cannot be accurately determined.

A more effective way of triaging patients for acute or delayed catheterization is needed. In the future, a combination of bedside clinical skills, continuous ischemia monitoring, and rapid CK-MB analysis will allow more accurate use of acute catheterization. Until then, cardiac catheterization during the first 24 hours is necessary to definitively document infarct vessel patency in AMI patients.

CONCLUSION

The primary message from clinical trials of thrombolytic therapy to date is that the practitioner must be prepared for continuing change. Advances are being made in so many areas simultaneously that clinicians must stay abreast of the major issues as they evolve. Promising improvements in our ability to impact platelet function and thrombin generation may lead to a great increase in the ability of pharmacologic therapy to achieve early patency and stability of the infarct artery. On the surface these advances would seem to obviate the need for invasive intervention. Alternatively, however, these changes could make the environment for mechanical intervention much safer and more effective. Finally, better methods of monitoring patients will allow for more effective individualization of therapy.

The overriding message to the clinician is that achieving patency of the infarct-related artery is a vital part of the strategy for the care of the patient with AMI. Every practitioner caring for patients with AMI should develop a plan, taking into account the current data and resources available in the specific community setting, in order to achieve reperfusion whenever possible.

REFERENCES

1. ISIS-2 Second International Study of Infarct Survival Collaborative Group: Randomised trial of intravenous streptokinase, oral aspirin, both, or neither among 17,187 cases of suspected acute myocardial infarction. ISIS-2. Lancet 1988;2:349-360.

2. Braunwald E: Myocardial reperfusion, limitation of infarct size, reduction of left ventricular dysfunction, and improved survival. Circulation 1989;79;441-444.

3. Califf RM, Harrelson-Woodlief SL: At home thrombolysis. J Am Coll Cardiol 1990;15:937-939.

4. Weaver WD, Eisenberg MS, Martin JS, et al: Myocardial infarction triage and intervention project-phase 1: patient characteristics and feasibility of prehospital initiation of thrombolytic therapy. J Am Coll Cardiol 1990;15:925-931.

5. Ohman EM, Sigmon KN, Califf RM: Is diagnostic certainty essential for the use of thrombolytic therapy during myocardial infarction in the 1990's? Circulation 1990;82:1073-1075.

6. The I.S.A.M. Study Group: A prospective trial of intravenous streptokinase in acute myocardial infarction. N Engl J Med 1986;314:1465-1471.

7. The GISSI Protocol: Effectiveness of intravenous thrombolytic treatment in acute myocardial infarction. Lancet 1986;2:397-401.

8. ASSET Study Group: Trial of tissue plasminogen activator for mortality reduction in acute myocardial infarction. Lancet 1988;2:525-530.

9. AIMS Trial Study Group: Effect of intravenous APSAC on mortality after acute myocardial infarction: Preliminary report of a placebo-controlled clinical trial. Lancet 1988;2:545-549.

10. Reimer KA, Lowe JE, Rasmussen MM, et al: The wavefront phenomenon of ischemic cell death. 1. Myocardial infarct size versus duration of coronary occlusion in dogs. Circulation 1977;56:786-794.

11. Yusuf S, Collins R, Peto R, et al: Intravenous and intracoronary fibrinolytic therapy in acute myocardial infarction: Overview of results on mortality, reinfarction and side-effects from 33 randomized controlled trials. Eur Heart J 1985;6:556-585.

12. Fortin DF, Califf RM: Long term survival from acute myocardial infarction: Salutary effect of an open coronary vessel. Am J Med 1990;88:9N-15N.

13. Yusuf S, Wittes J, Friedman L, et al: Overview of results of randomized clinical trials in heart disease. JAMA 1988;260:2088-2093.

14. Yusuf S, M.R.C.P., Phil D, et al: Reduction in infarct size, arrhythmias and chest pain by early intravenous beta-blocker in suspected acute myocardial infarction. Circulation 1983;67:I32-I41.

15. Stone GW, Rutherford BD, McConahay DR, et al: Direct coronary angioplasty in acute myocardial infarction: Outcome in patients with single vessel disease. J Am Coll Cardiol 1990;15:534-543.

16. Neuhaus KL, Tebbe U, Gottwik M, et al: Intravenous recombinant tissue plasminogen activator (rt-PA) and urokinase in acute myocardial infarction: Results of the German Activator Urokinase Study (GAUS). J Am Coll Cardiol 1988;12:581-587.

17. Mathey DG, Schofer J, Sheehan FH, et al: Intravenous urokinase is acute myocardial infarction. Am J Cardiol 1985;55:878-882

18. Wall TC, Phillips HR, Stack RS, et al: Results of high dose intravenous urokinase for acute myocardial infarction. Am J Cardiol 1990;65:124-131.

19. Schaer DH, Ross AM, Wasserman AG: Reinfarction, recurrent angina, and reocclusion after thrombolytic therapy. Circulation 1987;76:II57-II62.

20. The GISSI-2 Protocol: GISSI-2; A factorial randomised trial of alteplase versus streptokinase and heparin versus no heparin among 12,490 patients with acute myocardial infarction. Lancet 1990;2:65-71.

21. The International Study Group: In hospital mortality and clinical course of 20,891 patients with suspected acute myocardial infarction randomised between alteplase and streptokinase with or without heparin. Lancet 1990;2:71-75.

22. Hsia J, Hamilton WP, Kleiman N, et al: A comparison between heparin and low-dose aspirin as adjunctive therapy with tissue plasminogen activator for acute myocardial infarction. N Engl J Med 1990;323:1433-1437.

23. Bleich SD, Nichols T, Schumacher R, et al: Effect of heparin on coronary artery patency after thrombolysis with tissue plasminogen activator in acute myocardial infarction. Am J Cardiol 1990;66:1412-1417.

24. Califf RM, Topol EJ, Stack RS, et al: An evaluation of combination thrombolytic therapy and timing of cardiac catheterization in acute myocardial infarctions: Results of the TAMI 5 randomized trial. Circulation 1990, in press.

25. Wall TC, Topol ET, Genge BS, et al: The TAMI-7 trial of accelerated plasminogen activator dose regimens for coronary thrombolysis. Circulation 1990;82(4, suppl III), abstract.

26. Grines CL, Nissen SE, Booth DC, et al: A new thrombolytic regimen for acute myocardial infarction using combination half dose tissue type plasminogen activator with full dose streptokinase: A pilot study. J Am Coll Cardiol 1989;14:573-580.

27. Grines CL, Nissen SE, Booth DC, et al: A prospective, randomized trial comparing combination half dose tPA with streptokinase to full dose tPA in acute myocardial infarction: Preliminary report. J Am Coll Cardiol 1990;i:4A (abstract).

28. Topol EJ, Califf RM, George BS, et al: Coronary arterial thrombolysis with combined infusion of recombinant tissue-type plasminogen activator and urokinase in patients with acute myocardial infarction. Circulation 1988;77:1100-1107.

29. Jalihal S, Morris GK: Antistreptokinase titres after intravenous streptokinase. Lancet 1990;335:184-190.

30. Smalling RW, Schumacher R, Morris D, et al: Improved infarct-related arterial patency after high dose, weight-adjusted, rapid infusion of tissue-type plasminogen activator in myocardial infarction: Results of a multicenter randomized trial of two dosage regimens. J Am Coll Cardiol 1990;15:915-921.

31. Neuhaus KL, Feuerer W, Jeep-Tebbe S, et al: Improved thrombolysis with a modified dose regimen of recombinant tissue-type plasminogen activator. J Am Coll Cardiol 1989;14:1566-1569.

32. Tebbe U, Tanswell P, Seifried E, et al: Single-bolus injection of recombinant tissue-type plasminogen activator in acute myocardial infarction. Am J Cardiol 1989;64:448-453.

33. Tranchesi B, Verstraete M, Vanhove PH, et al: Intravenous bolus administration of recombinant tissue plasminogen activator to patients with acute myocardial infarction. Coronary Artery Disease 1990;1:83-88.

34. Lew AS, Cercek B, Lewis BS, et al: Efficiency of a two-hour infusion of 150-mg tissue plasminogen activator in acute myocardial infarction. Am J Cardiol 1987;60:1225-1229.

35. McKendall GR, Attbaro M, Drew TM, et al: Improved infarct artery patency using a new modified regimen of t-PA; results of the pre-hospital administration of t-PA (PATS) pilot trial (abstract). J Am Coll Cardiol 1989;15:3A (abstract).

36. Khan MI, Hackett DR, Andreotti F, et al: Effectiveness of multiple bolus administration of tissue-type plasminogen activator in acute myocardial infarction. Am J Cardiol 1990; 65:1051-1056.

37. O'Connor CM, Califf RM, Massey EW, et al: Stroke and acute myocardial infarction in the thrombolytic era: Clinical correlates and long-term prognosis. J Am Coll Cardiol 1990;16:533-540.

38. Tiefenbrunn AJ, Ludbrook PA: Coronary thrombolysis -it's worth the risk. JAMA 1989; 261:2107-2108.

39. Califf RM, O'Neil W, Stack RS, et al: Failure of simple clinical measurements to predict perfusion status after intravenous thrombolysis. Ann Intern Med 1988;108:658-662.

40. Krucoff MW, Wagner NB, Pope JE, et al: The portable programmable microprocessor-driven real-time 12-lead electrocardiographic monitor: A preliminary report of a new device for the noninvasive detection of successful reperfusion or silent coronary reocclusion. Am J Cardiol 1990;65:143-148.

41. Ohman EM, Christenson RH, Sigmon KN, et al: Noninvasive detection of reperfusion after thrombolysis using rapid CK-MB analysis. Circulation 1990;82:(4, suppl III), abstract.

42. Trip MD, Cats VM, Vreeken J, et al: Platelet hyperreactivity and prognosis in survivors of myocardial infarction. N Engl J Med 1990;322:1549-1554.

43. Fitzgerald DJ, Catella F, Roy L, et al: Marked platelet activation in vivo after intravenous streptokinase in patients with acute myocardial infarction. Circulation 1988;77:142-150.

44. Mickelson JK, Simpson PJ, Cronin M, et al: Antiplatelet antibody (7E3 F(ab')2) prevents rethrombosis after recombinant tissue-type plasminogen activator-induced coronary artery thrombolysis in a canine model. Circulation 1990;81:617-627.

45. Forman MB, Puett DW, Wilson HW, et al; Beneficial long-term effect of intracoronary perfluorochemical on infarct size and ventricular function on a canine reperfusion model. J Am Coll Cardiol 1987;9:1082-1090.

46. Schaer GL, Karas SP, Santoian EC, et al: Reduction in reperfusion injury by blood-free reperfusion after experimental myocardial infarction. J Am Coll Cardiol 1990;15:1385-1393.

47. The TIMI Study Group: Comparison of invasive and conservative strategies after treatment with intravenous tissue plasminogen activator in acute myocardial infarction. N Engl J Med 1989;320:618-627.

48. Califf RM, Harrelson-Woodlief L, Topol EJ: Left ventricular ejection fraction may be non-viable as an endpoint of thrombolytic therapy comparative trials. Circulation 1990; 82:1847-1853.

Chapter 7

NON-THROMBOLYTIC PHARMACOLOGIC THERAPY FOR ACUTE MYOCARDIAL INFARCTION

Cindy L. Grines

INTRODUCTION

The mortality reduction accomplished by thrombolytic therapy for acute myocardial infarction (AMI) has generated considerable excitement in the medical community and lay public. However, only 20-30% of AMI patients are appropriate candidates for thrombolytic therapy.[1] Since the majority of AMI patients cannot be treated with thrombolytic agents and since thrombolytic therapy reduces mortality by only 30%, other medical therapies will continue to play an important role. In patients not undergoing reperfusion therapy, drugs which alter the balance of myocardial oxygen supply and demand reduce infarct size and prolong survival.[2] Conventional antianginal drugs may widen the window of myocardial viability by reducing oxygen demand, allowing thrombolytic therapy to be given later in the course of an infarction. In addition, pharmacologic agents may prevent complications of thrombolytic therapy such as reperfusion injury, arrhythmias, reinfarction or thrombus formation.

ACUTE THERAPY TO LIMIT INFARCT SIZE

Although reperfusion therapy reduces infarct size, its effectiveness is time-dependent with the greatest benefit occurring within the first four hours of symptom onset.[3,4] Theoretically, pharmacologic agents which reduce myocardial oxygen demand or improve collateral blood flow might widen the window of opportunity for administration of thrombolytic drugs. In addition, these agents may be effective in reducing infarct size in patients who are not candidates for thrombolytic therapy. Infarct size and early impairment of ventricular function are important determinants of prognosis in patients with AMI.[5] Numerous attempts to modify infarct size have been made over the past two decades. Although interventions that restore perfusion, reduce myocardial oxygen requirements, affect anaerobic metabolism, or blunt the effects of reperfusion injury by oxygen free radicals reduce infarct size in animals, it has been difficult to reproduce these results in humans. This is due in part to the wide variations in human heart rate, blood pressure, extent of coronary disease (including degree of occlusion and states of collateral flow), infarct size, and time of treatment, as well as difficulty in accurately measuring infarct size.

Nitrates

The use of nitroglycerin therapy may favorably alter the balance of myocardial oxygen supply and demand by a variety of mechanisms including a reduction in left ventricular end-diastolic pressure which may in turn improve subendocardial ischemia. These agents also lower afterload by decreasing peripheral vascular resistance and blood pressure which may contribute to a reduction in myocardial oxygen demand. In addition, it is thought that nitrate therapy may enhance collateral blood flow to the ischemic zone.

Intravenous nitroglycerin has been demonstrated to affect infarct size in a variety of clinical studies. Derrida et al[6] reported that IV nitroglycerin resulted in a greater reduction in ST-segment elevation and less regression of R waves compared to control patients. Furthermore, in patients with heart failure, fewer arrhythmias and enhanced survival were observed in the nitroglycerin-treated group. Bussmann et al[7] reported a decrease in infarct size as measured by CPK in the nitroglycerin-treated group. In a prospective randomized trial Becker et al[8] demonstrated that treatment with intravenous nitroglycerin for 48 hours followed by topical nitroglycerin for 72 hours enhanced myocardial perfusion on thallium scintigraphy. These benefits occurred primarily in patients who were treated with nitrates within 10 hours from symptom onset.[8,9] Jaffe et al[10] randomized 85 patients to 24 hours of nitroglycerin versus placebo. Nitroglycerin infusion was initiated at a mean of 6 hours from chest pain onset with a goal to lower blood pressure by 10% or until a maximum dose of 200 µg/min was achieved. In these patients, creatine phosphokinase (CPK) was 37% lower in the nitroglycerin treated group, but only in the subgroup of patients with inferior AMI. Jugdutt and Warnica evaluated the effect of prolonged low dose intravenous nitroglycerin compared to placebo in 310 patients with AMI.[11] Nitroglycerin was titrated to reduce mean blood pressure by 10% in normotensive patients and up to 30% in hypertensive patients, but not below a mean arterial pressure of 80 mm Hg. The infusion was maintained for 39 hours. Nitroglycerin therapy proved to be safe and resulted in a smaller infarct size as measured by lower CPK, less regional left ventricular dysfunction, better global ejection fraction, less infarct expansion (as assessed by serial two-dimensional echocardiograms), better functional status, and fewer in-hospital complications such as congestive heart failure, left ventricular thrombus and cardiogenic shock. Furthermore, in the subgroup of patients with anterior myocardial infarction, mortality was reduced in the nitroglycerin-treated group.

Yusuf et al[12] pooled the results from 10 trials of intravenous nitroglycerin and nitroprusside involving 2,000 patients with AMI. The reduction in mortality in six trials with nitroglycerin[7,9,11,13-15] (Table 1) appeared to be somewhat greater than that observed with nitroprusside. Although separately the individual trials were too small to provide a reliable estimate of the effect of treatment on mortality, collectively there was a 35% reduction in mortality in patients treated with nitrate therapy.

Intravenous nitroglycerin, when given early (within 10 hours of chest pain onset), may reduce infarct size and mortality. However, adverse effects such as hypotension and tachycardia can occur. Therefore, this drug must only be given intravenously in patients who are continuously monitored in the coronary care unit. Nitrates should not be administered to patients who are hypotensive or who are possibly volume-depleted. As outlined in Table 2, intravenous nitroglycerin is usually started at a low dose, for example 20 µg/min, and increased every 2-5 minutes until symptoms are controlled or mean arterial pressure is decreased by 10%. At that point, a continuous infusion can be maintained. However, many patients rapidly develop tolerance to the drug, and increased doses may be required. Reduction in mean arterial pressure below 80 mm Hg should be avoided. If the patient develops reflex tachycardia, intravenous fluids

Table 1. *Mortality reduction in randomized trials of intravenous nitroglycerin therapy in AMI*

| Study | Follow-up | Deaths/Number Randomized | | P value |
		Nitrate	Control	
Chiche et al[13]	hospital	3/50 (6%)	8/45 (18%)	NS
Bussman et al[7]	18 mo	4/31 (13%)	12/29 (41%)	< 0.02
Flaherty et al[9]	3 mo	11/56 (20%)	11/48 (23%)	NS
Nelson et al[14]	hospital	0/14 (0%)	0/14 (0%)	NS
Jaffe et al[10]	hospital	4/57 (7%)	2/57 (4%)	NS
Lis et al[15]	4 mo	5/64 (8%)	10/76 (13%)	NS
Jugdutt et al[11]	3 mo	24/154 (16%)	44/156 (28%)	< 0.01
Pooled data		51/426 (12%)	87/425 (20.5%)	< 0.001

Adapted from Yusuf et al[12]

Table 2. *Dosing of pharmacologic agents during acute myocardial infarction*

Drug	Dose	Contraindications
Thrombolytic Agents		
Streptokinase	1.5 MU/1 hr IV	Active or recent bleeding, stroke, surgery, severe hypertension
t-PA	100 mg/3 hr IV	
APSAC	30 U bolus IV	
Anticoagulant/Antiplatelet Agents		
Aspirin	2-5 grains po or chewed daily	Active bleeding
Heparin	5-10,000 U bolus followed by 1000 U/hr IV to maintain PTT 1.5-2 x control	
Analgesics		
Morphine	2-10 mg IV	Obtundation, hypotension, hypoventilation
Meperidine	25-50 mg IV	
Nitrates		
Nitroglycerin	20 µg/min; increase by 20 µg/min Q 5 min if blood pressure stable	Volume depletion, hypotension
ß-Blockers		
Metoprolol	5 mg IV Q 2 min x 3 then 50-100 mg po BID, as tolerated	Bradycardia/heart block, hypotension, heart failure, bronchospasm
Atenolol	5-10 mg IV, then 100 mg po QD	
Calcium Antagonists		
Diltiazem	60 mg po Q 6 h	Bradycardia/heart block, pulmonary congestion (for non-Q wave AMI

should be administered and the dose of nitrate therapy decreased. Once the patient stabilizes, one can easily switch to oral preparations by slowly withdrawing intravenous therapy.

Calcium Channel Blockers

The rationale for using calcium channel blockers to limit infarct size is based on the ability of these agents to reduce blood pressure and myocardial contractility, thus decreasing myocardial oxygen demand. Certain calcium antagonists also slow the heart rate, which can reduce myocardial oxygen demand. Furthermore, calcium antagonists may increase collateral flow to the ischemic region and prevent coronary artery spasm. Theoretically, slowing the influx of calcium into injured myocardial cells may also be important for reducing reperfusion injury.

Despite many potential benefits, no clinical evidence suggests that calcium antagonists, used as primary therapy, limit infarct size. The Nifedipine Angina Myocardial Infarction Study analyzed 105 patients with threatened AMI and 66 patients with confirmed AMI.[16] Patients were randomized to nifedipine 120 mg per day orally or placebo, with randomization occurring a mean of 4.6 hours from symptom onset. This study demonstrated that nifedipine was unable to prevent progression to myocardial infarction, which occurred in 75% in both groups, and unable to reduce infarct size. Furthermore, a disturbing trend toward an increased mortality rate was observed in patients treated with nifedipine. The Norwegian Nifedipine Trial treated AMI patients within six hours of symptom onset.[17] Patients were randomized to nifedipine 120 mg per day or placebo, and therapy was continued for six weeks. There was no difference in mortality between the two groups. The Danish Verapamil Study randomized 3500 patients to placebo or verapamil at a dose of 0.1 mg/kg IV and oral therapy at 120 mg tid for 6 months.[18] Fifteen hundred of these patients had a documented myocardial infarction. There was no difference in reinfarction or mortality at 6- or 12-month follow-up. Patients randomized to verapamil therapy, however, had a twofold increase in the incidence of second or third degree heart block. A study conducted in France randomized patients to diltiazem or placebo within six hours of symptom onset.[19] Although there was no difference in peak CPKs, serial thallium scans demonstrated smaller perfusion defects in patients who were treated with diltiazem.

Yusuf et al[2] reviewed all trials of calcium channel blockers and noted that in no study was a reduction in mortality, morbidity, or enzyme release observed. This review involved four studies with nifedipine and two with verapamil involving more than 6,000 patients. The use of nifedipine (without β-blockers) in one trial of unstable angina was associated with an increase in incidence of myocardial infarction. These data demonstrate that nifedipine and probably verapamil are not likely to result in reduction in infarct size if administered during the acute phase of myocardial infarction.

Intravenous β-Blockers

The use of intravenous β-blockade during AMI has been studied extensively.[2,20] The rationale for the use of β-blockers is based on animal studies in which injured myocytes that were exposed to a relatively high concentration of catecholamines had increased numbers of β-adrenergic receptors. Beta-blockade may counter the adverse effects of catecholamines while reducing myocardial oxygen demand by lowering heart rate, blood pressure, and myocardial contractility. Reduction in heart rate may also result in improvement in perfusion since coronary flow occurs primarily during diastole. In the canine model, β-blockade selectively improved subendocardial blood flow. Therefore, if the subendocardium is the area initially involved in ischemia or infarction, selective improvement in subendocardial flow may be beneficial. The anti-catecholamine effect of β-blockers inhibits the shift in myocardial metabolism from glucose to free fatty acids, resulting in an increase in ATP formation. Therefore, β-blocking agents have several potential beneficial effects if administered during the acute phase of myocardial infarction.

In a clinical study conducted by the First International Collaborative Study Group, intravenous timolol was administered at a mean of 3.5 hours from chest pain onset and continued intravenously for the first 24 hours, with oral timolol thereafter.[21] Patients treated with timolol experienced a reduction in myocardial ischemia and infarct size as measured by the degree of ST-segment elevation and peak CPKs.

The First International Study of Infarct Survival (ISIS-I) randomized 16,000 patients to either atenolol or placebo.[22] Atenolol 5 mg was given twice intravenously, followed by 100 mg orally every day for 7 days. Although no reduction in infarct size occurred, by 24 hours there was a 30% reduction in mortality in the atenolol group. At one week this difference was reduced to 15% (3.9% mortality in atenolol group compared to 4.6% in control group, p < 0.04). It was originally postulated that the decreased mortality was due to a reduction in malignant arrhythmias; however, most recently the ISIS investigators reported that early β-blockade might prevent early cardiac rupture.[23] Although the GISSI trial did not prospectively randomize patients to β-blockade, patients who had been receiving β-blockers for clinical reasons also had a reduced incidence of cardiac rupture.[3] Intravenous β-blockade may reduce hypercontractility of noninfarcted tissue and improve dyskinesis of the infarct zone, which may in part account for the reduction in cardiac rupture.[24]

In 1985, Yusuf et al[25] provided an overview of the randomized trials incorporating β-blockade during AMI. Data from 27 trials of intravenous β-blockade, most of which were obtained on patients treated within six hours of symptom onset, suggested that levels of cardiac enzymes were reduced by approximately 20%. This appeared to be true in patients who were treated early and was unrelated to whether the β-blocking agent possessed cardioselectivity, membrane stabilizing activity, or intrinsic sympathomimetic activity. Electrocardiographic benefits, such as preservation of the R wave and reduction in the development of Q waves, have occurred with a number of agents including atenolol, propranolol, and timolol. These data suggest that infarct size may be reduced by early intravenous β-blockade. Furthermore, pooled data from 27 randomized trials suggest that acute treatment with intravenous β-blockade may reduce in-hospital mortality by 13% (p = 0.02).[25]

A reduction in ventricular arrhythmias may be an additional beneficial effect of early intravenous β-blockade. Ryden et al[26] reported a significant reduction in ventricular fibrillation during hospitalization in their study of IV metoprolol (17/698 control patients compared to 6/697 treated patients). Norris et al[27] reported a reduction in ventricular fibrillation from 14/371 in the control group to only 2/364 in propranolol-treated patients. The antiarrhythmic properties of β-blockade as well as reduction in infarct size may explain the observed reduction in ventricular fibrillation.

Patients who may benefit from acute administration of β-blocking agents include those who present within the first six hours of symptom onset, particularly in the presence of a hyperdynamic state (elevated heart rate, blood pressure, continued chest pain). Beta-blockade should be avoided in patients with bradycardia, hypotension, congestive heart failure, and bronchospasm. Metoprolol is the most commonly used intravenous β-blocker in the United States. A dose of 5 mg every 2 minutes up to 15 mg is given intravenously followed by 50-100 mg po bid (Table 2).

In summary, although intravenous thrombolytic therapy reduces early mortality by about 30%, there is also fairly convincing evidence that intravenous β-blockade may limit infarct size and reduce mortality by approximately 15%. Beta-blocking agents may also reduce the incidence of early ventricular fibrillation. Unfortunately, due to potential side effects of β-blockers, only 50-60% of AMI patients may be eligible for treatment.[28] Pooled data on intravenous nitrates also suggests a moderate reduction in infarct size and improvement in survival. Trials of early administration of calcium antagonists have not suggested a reduction in infarct size or mortality; therefore, acute administration in the early hours of myocardial infarction is not recommended. As shown in Table 3, intravenous β-blockade and/or intravenous nitroglycerin therapy should be considered for use during the early hours of AMI. Presumably because these agents act by reducing myocardial oxygen demand while thrombolytic therapy increases blood supply, their combined use may be complementary.

IN-HOSPITAL THERAPY FOR PREVENTION OR TREATMENT OF EARLY COMPLICATIONS

In the absence of appropriate therapy, patients who survive their initial infarction may succumb to the early complications of reinfarction, stroke, or pulmonary embolism. Reinfarction or clinically apparent reocclusion is associated with a high in-hospital mortality, ranging from 17-28% compared to only 2-8% in patients without reinfarc-

Table 3. *Beneficial effects of pharmacologic agents for myocardial infarction*

Limitation of Infarct Size (Acute Phase)

Thrombolytic agents

β-blockers

Nitroglycerin

Prevention of In-Hospital Complications

β-blockers

Aspirin

Anticoagulants

Diltiazem in non-Q wave MI

Long-Term Secondary Prevention

β-blockers

Aspirin

tion.[29,30] Although thrombolytic therapy has resulted in a reduction in mortality, the frequency of recurrent ischemia and reinfarction is greatly increased compared to patients who did not receive reperfusion therapy.[31] After successful thrombolytic reperfusion, a high grade coronary stenosis remains in most cases and may be responsible for the recurrent ischemic events. Since reinfarction may be due to rethrombosis, coronary artery spasm, or an increase in myocardial oxygen demand, a variety of pharmacologic agents have been studied in this setting.

Left ventricular mural thrombi are common in patients dying of myocardial infarction. Thrombus formation is more common in patients with large anterior or apical transmural infarctions, and occurs in a dyskinetic area of the ventricle. Mural thrombi can be recognized antemortem by 2-D echocardiography and are found in one-third of patients with anterior AMI. The incidence of embolic cerebrovascular accidents ranges from 4-27% in patients with mural thrombi.[20]

Bed rest and heart failure predispose to venous thrombosis and subsequent pulmonary embolism in patients with AMI. In one autopsy study, major pulmonary emboli were present (although not always responsible for a fatal outcome) in 11% of patients dying of AMI. Several decades ago, at a time when patients with AMI were subjected to prolonged periods of bed rest, significant pulmonary embolism was found at autopsy in more than 20% of patients with AMI.

Beta-Blockers

Data on in-hospital reinfarction are available for the majority of patients enrolled in the ISIS-I trial.[22] Reinfarction occurred in 148/5900 (2.5%) atenolol-treated patients compared to 161/5923 (2.7%) patients in the control group. In the MIAMI trial, as well as other intravenous trials, a slight reduction in reinfarction was observed in patients treated with β-blockade. Overall, these data suggest a slight reduction of about 16% ± 7% in the odds of in-hospital reinfarction with the use of intravenous β-blockers.[25]

Until recently, there was limited data to support the combined use of β-blockers and thrombolytic drugs. The TIMI Phase II trial treated 3262 patients with intravenous tissue plasminogen activator.[28] A subgroup of 1390 patients were eligible for intravenous β-blockade and were randomized to receive either 15 mg of intravenous metoprolol followed by oral metoprolol, or to late treatment with oral metoprolol begun on day six. In-hospital and six-week mortality and left ventricular function were identical in the two groups. However, the incidence of reinfarction and recurrent ischemia was reduced in patients treated with early intravenous β-blockade. Paradoxically, the six-week mortality was reduced only in low-risk subgroups and was slightly increased in higher risk subgroups. According to the TIMI investigators, intravenous metoprolol was of value only in uncomplicated, first inferior infarcts or in younger patients. This is in contradistinction to other trials in which higher risk patients appeared to benefit most from pharmacologic interventions. Therefore, the precise role of β-blockade in the prevention of early reinfarction remains controversial.

Calcium Channel Blockers

In the Danish verapamil trial, 1400 patients were randomized to either placebo or verapamil therapy, initially intravenously followed by 360 mg per day orally.[18] Thirty percent of patients who were randomized to verapamil withdrew because of side effects including heart block and congestive heart failure. No difference in the frequency of reinfarction between the two groups was observed.

Four thousand patients were studied in the Trial of Reinfarction with Early Nifedipine Therapy (TRENT).[32] There was no significant difference in mortality between those assigned to nifedipine (10%) and those assigned to placebo (9.2%). The Holland Inter-University Nifedipine/Metoprolol Trial (HINT)[33] randomized patients with unstable angina or suspected AMI to nifedipine or metoprolol. When nifedipine was compared to the combination of nifedipine and metoprolol, nifedipine alone increased risk of myocardial infarction.

Since patients with non-Q wave myocardial infarction have a greatly increased risk of reinfarction, Gibson et al[34] studied 576 patients with non-Q wave AMI. These patients were randomized to either diltiazem 90 mg every 6 hours or placebo and followed closely for 14 days. The diltiazem-treated group experienced a 50% reduction in recurrent myocardial infarction (5.2% in the diltiazem group compared to 9.3% in the control group). In addition, there was a 50% reduction in post-AMI angina. Therefore, it appeared that diltiazem was effective at preventing recurrent angina and early reinfarction in patients with non-Q wave AMI.

The Multicenter Diltiazem Postinfarction Trial[35] randomized 2600 patients with Q wave and non-Q wave myocardial infarction to placebo or diltiazem 240 mg/day and followed all patients for one year. Overall, diltiazem did not have a beneficial effect in the patients studied. Moreover, in the subgroup with evidence of pulmonary congestion on chest x-ray prior to randomization (20% of the population), there was an increase in mortality in diltiazem-treated patients. In patients with no evidence of congestive heart failure (approximately 80%) and who received diltiazem, decreased morbidity and mortality was apparent in both Q wave and non-Q wave infarctions.

In conclusion, diltiazem is the only calcium channel blocker shown to decrease the incidence of reinfarction when given during the hospital phase of therapy for non-Q wave infarctions. However, diltiazem given during the hospital phase of therapy is detrimental in AMI patients with evidence of congestive heart failure but may be cardioprotective in patients with no evidence of heart failure. Verapamil and nifedipine have not been shown to decrease morbidity or mortality compared to placebo. Therefore, when considering the use of a calcium channel blocker during non-Q wave AMI, diltiazem is the drug of choice. Since reinfarction frequently occurs within the first few hospital days in these patients, oral diltiazem therapy should be initiated early. However, its use should be avoided in patients with second or third degree heart block, heart rates less than 50, or pulmonary congestion on chest x-ray.

Anticoagulation

Many clinical studies performed over the past decade have examined the role of full dose anticoagulation (heparin and warfarin) after AMI. Until recently, no clinical evidence has supported the use of these agents as primary interventional therapy to reduce infarct size, salvage myocardium, or improve survival.[36] However, these agents have clearly reduced or prevented the morbidity and mortality associated with thromboembolic complications of AMI.

Heparin Therapy

Clinical studies have indicated that low dose heparin (5,000 units subcutaneously every 8-12 hours) may prevent the development of deep venous thrombosis. Three randomized clinical trials have demonstrated that low dose heparin reduces the incidence of deep venous thrombosis in AMI patients from 23% to 4% without an increased risk of bleeding complications.[37-39] Mini-dose heparin therapy was started within 12 hours of the onset of symptoms and continued for approximately 10 days.

Left ventricular mural thrombus formation usually occurs within the first five days after AMI. Most systemic emboli occur within the first three months after AMI in patients with a mural thrombus, and the risk of embolization appears to be greater if the thrombus is mobile and protrudes into the left ventricular cavity. Most thrombi appear to resolve or organize within three months, at which time their potential for embolization decreases.[40] In studies that have examined patients with documented mural thrombi, anticoagulant therapy reduced the overall incidence of systemic emboli from 5% to less than 1%.[41] Recent studies have demonstrated that high doses of subcutaneous heparin (12,500 units q 12h) were effective in preventing left ventricular mural thrombus formation in patients with acute anterior wall MI, with a very low incidence of bleeding complications.[42]

Many clinicians believe that heparin is essential for prevention of coronary reocclusion after successful thrombolytic therapy. This belief is based on the premise that a high grade stenosis with residual thrombus remains in the majority of patients after thrombolytic therapy. The fact that approximately 20% of vessels opened by thrombolytic therapy demonstrated early reocclusion led to a number of investigations to determine the optimal approach for prevention of reocclusion. In patients with unstable angina, heparin has been shown to be beneficial at reducing chest pain and preventing progression to myocardial infarction.[43,44] Therefore, it was thought that heparin might prevent recurrent ischemic events after the acute phase of myocardial infarction.

Fuster and Chesebro have reviewed the use of antithrombotic therapy during AMI.[45] A meta-analysis of six randomized trials found that the in-hospital use of anticoagulants reduced early mortality and reinfarction when compared to placebo. The SCATI trial recently randomized 711 patients with AMI to receive high dose subcutaneous heparin or no heparin, regardless of whether they received thrombolytic therapy.[42] In patients who received streptokinase, transient ischemic episodes were reduced in the heparin group (14.2%) compared with patients not receiving heparin (19.6%). Preliminary data also suggest that reocclusion and recurrent ischemia after tissue plasminogen activator are greatly increased in the absence of heparin.[46] The International t-PA/Streptokinase Mortality Trial and its constituent Italian GISSI-2 study randomized 20,000 patients to receive either t-PA or streptokinase with a second randomization to heparin (12,500 U subcutaneous twice daily starting 12 hours after thrombolytic therapy) or no heparin therapy.[47,48] Streptokinase and t-PA appeared to be equally effective in preventing in-hospital death. Heparin had no effect on survival, incidence of stroke, or other clinical events, but did result in a slight increase in the incidence of major bleeding complications. The use of delayed subcutaneous heparin has led some physicians to question whether the results of this study are relevant to the management of AMI patients in the United States where early intravenous heparin is used frequently. Therefore, the timing, route of administration, the duration, or even the need for heparin after thrombolytic therapy remains controversial.

On the basis of these studies, our approach to anticoagulant therapy after AMI is as follows: in the absence of active bleeding, all patients receive mini-dose heparin (5,000 units subcutaneously q 12h) until ambulatory. Patients who have been treated with thrombolytic therapy or angioplasty for AMI are routinely treated with intravenous heparin for 5-7 days, adjusted to maintain the PTT at 1.5-2 times control. We administer heparin immediately in patients who receive t-PA therapy, but delay therapy for 6-24 hours in patients who have been treated with systemic fibrinolytic agents such as streptokinase or APSAC. To prevent thromboembolic complications, high dose intravenous heparin is also routinely utilized in patients with large anterior infarctions, atrial fibrillation, history of previous emboli, or severe congestive heart failure. In patients with mural thrombus documented by 2-D echocardiography, heparin is followed by warfarin therapy for 3-6 months, adjusted to maintain the prothrombin time 1.5 times normal. At the end of six months, the mural thrombus has usually resolved or become laminated and endothelialized, allowing safe discontinuation of warfarin. In patients at lower or average risk, aspirin is given and continued after heparin is stopped (see below).

Antiplatelet Therapy

Like anticoagulants, antiplatelet agents have been extensively studied in AMI patients. Several placebo-controlled trials, the majority of which enrolled patients several weeks after AMI, have been performed to determine the efficacy of antiplatelet agents in secondary prevention.[49] Studies performed during the acute ischemic phase have been limited. Two randomized, placebo-controlled clinical trials have demonstrated that aspirin administered to patients with unstable angina reduces the incidence of progression to myocardial infarction and death by 50%.[50,51] The dose of aspirin used in these trials ranged from 324 mg per day to 324 mg qid. Aspirin is clearly effective in preventing mortality and morbidity associated with progression of unstable angina to AMI.

The ISIS-II trial enrolled 17,000 patients with suspected myocardial infarction and randomized them to either placebo, aspirin alone, streptokinase alone, or streptokinase plus aspirin.[4] Aspirin was given within 24 hours of chest pain onset, administered as a 160 mg dose chewed immediately and continued for four weeks. When compared to placebo, the aspirin group had a decreased mortality at five weeks. The combination of streptokinase and aspirin was associated with fewer reinfarctions (1.8% vs. 2.9%), strokes (0.6% vs. 1.1%), and deaths (8% vs. 13.2%) compared to placebo. This difference remained significant after a median of 15 months follow-up. Therefore, unless a contraindication exists, our approach is to administer 5 grains of chewable aspirin immediately, followed by 5 grains of oral aspirin each day continued indefinitely in all AMI patients.

Pharmacologic Management of Heart Failure

Following AMI, prognosis is related directly to the degree of left ventricular dysfunction.[5] Treatment for left ventricular dysfunction is therefore quite important. In the setting of acute pulmonary edema, diuretic therapy is clearly indicated. A low dose (eg, 20 mg furosemide IV) should be given and its effects monitored over the next several minutes. If a Swan-Ganz catheter is in place, a pulmonary capillary wedge pressure of less than 20 mm Hg is desirable. Vasodilators such as intravenous nitroglycerin or nitroprusside decrease the pulmonary capillary wedge pressure, decrease afterload, and improve the cardiac output; therefore, they are effective in the management of heart failure. Beta-adrenergic agonists such as dobutamine should be initiated only if a high pulmonary capillary wedge pressure in association with a very low cardiac output is documented. The usual dose of dobutamine is 5 µg/kg/min initially, increasing to 20 µg/kg/min as necessary. In order to determine appropriate treatment, hemodynamic monitoring including Swan-Ganz catheterization and arterial line placement is mandatory. Frequently, patients with volume depletion present with hypotension, and without hemodynamic monitoring they might be inappropriately managed as "cardiogenic shock."

Ongoing clinical trials are investigating the possibility that early treatment of left ventricular dysfunction might improve prognosis after AMI. However, the results of these trials are not yet available. Two clinical trials, not involving AMI patients, have demonstrated that vasodilators may have a beneficial effect. In patients with chronic congestive heart failure, The Veterans Administration Cooperative Trial demonstrated improvement in survival with the use of a combination of hydralazine and nitrates.[52] The following year the CONSENSUS trial demonstrated that treatment with the angiotensin-converting enzyme (ACE) inhibitor, enalapril, prolongs survival in patients with severe congestive heart failure.[53]

The use of ACE inhibitors in asymptomatic patients after AMI was assessed by Pfeffer et al[54] in a pilot study of anterior AMI with depressed left ventricular function. In this randomized, placebo-controlled trial, captopril therapy produced a significant reduction in left ventricular end-diastolic pressure and mean pulmonary artery pressure, and prevented a late increase in left ventricular end-diastolic volume.

In summary, management of a patient with congestive heart failure in the early infarction period should include oxygen, diuretics and vasodilators, specifically intravenous nitroglycerin. Beta-adrenergic agonists such as dobutamine should be reserved for patients with a very low cardiac output in the absence of a high systemic vascular resistance. Later during hospitalization, ACE inhibitors and nitrate/hydralazine combinations may be useful since they have been shown to prolong survival in patients with chronic congestive heart failure. Although initial results using prophylactic ACE inhibitors after AMI are encouraging, their exact role is still undetermined.

SUMMARY

Effective alternative therapy is available for patients in whom thrombolytic therapy is contraindicated. Furthermore, conventional medical therapy may have added beneficial effects when used concomitantly with thrombolytic drugs. All patients with AMI should be considered for immediate thrombolytic therapy, IV nitroglycerin, and IV β-blockade to reduce infarct size. To prevent in-hospital complications (arrhythmias, reinfarction and thromboembolic events), therapy with β-blockers, aspirin, anticoagulants, and in selected patients, diltiazem should be considered. This intensive pharmacologic approach should result in major reductions in morbidity and mortality after AMI.

REFERENCES

1. Grines CL, DeMaria AN: Optimal utilization of thrombolytic therapy for acute myocardial infarction: Concepts and controversies. J Am Coll Cardiol 1990;16:223-231

2. Yusuf S: The use of beta-adrenergic blocking agents, IV nitrates and calcium channel blocking agents following acute myocardial infarction. Chest 1988;93:25S-28S.

3. Gruppo Italiana per lo Studio della Streptochinasi nell'Infarto Miocardico (GISSI): Effectiveness of intravenous thrombolytic treatment in acute myocardial infarction. Lancet 1986;i:349-360.

4. ISIS-2 (Second International Study of Infarct Survival) Collaborative Group: Randomised trial of intravenous streptokinase, oral aspirin, both, or neither among 17,187 cases of suspected acute myocardial infarction: ISIS-2. Lancet 1988;II:349-360.

5. Multicenter Post-Infarction Research Group: Risk stratification after myocardial infarction. N Engl J Med 1983;309:331-336.

6. Derrida JP, Sal R, Chiche P: Favorable effects of prolonged nitroglycerin infusion in patients with acute myocardial infarction. Am Heart J 1978;96:833.

7. Bussmann WD, Passek D, Seidel W, et al: Reduction of CK and CK-MB indexes of infarct size by intravenous nitroglycerin. Circulation 1981;63:615-622.

8. Becker LC, Bulkley BH, Pitt B: Enhanced reduction of thallium 201 defects in acute myocardial infarction by nitroglycerin treatment: Results of a prospective randomized trial. Clin Res 1978;26:219A.

9. Flaherty JT, Becker LC, Bulkley BH, et al: A randomized prospective trial of IV nitroglycerin in patients with acute myocardial infarction. Circulation 1983;68:576-688.

10. Jaffe AS, Geltman EM, Tiefenbrunn AJ, et al: Reduction of infarct size in patients with inferior infarction with IV glyceryl trinitrate. A randomized study. Br Heart J 1983;49:452-460.

11. Jugdutt BI, Warnica JW: Intravenous nitroglycerin therapy to limit myocardial infarct size, expansion, and complications. Effect of timing, dosage and infarct location. Circulation 1988;78:906-919.

12. Yusuf S, Collins R, MacMahon S, et al: Effect of intravenous nitrates on mortality in acute myocardial infarction: An overview of the randomised trials. Lancet 1988;1:1088-1092.

13. Chiche P, Baligadoo SJ, Derrida JP: A randomized trial of prolonged nitroglycerin infusion in acute myocardial infarction. Circulation 1979;59,60(II):II-165 (abstract).

14. Nelson GIC, Silke B, Ahuja RC, et al: Haemodynamic advantages of isosorbide dinitrate over furosemide in acute heart-failure following myocardial infarction. Lancet 1983;1:730-733.

15. Lis Y, Bennett D, Lambert G, et al: A preliminary double-blind study of IV nitroglycerin in acute myocardial infarction. Intensive Care Med 1984;10:179-184.

16. Muller JE, Morrison J, Stone PH, et al: Nifedipine therapy for patients with threatened and acute myocardial infarction: A randomized, double-blind, placebo-controlled comparison. Circulation 1984;69:740-747.

17. Sirnes PA, Overskeid K, Pedersen TR, et al: Evolution of infarct size during the early use of nifedipine in patients with acute myocardial infarction: The Norwegian Nifedipine Multicenter Trial. Circulation 1984;70:638-644.

18. The Danish Study Group on Verapamil in Myocardial Infarction: Verapamil in acute myocardial infarction. Eur Heart J 1984;5:516-528.

19. Zannad F, Amor M, Karcher G, et al: Effect of diltiazem on myocardial infarct size estimated by enzyme release, serial thallium-201 single-photon emission computed tomography and radionuclide angiography. Am J Cardiol 1988;61:1172-1177.

20. Pasternak RC, Braunwald E, Sobel BE: Acute myocardial infarction, in Braunwald E (ed), *A Textbook of Cardiovascular Medicine.* Philadelphia, WB Saunders Co., 1988, p 1222.

21. The International Collaborative Group: Reduction of infarct size with the early use of timolol in acute myocardial infarction. N Engl J Med 1984;310:9.

22. ISIS-1 (First International Study of Infarct Survival) Collaborative Group: Randomized trial of intravenous atenolol among 16,027 cases of suspected acute myocardial infarction: ISIS-1. Lancet 1986;2:57-66.

23. ISIS-1 (First International Study of Infarct Survival) Collaborative Group: Mechanisms for the early mortality reduction produced by beta-blockade started early in acute myocardial infarction. Lancet 1988;1:921-923.

24. Grines CL, Booth DC, Gash DL, et al: Effects of parenteral beta-blockade on infarct and noninfarct zone function following successful reperfusion in man. Circulation 1989;80: II-114 (abstract).

25. Yusuf S, Peto R, Lewis J, et al: Beta blockade during and after myocardial infarction: An overview of the randomized trials. Prog Cardiovasc Dis 1985;27:335-371.

26. Ryden L, Arniego R, Arman K, et al: A double blind trial of metoprolol in acute myocardial infarction: Effects on ventricular tachycardia. N Engl J Med 1983;308:614-618.

27. Norris RM, Brown MA, Clarke ED, et al: Prevention of ventricular fibrillation during acute myocardial infarction by intravenous propranolol. Lancet 1984;2:883-886.

28. The TIMI Study Group: Comparison of invasive and conservative strategies after treatment with intravenous tissue plasminogen activator in acute myocardial infarction. Results of the Thrombolysis In Myocardial Infarction (TIMI) Phase II Trial. N Engl J Med 1989;320:18-27.

29. Marmor A, Sobel BE, Roberts R: Factors presaging early recurrent myocardial infarction ("extension"). Am J Cardiol 1981;48:603-610.

30. Theroux P, Bosch X, Pelletier GB, et al: Clinical importance of early ischemia after acute myocardial infarction (AMI). J Am Coll Cardiol 1986;7:66A.

31. Schaer DH, Ross AM, Wasserman AG: Reinfarction, recurrent angina, and reocclusion after thrombolytic therapy. Circulation 1987;76:II-57-II-62.

32. Wilcox RG, Hampton JR, Banks DC, et al: Trial of early nifedipine treatment in patients with suspected myocardial infarction (the TRENT study). Br Heart J (Clin Res) 1986;55 :506.

33. Holland Interuniversity Nifedipine/Metoprolol Trial (HINT) Research Group: Early treatment of unstable angina in the coronary care unit: A randomized, double blind, placebo controlled comparison of recurrent ischemia in patients treated with nifedipine or metoprolol or both. Br Heart J 1986;56:400-413.

34. Gibson RS, Boden WE, Theroux P, et al: Diltiazem and reinfarction in patients with non-Q-wave myocardial infarction. N Engl J Med 1986;315:423-429.

35. The Multicenter Diltiazem Postinfarction Trial Research Group: The effect of diltiazem on mortality and reinfarction after myocardial infarction. N Engl J Med 1988;319:385-392.

36. Chalmers TC, Matta RJ, Smith H Jr, et al: Evidence favoring the use of anticoagulants in the hospital phase of acute myocardial infarction. N Engl J Med 1977;297:1091-1096.

37. Handley AJ: Low-dose heparin after myocardial infarction. Lancet 1972;2:623-624.

38. Wray R, Maurer B, Shillingford J: Prophylactic anticoagulant therapy in the prevention of calf-vein thrombosis after myocardial infarction. N Engl J Med 1973;288:815-817.

39. Handley AJ, Emerson PA, Fleming PR: Heparin in the prevention of deep vein thrombosis after myocardial infarction. Br Med J 1972;2:436-438.

40. Reutyak GE, O'Rourke RA: Acute myocardial infarction: Current concepts of pathophysiology and therapy. Baylor Cardiology Series 1987;10(4):5-26.

41. Handshoe R, Nissen S, Smith MD, et al: Mural thrombi: Role of two-dimensional echocardiography in diagnosis and management. Cardiovasc Rev Rep 1986;7:183-196.

42. The SCATI (Studio sulla Calciparina nell'Angina e nella Trombosi Ventricolare nell'Infarto) Group: Randomised controlled trial of subsctaneous calcium-heparin in acute myocardial infarction. Lancet 1989;1:182-186.

43. Telford AM, Wilson C: Trial of heparin versus atenolol in prevention of myocardial infarction in intermediate coronary syndrome. Lancet 1981;1:1225-1228.

44. Theroux P, Ouimet H, McCans J, et al: Aspirin, heparin or both to treat acute unstable angina. N Engl J Med 1988;319:1105-1111.

45. Fuster V, Chesebro J: Antithrombotic and lipid lowering therapy in follow-up for acute myocardial infarction. Choices Cardiol 1989;3(2):10-12.

46. Ross AM, Hsia J, Hamilton W, et al: Heparin versus aspirin after recombinant tissue plasminogen activator therapy in myocardial infarction: A randomized trial. J Am Coll Cardiol 1990;15:64A (abstract).

47. GISSI-2: A factorial randomised trial of alteplase versus streptokinase and heparin versus no heparin among 12490 patients with acute myocardial infarction. Lancet 1990;336:65-71.

48. The International Study Group: In-hospital mortality and clinical course of 20891 patients with suspected acute myocardial infarction randomised between alteplase and streptokinase with or without heparin. Lancet 1990;336:71-75.

49. Friedewald WT, Furberg CD, May GS: Aspirin and myocardial infarction. Cardiovasc Rev Rep 1984;5:1285-1289.

50. Lewis HD Jr, Davis JW, Archibald DG, et al: Protective effects of aspirin against acute myocardial infarction and death in men with unstable angina: Results of a Veterans Administration cooperative study. N Engl J Med 1983;309:396-403.

51. Cairns JA, Gent M, Singer J. et al: Aspirin, sulfinpyrazone, or both in unstable angina. N Engl J Med 1985;313:1369-1375.

52. Cohn JN, Archibald DG, Tresche S: Effect of vasodilator therapy on mortality in chronic congestive heart failure. Results of a Veterans Administration cooperative study. N Engl J Med 1986;314:1547.

53. CONSENSUS Trial Study Group: Effects of enalapril on mortality in severe congestive heart failure. Results of the Cooperative North Scandinavian Enalapril Survival Study (CONSENSUS). N Engl J Med 1987;316:1429-1435.

54. Pfeffer MA, Lamas GA, Vaughn PE, et al: Effect of captopril on progressive ventricular dilation after anterior MI. N Engl J Med 1988;319:80-86.

THROMBOLYTIC AGENTS

Section III

Chapter 8

BLOOD AND VASCULAR EFFECTS OF THROMBOLYTIC AGENTS

Victor J. Marder

INTRODUCTION

Thrombolytic therapy regularly induces striking changes in blood coagulation. Despite unique biochemical properties, dose requirements and temporal distinctions in hemostatic response for streptokinase (SK), urokinase (UK), single chain urokinase (pro-urokinase, scu-PA), tissue plasminogen activator (rt-PA), and acylated plasminogen streptokinase activator complex (APSAC), all of these plasminogen activators result in generally similar changes in laboratory assays of coagulation, platelet, and fibrinolytic activities.[1] Furthermore, vascular and clinical effects also appear to be equivalent, justifying attention to the general implications of in vitro tests for thrombolytic therapy. This report summarizes the implications of blood fibrinolytic assay results on the clinical manifestations of bleeding and on the vascular effects of reperfusion and reocclusion.

Changes in Coagulation Status During Thrombolytic Therapy

The coagulation status of the blood resulting from thrombolytic treatment can be arbitrarily divided into three overlapping phases of variable duration but distinct hemostatic potential (Table 1). Initial exposure of blood to fibrinolytic agents is associated with alterations that suggest an activated state, due either to direct action of the plasminogen activator or to indirect effects of plasmin formation or thrombin exposure. The characteristic findings include an exaggerated response of platelets to agonists[2] and evidence of fibrinogen to fibrin conversion reflected by increased blood fibrinopeptide concentration.[3] Both effects are transient and dissipate after a short interval of perhaps 15-60 minutes. The implications of these hypercoagulable changes relate mostly to the potential for vascular reocclusion that may follow successful

Table 1. *Changes in coagulation status during and after thrombolytic treatment*

Treatment		Characteristic laboratory values	Potential hemostatic effect
Phase	Duration		
Early	First 15-60 minutes	Increased platelet reactivity Fibrinopeptide cleavage	Hypercoagulable
Sustained (during and immediately after treatment)	4-8 hours	Rapid lysis time Decreased plasma fibrinogen Impaired platelet aggregation and long bleeding time	Hypocoagulable
Recovery	24-36 hours	Normalization of lysis time, fibrinogen, platelet function, and bleeding time	Return to pre-treatment state

reperfusion, an event that occurs in up to 20% of patients with acute myocardial infarction.[1]

The early hypercoagulable state is usually supplanted by a more dominant and longer-lasting hypocoagulable state during the remainder of the fibrinolytic infusion and for variable intervals following treatment. Aspects of laboratory measurements may reflect both the hyper- and the hypocoagulable states at the same time in a given patient, and the degree and duration of such changes will necessarily depend upon the type of activator, dosage and duration of infusion. The half-life of each activator varies considerably from about 5 minutes for rt-PA to more than 60 minutes for APSAC. This property dictates the length of time that an infusion is needed to induce thrombolysis and also controls the rate of clearance of activator after the infusion is stopped. Still, the overall duration of this second ("sustained") phase is roughly the same for all activators, about 4-8 hours. The characteristic changes are a rapid lysis time (secondary to the presence of activator in blood), a decrease in plasma fibrinogen (secondary to plasmin degradation), and impaired platelet aggregation and prolongation of the bleeding time (secondary to several factors, including plasma fibrinogen and platelet membrane receptor degradation).[4,5] The plasma "lytic state"[6] has relevance primarily for its potential contribution to bleeding complications.

Once plasminogen activator is cleared from the circulation, a progressive recovery of deranged coagulation and fibrinolytic components to pre-treatment status follows. This 24-36 hour duration depends on physiologic responses of marrow hemopoiesis and hepatic protein synthesis to regenerate intact platelets and fibrinogen, respectively. These recovery processes are largely independent of the type of activator used for therapy. The potential clinical consequence of this recovery to normal blood hemostatic function relates mostly to a risk of hemorrhage in the post-treatment period in association with vascular injury, for example, during coronary artery bypass graft surgery or angioplasty. The blood and vascular effects of plasminogen activator infusion are illustrated in Figure 1.

RELEVANCE OF LABORATORY CHANGES FOR BLEEDING AND FOR REPERFUSION/REOCCLUSION

Bleeding Complications

The relevance of laboratory changes has been studied most extensively for possible association with bleeding complications. Several lines of evidence suggest that changes in coagulation and/or fibrinolytic values are not useful in predicting bleeding events. First, most hemorrhage occurs in regions of vascular injury, for example at sites of femoral artery catheterization for coronary angiography. Such observations reinforce the concept that vascular injury rather than hemostatic changes causes hemorrhage during fibrinolytic therapy, regardless of the agent utilized. Second, a comparison of nadir fibrinogen concentrations in patients with or without bleeding shows no correlation after streptokinase[7,8] and only a weak correlation of marginal biologic significance after rt-PA.[8] Notable are those patients with a low fibrinogen who do not bleed and those a with relatively high fibrinogen value who do bleed, indicating that individual laboratory determinations are not predictive for bleeding in a given patient. The TAMI-1 data[9] for rt-PA also show that the decrease and nadir fibrinogen values are marginally different and the peak concentration of degradation products is not statistically or biologically different in patients with or without major non-surgical bleeding. Interestingly, a higher concentration of rt-PA antigen occurs in patients who do bleed, compatible with a dose-response relationship of this activator on hemostatic plugs. A rationale exists to suggest that surgery would be safer after completion of rt-PA than after SK, since fibrinogen falls less strikingly during treatment with the former and rt-PA disappears more quickly from the blood than does SK. Evidence

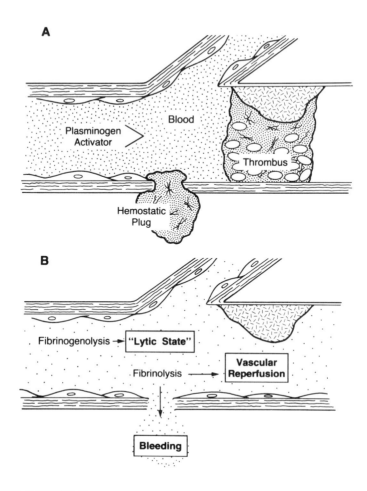

Figure 1. *Schematic illustration of the three principal sites of action of plasminogen activators. Upon degradation of fibrin and disintegration of platelet aggregates, the thrombus fragments and progressively diminishes until the vessel is reperfused. Lysis of hemostatic plugs occurs concomitantly with lysis of the thrombus, inducing a bleeding risk through the now patent vessel. The major plasma substrate of plasmin is fibrinogen, the pathologic result being a hypocoagulable plasma ("lytic state") manifest, for example, by a decrease in fibrinogen concentration. This defective hemostatic condition may be beneficial, by impeding vascular rethrombosis, or harmful, by exaggerating the severity of bleeding from sites of hemostatic plug disintegration. Rethrombosis can occur at the site of original thrombus formation, through a combination of local forces (plaque exposure, thrombus-associated thrombin, flow disturbances) and systemic changes of hypercoagulability. This figure is reproduced with permission from Marder VJ, Sherry S: Thrombolytic therapy: current status. New Engl J Med 1988;318:1512-1520.*

suggests that bleeding occurs after both agents. In the TIMI-IIA study,[10] a greater proportion of patients who had angioplasty immediately after receiving rt-PA needed transfusion than did those who had angioplasty one or two days later. This time-dependent recovery of normal hemostasis after rt-PA treatment parallels that occurring after SK therapy, in which surgery performed soon after treatment produced bleeding complications.[11] Direct comparisons of agents under these circumstances have not yet been reported.

Third, the TIMI-I comparison of rt-PA with SK[8] shows that the mean fibrinogen concentration itself does not predict bleeding. Fibrinogen fell to below 100 mg/dL in 30% of patients receiving SK, as opposed to only 3% of patients receiving rt-PA. Yet, the incidence of bleeding, whether overall (33% vs. 31%) or major (15% vs. 16%) was identical for rt-PA and SK. Additionally, the incidence of severe bleeding complications in large mortality trials[12-14] with few invasive procedures is similar using SK, rt-PA and APSAC: 0.6-2.0% in treated patients versus 0.3-1.8% of controls, despite differences in plasma fibrinogen concentration induced by each agent.

Recent interest in platelet function as a predictor of bleeding has utilized the bleeding time in patients treated with rt-PA.[15] The mean bleeding time was prolonged from 6 to 9 minutes at 90 minutes after the start of rt-PA treatment, and most of the patients who did not bleed had shorter values than the nine minute mean bleeding time, while half of those with spontaneous bleeding had prolonged bleeding times. Still, individual bleeding time values do not allow accurate prediction of bleeding in the individual patient, since three patients with excessive prolongations of 15 minutes or longer did not have bleeding complications. More studies are needed to evaluate the bleeding time, especially in studies comparing different plasminogen activators.

Reperfusion/Reocclusion

Correlation of laboratory change with thrombolysis also has been generally unimpressive. Laboratory evidence of a lytic state appears to coincide with, and perhaps be necessary in order to achieve, successful coronary artery reperfusion.[16] A minimal dose for UK,[17] rt-PA,[18] and APSAC[19] probably exists as well, below which insufficient thrombolysis is attained. While such subtherapeutic dosages may well induce minimal or non-detectable changes in plasma fibrinogen, dosages of any of the plasminogen activators which produce consistent vascular reperfusion appear also to produce the lytic state, even with the use of relatively "fibrin specific" agents such as rt-PA.[20]

At these "therapeutic" dosages, almost all patients have some degree of lytic state demonstrable. However, just as for bleeding complications, a weak or no correlation exists between the extent of the lytic state and the extent of clot dissolution. This lack of correlation has been noted for deep vein thrombosis using SK,[7] pulmonary embolism using UK,[21] and coronary artery thrombosis using rt-PA.[9] The latter study failed to show any biologically important distinction in initial fibrinogen concentration, drop in plasma fibrinogen, nadir fibrinogen concentration or fibrinogen degradation product concentration in patients with or without successful reperfusion.

The explanation for this lack of correlation between clot lysis and changes in blood coagulation is to be found in the thrombus structure itself. Factors such as platelet content, concentration of fibrin-bound inhibitors and degree of fibrin polymer chain crosslinking,[22] can certainly contribute to the resistance or vulnerability of a thrombus to fibrinolytic agents. This thrombus-oriented view of successful reperfusion considers quantitative changes in the blood as a related but independent reaction, just as the reaction occurring in the hemostatic plug is independent of quantitative blood changes (Figure 1).[23]

Contrary to the apparently independent reactions controlling the degree of the lytic state, vascular reperfusion, and clinical bleeding, the reocclusion phenomenon may be directly influenced by blood changes. First, the TAMI-1 results indicate that the change in fibrinogen concentration (from pre-treatment levels to nadir) negatively correlates with reocclusion, the lower rates associated with greater drops in fibrinogen and with higher concentrations of degradation products.[9] Second, an analysis of fibrinogen concentration in patients with coronary artery reocclusion after rt-PA[24] administration suggests that a lower fibrinogen concentration is associated with a lower reocclusion rate. Third, reocclusion is more common with rt-PA than with SK,[25] perhaps in part related to the more profound hypocoagulable state induced by SK. That this correlation is not due to a straightforward coagulation defect is suggested by the inability of heparin to prevent post-rt-PA reocclusion[26] and by the striking effect of antiplatelet agents such as aspirin to reduce reinfarction after SK treatment of myocardial infarction[14] or by monoclonal antibody again glycoprotein IIb/IIIa to keep experimental models of reperfused coronary arteries patent after rt-PA.[27] A summary of the clinical relevance of blood coagulation tests during thrombolytic treatment is shown in Table 2.

SUMMARY

Changes in laboratory reflections of thrombolytic treatment occur in almost every patient treated with therapeutic dosages of any of the currently available plasminogen activators. These changes vary in degree according to the activator utilized, but individual and even mean values are poorly predictive of bleeding complications or successful thrombolysis. Bleeding is associated with prior vascular injury, and susceptibility to thrombolysis depends greatly on thrombus architecture, accessibility and structure. Vascular reocclusion/reinfarction may correlate with the degree of fibrinogen decrease, the latter hypocoagulable state perhaps inhibiting local vascular conditions that predispose to thrombosis.[28]

144

Table 2. *Clinical relevance of blood coagulation tests during thrombolytic therapy*

Effect in the blood	Hemorrhagic complications	Therapeutic thrombolysis	Reocclusion/ reinfarction
Standard treatment:			
High-dose streptokinase causes a 20 to 80% drop in plasma fibrinogen in > 90% of patients.	Bleeding does not correlate with fibrinogen concentration.	No biologically-important correlation with fibrinogen.	Residual risk reduced by half with aspirin.
Fibrin-specific agents:			
t-PA regularly causes a drop in fibrinogen, less than with streptokinase.	Equal bleeding risk for t-PA as for streptokinase.	Greater thrombolysis with "older" thrombi, equal for fresh clots (< 3 hours).	Higher rate than with SK.
Third-generation:			
New activators with greater fibrin specificity may spare plasma fibrinogen.	Hemostatic plugs should still be vulnerable to lysis.	Theoretically possible without lytic state.	Expectation for high rate, requiring adjunct anti-thrombotic treatment.
Regional infusion:			
High local concentration and relatively small effect in the blood.	Even minimal effects in the blood associated with bleeding.	Higher rates of reperfusion possible.	Still may occur without adjunct antithrombotic treatment.

REFERENCES

1. Marder VJ, Sherry S: Thrombolytic therapy: Current status. New Engl J Med 1988;318: 1512-1520.

2. Fitzgerald DJ, Catella F, Roy L, FitzGerald GA: Marked platelet activation in vivo after intravenous streptokinase in patients with acute myocardial infarction. Circulation 1988; 77:142-150.

3. Eisenberg PR, Sherman LA, Jaffe AS: Paradoxic elevation of fibrinopeptide A after streptokinase: evidence for continued thrombosis despite intense fibrinolysis. J Am Coll Cardiol 1987;10:527-529.

4. Owen J, Friedman KD, Grossman BA, et al: Quantitation of fragment X formation during thrombolytic therapy with streptokinase and tissue plasminogen activator. J Clin Invest 1987;79:1642-1647.

5. Loscalzo J, Vaughan DE: Tissue plasminogen activator promotes platelet disaggregation in plasma. J Clin Invest 1987;79:1749-1755.

6. Alkjaersig N, Fletcher AP, Sherry S: The mechanism of clot dissolution by plasmin. J Clin Invest 1959;38:1086-1095.

7. Marder VJ, Soulen RL, Atichartakarn V, et al: Quantitative venographic assessment of deep vein thrombosis in the evaluation of streptokinase and heparin therapy. J Lab Clin Med 1977;89:1018-1029.

8. Rao AK, Pratt C, Berke A, et al: Thrombolysis in myocardial infarction (TIMI) trial — Phase I: Hemorrhagic manifestations and changes in plasma fibrinogen and fibrinolytic system in patients treated with recombinant tissue plasminogen activator and streptokinase. J Am Coll Cardiol 1988;11:1-11.

9. Stump DC, Califf RM, Topol EJ, et al: Pharmacodynamics of thrombolysis with recombinant tissue-type plasminogen activator. Correlation with characteristics of and clinical outcomes in patients with acute myocardial infarction. Circulation 1989;80:1222-1230.

10. The TIMI Research Group. Immediate vs delayed catheterizations and angioplasty following thrombolytic therapy for acute myocardial infarction: TIMI IIA results. JAMA 1988;260:2849-2858.

11. Marder VJ: Comparison of thrombolytic agents: Selected hematologic, vascular and clinical events. Eminase Symposium Proceedings. Am J Cardiol 1989;64:2A-7A.

12. Wilcox RG, von der Lippe G, Olsson CG, et al: Trial of tissue plasminogen activator for mortality reduction in acute myocardial infarction: Anglo-Scandinavian Study of Early Thrombolysis (ASSET). Lancet 1988;2:525-530.

13. AIMS Trial Study Group. Effect of intravenous APSAC on mortality after acute myocardial infarction: Preliminary report of a placebo-controlled clinical trial. Lancet 1988; 1: 545-549.

14. ISIS-2 (Second International Study of Infarct Survival) Collaborative Group. Randomised trial of intravenous streptokinase, oral aspirin, both, or neither among 17,187 cases of suspected acute myocardial infarction: ISIS-2. Lancet 1988;2:349-360.

15. Gimple LW, Gold HK, Leinbach RC, et al: Correlation between template bleeding times and spontaneous bleeding during treatment of acute myocardial infarction with recombinant tissue-type plasminogen activator. Circulation 1989;80:581-588.

16. Rothbard RL, Fitzpatrick PG, Francis CW, et al: Relationship of the lytic state to successful reperfusion with standard- and low-dose intracoronary streptokinase. Circulation 1985;71:562-570.

17. Fletcher AP, Alkjaersig N, Sherry S: The maintenance of a sustained thrombolytic state in man. I. Induction and effects. J Clin Invest 1959;38:1096-1110.

18. Collen D, Topol EJ, Tiefenbrunn AJ, et al: Coronary thrombolysis with recombinant tissue-type plasminogen activator: A prospective, randomized placebo-controlled trial. Circulation 1984;70:1012-1017.

19. Marder VJ, Rothbard RL, Fitzpatrick PG, Francis CW: Rapid lysis of coronary artery thrombi with anisoylated plasminogen:streptokinase activator complex: treatment by bolus intravenous injection. Ann Intern Med 1986;104:304-310.

20. Korninger C, Collen D: Studies on the specific fibrinolytic effect of human extrinsic (tissue-type) plasminogen activator in human blood and in various animal species in vitro. Thromb Haemost 1981;46:561-565.

21. The Urokinase Pulmonary Embolism Trial: A National Cooperative Study. Circulation 1973;47(suppl II):II-1-II-108.

22. Francis CW, Marder VJ: Increased resistance to plasmic degradation of fibrin with highly crosslinked -polymer chains formed at high factor XIII concentrations. Blood 1988; 71: 1361-1365.

23. Marder VJ: The use of thrombolytic agents: Choice of patient, drug administration, laboratory monitoring. Ann Int Med 1979;90:802-808.

24. Johns JA, Gold HK: Management of coronary reocclusion following successful thrombolysis. In: Topol EJ, ed. Acute Coronary Intervention. New York: Alan R. Liss, 1988:95-106.

25. Chesebro JH, Knatterud G, Roberts R, et al: Thrombolysis in Myocardial Infarction (TIMI) Trial, Phase I: a comparison between intravenous tissue plasminogen activator and intravenous streptokinase: clinical findings through hospital discharge. Circulation 1987;76:142-154.

26. Johns JA, Gold HK, Leinbach RC, et al: Prevention of coronary artery reocclusion and reduction in late coronary artery stenosis after thrombolytic therapy in patients with acute myocardial infarction. A randomized study of maintenance infusion of recombinant human tissue-type plasminogen activator. Circulation 1988;78:546-556.

27. Coller BS: Platelets and thrombolytic therapy. New Engl J Med 1990;322:33-42.

28. Francis CW, Markham RE Jr, Barlow GH, et al: Thrombin activity of fibrin thrombi and soluble plasmic derivatives. J Lab Clin Med 1983;102:220-230.

Chapter 9

REVIEW OF ANISTREPLASE (APSAC) FOR ACUTE MYOCARDIAL INFARCTION

Jeffrey L. Anderson

BIOCHEMISTRY AND PRECLINICAL EVALUATION

History

Anistreplase is a "designer compound" synthesized by chemists at Beecham Laboratories (London, United Kingdom). They speculated that temporary masking of the catalytic center of the plasminogen-streptokinase activator complex might confer functional advantages over streptokinase as a thrombolytic agent for clinical practice. Acylation was accomplished with a number of groups, and the anisoylated compound was selected for further development. This novel approach to chemical modification of plasminogen-streptokinase activator complexes was patented in 1979 and published by Smith et al in 1981.[1] Preclinical and clinical studies followed shortly thereafter, leading to approval of anistreplase for clinical application in acute myocardial infarction (AMI) in several countries in the late 1980s, including the United States.[2]

Nomenclature and Chemical Structure

Anistreplase is the proper name for the plasminogen activator frequently identified in the literature by the common name anisoylated plasminogen-streptokinase activator complex (APSAC). Anistreplase has a molecular weight of 131,000 daltons. APSAC represents the para-anisoylated derivative of human lys-plasminogen complexed in a 1:1 molar ratio with streptokinase.[1] Removal of a small N-terminal peptide converts human glu-plasminogen to lys-plasminogen. The serine residue residing in the center of the active site on lys-plasminogen is then anisoylated to form APSAC (Figure 1).

Eminase (Anistreplase)
Anisoylated (lys) - Plasminogen Streptokinase Activator Complex (APSAC)

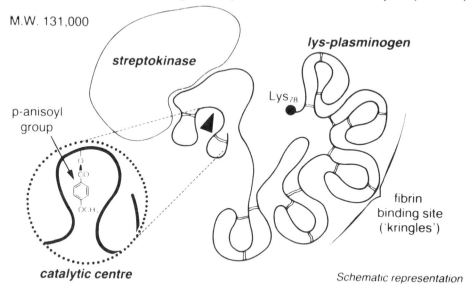

Figure 1. *Structure of anistreplase. Courtesy of H. Ferres, Beecham Laboratories.*

Chemical Preparation and Properties

Anistreplase is prepared by reacting streptokinase and human lys-plasminogen in the presence of an excess of the acylating agent 4-amidinophenyl 4^1-anisate hydrochloride (APAN).[1,3] Acylation is specific for the active site of the plasminogen molecule; there is little, if any, indiscriminate acylation of other parts of the activator molecule. In its protected acyl-form, anistreplase is a pro-enzyme that is inactive and stable in lyophilized form for at least one year at 5° C. When placed in aqueous solution, deacylation occurs by a simple ester hydrolysis process which follows pseudo-first-order kinetics in a temperature-dependent fashion. Products of this deacylation reaction are p-anisic acid and the free lys-plasminogen streptokinase activator complex in equimolar amounts. Deacylation occurs at approximately equal rates in free plasma and when bound to fibrin in clot. The free activator complex displays potent enzymatic activity in promoting the formation of the active fibrinolytic enzyme plasmin from its proenzyme plasminogen. Biologic activity of anistreplase is expressed in units specific to APSAC, and was initially selected so that one unit corresponded to the activity of 1 mg of drug. The commonly used clinical dosage of 30 units of anistreplase corresponds to approximately 1.1 million units of streptokinase.

PHARMACOLOGY AND PRE-CLINICAL EVALUATION

Pharmacologic Objectives

Streptokinase has certain disadvantages when given intravenously as a thrombolytic agent.[1-3] In order to achieve an activator complex with improved properties, anistreplase was synthesized with the major pharmacologic and clinical objectives shown in Table 1.

Streptokinase when injected intravenously rapidly forms a complex with glu-plasminogen in a 1:1 molar ratio. The streptokinase-plasminogen complex is then subject to immediate and rapid degradation by plasmin antiactivators. Vigorous but nonspecific systemic fibrinogenolysis and plasminemia occur simultaneously.

In the acyl-form, the modified activator shows substantial attenuation of rates of nonspecific systemic neutralization by plasmin inhibitors and antiactivators and degradation by autodigestion.[4-6] This results in prolonged generation and persistence of fibrinolytic activity. However, the fibrin binding sites on plasminogen are not adversely affected by acylation.[7] Furthermore, in its lys-form, plasminogen shows greater fibrin affinity than in the native glu-form.[8] Thus, fibrin affinity is present immediately upon APSAC injection, and circulating anistreplase is bound avidly to the fibrin clot.[2,9] Because the entire dose of drug is injected essentially as a bolus, a high concentration gradient between plasma and clot is rapidly achieved, also favoring diffusion of activator into thrombus.[9,10]

Table 1. *Key objectives in the synthesis of anistreplase*

Synthesis of Anistreplase:

Pharmacologic Objectives

– Simpler administration

– Longer plasma half-life

– Enhanced fibrin (thrombus) affinity

Clinical Expectations

– Easier patient management

– Prolonged action without prolonged administration

– Sustained action during period of high risk for early reocclusion

---

Adapted from H. Ferres, Beecham Laboratories.

Tolerance of much more rapid injection of activator complex in the inactive, acyl-form, than of an active form of drug was also anticipated because of attenuation of the generation of plasmin and bradykinin (kallikrein system activation), believed to be responsible for the precipitous hypotension associated with rapid injections of streptokinase. Pre-clinical testing was directed at demonstrating whether these and other pharmacologic objectives in the synthesis of anistreplase had been achieved.

Effect of Acylation on Systemic Plasmin/Kallikrein Flux and Hemodynamic Effects

Rapid injection of potent plasminogen activators may cause excessive lowering of blood pressure by rapid generation of plasmin, which converts prekallikrein to kallikrein, resulting in the formation of bradykinin, a potent vasodilator. To see whether acylation dampens this response, allowing bolus injection of activator without hemodynamic compromise, Green et al[11] injected dogs with equivalent doses of streptokinase-plasminogen (comparable to a 2,000,000 IU dose of streptokinase in humans) and anistreplase (50 U) as intravenous boluses (Figure 2). Profound hypotension, charac-

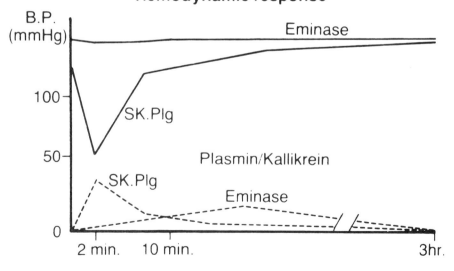

Figure 2. *Hemodynamic response to bolus doses of streptokinase-plasminogen (SK.Plg) versus anistreplase (Eminase) and plasmin/kallikrein flux in dogs (from Green et al [11]). Courtesy of Beecham Laboratories, H. Ferres.*

terized by 50% average reductions in mean blood pressure, developed within three minutes of streptokinase boluses in association with abrupt generation of large quantities of plasmin-kallikrein. Blood pressure was unaffected by anistreplase, which was associated with marked attenuation of the rate and peak of plasmin and kallikrein generation.

Clearance Rates of Fibrinolytic Potential in Animal Models, Plasma, and Patients

Dramatic gains in persistence rates of total potential fibrinolytic activity (activity resulting from both acylated and nonacylated forms) were confirmed by in vivo measurements in several animal species.[2,6] In guinea pigs, acylation increased plasma clearance half-life from 1.5 to 92 minutes, in rabbits from 2.5 minutes to 47 minutes, and in dogs to 60 minutes.

In humans, increases have been proportionately less but directionally similar. In human plasma, the half-life of fibrinolytic activity has been found to be about 90-120 minutes for anistreplase,[2,6,12,13] compared with 20-30 minutes for streptokinase,[2,13-16] measured both in vitro[17] (Figure 3) and in vivo[5,16] (Figure 4).

The half-life for deacylation is similar to the half-life for fibrinolytic activity, suggesting that deacylation is the limiting step in clearance.[2] Deacylation rates have

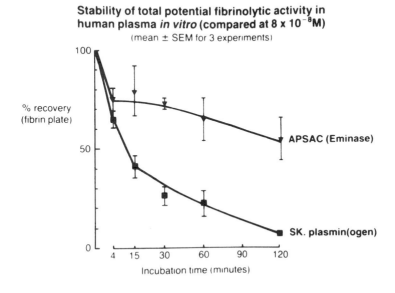

Figure 3. *Persistence of fibrinolytic activity in human plasma after anistreplase (APSAC) and streptokinase (SK) – plasminogen. Figure Courtesy of H. Ferres, Beecham Laboratories. From Fears et al,[17] with permission of Drugs.*

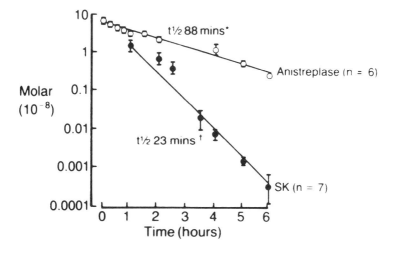

Figure 4. *Pharmacokinetics of anistreplase and streptokinase (SK) in acute myocardial infarction patients. Courtesy of H. Ferres, Beecham Laboratories.*
* *Been et al[5]*
† *Mentzer et al[16]*

been measured in glycerol-containing buffer,[1] nonglycerated buffer, plasma, whole blood, and plasma clots.[7] In these studies, a deacylation half-life of about 40 minutes was determined in buffer,[1] and longer half-lives of 105 minutes at 37° C in human plasma, about 120 minutes in clotted human plasma, and almost 150 minutes in phosphate-buffered albumin.[12] These studies also suggest that acylation was protective against plasma inhibitors of activator activity, proteolytic autodegradation, and rapid hepatic clearance.

Values obtained for the clearance half-life of total fibrinolytic activity in patients with AMI are similar to those obtained in vitro for treatment with both anistreplase and streptokinase (ie, 90-105 minutes for anistreplase[5,13] and 18-23 minutes for streptokinase).[15,16] This suggests that clearance of activator activity from the circulation is largely determined by processes assessed in vitro. As determined by its clearance half-life, anistreplase generates plasma fibrinolytic therapy for about 4-6 hours. However, substantially longer periods of time (1-2 days) are required for the liver to regenerate plasma factors depleted by fibrinolytic activity, such as fibrinogen, α_2-antiplasmin, and plasminogen.[18-20]

Improved Fibrin Binding Properties

The fibrin binding capacity of lys-APSAC (anistreplase), glu[1]-APSAC, and SK-glu[1]-plasmin(ogen) were evaluated by assessing uptake of radiolabeled compounds into preformed human plasma clots in vitro.[8] At the end of 30 minutes, uptake of lys-APSAC was 0.5 picomoles, compared with 0.3 picomoles for glu-APSAC or SK-glu-plasmin(ogen) (p < 0.05) (Figure 5). Additional experiments showed that the significantly increased uptake of ^{125}I-radiolabeled proteins was due to differential binding of lys- versus glu-plasminogen, rather than acyl versus nonacyl forms.[8]

The fibrin binding capacity of anistreplase has also been compared to that of tissue plasminogen activator (rt-PA), which is known to have strong fibrin affinity, and urokinase, known to have little fibrin affinity.[2,9,21] The relative order of continuing accumulation into clot was: APSAC = rt-PA > lys-plasminogen > urokinase. The formation of an acylated, stabilized activator complex thus conferred additional fibrin binding to lys-plasminogen.

Fibrin Semiselectivity

The structure of anistreplase suggests the possibility of fibrin semi-selective plasminogen activation by binding to clot followed by activation at the site of clot upon deacylation. In clinical practice, little systemic lytic effect has been observed with small doses of anistreplase (≤ 7.5 mg), but at doses used clinically (30 mg = 30 U), substantial systemic as well as thrombus-related deacylation occurs in association with substantial systemic (lytic) effects.[4,18-20,22,23] These effects were comparable to those of equivalent doses of streptokinase (1,000,000 to 1,500,000 IU).

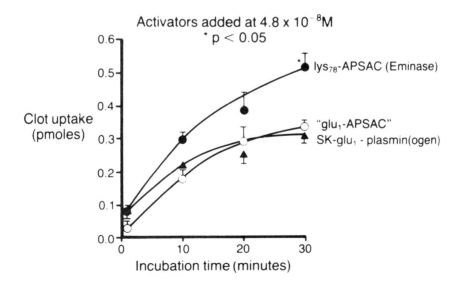

Figure 5. *Uptake into plasma clots of anistreplase (APSAC), glu-APSAC, and streptokinase (SK)-glu-plasminogen in vitro. Data reproduced from ref 8. Figure courtesy of H. Ferres, Beecham Laboratories.*

Thrombolytic Efficiency

In a guinea pig in vivo pulmonary embolism model, the dose response curve for anistreplase was shown to be shifted substantially to the left of that for streptokinase-plasmin (15 times more potent) when both agents were given as a bolus.[2] This differential may be attributed to greater bioavailability at the site of thrombus, resulting from the longer-lasting activity of anistreplase and its superior properties of fibrin binding and clot retention.[2] Immersion of preformed human thrombi for one minute in plasma containing equivalent concentrations of anistreplase, streptokinase, and urokinase, followed by observations of clot lysis for over five hours, also suggested superior clot retention and sustained activity for anistreplase (60% eventual thrombolysis vs. 10% for urokinase and streptokinase).[2]

Comparisons of thrombolytic efficiency of various thrombolytic agents are complicated by the varying potential for activation by heparin and fibrin.[24] When comparisons are made, conditions for heparin and fibrin need to be defined and optimized. The net fibrinolytic efficiency has been shown to be equivalent for anistreplase in the presence of fibrin and rt-PA in the presence of fibrin and heparin in vitro experiments.[24]

Stability and Molecular Integrity in Plasma

The integrity and stability of the anisoylated plasminogen-streptokinase molecule has been shown in two ways. First, tritium-labeling experiments have shown that the streptokinase moiety in anistreplase does not dissociate and exchange with non-acylated plasminogen in the bloodstream when tested over a period of at least one hour at 37° C.[25] Second, streptokinase-plasmin[ogen] activates not only free plasminogen but also causes autodigestion of the plasminogen-streptokinase activator complex itself. This "autodigestion process" can be examined by SDS-polyacrylamide gel electrophoresis. Such electrophoretic analysis has shown that acylation of plasminogen-streptokinase renders the active complex less susceptible to fast auto-proteolytic degradation.[6]

Summary of Preclinical Pharmacology and Pharmacokinetics

Results of preclinical evaluation from in vitro experiments and animal models have suggested that the proposed pharmacologic objectives of the chemical synthesis (Table 1) were largely achieved.[2,10] Bolus injection is possible without causing precipitous hypotension;[11] substantial lengthening in plasma half-life of total potential fibrinolytic activity was achieved (averaging 1.5-2 hours);[6] and enhanced fibrin (thrombus) affinity has been demonstrated.[8] In addition, acylation of the active site does not interfere with the high fibrin-binding capacity of the complex.[8,9] Attenuated systemic activation of the fibrinolytic system at low (but not high) doses is observed, compared with strepto-kinase.[22] Acylation provides partial protection against autodigestion,[6] is associated with molecular integrity (streptokinase component does not exchange with free plasminogen in human plasma),[6] substantially prolongs the persistence of plasminogen activator activ-ity,[5] and is associated in various animal species with increased thrombolytic efficacy.[2]

CLINICAL TRIALS EVALUATION

Endpoints for Assessment

The primary efficacy endpoints for the assessment of thrombolytic agents, including anistreplase, in AMI have included: 1) coronary artery reperfusion/patency; 2) left ventricular function/infarct size; and 3) mortality. Comparisons have been made against both placebo/nonthrombolytic therapy controls and, in many recent studies, positive controls with other (standard) thrombolytic regimens. Safety endpoints of most concern have been bleeding events, particularly serious events such as intracran-ial hemorrhage. Hypotensive reactions and potential allergic reactions and anaphy-laxis have also been assessed.

Effects on Reperfusion and Patency

Current evidence from thrombolytic trials supports the patent artery hypothesis; ie, early reestablishment and maintenance of coronary blood flow are central to the clinical benefits of thrombolysis.[26] Patient groups in which reperfusion has been achieved and maintained have consistently shown reduced mortality (although with higher risk of recurrent ischemia) than groups in which reperfusion has not been established.[27-30] Other beneficial effects of thrombolytic therapy have been suggested, such as reduction in blood viscosity with improvement of microvascular flow,[10] but the clinical importance of this and other effects has not been demonstrated.

Reperfusion and patency have specific and differing definitions. Reperfusion (recanalization) refers to reestablishment of flow. This requires a pre-treatment angio-gram to document coronary occlusion (generally defined as TIMI Grade 0 [absent] or 1 [minimal] flow).[31] Reperfusion is then documented as reestablishment of flow at a specific time after treatment, by convention most commonly at about 90 minutes. Patency refers to the angiographic documentation of post-treatment coronary flow, again at ≥ 90 minutes, but with patient entry based on clinical and electrocardio-graphic criteria rather than on coronary angiography. Patency rates generally exceed reperfusion rates by 10-20%, because this proportion of patients presenting within about six hours of clinical onset of AMI show residual blood flow (probably due to spontaneous reperfusion) in the infarct-related artery at the time of presentation.[30,32,33] Patients with even a small amount of residual antegrade flow in the infarct-related artery show substantially higher reperfusion rates post-treatment than those with total occlusion.[34]

Initial clinical trial experience and dose selection

Anistreplase shows efficacy similar to that of streptokinase when administered by the intracoronary route. Kasper et al[35] observed reperfusion in 15 of 22 patients (68%) at a mean of 42 ± 37 minutes after initiating thrombolytic therapy by the intracoronary route. However, the unique features of anistreplase relate to intravenous administration, which has been the route of administration in most of the other clinical trials.[5,18,36-41] A variety of different doses and different study designs were used in these trials. A pooled analysis (n = 160) of rates of coronary perfusion (generally patency rates) from these early trials using different doses showed a dose response relationship, with inadequate response rates (21% perfusion) at doses which cause little systemic fibrinogenolysis [5-10 U], intermediate response rates at 15-20 U (49% response), and optimal rates at 25-30 U (70% perfusion).[42] The vast majority of the patients in subsequent trials have received a 30 U dose of anistreplase.

Reperfusion potential of anistreplase and placebo

A double-blind, placebo controlled, randomized reperfusion comparison of anistreplase (30 U/2-5 minutes) and placebo was performed in 40 patients with AMI.[43] Pretreatment angiography documented coronary occlusion in 29 patients, qualifying them for randomization and treatment, which was performed at a mean of 3.4 hours (2.1-6.0) after the onset of symptoms. At the 90 minute post-treatment angiographic endpoint, reperfusion had occurred in 9 of 16 patients (56%) given anistreplase and in only 1 of 13 (8%) given placebo (p < 0.01). Anistreplase was well tolerated, and clinical outcome appeared better with thrombolytic therapy. Because of rapidly accumulating evidence from concurrent studies that reperfusion therapy is associated with patient benefit,[29,30,44-46] subsequent trials, particularly in the United States, have generally used a positive treatment control rather than placebo.

Reperfusion trials comparing IV anistreplase with intracoronary streptokinase

Until November 1987, only intracoronary (IC) thrombolytic therapy (with streptokinase or urokinase) had been approved by the United States Food and Drug Administration for the therapy of AMI. Thus, intracoronary streptokinase was selected as a positive comparative regimen for two key reperfusion studies of anistreplase, one in the United States[34] and one in the Netherlands.[47]

United States Comparative Reperfusion Study: A multicenter United States reperfusion study group, subsequently known as TEAM-1 (**T**hrombolytic **T**rials of **E**minase in **A**cute **M**yocardial-Infarction) compared the reperfusion potential of intravenous (IV) anistreplase and intracoronary (IC) streptokinase (SK), administered according to FDA approved dosing recommendations (TEAM-1 study). Patients were included who had clinical and ECG criteria for AMI, were aged 76 years or less, and could be angiographically studied and treated within six hours of the onset of symptoms. A total of 240 consenting patients with documented coronary occlusion (flow Grade 0 or 1) qualified for randomization and were treated at a mean 3.4 hours, range 0.4-6.0, after symptom onset with either IV anistreplase (30 U/2-4 minutes) or intracoronary SK (20,000 U bolus, then 2,000 U/min/60 minutes). Both groups received heparin for $\geq$ 24 hours. Reperfusion success, defined as the advancement of Grade 0 or 1 flow to Grade 2 or 3 flow (at 60 minutes for IC and 90 minutes for IV therapy) was 51% for anistreplase (59 of 115) and 60% for IC SK (67 of 111, p = 0.18). Reocclusion rates at 24 hours in successfully treated patients were low.

A striking dependence of 60-90 minute success on the time from symptom onset to patient entry was observed (Figure 6).[34] Anistreplase achieved a 60% reperfusion rate if given within 4 hours, identical to that of IC SK. If given between 4-6 hours after onset, IV therapy (but not IC therapy) was less successful (33% reperfusion) at the 90 minute endpoint. The success of therapy was also significantly related to initial coronary angiographic flow grade (Figure 7).[34] If even a trickle of flow around the clot

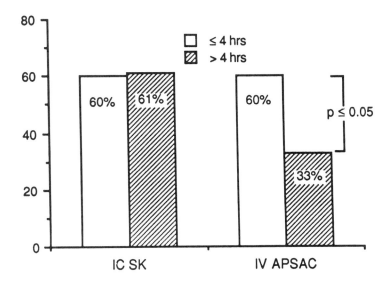

Figure 6. *Early reperfusion success (Y axis, in percent) achieved in AMI patients treated earlier ($\leq$ 4 hrs) or later (> 4 hrs) after symptom onset after either intracoronary streptokinase (IC SK) or intravenous anistreplase (IV APSAC) in the TEAM-1 study. From Anderson et al,[34] with permission of J Am Coll Cardiol.*

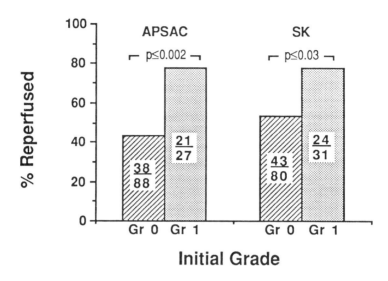

Figure 7. *Relation of early reperfusion success to initial (pre-treatment) coronary flow grade for intravenous anistreplase (APSAC) and intracoronary streptokinase. From Anderson et al,[34] with permission of J Am Coll Cardiol.*

(grade 1) was present at pretreatment angiography, the success rate increased by about 25-35% compared to patients with no flow (grade 0) before treatment with intracoronary or intravenous thrombolytic therapy.

The rate of achieving reperfusion for IV compared with IC therapies is shown in Figure 8. The mean time to reperfusion was 31 ± 17 minutes (mean $\pm$ SD) after IC, and 43 ± 23 minutes after IV therapy.[34] The 12 minute differential, while statistically significant, is not clinically important, because of the additional time required in catheterization to enable delivery of IC drug. A plateau in reperfusion rates occurs by 45-60 minutes during IC therapy, but is not yet reached at the 90 minute endpoint for IV therapy, suggesting that even later assessment may be necessary to demonstrate maximal (optimal) effects of IV drug (anistreplase).

Rapid injections of IV anistreplase were generally well tolerated, although a modest transient decrease in blood pressure was observed (median decline of 10 mm Hg at 3 minutes). Anistreplase in a dose of 30 U caused substantial systemic lytic effects. Plasma fibrinogen levels decreased to 32% of pretreatment controls at 90 minutes, and plasminogen levels to 22%.[34] Both levels gradually increased back to within 20% of baseline by 24-48 hours. Adverse bleeding events after the larger relative doses of anistreplase were somewhat greater than after IC SK, but no intracranial hemorrhages occurred, and changes in hematocrit at 24 hours did not differ between the two groups. Mortality rates were low: 4% in the anistreplase and 8% in

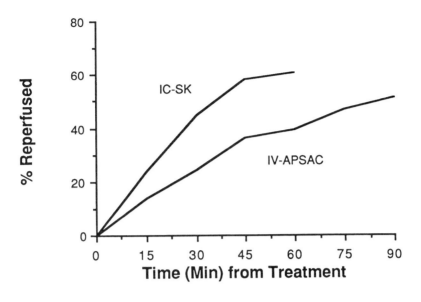

Figure 8. *Rate of reperfusion as a function of time after beginning intracoronary (IC) or intravenous (IV) lytic therapy. From Anderson et al,[34] with permission of J Am Coll Cardiol.*

the streptokinase group. Additional interventions were given as necessary (97 of 240 patients) and were well tolerated.

Dutch Comparative Study of Anistreplase and IC Streptokinase: In a multicenter Dutch reperfusion study, Bonnier et al[47] compared the efficacy of anistreplase (30 U/5 min) and IC streptokinase, given at a higher infusion rate (about 250,000 U/1 hour) than in the TEAM-1. Patients with clinical and ECG criteria of AMI were angiographically studied within four hours, and a total of 85 with initial coronary occlusion (grade 0, 1) were entered and treated at a mean of 2.4 hours after symptom onset. Reperfusion was achieved in 23 of 36 patients (64%) by anistreplase and 25 of 37 patients (68%) after IC streptokinase at the endpoint of 90 minutes (p = NS). Repeat angiography at 24 hours showed a low reocclusion rate (anistreplase = 1/22, SK = 3/23). Therapy was well tolerated in both groups, and no intracranial or other serious bleeding was observed.

Summary of controlled reperfusion studies: An overview of reperfusion studies with anistreplase is shown in Table 2.[42,48] Two major studies combined with five

Table 2. *Overview of reperfusion/patency and reocclusion/ reinfarction after anistreplase*

Variable	No. Studies	No. Pts.	Result % (n)
1. Reperfusion			
(90 min)	5	177	55.4 (98)
2. Early Patency			
at about 90 min			
(0.5 - 6 hr)	7	513	73.3 (376)
3. Late Patency			
at about 4 days			
(1-14 days)	3	187	80.0 (149)
4. Reocclusion			
within 1-3 days	8	289	3.1 (9)
5. Reinfarction	all		
in-hospital	available	1,058	
a. Early (<1-3 d)			3.7 (39)
b. Anytime			8.5 (90)

Modified after Anderson JL: Summary of clinical trials program for evaluation of anistreplase. Clin Cardiol 1990;13(suppl V):V-33. (Also see references 40, 42, 48)

smaller studies in 177 patients show a reperfusion rate of 55.4%. Limiting evaluation to patients treated within four hours, reperfusion rates of 60-65% may be expected, similar to that achieved with IC streptokinase, which is believed to provide near optimal reperfusion rates in AMI, and substantially greater than spontaneous early reperfusion rates seen after placebo (< 10%).[30,43] The studies also showed good safety and tolerance and much greater ease of administration than IC therapy with catheterization. The reperfusion results with anistreplase[34,47] can be compared indirectly with those of streptokinase and rt-PA from the U.S. TIMI study.[31] Overall reperfusion rates in TIMI were 31% for streptokinase and 60% for rt-PA. Restricting analysis to therapy given within 4 hours, streptokinase reperfused 44% and anistreplase 60% of patients.

Patency studies with anistreplase

Comparisons with streptokinase and heparin: Data available in 1989 from seven patency studies using anistreplase and follow-up angiography (at a mean of about 90 min) are reviewed in Table 2.[42,48] The overall patency rate was 73.3% (376 of 513 patients). Three studies were observational (no concurrent controls), and four used intravenous streptokinase as a positive control. Direct patency comparisons of anistreplase with streptokinase and rt-PA have been or are being performed. Two of the largest completed comparative trials will be summarized.

French comparative study of anistreplase in streptokinase: In a preliminary report of an open-design multicenter study[49] and subsequently updated,[42] 116 patients with AMI and symptoms of < 6 hours duration were randomized to therapy with either anistreplase (30 U/2-5 min) or SK (1.5 million U/60 min). Mean time to treatment was 2.8 hours. Post treatment angiography, performed at an average of about 90 minutes, allowed determination of patency status in 107 patients. Overall patency (Grade 2/3 flow) was 72% (30/54) in the anistreplase group and 53% (28/53) in the SK group (p = 0.05). These reperfusion rates compared quite closely to those reported by Verstraete et al[50] for the comparison of IV recombinant rt-PA vs. IV SK in a European cooperative study (patency rates of 70% and 55%, respectively).

United States comparative trial: A larger patency trial of IV anistreplase and IV SK has been completed in the United States, and a preliminary report of an interim analysis of 328 of 370 entered patients has been presented.[51] The study was randomized and double blind. Drug regimens included anistreplase, 30 U/2-5 min, and SK, 1.5 million U/1 hr. The study enrolled patients of age < 76 years with symptoms of AMI ≤ 4 hours duration with diagnostic ECG criteria (ST elevation). Angiographic evaluation of patency occurred at a mean of 2.4 hours after initiation of therapy. In the preliminary analysis, overall patency rates were high and similar for the two regimens (73%, 74%, respectively). However, a higher percentage of patients had grade 3 (complete) flow after anistreplase (61% vs. 52%).

These studies and the overview analysis consistently show patency rates of 70-75% after anistreplase. Patency rates reported after streptokinase have been more variable but have generally been lower in rate or grade of patency than after anistreplase, which is easier to administer.

Late patency after anistreplase vs. heparin

Long term clinical outcome following hospital discharge appears to be predicted by patency at hospital discharge.[26-29] Late patency may differ from early (90 min) patency because of the continuing process of reperfusion balanced against the opposing process of reocclusion. In a review of three studies,[48,49,52] late patency after anistreplase was determined at 1-14 days (median = 4), and averaged 80% (149/187 patients) (Table 2). In two studies, patients were randomized to control therapy with heparin. Late patency was significantly less after heparin (40%, 61 of 154 patients, p < 0.001).[48,52] In one study, late patency after streptokinase was 89% (24/27), similar to that after anistreplase (92%, 25/27).[49] Thus, these studies of late patency confirm the superiority of thrombolytic therapy over heparin. Late net patency rates actually tend to be higher than early rates for anistreplase and also for SK, which appears to "catch up" over time.

Rates of Reocclusion and Reinfarction After Anistreplase

Reocclusion is an important morbid event, leading to loss of clinical benefit of early reperfusion. Despite this, less information is generally available on reocclusion rates after thrombolytic therapy than on reperfusion/patency rates. Reocclusion assessment requires a second angiographic study. Also, many exclusions prevent reocclusion assessment because of early interventions such as angioplasty and surgery, often performed for varying indications. Despite these difficulties, information on reocclusion within 1-3 days after initially successful anistreplase therapy is available for 289 patients evaluated in several clinical studies[34,40,47,49,51-53] (Table 2). Angiographic reocclusion was documented in only 9 (3.1%). In six trials, intravenous streptokinase was used as the comparison agent. Among 181 patients given IV SK, reocclusion was noted in 8 (4.4%).

Clinical reinfarction during hospitalization after anistreplase therapy can be summarized for a much larger patient base (n = 1058)[48] (Table 2). The diagnosis of reinfarction was made by individual clinical investigators, based on clinical, ECG, and enzymatic criteria. Early hospital reinfarction (within 1-3 days) was noted in 3.7% (39 patients), and reinfarction occurring any time during the hospitalization was reported in 8.5% (90 patients).

These rates of reocclusion and reinfarction after anistreplase are low and compare favorably with those reported for other agents. In the TIMI study,[54] 24% of patients (15 of 69) successfully treated with rt-PA showed reocclusion when studied at the time of hospital discharge, compared with 14% (4 of 29) who responded to SK and were restudied. Clinical reinfarction during hospitalization occurred in 13% and 12% of these groups, respectively. Similarly, for a study comparing urokinase and rt-PA, reocclusion occurred in 7% after urokinase and 12% after rt-PA.[55]

ARMS (Anistreplase **R**eperfusion and Reocclusion **M**ulticenter **S**tudy), an open, multicenter trial of anistreplase (30 U), was specifically designed to study reocclusion in 156 AMI patients successfully treated with anistreplase within 4 hours of symptom onset and evaluated angiographically at 90 minutes and again at 24 hours.[53] Results were evaluated initially by the investigator and subsequently by an independent reviewer, with similar results. Initial patency was observed in 71-73%. Ninety-six percent (102/106) of initially patent arteries remained patent at the 24-hour angiogram, and only 4 (4%) became reoccluded.

Effects on Left Ventricular Function and Myocardial Infarct Size

The potential of anistreplase to reduce myocardial infarct size and improve left ventricular function has been investigated in a French multicenter study by Bassand et al.[52] In this double blind, parallel group study, 231 patients with AMI were randomized and treated within 5 hours of the onset of symptoms with either anistreplase (30 U/5 min) or heparin (5,000 IU bolus). Heparin was reintroduced in both groups four hours after initial therapy. Left ventricular ejection fraction (EF) was measured during the first and third weeks after treatment (in the first week [mean 4 ± 1 day] by contrast angiography, in the third week [19 ± 3 days] by radionuclide ventriculography). Infarct size was assessed in the third week by thallium SPECT (single photon emission computed tomography) using a method validated in animal studies and in previous clinical trials. All test interpretations were performed in a blinded fashion.

Within the first week following treatment, EF measured by contrast ventriculography had significantly diverged in favor of anistreplase by six percentage points:

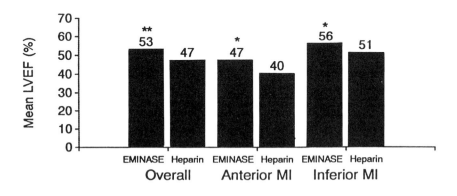

Figure 9. *Contrast left ventricular function in AMI patients at a mean of 4 days after anistreplase (Eminase) or heparin.*
  * $p \leq 0.05$
  ** $p \leq 0.01$
Adapted from Bassand et al.[52] Courtesy of H. Eckerson, Beecham Laboratories.

EF = 53% (anistreplase) vs. 47% (heparin), p < 0.01 (Figure 9). Ejection fraction was significantly higher after anistreplase in both the anterior infarct group (47% vs. 40%) and the inferior group (56% vs. 51%). Infarct related arteries were patent in 77% of anistreplase vs. 36% of heparin patients (p < 0.01).

Infarct size assessed after the acute phase (during the third week following MI) was substantially reduced in the anistreplase group by 31% overall (Figure 10). Reduction in the anterior infarct group (33%) was greater than in the inferior infarct group (16%). A significant difference in radionuclide ejection fraction between the anistreplase and heparin groups was also shown during the third week, although the difference was more modest (4 percentage points) and was significant only for the anterior infarct group (6 point differential). A significant inverse relationship was found linking tomographic (SPECT) infarct size and radionuclide left ventricular ejection fraction during the third week after AMI.

These favorable effects on left ventricular function after anistreplase are similar to those reported for studies of streptokinase and rt-PA, where a 2-8 percentage point advantage to lytic therapy has been shown,[44,56-64] and where measured, a 20-30% reduction in infarct size.[57,63]

In a separate German study,[65] anistreplase therapy was associated with a more than 50% reduction in mortality (from 12% to 5%), but convalescent radionuclide ejection fraction did not differ significantly in survivors in the two groups. Variability has also been observed in results of studies with streptokinase and rt-PA.[44,56-64,66] Because dying patients invariably have very low ejection fractions, the exclusion

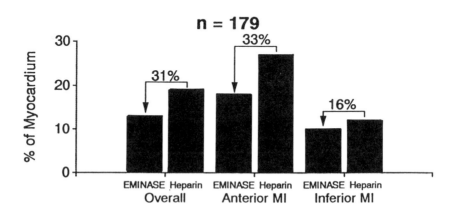

Figure 10. *Infarct size, measured by thallium scintigraphy, after anistreplase (Eminase) or heparin measured in third week.*
n = 179
Adapted from Bassand et al.[52] Courtesy of H. Eckerson, Beecham Laboratories.

from assessment of over twice as many of these patients in the control (heparin) group may have biased the study results in favor of heparin.[65] Also, ventriculography was performed at many individual centers, introducing the possibility of technical variation in results. Of course, improvement in survival in treated patients is a highly important result, whatever the mechanism.[26]

Effects of Anistreplase on Post-Infarction Mortality

Although early trials with anistreplase were too small to assess mortality effects, pooling early controlled trials into an overview provided strong suggestive evidence for a substantial mortality benefit.[40] In these trials, 708 patients received nonthrombolytic control therapy, and 1,386 patients received anistreplase (more than 85% received 30 U). Early mortality (in-hospital or within one month) was 6.1% (85 patients) in the anistreplase group and 12.3% (87 patients) after standard therapy. These differences were highly significant ($p < 0.001$) but as with other meta-analyses, should be viewed with caution and used to generate hypotheses to be tested prospectively, as was done in the AIMS trial (anistreplase intervention mortality study).[67]

The AIMS trial

AIMS (**A**nistreplase **I**ntervention **M**ortality **S**tudy), a multicenter trial from the United Kingdom, has recently confirmed the substantial mortality benefit of anistreplase therapy in patients presenting within six hours of the onset of AMI symptoms and treated with anistreplase or placebo, along with heparin, subsequent warfarin, and other standard therapy (ie, β-blockade with timolol), and followed for mortality outcome at one month and one year. AIMS intended to recruit 2,000 patients but was stopped at the second interim analysis by the safety monitoring board (after 1,004 patients had been analyzed), because of substantial mortality differences in favor of thrombolytic therapy. In this analysis of 1,004 patients, 30-day mortality was 6.4% (32 patients) in the anistreplase group, compared with 12.2% (61 patients) in the placebo group ($p = 0.0016$).[67] This mortality reduction of 48% is the most auspicious for a single agent reported to date.[68]

At the time the decision to stop AIMS was made, 1,258 patients had been entered. The result of a final analysis of all 1,258 patients has recently been presented, confirming results of the interim analysis (Figure 11, Tables 3-5).[69,70] Mortality risk at 30 days was 6.4% (40/624) in the anistreplase group, and 12.1% (77/634) ($p = 0.0006$) in the placebo group, representing a 47% risk reduction or a 50.5% odds reduction (95% confidence interval, 26.1-66.8%) (Table 3). After one year, 69/624 (11.1%) anistreplase patients and 113/634 (17.8%) placebo patients had died ($p = 0.0007$), a 38% risk reduction or 42.7% odds reduction (confidence interval 20.9-58.5%). As shown

Table 3. *Anistreplase intervention mortality study (AIMS): mortality effects by treatment groups*

| | Mortality % (n) | | | |
| | 30 days | | 1 year | |
Group	Anistreplase	Placebo	Anistreplase	Placebo
I. Overall (n = 1258)	12.1%(77/634)	6.4%(40/624)	17.8%(113/634)	11.1% (69/624)
II. Time to therapy (predefined)				
< 4 hrs (n = 828)	9.9%	5.3%	16.2%	9.2%
4-6 hrs (n = 400)	14.7%	8.2%	19.6%	14.3%
> 6 hrs (n = 27)	40.0%	16.7%	40.0%	25.0%
III. Age				
< 55 yrs	3.8%	3.1%	9.2%	7.6%
55-64 yrs	12.0%	6.8%	19.5%	11.4%
> 64 yrs	30.6%	12.1%	33.1%	17.2%
IV. Infarct site				
Anterior	17.5%	9.6%	25.0%	14.7%
Inferior	7.8%	3.4%	12.0%	7.6%
V. Previous MI				
Yes	21.2%	11.7%	27.4%	21.4%
No	10.2%	5.4%	15.8%	9.0%
VI. Gender				
Male	—	—	16.5%	11.5%
Female	—	—	23.9%	9.1%

Data from Julian[69]

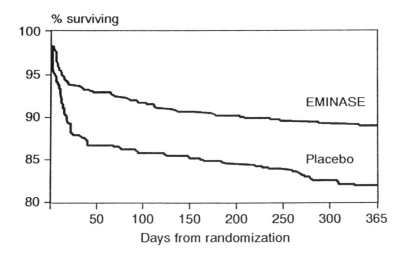

Figure 11. *One-year survival curve of myocardial infarction patients randomly assigned to treatment with anistreplase (Eminase) or placebo in the AIMS. Adapted from reference 70, with permission of Lancet.*

in Figure 11, the absolute differential mortality benefit of anistreplase (about 6%) established by 6 weeks was maintained or increased during the one-year follow-up.

Of note was the observation that mortality benefits extended to all subgroups tested, including those with early and later times to treatment (0-4 vs. 4-6 hours), younger and older patients, inferior (56% risk reduction) as well as anterior (45% risk reduction) infarction, those with as well as without previous infarction, and both genders (Table 3).

AIMS also allowed the assessment of side effects of infarction and treatment to be assessed within a large placebo controlled population[71] (Table 4,5). It should be noted that AIMS required diagnostic ECG entry criteria to be met, and 93% of ECGs analyzed retrospectively fulfilled these criteria. Infarction was independently confirmed by elevation in enzymes in 80%; 75% developed Q wave infarction; and 98% of each treatment group had enzymatic and/or electrocardiographic changes diagnostic of AMI. As in other large mortality studies,[44-46,72] reductions in several adverse complications of AMI were observed, including shock, cardiac arrest, myocardial rupture, heart failure, ventricular fibrillation, and pericarditis (Table 4). As expected, treatment slightly increased the risk of reinfarction in the hospital (1.4 percentage point differential) within the first year after discharge (1.0 point differential). As expected, other ventricular arrhythmias ("reperfusion" arrhythmias), hypotension, and supraventricular arrhythmias were observed somewhat more frequently in the treated group. Anaphylaxis (nonfatal) occurred in only four treated patients (0.6%), and other "allergic" phenomenon such as pruritus, fever/chills, etc., were actually

Table 4. *Nonhemorrhagic complications after acute myocardial infarction by treatment in AIMS*

Event (n)	Anistreplase (n = 624)	Placebo (n = 634)	Absolute change (%)*
Shock	16	29	2.0%
Cardiac arrest (died)	26	37	1.7%
Sudden death (< 1 yr)	13	21	1.2%
Cardiac rupture	5	13	1.2%
Heart failure	131	154	3.3%
Pericarditis	43	98	8.6%[†]
Ventricular fibrillation	41	46	0.7%
Ventricular tachycardia	96	67	− 5.1%
Hypotension			
(SBP < 80 mmHg)	55	31	− 0.7%
Anaphylaxis	4	0	− 0.6%
Pruritus/rash	11	17	0.9%
Reinfarction			
In-hospital	38	30	− 1.4
Post-hospital (to 1 yr)	29	23	− 1.0

* Positive percent indicates reduced events per 100 treated patients by anistreplase; negative number indicates increased event rate.
† $p < 0.001$
Data from Fox[71]

more frequently reported in the placebo group. Premedication (ie, with hydrocortisone) had no effect on the incidence of these minor reactions.

As expected, hemorrhage was observed more frequently after thrombolytic therapy (Table 5). These were primarily at puncture sites, although gastrointestinal bleeding, hematuria, and hemoptysis were all somewhat more common with treatment. Transfusions, however, were given to only five patients in each group, and changes in hemoglobin did not differ by treatment.

Table 5. *Hemorrhagic and CNS complications after acute myocardial infarction by treatment in AIMS*

Event	Anistreplase (n=624)	Placebo (n=634)	Absolute change (%)*
Hemorrhage (any)	86	26	– 9.7[†]
Puncture site	46	6	– 6.4[†]
Gastrointestinal	19	9	– 1.6
Hematuria, epistaxis	30	5	– 4.0[†]
Transfusion	5	5	0.0
Stroke	8	5	– 0.5
Stroke + TIA	13	5	– 1.0
Onset < 24 hr	5	0	– 0.8
1-30 days	4	4	0.0
1-12 months	4	1	– 0.5
Disability	2	1	– 0.2
Death	4	3	– 0.2

* Positive percent indicates reduced events per 100 treated patients by anistreplase; negative number indicates increased event rate.
† $p < 0.001$
Data from Fox[71]

Intracranial hemorrhage is a key safety variable. Overall, 8 strokes were reported in the anistreplase group and 5 in the placebo group, a difference of 0.5 percentage points. Adding symptoms of transient cerebral ischemia to stroke gives an incidence of 13 vs. 5 (absolute difference, 1.0%) (Table 5). An excess in cerebral events occurred within the first 24 hours (5 vs. 0). However, deaths from stroke were similar (4 vs. 3) in the two groups. A differential risk of strokes/intracranial hemorrhage of about 0.5% is in keeping with the range of risk reported for rt-PA and streptokinase.

Overview of mortality trials of anistreplase, rt-PA, and streptokinase

Yusuf et al recently reviewed published data from acceptably controlled trials for anistreplase (9 trials, 2,000 patients), rt-PA (5 trials, 6,500 patients),[73] and streptokinase (31 trials, 41,000 patients). Overall, reductions in early mortality after SK averaged 24% (CI 20-33); after rt-PA, 26% (CI 11-39); and after anistreplase, 52% (CI 33-65). The majority of these trials did not require aspirin as part of the regimen. Because of the overlapping confidence intervals and differing patient populations and study designs, however, direct comparative trials using standardized entry criteria and standard concomitant therapies will be required to firmly establish any differential in mortality benefit among these agents. Such a trial (ISIS-3) is currently underway.

OVERALL SAFETY PROFILE OF ANISTREPLASE

Safety experience with anistreplase in clinical trials has been summarized[40] and recently updated.[42] This adverse event summary results from experience gained in nearly 7,000 patients, 5,275 of whom have received anistreplase (about 90% received the standard dose of 30 U/2-5 min. Safety data from the pivotal AIMS study have already been summarized (Tables 4 and 5). Important aspects of safety to be reviewed include: 1) bleeding events; 2) changes in clotting parameters and hemoglobin concentrations; 3) cerebral vascular accidents; and 4) anaphylactoid reactions.

Bleeding Events

Overall, hemorrhagic events were reported in 14.6% of patients (Table 6). The most frequent event was puncture site hemorrhage or hematoma, occurring in 5.7% of the patients. Hemorrhagic events were reported as severe in only 1.6% of patients, however. Not surprisingly, the incidence of hemorrhagic events is higher in studies incorporating invasive (angiographic) techniques than in noninvasive studies, 22% vs. 13%. The difference between these is accounted for by a higher incidence of puncture site hemorrhages in invasive studies (14.5% vs. 5.0%). Severe bleeding was reported in 3.1% vs. 2.0% of these studies, respectively.

Using a fall in hemoglobin greater than 4 grams/dL as evidence for a major hemorrhagic event, a small and similar number of affected patients studied in non-invasively controlled trials were identified: 3.5% in the anistreplase group and 3.7% in the control (usually heparin) groups, respectively. As noted above for the AIMS, only a small percentage of patients (less than 1%) received transfusions in large studies in the United Kingdom.

Changes in Hematologic Parameters

Changes in hematologic (clotting) parameters are of interest to the assessment of thrombolytic therapy. Changes in plasma fibrinogen were measured in two major reperfusion trials of intravenous anistreplase.[34,47] A large fall in fibrinogen was initially observed, with trough levels reached by 90 minutes after dosing and with return

172

to baseline by 48 hours. Specifically, in the TEAM-1 study (n = 110), fibrinogen fell to 32% of control, plasminogen to 22%, and α_2-antiplasmin to 18% of control. At 24 hours these values had returned to 79%, 45%, and 65% of control, respectively.

Although such reductions in clotting factors may potentially increase bleeding risks, and were the motivation for development of more fibrin-specific agents (such as rt-PA and pro-urokinase), subsequent trial experience suggests that non-specificity may not increase bleeding appreciably[54] and may also be of benefit.[10] Fibrinogenolysis reduces the viscosity of blood and may improve capillary perfusion, particularly in beds with low perfusion pressure, such as in the zone of myocardial infarction. In addition, the platelet activating effects of thrombolytic agents (which expose sites for blood aggregation on platelet membranes) may be counterbalanced by the generation of fibrinogen degradation products (FDPs) by the nonfibrin selective agents (anistreplase, streptokinase, urokinase) to a greater extent than by fibrin selective drugs (rt-PA), which have high reported associated reocclusion rates.[54,55] Furthermore, depletion of fibrinogen, and hence fibrin, reduces the ability of activated platelets to aggregate and hence to form the nidus for a reocclusive thrombus. Moreover, the

Table 6. *Overview of reported hemorrhagic events after anistreplase administration*

	Type of Study	
	Invasive (n = 289)	Non-invasive (n = 1246)
I. Invasive/non-invasive studies		
A. All hemorrhagic events	64 (22.1%)	163 (13.1%)
B. Puncture site hemorrhage/hematoma	42 (14.5%)	62 (5.0%)
C. Hemorrhage, other sites	28 (9.7%)	133 (10.7%)
II. All studies	**Cumulative experience (n=5275)**	
A. All hemorrhagic events	769 (14.6%)	
B. Puncture site hemorrhage/hematoma	299 (5.7%)	
C. Hemorrhage, other sites	538 (10.2%)	
D. Severe events (investigator experience)	87 (1.6%)	

safety profile with respect to hemorrhage is not different for fibrin selective and nonfibrin selective agents.[54]

Risk of Cerebral Vascular Accidents

The overall incidence of cerebral vascular accident occurring any time after anist-replase was 0.99% versus 0.80% after nonthrombolytic therapy (Table 7). Analyzing the event rate as a function of time from treatment, an excess was noted after an-istreplase for events occurring within 7 days of treatment, and a reverse trend was seen after 7 days. A similar finding was noted for streptokinase in the ISIS-2 study.[46] When analyzed by etiology, cerebral vascular accidents were identified as hemor-rhagic in 0.3% of anistreplase treated patients and no nonthrombolytic patients. A similar and low percentage (0.15%) in the two groups had nonhemorrhagic strokes. Etiology was unknown in about 0.2% of patients in each group. The differential risk of stroke was 0.4% within the first seven days of therapy after anistreplase but only 0.19% overall. These figures for stroke incidence are in the range of those reported in various studies of rt-PA and streptokinase.[44-46,54,61,72-74]

The impact on severe hemorrhagic events of adding aspirin to anistreplase has also been assessed by retrospective review.[42] A similar incidence of hemorrhage and possible intracranial hemorrhage was reported with or without aspirin (Table 8). In these trials, the use of aspirin was neither specifically indicated (and no specific regimen defined) nor contraindicated. Future trials (ISIS-3) will provide more com-plete information on combined anistreplase and aspirin therapy.

Table 7. *Cerebrovascular accidents after anistreplase or non-thrombolytic therapy*

Time of occurrence and etiology	Anistreplase (n = 5275)	Non-thrombolytic therapy (n = 1249)
I. ≤ 7 days	38 (0.72%)	4 (0.32%)
A. Hemorrhagic	18 (0.34%)	0 (0)
B. Non-hemorrhagic	8 (0.15%)	2 (0.16%)
C. Unknown	12 (0.23%)	2 (0.16%)
D. Possibly hemorrhagic (A + C)	30 (0.57%)	2 (0.16%)
II. > 7 days	14 (0.27%)	6 (0.48%)
III. Overall (I + II)	52 (0.99%)	10 (0.80%)

Adapted from Cregeen[42]

Table 8. *Hemorrhagic events after anistreplase with or without aspirin*

	With Aspirin	Without Aspirin
Any severe event	15/453 (3.3%)	54/1389 (3.9%)
CVA of hemorrhagic or unknown etiology	4/453 (0.88%)	12/1389 (0.86%)

CVA = cerebrovascular accident
Adapted from Cregeen[42]

Risk of Allergy/Anaphylaxis

The incidence of anaphylactoid reactions following anistreplase has been very low. Eleven cases have been reported by investigators as representing possible anaphylaxis, anaphylactic reaction, or anaphylactoid shock.[42] This 0.2% incidence with anistreplase (11 of 5,275 patients) is similar to the 0.3% incidence found in patients treated in parallel with streptokinase (1 of 327). As noted above for AIMS, other minor reactions designated as possibly allergic have not been shown to be increased in treated versus untreated AMI patients, and premedication (eg, with hydrocortisone or diphenhydramine) has not affected the incidence of these reactions.[42]

ANISTREPLASE AND ANCILLARY THERAPIES (MEDICAL AND MECHANICAL)

Ancillary Medical Therapies

Whether additional mortality benefit may be achieved by combining aspirin with anistreplase, as was recently shown for streptokinase,[46] remains to be demonstrated. Such a combined regimen is being tested in the ongoing ISIS-3 study. However, information available (Table 8) suggests that, as with streptokinase, combined therapy is feasible with low anticipated additional risk. Heparin has been administered after anistreplase, as after other agents, in a high percentage of patients in clinical trials. Thus, safety figures generally relate to combined therapy with anistreplase followed by heparin. The specific benefit/risk of heparin combined with anistreplase (and streptokinase and rt-PA) is being evaluated in the ongoing ISIS-3 study. Information about heparin is also available for streptokinase and rt-PA from the recently completed GISSI-2 trial. Short-term anticoagulation (warfarin for 90 days) and long-term β-blockade (timolol) were administered to patients without contraindications in the AIMS, and were associated with a favorable outcome at one year. Intravenous β-blockade was not specifically tested

175

in AIMS, but afforded additional benefit when added to rt-PA therapy in the TIMI-2 trial.[75,76]

Mechanical Interventions (Angioplasty, Surgery)

Mechanical interventions following thrombolytic therapy during hospitalization are common, particularly in the United States. Evaluation of the outcome of patients undergoing mechanical procedures indicates a favorable interaction between anistreplase and subsequent angioplasty or surgery, with no unanticipated safety or efficacy problems.[34,42] In the TEAM-1, study 155 patients (81 anistreplase treated, 74 streptokinase treated) had mechanical interventions (angioplasty, guidewire probe, surgery) or additional thrombolytic therapy.[34] Some had more than one intervention. Nineteen anistreplase and 17 SK patients underwent bypass grafting, 7 and 10, respectively, within 48 hours. One hundred nine underwent balloon angioplasty; 58 after anistreplase and 51 after streptokinase. The majority of interventions (55 with anistreplase, 47 with SK) occurred within 48 hours of therapy; 33 and 32 of these, respectively, occurred within two hours of therapy. Efficacy data were not collected prospectively, but safety data were available for comparison. No patients experienced adverse events potentially increased by angioplasty (dissection, embolic, thrombotic events). The frequency of conduction disorders and arrhythmias in these patients was similar to the frequency in the overall population (21%). All five deaths after angioplasty were in the streptokinase group. None of these appeared related to angioplasty. From these data it appears that patients treated with anistreplase tolerated angioplasty, including early emergency angioplasty (within two hours of therapy), with no increased risk. Bypass surgery increased, as expected, the frequency of transfusions (from 12-14% to 21-23%), but the differential was similar for both agents and not different than expected, based on other thrombolytic trials. Thus, if necessary, early balloon angioplasty and surgery may be performed with reasonable safety.

Aggressive Versus Conservative Management Strategies

An additional question is whether patient outcome is improved (or impaired) by the *routine* application of coronary angiography and, where significant stenosis remains, by prophylactic angioplasty. Such an approach has been shown to be associated, if anything, with a worse outcome than a conservative approach in at least three major studies using rt-PA.[75-78] The SWIFT study (**S**hould **W**e **I**ntervene **F**ollowing Thrombolysis?)[79] was designed to answer this question for the non-fibrin selective agent, anistreplase. SWIFT entered 933 patients and randomized 833 to either a conservative approach (n = 397) or an invasive approach (n = 377). Angiography, as in the TIMI-2B study,[76] was undertaken an average of 1-2 days after therapy. The infarct-related artery was patent in 68% of the 256 patients, and angioplasty was undertaken in 134, with initial success in 88%. Bypass surgery was performed in 42 patients, for a 47% intervention rate in the invasive group (the rate of angioplasty in the noninvasive group was 11%). In-hospital and three-month mortality were low in both groups, but the trend favored conventional care over the intervention group (3.2% vs. 4.8% three month mortality, p = 0.3). Furthermore, there was no difference in the three-month ejection fraction, although marginally less angina was present in the intervention group. Hospital stay was longer in the invasive group. Thus, results of SWIFT for anistreplase are similar to those of studies for rt-PA.[75-78] The answer to the question of SWIFT, "Should we intervene following thrombolysis?" appears to be, "only if we have to" (De Bono).[79]

INDICATIONS/CONTRAINDICATIONS/PRECAUTIONS

Recent clinical trials support the use of anistreplase in patients with AMI aged 75 years or less, presenting within six hours of symptom onset, and without contraindications to thrombolytic therapy. The establishment of a diagnosis of AMI should be made by electrocardiographic and clinical criteria. In these patients, anistreplase is indicated for: 1) reestablishment of coronary blood flow (reperfusion/patency); 2) reduction in infarct size; 3) improvement in left ventricular function; and 4) improvement in survival (reduced mortality). Precautions and contraindications to anistreplase are essentially identical to those for streptokinase.

Bleeding

As noted above, bleeding represents the most common adverse event following thrombolytic therapy. Hemorrhagic events can be expected in about 15% of patients studied invasively and 10% of patients studied non-invasively. About two-thirds of bleeding occurs at vascular puncture sites. The risk of stroke is about 1% following thrombolytic therapy (a somewhat similar percentage, about 0.8%, is also present without lytic therapy). The mechanism of stroke, however, is often intracranial hemorrhage after thrombolytic therapy, occurring in about 0.5% (0.3-0.6%) of treated patients, and is roughly similar to that of other agents.

Possible Allergic Events

The streptokinase contained in anistreplase is antigenic; however, anaphylactoid reactions have occurred in only about 0.2% of patients and have responded to standard symptomatic therapy without fatality.

Purpuric skin rashes have also been reported (about 1% incidence). More commonly, fever, flushing, and chills have been observed (about 5% of patients), but these symptoms may also occur in untreated, rt-PA-treated, and urokinase-treated[31,54,72,80]

177

patients. Premedication with corticosteroids or antihistamines, although commonly used, has not been shown to be of prophylactic benefit and is not required.

Antigenicity may have greater implications for efficacy on reuse. Titers of blocking antibodies high enough to affect efficacy for the doses of SK and anistreplase currently recommended rarely exist in untreated patients, but often develop by five days after treatment and may persist for at least a year.[81,82] Thus, reuse of SK and anistreplase should probably be avoided, if possible, for at least 1-2 years.

Hypotension

Anistreplase, like streptokinase, can cause hypotension. By activating plasmin, bradykinin, a potent vasodilator, is produced. The more gradual production of plasmin and bradykinin production by anistreplase, however, allows anistreplase to be given by bolus injection. Some lowering of blood pressure both initially[34] and over a 24-hour period may still be observed.[71] Modest reductions in blood pressure and afterload may, in fact, be beneficial. However, more severe (although transient) hypotension is occasionally observed, most commonly at 5-15 minutes after injection. This may be treated by postural measures, intravenous fluids, and (very rarely) pressor agents. Some transient clinical hypotension has been reported in 10-20% of patients.[34] In one comparative study,[34] median reductions of blood pressure of 10 mm Hg were observed directly following anistreplase injection (at 2-5 minutes), compared with 5 mm Hg after the initiation of low dosage IC streptokinase.

DOSAGE AND ADMINISTRATION

How Supplied

Anistreplase is marketed in vials of lyophilized powder containing 30 U (about 30 mg). Reconstitution is achieved by injecting 5 ml of sterile water or saline into the 30 U vial and gently rolling or tilting to effect dissolution without causing excessive foaming. After allowing a moment for air bubbles to disperse, the solution is injected slowly over 2-5 minutes through a dedicated intravenous line with constant monitoring of blood pressure and the electrocardiogram. After reconstitution, anistreplase should be given within 30 minutes. The maximum hypotensive effect of anistreplase generally occurs within 5-15 minutes.

Although the need for concurrent heparin has not been demonstrated, most patients have received subsequent heparin therapy beginning about 4-6 hours later or when the partial thromboplastin or thrombin times fall to less than 2-2.5 times the upper limit of normal. Because the fibrinolytic effect of anistreplase persists for at least 4-6 hours and the nadir of circulating fibrinogen also occurs at that time,[18] it appears reasonable to withhold heparin until then, and then begin empirically, often at a dose of 750-1,000 U/hr, with adjustment after four hours to maintain the PTT at 1.5-2 times the upper normal range, generally for 1 to 4 days.

Based on the ISIS-2 study[46] and observational data presented for anistreplase, it also appears reasonable to consider the concurrent use of aspirin. The optimal initial aspirin dose is unknown, but the ISIS-2 dose of 160 mg (for example, 2 x 80 mg chewable tablets) may be given on patient presentation. Thereafter, 160-325 mg per day may be administered. (For example, one enteric-coated aspirin [325 mg] may be given daily during hospitalization, then continued during outpatient therapy for at least six weeks to indefinitely). When not initiated simultaneously with anistreplase and heparin, aspirin may be started prior to discontinuing heparin therapy and then continued chronically. Concurrent therapy with other drugs commonly used in patients with AMI (ie, lidocaine, nitroglycerin, β-blockers) has been given frequently without difficulty.

Marketing Approval and Cost

Anistreplase received U.S. FDA approval in December 1989, and has been marketed in the U.S. since January 1990. The pharmacy cost of anistreplase is about $1,700 per 30 U dose.

REFERENCES

1. Smith RAG, Dupe RJ, English PD, Green J. Fibrinolysis with acyl-enzymes: a new approach to thrombolytic therapy. Nature 1981;290:505-508.

2. Ferres H. Pre-clinical pharmacological evaluation of Eminase (APSAC). Drugs 1987;33 (suppl 3):33-50.

3. Fears R. Development of anisoylated plasminogen-streptokinase activator complex from the acyl enzyme concept. Seminars in Thrombosis and Hemostasis 1989;15:129-139.

4. Nunn B, Esmail A, Fears R, Ferres H, Standring R. Pharmacokinetic properties of an-isoylated plasminogen streptokinase activator complex and other thrombolytic agents in animals and in humans. Drugs 1987;33(suppl 3):88-92.

5. Been M, de Bono DP, Muir AL, Boulton FE, Fears R, Standring R, Ferres H. Clinical effects and kinetic properties of intravenous APSAC - anisoylated plasminogen - strepto-kinase activator complex (BRL 26921) - in acute myocardial infarction. International J Cardiol 1986;11:53-61.

6. Standring R, Fears R, Ferres H. The protective effect of acylation on the stability of APSAC (Eminase) in human plasma. Fibrinolysis 1988;2:157-163.

7. Fears R. Binding of plasminogen activators to fibrin: characterization and pharmacolog-ical consequences. Biochem J 1989;261:313.

8. Fears R, Ferres H, Standring R. Pharmacological comparison of anisoylated lys-plasmin-ogen streptokinase activator complex with its glu-plasminogen variant and streptokinase-glu-plasminogen: binding to human fibrin and plasma clots. Fibrinolysis 1989;3:93.

9. Fears R, Standring R, Ferres H. Evidence for a continuing accumulation of APSAC (Anisoylated plasminogen streptokinase activator complex) by human clots: comparison with the binding of other plasminogen activators and plasminogen. Fibrinolysis 1987; 1:215-223.

10. Sherry S. Pharmacology of anistreplase. Clin Cardiol 1990;13(suppl V):V-3 to V-10.

11. Green J, Dupe RJ, Smith RAG, Harris GS, English PD. Comparison of the hypotensive effects of streptokinase (human)-plasmin activator complex and BRL 26921 (anisoylated streptokinase-plasminogen activator complex) in the dog after high dose bolus adminis-tration. Thromb Res 1984;36:2936.

12. Ferres H, Hibbs M, Smith RAG. Deacylation studies in vitro on anisoylated plasminogen streptokinase activator complex. Drugs 1987;33(suppl 3):80-82.

13. Fears R, Ferres H, Glasgow E, Greenwood HC, Standring R. Comparison of fibrinolytic and amidolytic methods for the measurement of streptokinase pharmacokinetics with acute myocardial infarction. Fibrinolysis 1989;3:175.

14. Doenecke P, Schwerdt H, Hellsten P, et al. Bolus injection of anisoylated plasminogen-streptokinase activator complex (BRL 26921): a new approach to intravenous thrombo-lytic treatment of acute myocardial infarction. Klin Wochenschr 1986;64:682-687.

15. Martin M. Streptokinase in chronic arterial disease. CRC Press, 1982.

16. Mentzer RL, Budzynski AZ, Sherry S. High-dose, brief-duration intravenous infusion of streptokinase in acute myocardial infarction: description of effects in circulation. Am J Cardiol 1986;57:1220-1226.

17. Fears R, Ferres H, Standring R. The protective effect of acylation on the stability of anisoylated plasminogen streptokinase activator complex in human plasma. Drugs 1987; 33(suppl 3):57-63.

18. Marder VJ, Rothbard RL, Fitzpatrick PG, Francis CW. Rapid lysis of coronary artery thrombi with anisoylated plasminogen-streptokinase activator complex: treatment by bolus intravenous injection. Ann Intern Med 1986;104:304-310.

19. Monassier JP (on behalf of the IRS II Study Group), Hanssen M. Hematological effects of anisoylated plasminogen streptokinase activator complex and streptokinase in patients with acute myocardial infarction: interim report of the IRS II study. Drugs 1987;33(suppl 3):247-252.

20. Samama M, Conard J, Verdy E, et al. Biological study of intravenous anisoylated plasminogen streptokinase activator complex in acute myocardial infarction. Drugs 1987;33 (suppl 3):268-274.

21. Fears R, Ferres H, Standring R. Evidence for the progressive uptake of anisoylated plasminogen streptokinase activator complex by clots in human plasma in vitro. Drugs 1987;33(suppl 3):51-56.

22. Marder JV, Kinsalle PA, Brown MJ. Fibrinogen concentration and coronary artery reperfusion after intravenous anisoylated plasminogen streptokinase activator complex or intracoronary streptokinase therapy. Drugs 1987;33(suppl 3):237-241.

23. Fears R, Green J, Smith RAG, et al. Induction of a sustained fibrinolytic response by BRL 26921 in vitro. Thromb Res 1985;38:251-260.

24. Fears R. Kinetic studies on the effect of heparin and fibrin on plasminogen activators. Biochem J 1988;249:77-81.

25. Smith RAG. Non-exchange of streptokinase from anisoylated plasminogen streptokinase activator complex and other acylated streptokinase-plasminogen complexes. Drugs 1987; 33(suppl 3):75-79.

26. Braunwald E. Myocardial reperfusion, limitation of infarct size, reduction of left ventricular dysfunction, and improved survival. Should the paradigm be expanded? Circulation 1989;79:441-444.

27. Marder VJ, Francis CW. Thrombolytic therapy for acute transmural myocardial infarction: intracoronary versus intravenous. Am J Med 1984;77:921-927.

28. Kennedy JW, Gensini GG, Timmis GC, et al. Acute myocardial infarction treated with intracoronary streptokinase: a report of the society for cardiac angiography. Am J Cardiol 1985;55:871-877.

29. Kennedy JW, Ritchie JL, Davis KB, et al. The Western Washington Randomized Trial of intracoronary streptokinase in acute myocardial infarction: a 12-month follow-up report. N Engl J Med 1985;312:1073-1078.

30. Simoons ML, Serruys PW, Van den Brand M, et al. Improved survival after early thrombolysis in acute myocardial infarction: a randomized trial of the Interuniversity Cardiology Institute in the Netherlands. Lancet 1985;2:578-581.

31. Chesebro JH, Knatterud G, Roberts R, et al. Thrombolysis in myocardial infarction (TIMI) trial, phase I: a comparison between intravenous tissue plasminogen activator and intravenous streptokinase. Circulation 1987;76:142-154.

32. DeWood MA, Spores J, Notske R, Mouser LT, Burroughs R, Golden MS, Lang HT. Prevalence of total coronary occlusion during the early hours of transmural myocardial infarction. N Engl J Med 1980;303:897-902.

33. Anderson JL, Marshall HW, Bray BE, Lutz JR, Frederick PR, Yanowitz FG, Datz FL, Klausner SC, Hagan AD. A randomized trial of intracoronary streptokinase in the treatment of acute myocardial infarction. N Engl J Med 1983;308:1312-1318.

34. Anderson JL, Rothbard RL, Hackworthy RA, Sorensen SG, Fitzpatrick PG, Dahl CF, Hagan AD, Browne KF, Symkoviak GP, Menlove RL, Barry WH, Eckerson HW, Marder VJ, for the APSAC Multicenter Investigators. Multicenter reperfusion trial of intravenous anisoylated plasminogen streptokinase activator complex (APSAC) in acute myocardial infarction: controlled comparison with intracoronary streptokinase. J Am Coll Cardiol 1988;11:1153-1163.

35. Kasper W, Erbel R, Meinertz T, et al. Intracoronary thrombolysis with an acylated streptokinase plasminogen activator (BRL 26921) in patients with acute myocardial infarction. J Am Coll Cardiol 1984;4:357-362.

36. Hillis WS, Hornung RS. The use of BRL 26921 (APSAC) as fibrinolytic therapy in acute myocardial infarction. Eur Heart J 1985;6:909-912.

37. Been M, De Bono DP, Muir AL, et al. Coronary thrombolysis with intravenous anisoylated plasminogen-streptokinase complex BRL 26921. Br Heart J 1985;53:253-259.

38. Ikram S, Lewis S, Buckwall C, et al. Treatment of acute myocardial infarction with anisoylated plasminogen streptokinase activator complex. Br Med J 1986;293:786-789.

39. Kasper W, Meinertz T, Wollschlager H, et al. Coronary thrombolysis during acute myocardial infarction by intravenous BRL 26921, a new anisoylated plasminogen-streptokinase activator complex. Am J Cardiol 1986;58:418-421.

40. Johnson ES, Cregeen RJ. An interim report of the efficacy and safety of anisoylated plasminogen streptokinase activator complex (APSAC). Drugs 1987;33(suppl 3):298-311.

41. Jackson D. Summary of early clinical experience with anisoylated plasminogen streptokinase activator complex in the treatment of acute myocardial infarction. Drugs 1987;33 (suppl 3):104-111.

42. Cregeen R. Report to the US FDA Advisory Committee, Bureau of Biologies. Anistreplase review meeting, Oct 31, 1989, Bethesda, MD.

43. Timmis AD, Griffin B, Crick JCP, Sowton E. APSAC in acute myocardial infarction: a placebo-controlled arteriographic coronary recanalization study. J Am Coll Cardiol 1987; 10:205-210.

44. ISAM Study Group. A prospective trial of intravenous streptokinase in acute myocardial infarction (ISAM): mortality, morbidity, and infarct size at 21 days. N Engl J Med 1986; 14:1465-1471.

45. Gruppo Italiano per lo Studio della Streptochinasi nell'Infarcto Miocardico (GISSI): effectiveness of intravenous thrombolytic treatment in acute myocardial infarction. Lancet 1986;1:397-401.

46. ISIS-2 Collaborative Group. Randomized trial of intravenous streptokinase, oral aspirin, both, or neither among 17,187 cases of suspected acute myocardial infarction: ISIS-2. Lancet 1988;2:349-360.

47. Bonnier HJRM, Visser RF, Klomp HD, Hoffman HMJL, and the Dutch Invasive Reperfusion Study Group. Comparison of intravenous anisoylated plasminogen streptokinase activator complex and intracoronary streptokinase in acute myocardial infarction. Am J Cardiol 1988;62:25-30.

48. Cregeen RJ. Clinical studies of Eminase in patients with myocardial infarction: summary of the phase III efficacy data. Beecham Pharmaceuticals Report, May 1988.

49. Brochier ML, Quilliet L, Kulbertus H, Materne P, Latac B, Cribier A, Monassier JP, Sacrez A, Favier JP. Intravenous anisoylated plasminogen streptokinase activator complex versus intravenous streptokinase in evolving myocardial infarction: preliminary data from a randomized multicentre study. Drugs 1987;33(suppl 3):140-145.

50. Verstraete M, Bernard R, Bory M, Brower RW, Collen D. Randomized trial of intravenous recombinant tissue-type plasminogen activator versus intravenous streptokinase in acute myocardial infarction. Lancet 1985;1:842-847.

51. Anderson JL, Hackworthy RA, Sorensen SG, Browne KF, Dale HT, Leja F, Dangoisse V, Marder VJ, and the TEAM Investigators. Comparison of intravenous anistreplase (APSAC) and streptokinase in acute myocardial infarction: interim report of a randomized, double-blind patency study. Circulation 1989;80 (Part II), II-420 (abstract #1669).

52. Bassand J-P, Machecourt J, Cassagnes J, Anguenot T, Lusson R, Borel E, Peycelon P, Wolf E, Ducellier D, for the APSIM Study Investigators. Multicenter trial of intravenous anisoylated plasminogen streptokinase activator complex (APSAC) in acute myocardial infarction: effects on infarct size and left ventricular function. J Am Coll Cardiol 1989; 13:988-997.

53. Relik-Van Wely L, Visser RF, Van der Pol JMJ, et al. The angiographically assessed potency and reocclusion in patients treated with APSAC for acute myocardial infarction (AMI): final data of the ARMS Study. Eur Heart J 1989;10(suppl):199 (abstract #983).

54. Rao AK, Pratt C, Berke A, Jaffe A, Ockene I, Schreiber TL, Bell WR, Knatterud G, Robertson TL, Terrin ML for the TIMI Investigators. Thrombolysis in myocardial infarction (TIMI) trial-phase I: hemorrhagic manifestations and changes in plasma fibrinogen and the fibrinolytic system in patients treated with recombinant tissue plasminogen activator and streptokinase. J Am Coll Cardiol 1988;11:1-11.

55. Califf RM, Topol EJ, George BS, et al. TAMI 5: a randomized trial of combination thrombolytic therapy and immediate cardiac catheterization. Circulation 1989;80:II-420 (abstract).

56. White HD, Norris RM, Brown MA, et al. Effect of intravenous streptokinase on left ventricular function and early survival after acute myocardial infarction. N Engl J Med 1987;317:850-855.

57. Simoons ML, Serruys PW, Van den Brand M, et al. Early thrombolysis in acute myocardial infarction: limitation of infarct size and improved survival. J Am Coll Cardiol 1986; 7:717-728.

58. Serruys PW, Simoons ML, Suryapranta H, et al. Preservation of global and regional left ventricular function after early thrombolysis in acute MI. J Am Coll Cardiol 1986;7: 729-742.

59. Guerci AD, Gerstenblith G, Brinker JA, et al. A randomized trial of intravenous tissue plasminogen activator for acute myocardial infarction with subsequent randomization to elective coronary angioplasty. N Engl J Med 1987;317:1613-1618.

60. O'Rourke M, Norris R, (for the TICO Group). Improved LV ejection fraction at 21 days following coronary occlusion treated by early intravenous rt-PA infusion (abstract). J Am Coll Cardiol 1988;11(suppl A):105A.

61. Van de Werf F, Arnold AER. Intravenous tissue plasminogen activator and size of infarct, left ventricular function, and survival in acute myocardial infarction. Br Med J 1988; 297:1374-1379.

62. Armstrong PW, Baigrie RS, Daly PA, et al. Tissue plasminogen activator: Toronto (TPAT) placebo-controlled randomized trial in acute myocardial infarction. J Am Coll Cardiol 1989;13:1469-1476.

63. Kennedy JW, Martin GV, Davis KB, et al. The Western Washington intravenous streptokinase in acute myocardial infarction randomized trial. Circulation 1988;77:345-352.

64. National Heart Foundation of Australia Coronary Thrombolysis Group. Coronary thrombolysis and myocardial salvage by tissue plasminogen activator given up to 4 hours after onset of myocardial infarction. Lancet 1988;1:203-207.

65. Meinertz T, Kasper W, Schumacher M, et al. The German multicenter trial of anisoylated plasminogen streptokinase activator complex versus heparin for acute myocardial infarction. Am J Cardiol 1988;62:347-351.

66. Spann JF, Sherry S. Coronary thrombolysis for evolving myocardial infarction. Drugs 1984;28:465-483.

67. AIMS Trial Study Group. Effect of intravenous APSAC on mortality after acute myocardial infarction: preliminary report of a placebo-controlled clinical trial. Lancet 1988;1: 545-549.

68. Editorial. Thrombolytic therapy for acute myocardial infarction-Round 2. Lancet 1988;1: 565-5566.

69. Julian D. Final report of the AIMS study: efficacy data. Clin Cardiol 1990;13(suppl V): V-20 to V-21.

70. AIMS Trial Study Group. Long-term effects of intravenous anistreplase in acute myocardial infarction: final report of the AIMS study. Lancet 1990;335:427.

71. Fox KA. Final report of the AIMS study: safety data. Clin Cardiol 1990;13(suppl V):V-22 to V-26.

72. Wilcox RG, Lippe GV, Olsson CG, Jensen G, Skene AM, Hampton JR, for the ASSET Study Group. Trial of tissue plasminogen activator for mortality reduction for acute myocardial infarction: Anglo-Scandinavian study of early thrombolytic therapy (ASSET). Lancet 1988;2:525-533.

73. Yusuf S, Wittes J, Friedman L. Overview of results of randomized clinical trials in heart disease: I. Treatments following myocardial infarction. JAMA 1988;260:2088-2093.

74. Braunwald E, Knatterud GL, Passamani ER, Robertson TL. Announcement of protocol change in thrombolysis in myocardial infarction trial (letter). J Am Coll Cardiol 1987; 9:467.

75. The TIMI Research Group. Immediate vs delayed catheterization and angioplasty following thrombolytic therapy for acute myocardial infarction: TIMI II-A results. JAMA 1988; 260:2849-2858.

76. The TIMI Study Group. Comparison of invasive and conservative strategies after treatment with intravenous tissue plasminogen activator in acute myocardial infarction: results of the thrombolysis in myocardial infarction (TIMI) phase II trial. N Engl J Med 1989;320:618-627.

77. Topol EJ, Califf RM, George BS, et al. A randomized trial of immediate versus delayed elective angioplasty after intravenous tissue plasminogen activator in acute myocardial infarction. N Engl J Med 1987;317:581-588.

78. Simoons ML, Betriu A, Col J et al. Thrombolysis with tissue plasminogen activator in acute myocardial infarction: no additive benefit from immediate coronary angioplasty. Lancet 1988;1:197-202.

79. De Bono DP. For the SWIFT Investigators. Should we intervene following thrombolysis? The SWIFT study of intervention versus conservative management after anistreplase thrombolysis. Eur Heart J 1989;10(suppl):253 (abstract #1318).

80. Goldhaber SZ, Kessler CM, Heit J, et al. Randomized, controlled trial of recombinant tissue plasminogen activator versus urokinase in the treatment of acute pulmonary embolism. Lancet 1988;2:293-298.

81. Fears R, Ferres H, Hibbs M, Standring R. Consequences of antibody binding in vitro on the pharmacological properties of anisoylated plasminogen streptokinase activator complex. Drugs 1987;33(suppl 3):64-68.

82. Hoffman JJML, Fears R, Bonnier JJRM, Standring H, Ferres H, De Swart JBRM. Significance of antibodies to streptokinase in coronary thrombolytic therapy with streptokinase or APSAC. Fibrinolysis 1988;2:203.

Chapter 10

STREPTOKINASE IN ACUTE MYOCARDIAL INFARCTION

Jeffrey L. Anderson
Bruce R. Smith

HISTORICAL PERSPECTIVE

Streptokinase (SK) was the first thrombolytic agent discovered and developed for clinical use. It is also the most extensively studied agent and represents the standard with which other agents are compared. Despite the development of other thrombolytic agents with differing properties, SK remains an important therapeutic agent in the 1990s.

Streptokinase is a bacterial protein secreted into culture fluid during the growth phase of β-hemolytic streptococci cultures. Tillet and Garner first discovered the ability of filtrates of streptococcal cultures to lyse human clots in the early 1930s.[1] The subsequent characterization[2] and clinical application of SK have been reviewed by Sherry.[3,4] Early studies showed that SK, originally named streptococcal fibrinolysin,[2] forms a complex that acts on native plasminogen to form the active fibrinolytic enzyme plasmin.

The first successful clinical application of SK — liquefaction of a pleural clot — was reported in 1949.[5] Use of SK in AMI began in 1954,[3] with the first report of a patient series published in 1958.[6-8] Expanded studies of SK followed, and approval for use in the management of pulmonary embolism and deep venous thrombosis occurred in 1977.[4] The additional indications of arterial thrombosis and embolism, clotted external dialysis shunts, and, importantly, intracoronary (1982) and intravenous (1987) administration for AMI followed in subsequent years.

PROPERTIES

Chemistry

Streptokinase is a single-chain protein consisting of 415 amino acid residues with a molecular weight of 47,000 daltons.[9,10] It contains little carbohydrate and no disulfide bonds. The amino acid sequence of streptokinase is shown in Figure 1. Early preparations of SK were relatively impure, with some containing only about 10% active drug,

```
     1                        10                                    20
NH2-Ile-Ala-Gly-Pro-Glu-Trp-Leu-Leu-Asp-Arg-Pro-Ser-Val-Asn-Asn-Ser-Gln-Leu-Val-Val-
     21                       30                                    40
Ser-Val-Ala-Gly-Thr-Val-Glu-Gly-Thr-Asn-Gln-Asp-Ile-Ser-Leu-Lys-Phe-Phe-Glu-Ile-
     41                       50                                    60
Asp-Leu-Thr-Ser-Arg-Pro-Ala-His-Gly-Gly-Lys-Thr-Glu-Gln-Gly-Leu-Ser-Pro-Lys-Ser-
     61                       70                                    90
Lys-Pro-Phe-Ala-Thr-Asp-Ser-Gly-Ala-Met-Ser-His-Lys-Leu-Glu-Lys-Ala-Asp-Leu-Leu-
     81                       90                                    100
Lys-Ala-Ile-Gln-Glu-Gln-Leu-Ile-Ala-Asn-Val-His-Ser-Asn-Asp-Asp-Tyr-Phe-Glu-Val-
     101                      110                                   120
Ile-Asp-Phe-Ala-Ser-Asp-Ala-Thr-Ile-Thr-Asp-Arg-Asn-Gly-Lys-Val-Tyr-Phe-Ala-Asp-
     121                      130                                   140
Lys-Asp-Gly-Ser-Val-Thr-Leu-Pro-Thr-Gln-Pro-Val-Gln-Glu-Phe-Leu-Leu-Ser-Gly-His-
     141                      150                                   160
Val-Arg-Val-Arg-Pro-Tyr-Lys-Glu-Lys-Pro-Ile-Gln-Asn-Gln-Ala-Lys-Ser-Val-Asp-Val-
     161                      170                                   180
                              Leu
Glu-Tyr-Thr-Val-Gln-Phe-Thr-Pro-      -Asn-Pro-Asp-Asp-Asp-Phe-Arg-Pro-Gly-Leu-Lys-
                              Asp
     181                      190                                   200
Leu
    -Thr-Lys-Leu-Leu-Lys-Thr-Leu-Ala-Ile-Gly-Asp-Thr-Ile-Thr-Ser-Gln-Glu-Leu-Leu-
Asp
     201                      210                                   220
Ala-Gln-Ala-Gln-Ser-Ile-Leu-Asn-Lys-Asn-His-Pro-Gly-Tyr-Thr-Ile-Tyr-Glu-Arg-Asp-
     221                      230                                   240
Ser-Ser-Ile-Val-Thr-His-Asp-Asn-Asp-Ile-Phe-Arg-Thr-Ile-Leu-Pro-Met-Asp-Gln-Glu-
     241                      250                                   260
Phe-Thr-Tyr-Arg-Val-Lys-Asn-Arg-Glu-Gln-Ala-Tyr-Arg-Ile-Asn-Lys-Lys-Ser-Gly-Leu-
     261                      270                                   280
Asn-Glu-Glu-Ile-Asn-Asn-Thr-Asp-Leu-Ile-Ser-Leu-Glu-Tyr-Lys-Tyr-Val-Leu-Lys-Lys-
     281                      290                                   300
Gly-Glu-Lys-Pro-Tyr-Asp-Phe-Asp-Arg-Ser-His-Leu-Lys-Leu-Phe-Thr-Ile-Lys-Tyr-
     301                      310                                   320
Val-Asp-Val-Asp-Thr-Asn-Glu-Leu-Leu-Lys-Ser-Glu-Gln-Leu-Leu-Thr-Ala-Ser-Glu-Arg-
     321                      330                                   340
Asn-Leu-Asp-Phe-Arg-Asp-Leu-Tyr-Asp-Pro-Arg-Asp-Lys-Ala-Lys-Leu-Leu-Tyr-Asn-Asn-
     341                      350                                   360
Leu-Asp-Ala-Phe-Gly-Ile-Met-Asp-Tyr-Thr-Leu-Thr-Gly-Lys-Val-Glu-Asp-Asn-His-Asp-
     361                      370                                   380
Asp-Thr-Asn-Arg-Ile-Ile-Thr-Val-Tyr-Met-Gly-Lys-Arg-Pro-Glu-Gly-Glu-Asn-Ala-Ser-
     381                      390                                   400
Tyr-His-Leu-Ala-Tyr-Asp-Lys-Asp-Arg-Tyr-Thr-Glu-Glu-Glu-Arg-Glu-Val-Tyr-Ser-Tyr-
     401                      410
    Leu-Arg-Tyr-Thr-Gly-Thr-Pro-Ile-Pro-Asp-Asn-Pro-Asp-Asp-Lys-COOH
```

Figure 1. *Amino acid sequence of streptokinase. Reprinted with permission from Bell WR, Sasahara AA (eds):* Review of Thrombolytic Therapy and Thromboembolic Disease. *Glenview, Physicians & Scientists Publishing Co., Inc., 1989, p 6.*

and were poorly tolerated clinically. Current preparations have a purity of greater than 95% and are well tolerated.[3,4]

In solution, SK is stable in a pH range of 6 to 8 and is inactivated at pH less than 5 or greater than 9.[11,12] The activity of SK is quantified by its ability to lyse a standard blood clot. The United States (Christensen) unit (U) is equivalent to the International Unit (IU) and is the quantity of SK that will lyse a clot of defined weight in 10 minutes. One milligram of SK contains approximately 3100 IU of activity.[13] SK is available as a sterile, lyophilized powder; it is stable at room temperature and is diluted to appropriate specifications at the time of administration.

Pharmacology

Streptokinase produces fibrinolysis by activating the body's natural fibrinolytic system.[2,14,15] Streptokinase is not appreciably absorbed following oral or rectal dosing[16] and must be given parenterally. Immediately after administration, SK combines with circulating plasminogen, a proenzyme, in an equimolar ratio to form an activator complex (Figure 2). The SK-plasminogen activator complex then converts free plasminogen to the active fibrinolytic enzyme plasmin, which then acts on fibrin (or fibrinogen) to yield soluble fibrin(ogen) degradation products.[4] During this process

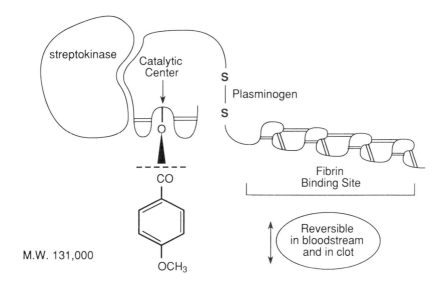

Figure 2. *Schematic representation of streptokinase-plasmin(ogen) activator complex. Reprinted with permission from Bell WR, Sasahara AA (eds):* Review of Thrombolytic Therapy and Thromboembolic Disease. *Glenview, Illinois, Physicians & Scientists Publishing Co., Inc., 1989, p 12.*

the SK-plasminogen complex is gradually converted to the SK-plasmin form, which retains activator activity. In vivo, the fibrinolytic activity of SK has a half-life of about 18 to 25 minutes[17-19] and shows monophasic elimination. Streptokinase is believed to be cleared by the reticuloendothelial system.[20]

Plasmin, the active fibrinolytic enzyme generated by the SK-plasminogen activator complex, is a nonspecific proteolytic agent that can digest fibrin, fibrinogen, prothrombin, and clotting factors V and VIII. When it is formed on a fibrin surface (through activation of fibrin-bound plasminogen), fibrinolysis occurs; when formed in plasma, fibrinogenolysis occurs. Details of the fibrinolytic reaction catalyzed by the plasminogen activators are provided in Chapter 8. In contrast to agents such as tissue plasminogen activator (t-PA) and pro-urokinase, which require the presence of fibrin for optimal activity ("fibrin-specificity"),[21] streptokinase (like urokinase) has substantial activity in the absence of fibrin and therefore has an increased propensity to activate circulating plasminogen ("non-specific" lytic activity). Despite this "non-specificity" of enzymatic activity, SK-plasmin(ogen) is an effective thrombolytic because it binds avidly to forming and preformed clots through binding sites on the activator complex and, once in the presence of fibrin, displays exceptionally high enzymatic efficiency, exceeding that of urokinase, pro-urokinase, and even t-PA.[22] The generation of circulating fibrinogen degradation products and the depletion of circulating fibrinogen, manifestations of the "nonspecific" actions of SK, were once viewed as a liability (possibly increasing bleeding risk), but are now viewed as usually beneficial, providing a long-acting anticoagulant effect that promotes ongoing clot removal and reduces the risk of reocclusion. Regeneration of fibrinogen and other clotting factors by the liver requires about 1 to 2 days after SK administration is completed.

Because SK is a foreign protein, it is antigenic. To the extent that preformed antibody is present, SK is complexed immediately after administration and its effect is neutralized. The recommended doses of SK (eg, 1.5 million IU IV) are almost always greatly in excess of the amounts required to neutralize these antibodies.[23] Recent streptococcal infection or, especially, recent SK administration (within 6 to 12 months), however, may induce exceptionally high levels of antistreptococcal antibodies.[24] Because of the possibility of reduced therapeutic activity or allergic reactions after previous dosing due to neutralizing antibodies, SK readministration is probably best avoided between about 5 days and 1 to 2 years of initial use. If repeat thrombolysis is required during this time window, nonantigenic drugs such as t-PA or urokinase may be considered.

APPLICATION OF STREPTOKINASE IN ACUTE MYOCARDIAL INFARCTION

Extensive clinical trial experience with SK in AMI is now available. Evaluations of thrombolytic regimens in these trials have assessed the following endpoints: 1) coronary reperfusion or recanalization (defined by pre- and posttreatment angiography) and/or patency (defined by posttreatment angiography only); 2) left ventricular function and/or myocardial infarct size; and 3) mortality. Trial experience has included both uncontrolled observations and controlled comparisons with placebo (or non-thrombolytic) therapy and with other thrombolytic regimens. Safety comparisons between differing treatment regimens are of additional importance and have included the risk of hemorrhagic events, transfusion requirements, and, especially, life-threatening events such as intracranial hemorrhage. These extensive clinical trial results reviewed below support the use of SK-containing regimens as a primary treatment approach to AMI.

Intracoronary SK Use in AMI

Reperfusion studies with intracoronary SK

The feasibility of recanalizing acutely occluded infarct-related arteries with intracoronary (IC) SK was reported by Rentrop et al in 1979.[25] In 1981 several studies from both Europe and the United States provided detailed accounts of the feasibility, safety, and clinical outcome after IC SK administration given in doses of 1,000 to 8,000 IU/min in AMI.[26-31] This experience together with subsequent and controlled studies[32-37] demonstrated the ability of IC SK to establish or maintain perfusion within 60 to 90 minutes of initiating therapy in an average of about 70 to 75% of patients.[33] In contrast, when no thrombolytic therapy was given (ie, placebo or nitroglycerin was administered), reperfusion rates of only 10 to 15% were observed during 1 to 2 hours of angiographic observations.[35-37] In the largest single controlled study, the Western Washington Trial,[36] 250 patients with AMI were randomized after baseline angiography (at a mean of about 4.6 hours after AMI onset) to IC SK or nitroglycerin infusion. Early reperfusion was observed in 69% of patients treated with IC SK (4,000 IU/minute over 1 hour) and in only 12% of control patients (p < 0.001).

These early studies of IC SK were performed before a clear distinction between patency and reperfusion study designs was make and before blinded and semiquantitative grading (ie, Thrombolysis in Myocardial Infarction [TIMI] system[38]) was established and consistently used as a standard for evaluation. In two more recent and relatively large studies in which IC SK was used as a positive control, a strict reperfusion (recanalization) study design was used and blinded, TIMI perfusion assessments were made.[39,40] In the TEAM study,[39] Anderson et al observed reperfusion (advancement of TIMI grade 0 or 1 to grade 2 or 3 perfusion) in 60% of AMI patients (67 of 111) treated at a mean of 3.4 hours after symptom onset and assessed after a 60 minute infusion of IC SK (20,000 IU bolus followed by a 2,000 IU/minute infusion). Bonnier et al[40] observed reperfusion (similarly defined) in 68% of AMI patients (25 of 37) treated at a mean of 2.4 hours after symptom onset with IC SK (250,000 IU over 1 hour, or about 4,000 IU/minute) and assessed after 90 minutes. The higher success rates of about 75% reported in earlier studies[33] may be explained by the inclusion in some studies of patients with subtotal occlusions ("patency" design) and the use of less stringent criteria for the determination of success. Differing patient populations, differing dose rates and durations of SK therapy, and differing times to initiation of therapy after AMI onset and to assessment of outcome also may have contributed to differences in study results. Taking these factors into account, IC SK therapy may be expected to be successful in establishing perfusion in about 60-70% of patients treated with 2,000 to 5,000 IU/minute and reassessed after 60-90 minutes using a strict "reperfusion" definition and in about 70-80% of patients using a "patency" definition (ie, including AMI patients with initially incompletely occluded as well as those with completely occluded arteries) .

Cardiac functional outcome after IC SK

Anderson et al[34] first showed a functional benefit after IC SK within a randomized, controlled study design. Thrombolytic therapy achieved patency in 79% of the SK group of 24 patients and was associated with relief of ischemic pain and prevention of progression of heart failure compared with the group given only standard, non-thrombolytic coronary care (n = 26). Left ventricular ejection fraction was similar on the day of admission in both patient groups but diverged by an average of 7 percentage points by day 10 in favor of the SK group (46% vs. 39%, p < 0.01). Cardiac enzymes peaked significantly earlier after SK, and the peak of the cardiac isoenzyme LDH-1 release curve tended to be lower. The electrocardiogram (ECG) evolved rapidly after thrombolysis, with ST segment elevations quickly declining toward baseline. By the end of hospitalization, adverse ECG changes including residual ST elevation, R wave loss and Q wave development, were less in the intervention than in the control group. Serial echocardiographic evaluations of wall motion and convalescent thallium-201 perfusion studies of infarct size also showed better results in the intervention group. Favorable long-term (two-year) trends in morbidity and mortality were also observed after the strategy of IC SK and heparin, followed by aspirin and the selected use of bypass surgery.[41]

Concurrent controlled studies assessing ventricular function from Michigan[35] and Washington[36] failed to demonstrate a beneficial effect of IC SK on left ventricular function. A key difference between these studies and the Utah study[34] was the average time of therapy after symptom onset: 5.4 hours[35] and 4.6 hours[36] versus 3.9 hours.[34] The impact of time to therapy on functional outcome was further suggested by a subsequent review of other studies of IC and intravenous (IV) SK.[42,43] In at least 12 studies in which SK infusions were begun within an average of 4 hours of symptom onset, significant improvement in regional function in the infarct zone was consistently observed; improvement in global ejection fraction was also reported in nine of these studies. In contrast, among the six studies in which SK was administered after more than 4 hours, none showed a beneficial effect on global function, and regional wall motion improved in only one.

Mortality effects of IC SK

Evidence for a mortality benefit of IC SK in AMI is strongly suggestive but not as definitive as for IV SK, probably because of the smaller numbers of patients treated and the greater time delays associated with the IC application of therapy. The largest United States controlled trial of IC SK, the Western Washington Trial, first suggested a mortality benefit.[36] It entered 250 patients after angiographic documentation of coronary occlusion and randomized them to therapy with IC SK or nitroglycerin. Early (30-day) mortality was 3.7% in the IC SK group and 11.2% in the control group (p = 0.02). After one year, mortality was 8.2% and 14.7%, respectively (p = 0.1). Within the SK group, one-year mortality was 2.5% among those achieving initial reperfusion compared with 16.7% in those with partial or no reperfusion (p < 0.01). Thus, mortality after SK was improved only in those achieving reperfusion, suggesting reperfusion to be the mechanism for mortality reduction. An early Dutch study[44] in 533 patients also suggested a mortality benefit of IC SK compared with control both at one month (5.9% vs. 11.7%, p < 0.03) and one year (8.6% vs. 15.9%, p < 0.001), although the study results for IC SK were confounded in that IV SK was the initial therapy in the last 117 patients. Yusuf et al[45,46] performed an overview (meta-analysis) of all controlled trials of IC SK. Nine trials entering a total of about 1,000 patients were identified and analyzed. Pooling the results of these studies yielded an 18% mortality reduction in the treatment group; however, the 95% confidence intervals were broad (44% reduction to 19% increase) and the results not statistically significant.

In summary, intracoronary SK probably has beneficial effects on mortality in AMI, but the more definitive mortality results for IV SK and its greater ease of administration has led to virtual abandonment of the IC route of therapy except in limited circumstances (eg, when small-dose use is desired in patients with relative contraindications to IV SK and to primary angioplasty). The overall clinical application and outcome of IC SK are summarized in Table 1.

Intravenous SK Use in AMI

Intravenous SK has been extensively studied in AMI, leading to approval for this indication in 1987.

Table 1. *Summary of application and clinical outcome of IC SK for AMI*

Usual IC Dose	
Loading:	10,000-20,000 IU
Maintenance:	5,000 IU/min (range, 2,000 to 6,000); infuse for 60 minutes, or 30 minutes after coronary recanalization
Expected Reperfusion Success:	60-70% (at 60-90 minutes)
Expected Patency Success:	70-80% (at 90 minutes)
LV Functional Improvement:	Yes, if given in < 4 hours after AMI onset No, if given after > 4 hours
Mortality Reduction:	18% (C.I. −19% to 44%)
Hematologic Effects:	Systemic lytic effects (fibrinogenolysis) usually occur, but are dose-dependent, and less than for larger dose IV SK
Advantages:	Achievement of high local concentrations of drug with less systemic effect; higher early reperfusion rates than IV SK
Disadvantages:	Requirement of cardiac catheterization, with added time loss, expense and complexity of IC administration and limited patient access to therapy

Early studies

Preparations containing SK were first given intravenously in the late 1950s.[3,6-8,47,48] In a pioneering study published in 1958, Fletcher and colleagues[6] reported that among 24 treated patients, those treated early appeared to show clinical improvement, whereas late treatment did not seem to affect clinical outcome. Many additional trials, both small and large in scope, were conducted over the next 2 decades,[47-50] including at least 17 controlled trials reported between 1966 and 1979.[14,50] These trials did not have a major impact on the practice of cardiology for a number of reasons: 1) pathologists did not agree that coronary thrombosis was the cause of AMI; 2) accurate methods of assessing coronary artery perfusion, infarct size, and left ventricular functional outcome were not in clinical use and most individual studies were too small to establish mortality benefits; 3) therapy was often delayed until many hours after the onset of symptoms, until AMI was "confirmed;" and, 4) concerns about bleeding complications of thrombolytic therapy were increasing. However, Stampfer et al[50] found that by pooling the results of eight major trials of acceptable design involving 3,275 patients, a significant reduction (20%) in early mortality could be shown. Even better results were found (26% mortality reduction, $p \leq 0.01$) after excluding the two studies that allowed very late enrollment (up to 72 hours).

After the role of coronary thrombosis was established[51,52] and the feasibility but also the limitations of IC SK were realized, contemporary interest in IV SK was reawakened. A sentinel contemporary study was performed by Schroder et al in 1983.[53] Short-term, high-dose IV infusions of SK caused reperfusion within 1 hour in 52% of patients (11 of 21) studied angiographically. Early total patency rate was 62%, and late patency (after 3 weeks) was 84%. Reperfusion occurred more frequently when treatment was given in less than 4 hours (67% rate) versus greater than 4 hours after symptom onset (33% rate). Subsequent studies reported a wide range of patency rates (55%-96%) and a wide but lower range of angiographically determined reperfusion rates (31-62%).[42,43,54] As noted earlier, patency rates, determined angiographically only after therapy, are typically 10-20% higher than reperfusion rates (determined by pre- and posttreatment angiography), because this percentage of patients with AMI demonstrate at least partially patent arteries even before therapy.[51]

Controlled IV SK trials of reperfusion/patency

Controlled reperfusion/patency trials of SK have usually involved positively controlled comparisons, primarily versus IC SK, IV t-PA, or IV anistreplase. In comparison with IC SK, reperfusion/patency rates after IV application were found to be variably lower,[55,56] even though IV therapy could be given earlier, but functional outcome was found to be equivalent or better than after IC application.[55,57] In the TIMI-1 study,[38] 290 patients were randomized and treated with IV SK (1.5 million IU/1 hour) or with IV t-PA (100 mg/3 hours). Reperfusion, the primary endpoint, was achieved at 90 minutes in 31% of patients given SK compared with 62% given t-PA ($p < 0.001$). Patency rates after 90 minutes were 43% for SK compared with 70% for t-PA patients ($p < 0.001$). Reperfusion success after SK was significantly time-dependent: only 24% achieved reperfusion when treated more than 4 hours after symptom-onset compared with 44% when treatment was given in 4 hours or less.

A European Cooperative Study[58] in 128 patients assessed patency 90 minutes after IV SK (1.5 million IU/1 hour) or t-PA (0.75 mg/kg over 90 min). Patency was achieved in 55% of SK and 70% of t-PA patients ($p < 0.06$). A French study[59] compared patency 90 minutes after IV SK (1.5 million IU/1 hour) or anistreplase (30 U/5 min) in 107 patients. Patency was achieved in 51% of SK and 70% of anistreplase patients ($p \leq 0.05$). In a more recent comparison of SK with anistreplase (TEAM-2)[60] in 370 patients, therapy was given after a mean of 2.6 hours of symptoms and patency assessed a mean of 2.3 hours later. Streptokinase achieved an early patency rate of 73%, which was similar to anistreplase, while the residual percent stenosis was quantitatively slightly less than that for anistreplase. The European PRIMI trial[61] compared SK with pro-urokinase in 401 patients. Therapy was begun within 4 hours (mean, 2.3 hours) of onset of symptoms. Patency at 60 minutes was 48% for SK and 72% for pro-urokinase ($p < 0.001$). Patency at the 90 minute endpoint was achieved in 64% of SK and 71% of pro-urokinase patients ($p = 0.15$). At later angiography (at 24-36 hours), patency rates were 88% and 85%, respectively ($p = NS$).

In summary, controlled trials suggest that patency rates after IV SK depend significantly on the time to treatment and the time of assessment.[21,38,61] In contemporary practice, when therapy is given after a mean of about three hours of symptoms, 90 minute patency rates of about $60 \pm 10\%$ can be expected. Treatment late after symptom onset results in much lower early rates of patency, probably a manifestation of increased resistance of older, more crosslinked fibrin clots to the actions of SK.[4] In comparison with other thrombolytics, IV SK achieves patency more slowly than t-PA, pro-urokinase, and probably anistreplase, as manifested by lower 90 minute patency rates, but SK "catches up" by 2 to 24 hours, achieving stable, plateau patency rates of 75-85%, similar to those of other agents. The extent to which achieving slower but eventually comparable recanalization affects functional or mortality outcomes after SK in comparison with other thrombolytics is uncertain and must be assessed by direct studies comparing these endpoints (see below).

Effects of IV SK on ventricular function and infarct size

Several trials have assessed the impact of SK administered an average of < 4 hours from AMI onset on left ventricular function and infarct size.[42,62] In a Dutch randomized study in 533 patients, SK was given as either IC SK or IV SK followed, if needed, by IV SK at early angiography,[44] and compared with control therapy without thrombolysis. (Treatment was begun at a median of 3.3 hours after symptom onset and achieved eventual patency in 85% of patients.) Left ventricular ejection fraction was better by 4 to 5 percentage points after the thrombolysis strategy than after control therapy, both at discharge ($48 \pm 15\%$ vs. $44 \pm 15\%$, $p \leq 0.03$) and at three months (50% vs. 45%, $p \leq 0.002$).[63] Infarct size, estimated by release of the cardiac enzyme α-hydroxybutyric dehydrogenase, was reduced by 30%: 51% in those admitted to the study within 1 hour of symptom onset, 31% in those entered between 1 and 2 hours, and 13% for those entered between 2 and 6 hours.[64] The ISAM trial[65] randomized 1,741 patients within six hours of AMI (average about 3.3 hours) to treatment with IV SK (1.5 million IU/1 hour) plus heparin and aspirin, or to placebo. Infarct size, determined by integrating creatine kinase MB isoenzyme time-activity curves, was reduced by 16% when therapy was begun within 3 hours of symptom onset. At ventriculography, performed at 3-4 weeks in 848 patients, left ventricular ejection fraction was 3.1 points higher in the SK group (56.9 vs. 53.8%, p ≤ 0.005).

In a trial carried out in New Zealand, White et al[66] randomized 219 patients with AMI at a mean of 3.0 hours from symptom onset to receive either IV SK (1.5 million IU/30 min) or placebo. Contrast angiographic assessment at 3 weeks showed a 6 percentage point better left ventricular ejection fraction after SK than after placebo (59% vs. 53%, p < 0.005). Mortality was also reduced by SK therapy. In the Western Washington Intravenous SK Trial,[67] 368 patients were randomized to IV SK (1.5 million IU/1 hour) or to standard care. Treatment was given within 6 hours (mean, 3.5) of AMI onset. Ejection fraction, determined at 10-14 days, was 3.6 percentage points higher after SK (54.3% vs. 50.7%, p = 0.056).

Thus, reductions in infarct size averaging about 15 to 30% and improvements in convalescent resting left ventricular function averaging 3 to 6 percentage points follow IV SK therapy when it is given within an average of ≤ 3 to 4 hours after the onset of symptoms; very early therapy (within 1 hour) leads to substantially greater salvage (50% infarct size reductions), whereas functional benefit is usually not found for therapy given more than an average of 4 hours after symptom onset.[42,43]

Functional outcome after SK has also been directly compared with that after t-PA. White et al[68] randomized 270 patients with ≤ 3 hours of ischemic pain to IV SK (1.5 million IU/30 min) or t-PA (100 mg/3 hours). Concomitant therapy included IV heparin, aspirin, and dipyridamole. Left ventricular function was assessed by contrast ventriculography at three weeks in 240 patients. Ejection fraction was identical in both groups (58%). Similarly, in the TIMI-1 comparison of streptokinase and t-PA, radionuclide ventriculography at discharge, performed in 229 patients, showed no significant difference in global ejection fraction, although the late recruitment in that study (mean, 4.8 hours) detracts from the importance of the functional comparison. Recently, the functional as well as mortality outcomes after SK and t-PA, given with and without concomitant subcutaneous heparin, were reported from the large Italian randomized study in 12,490 patients, GISSI-2.[69] Segmental and global left ventricular function were assessed by echocardiography. There was no difference in any functional endpoint between groups, including clinical heart failure, ejection fraction ≤ 35%, or myocardial segment injury ≥ 45%. Thus, the differences in the kinetics of coronary artery reperfusion between SK and t-PA, discussed above, do not appear to be translated into significant differences in left ventricular functional outcome.

Effects of IV SK on mortality

A wealth of clinical trial data have now firmly documented the beneficial effects of IV SK on postinfarction mortality. As reviewed by Yusuf et al,[45,46,62] at least 31 randomized trials of IV SK involving about 41,000 patients with suspected AMI have been reported in the past 25 years. An overview of all of these trials indicates that early mortality (at 2 to 5 weeks) is reduced by an average of 24% (odds reduction), from 12.8% to 10.0%. The 95% confidence interval for the mortality reduction is from 20% to 29%. About 25,000 patients were treated within 6 hours from symptom onset. In these patients, mortality reductions averaged 26%, with a confidence interval of 20% to 32%. Further review suggests that these benefits are maintained for at least 1 to 2 years.[70-72]

A pivotal mortality study in the current thrombolytic era was the ambitious Italian Group Study (GISSI).[70] In GISSI, the mortality effects of IV SK (1.5 million IU/1 hour) were compared with standard care in 11,806 patients entered within 12 hours of the onset of symptoms of suspected AMI. Overall, a risk reduction of 18% (or odds reduction of 19%) was observed at 21 days; mortality was 10.7% in the SK group compared with 13.0% in the control group (p < 0.002). Effects on relative mortality risk were also time dependent; they were not significant for treatment begun after 6 hours, but averaged 23% (p < 0.005) for therapy given within 3 hours, and impressively, 47% (p < 0.002) for treatment begun within 1 hour of symptom onset (Figure 3). For patients given therapy within 6 hours, an overall mortality benefit of 23% (odds reduction) was observed. A follow-up report by the Italian Study Group confirmed that the differences in mortality established by treatment within the first 3 weeks after AMI were maintained for at least 1 to 2 years.[71]

The Second International Study of Infarct Survival (ISIS-2)[72] is the most important single thrombolytic mortality trial to date. ISIS-2, coordinated in the United Kingdom, entered 17,187 patients in 417 hospitals within 24 hours (median, 5 hours) of the

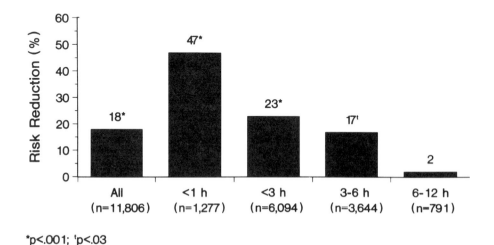

*p<.001; ʼp<.03

Figure 3. *Summary of mortality effects of IV SK from the GISSI-1 study. Data from reference 70, with permission.*

onset of suspected AMI into a double-blind, double-randomized study of 1) IV SK (1.5 million IU/1 hour) vs. placebo; and 2) oral aspirin (160 mg/day) vs. placebo. Vascular mortality was assessed at five weeks. Streptokinase alone and aspirin alone each yielded significant mortality benefits (Figure 4). Streptokinase reduced mortality by 25% (odds reduction), p < 0.0001; aspirin reduced mortality by 23% (p < 0.0001). The benefits of SK and aspirin were also additive; their combination yielded a mortality reduction of 42%, significantly better than that of either agent alone (p < 0.0001). As in GISSI, mortality effects in ISIS-2 were time dependent, although less so. Streptokinase reduced mortality by 43% when given within 1 hour of ischemic symptoms, 35% when given within 4 hours, and 17% when given between 5 and 24 hours (Figure 4). The benefit after 5 hours, although modest, was still significant (p ≤ 0.004). Impressively, when SK and aspirin were both given and treatment was begun within 4 hours, mortality was reduced by 53%. Differences in vascular and all-cause mortality produced by SK and aspirin remained highly significant after a median follow-up of 15 months.[72]

ISIS-2 was large enough to assess the effects of thrombolytic therapy in several AMI subgroups in which the benefits of therapy had been questioned based on inadequate or contradictory data from previous trials. These subgroups included the elderly (aged > 70 years old), inferior infarction patients, late-presenting (at > 4-6 hours) AMI patients, patients with previous AMI, females, and patients presenting with either hypotension or hypertension. Each of these subgroups benefitted from therapy in ISIS-2.[72] In no subgroup did SK have an adverse effect, although those presenting

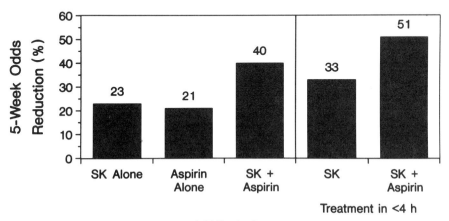

* n=17,187 patients with symptoms of AMI <24 h.

Figure 4. *Summary of key mortality results from the ISIS-2 study. Data from reference 72, with permission.*

with electrocardiographic ST segment depression showed no benefit. In ISIS-2, SK was associated with an excess of bleeding events requiring transfusions and with cerebral hemorrhage, but the incidence of these was very low, and, interestingly, the overall rate of strokes actually was lower. The modest excess risk of reinfarction after SK was avoided by the addition of aspirin.

Comparative mortality effects among thrombolytic agents

Because of differences in study design and patient populations, direct comparative trials are required to establish relative superiority of one thrombolytic agent over another. The first of these direct comparative trials, the GISSI-2/International Study, was recently published.[73] In this randomized study, therapy with SK (1.5 million IU/1 hour) was compared with t-PA (alteplase, 100 mg/3 hours), each with aspirin and with or without heparin, in 20,891 patients. Mortality at two weeks was similar in the two groups: 8.5% (SK) vs. 8.9% (t-PA), p = NS (Figure 5). The risk of stroke was slightly but significantly less after SK (0.9% vs. 1.3%), as was the risk of minor bleeding, but the risk of major bleeding events was slightly greater (0.9% vs. 0.6%). Heparin, begun 12 hours after the initiation of t-PA or SK and given subcutaneously (12,500 U q12 h) tended to benefit patients given SK but not t-PA. However, the heparin regimen has been criticized as suboptimal adjunctive therapy, especially for t-PA,[74] both because of the delay in its initiation and the dose and route of its application (subcutaneous instead of IV). For this reason, GISSI-2 has not been universally accepted as a defin-

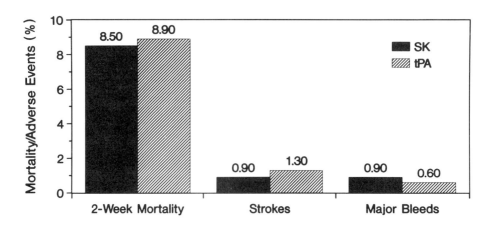

Figure 5. *Summary of key outcomes from the GISSI-2/International Study. Adapted from references 69 and 73*

itive comparison of SK with t-PA. The clinical application and outcome after IV SK are summarized in Table 2.

CONCOMITANT AND ADJUNCTIVE THERAPIES TO SK IN AMI

In general, other medications commonly used in AMI may be used in combination with SK. Specifically, nitroglycerin, β-blockade, aspirin, heparin, and lidocaine have been used safely and effectively together with thrombolytic therapy. Angioplasty and surgery have also been commonly performed for clinical indications after SK with acceptable safety.

Nitroglycerin

Prior to the thrombolytic era, nitroglycerin infusions were tested for potential beneficial effects on AMI morbidity and mortality. Although individual trials gave variable results, an overview of all randomized trial suggests benefit:[46] among 10 trials recruiting about 2,000 patients, mortality was reduced by 35% (95% confidence intervals, 18% to 49%). In the thrombolytic era, Rentrop et al specifically tested the effects of combining nitroglycerin infusions with IC SK in AMI in two randomized studies.[37,75] In the second, more definitive study,[75] a total of 393 patients were recruited and treated after a mean of 6.3 hours of symptoms with IC SK (2,000 IU/minute), IC nitroglycerin (0.01 mg/min), both, or neither (placebo), each given for a minimum of 75 minutes and for an additional 30 minutes after recanalization, for a maximum of 120 minutes. A significant beneficial interaction between SK and nitroglycerin was observed, resulting in a significant increase in ejection fraction (of 3.9 percentage points) only in the combined treatment arm (p < 0.001). Specifically, patients with collateral flow to an initially occluded coronary artery showed significant functional benefit with SK therapy, despite the late initiation of therapy, and this effect was potentiated by nitroglycerin. Thus, nitroglycerin, in addition to its known beneficial hemodynamic effects, may augment reperfusion-related improvement in myocardial function after SK and may extend the time-window of opportunity for achieving a beneficial functional effect in some patients.

Beta-blockers

Beta-blockade was tested extensively after AMI in the prethrombolysis era. Chronic oral therapy, begun during convalescence, was clearly shown to be of benefit.[46] Subsequently, trials of acute β-blocker therapy, usually beginning with IV administration, were undertaken. An overview of 27 of these trials in about 27,000 patients indicated a small but significant benefit (13% mortality reduction, 95% confidence interval 2% to 25%).[46] In ISIS-2, SK and SK plus aspirin resulted in approximately the same

Table 2. *Summary of application and clinical outcome of IV SK for AMI*

Usual IV Dose:	1.5 million IU infused over 1 hour
Expected Reperfusion Success:	50 ± 15% (at 90 minutes)
Expected Patency Success:	60 ± 10% (at 90 minutes) 75-85% (at 4 to 24 hours and beyond)
Functional Improvement (Therapy in < 4 hours):	
Increase in LV ejection fraction: Decrease in infarct size:	3 to 6 percentage points 15 to 30%
Mortality Reduction:	24% (C.I. = 20 to 29%)
If therapy given in < 6 hours: If given with aspirin:	26% (C.I. = 20 to 32%) 42%
Hematologic Effects:	Marked systemic lytic effects (fibrinogenolysis)
Advantages of IV Dosing:	Easy and rapid applicability; well-studied mortality benefits
Disadvantages of IV Dosing:	Lower (slower) rates of early reperfusion/ patency than IC

percentage mortality reductions in patients in whom IV β-blocker therapy was planned as in other patients.[72] Also, mortality after SK plus aspirin was 6.8% in patients receiving IV β-blockade and 8.1% in those not receiving β-blockade. However, this difference may have been due to patient selection bias (ie, selecting lower-risk patients for therapy), because the comparison with β-blocker therapy was not randomized. In the TIMI-2 study, a randomized comparison of immediate (IV followed by oral meto-prolol) versus delayed β-blockade was undertaken.[76] Immediate β-blockade reduced recurrent ischemic events and reinfarctions. Although t-PA was the thrombolytic used in TIMI-2, it appears reasonable to assume that a similar favorable interaction exists between acute β-blockade, given to appropriately selected patients, and thrombolysis with SK.

Aspirin

Clinical trials have confirmed a beneficial effect of aspirin, which has important antiplatelet effects, on morbidity and mortality in patients with unstable angina and with recent MI.[46,62] In patients with AMI, ISIS-2[72] demonstrated that oral aspirin (160 mg/day) reduces mortality when given alone (odds reduction 23%, p < 0.0001) and provides added benefit when combined with SK (odds reduction 42%, p < 0.0001). The five-week vascular mortality for combined aspirin and SK therapy was 8.0%, compared with 13.2% in patients receiving neither agent. Mortality reductions for aspirin, unlike SK, were largely independent of the time of treatment when begun within 24 hours of AMI. The prevention by aspirin of the excess rate of reinfarction after SK may explain in part its beneficial mechanism of action. Fortunately, the rate of serious adverse reactions, including major hemorrhagic events, did not appear to be significantly increased. The GISSI-2/International Study[69,73] provided an additional large, although uncontrolled clinical experience of combined aspirin and SK therapy. In GISSI-2, a similar low mortality rate was observed for patients receiving combined aspirin and SK therapy (8.5%) as was seen in ISIS-2 (8.0%). Based on these data, the routine use of aspirin (160-325 mg/day, beginning immediately and continuing indefinitely — at least for 6-12 weeks) together with SK for AMI is indicated, except in aspirin allergic or intolerant patients.

Heparin

The utility of routinely coadministering heparin with SK (and aspirin) is being definitively tested in the ISIS-3 study. Previous clinical study experience suggests an additional modest overall benefit for adjunctive heparin therapy, even though minor bleeding is increased. In ISIS-2,[72] cardiovascular mortality was 10.1% after SK without planned heparin, 9.0% after SK plus subcutaneous (SC) heparin, and 8.3% after SK plus planned IV heparin. After SK plus aspirin, these rates were 9.6% (no heparin), 7.6% (SC heparin), and 6.4% (IV heparin). Because the use of heparin was not randomized, these trends are suggestive but not definitive of benefit. In a pilot study preceding GISSI-2 (SCATI[77]), AMI patients receiving SK were also randomly assigned to receive SC heparin (n = 218) or no heparin (n = 215); aspirin was not given. Mortality was 4.5% in the heparin group versus 8.8% in the control group (p = 0.05). In the full-scale trial,[69,73] mortality after SK plus aspirin was 7.9% in the group (n = 5,101) randomized to SC heparin (12,500 U q12 h, beginning after 12 hours) and 9.2% in the control group (n = 5,205). The difference in favor of heparin was nominally significant but was interpreted cautiously.

Support for the use of IV heparin beginning simultaneously with IV SK has recently been provided.[78] The rationale for simultaneous use derives from the paradoxical increase in thrombin activity that has been observed during fibrinolytic therapy and its potential to impede thrombolysis. In a randomized trial in 39 patients, Melandri et al[78] found that *simultaneous* IV heparin reduced the estimated time to reperfusion after SK and reduced enzymatic infarct size as compared with heparin given after SK. In summary, SC or IV heparin may add modestly to the benefit of SK plus aspirin, associated with a modest[73] to moderate[65] excess risk of bleeding, based on incomplete trial data; additional important information will be forthcoming in the ISIS-3 and GUSTO trials.

Angioplasty and Surgery after SK

Angioplasty and coronary bypass surgery have frequently been performed for clinical indications at variable times after SK administration. In the authors' experience, if due consideration is given to the patient's hematologic status, these procedures may be performed with acceptable safety and with a favorable outcome.[34,39,57,60,79] It should be added that no benefit has been shown for the early (2 hours to 2 days) prophylactic use of angioplasty after the use of either fibrin selective[76,80] or non-selective[81] thrombolysis in well-designed trials. In a single controlled trial using SK, Erbel et al[82] randomized 162 AMI patients to receive SK alone (IC plus supplemental IV dosing) (group 1), or SK together with immediate coronary angioplasty (group 2). Reperfusion rates were 90% (group 1) versus 86% (group 2). In-hospital reocclusion rates were 20% (group 1) and 14% (group 2). Global ejection fraction was the same in both groups; regional wall motion improved in group 2 patients with anterior AMI. The results with combined IC SK and angioplasty were interpreted favorably by the authors, but are not regarded as providing compelling evidence for routinely adding angioplasty to SK, now usually given IV.

OTHER CARDIOVASCULAR APPLICATIONS OF SK

Other accepted cardiovascular indications for SK include acute pulmonary embolism, deep venous thrombosis, peripheral arterial thrombosis and embolism, and clotted external dialysis shunts.[4] In acute massive pulmonary embolism, SK may be administered as a 250,000 IU loading dose followed by an infusion of 100,000 IU/hour for 24 hours. In controlled studies, such therapy has been shown effective in reducing hemodynamic instability and improving pulmonary capillary perfusion.[83,84] In acute deep venous thrombosis, SK may be administered as a loading dose of 250,000 U, followed by an infusion of 100,000 IU/hour for up to 72 hours, until adequate venous blood flow is restored, as measured by noninvasive techniques. The rationale for use of SK within 1-2 days (maximum, 7-10 days) of onset of venous thrombosis is to rapidly resolve underlying thrombus and preserve venous valvular function, preventing later development of dependent venous insufficiency and its consequences.[85,86] SK may be used in a standard IV infusion regimen for therapy of thrombotic and embolic occlusion of peripheral arteries and grafts.[4] As in other conditions, SK works better on fresh clots (occlusion of < 48 hours duration) and when partial rather than complete occlusion is present. Local application through a vascular catheter, placed near the occluding clot, has become increasingly popular as an alternative to full-dose IV therapy. In this way, higher local concentrations of SK-activator complex can be achieved using lower infusion rates. The duration of therapy is tailored to the therapeutic response.

ADVERSE REACTIONS AND SAFETY ASSESSMENTS

The major safety concerns with SK include bleeding events (as with all thrombolytic agents), allergic reactions, and hypotension (Table 3).

Bleeding

Bleeding after thrombolytic therapy is now believed to be caused primarily by lysis of hemostatic plugs at sites of previous invasive procedures or internal vascular injury.[21] Depletion of circulating fibrinogen, although contributing to bleeding severity and duration, is probably not as important a factor as previously believed, as evidenced by the approximately similar bleeding risk with t-PA, a more fibrin-selective agent.[38,69,73,87] Bleeding occurs most frequently at cutaneous sites of vascular invasion, but serious although much less common events may occur internally, including intracranial hemorrhage. The reported incidence of bleeding varies widely. This may be due to a number of factors, including 1) variable thresholds for reporting; 2) variable use of invasive procedures; 3) differing doses and durations of therapy; 4) differing concomitant medical therapy (aspirin, heparin, etc.); 5) differing characteristics of patients studied (eg, age, blood pressure, gender, etc.); and 6) varying degrees of ascertainment (ie, ascertainment may be greater for small, carefully studied and single center trials; much less for very large, multicenter trials).

Table 3. *Summary of adverse reactions with IV SK*

Event	Percentage of patients at risk
Hemorrhage (any):	
1) Noninvasive studies	5-10%
2) Invasive studies	15-30%
Serious hemorrhage	2% (range, 1 to 4%)
Intracranial hemorrhage	$\leq 0.5\%$
Potential allergic reaction	2 to 5%
Anaphylaxis	$\leq 0.3\%$
Clinical hypotension	2 to 10% (usually transient)

Taking these factors into account, a general literature review and personal experience[60] suggests the following approximate risk of bleeding events after IV SK for AMI, using current protocols: 1) any drug-related hemorrhagic event: 5-10% for treatment without invasive procedures; 15-30% for treatment followed by or together with invasive procedures (ie, angiography, angioplasty); 2) serious hemorrhage (potentially life-threatening if untreated, requiring transfusions), 2% (range, 1-4%); and 3) intracranial hemorrhage, $\leq 0.5\%$. Intracranial hemorrhage, a devastating event, usually causes disability and may be fatal in up to half of cases; risk factors may include advanced age and hypertension.[88]

A few statistics from controlled trials on bleeding rates are useful. In the invasive TIMI-1 trial,[38] SK led to greater fibrinogen depletion than t-PA, as expected (57% vs. 26% reductions from control concentrations).[87] However, the incidence of any bleeding events (SK = 31%, t-PA = 33%) and of patients receiving transfusions (SK = 20%, t-PA = 22%) was similar.[87] In the TEAM-2 study,[60] which included delayed (1 day) catheterization, bleeding risk could be compared for SK (1.5 million U) and anistreplase (30 U, equivalent to 1.1 million SK U). Fibrinogen depletion was only slightly greater for SK than anistreplase, and bleeding events attributed to therapy (18% vs. 20%) and severe events (4% vs. 4%) occurred with similar frequency in both groups. The lower incidence of bleeding reported in such large trials as GISSI-1,[70] ISIS-2,[72] and GISSI-2[69,73] may be due, at least in part, to under-reporting, but these trials, especially the blinded ones such as ISIS-2 and ISIS-3, can give an estimate of *relative* bleeding rates of different regimens. In ISIS-2,[72] for example, bleeding, including intracranial hemorrhage, was somewhat higher after SK, but total stroke rate was similar after SK and placebo (about 1%), probably because of offsetting effects of SK on thrombotic and hemorrhage strokes. In GISSI-2,[69,73] stroke was slightly lower after SK (0.9%) than t-PA (1.3%), especially in the elderly (aged > 70 years).

The management of bleeding usually includes local measures and volume replacement.[89] Adjustment in dose or discontinuation of lytic therapy or heparin may need to be considered. Occasionally, blood products are required. Only rarely are antifibrinolytic agents such as aminocaproic acid (Amicar) needed. The risks of bleeding may increase as the duration of therapy increases, as for prolonged infusions for deep venous thrombosis or pulmonary embolism.[4] The risk decreases for lower dose rates and durations, such as for intracoronary regimens.[39]

Allergy

As a foreign antigen SK may provoke allergic reactions. However, these reactions are relatively uncommon and usually mild. Reactions that are possibly or presumably allergic in nature include mild-moderate fevers, chills/rigors, urticaria/rashes, flushing, pruritus, nausea/vomiting, and musculoskeletal pain. Because many of these reactions are common and nonspecific, they may be caused by something other than true allergy. Potentially allergic reactions occur with a reported incidence of about 2-5%.[60,73] Management is usually symptomatic and may include antihistamines and steroids. Prophylactic use of these medications has been advised by some, but the authors believe such routine use is unnecessary.[39,60,90] In GISSI-2,[69,73] SK and t-PA, which is a human recombinant protein and presumably nonantigenic, were directly compared in a large population. As expected, potentially allergic reactions were reported significantly more frequently after SK (1.7% incidence) than after t-PA (0.2%), but the incidence was still low. In contrast to allergic reactions, anaphylactoid reactions have been distinctly rare, with a reported incidence of $\leq 0.3\%$. Prompt therapy for these reactions usually leads to recovery.

Hypotension

In a canine model,[91] bolus injections of SK led to rapid and marked (50%) reductions in blood pressure that correlated with abrupt generation of the potent vasodilators plasmin and bradykinin in the circulation. In clinical studies, administration of SK at rates of > 750,000 IU/30 minutes has also been noted to cause transient hypotension in a significant percentage of patients (up to 30-50%),[92-94] with maximum effect at 15 minutes after instituting therapy.[92] During administration of a conventional SK dose of 1.5 million IU over 1 hour, mean blood pressure may be expected to decrease by an average of about 10 mm Hg, reaching a maximal effect by about 20 minutes.[60] In the blinded TEAM-2 study,[60] hypotension believed to be drug-related was reported in 8% of patients receiving SK compared with 5% receiving anistreplase. In the large but uncontrolled GISSI-2 study,[73] hypotension was reported in a small but significantly greater percentage of patients receiving SK (3.8%) compared with t-PA (1.7%). In summary, in clinical practice using recommended dosing, clinical hypotension due to SK may occur but is generally mild and managed easily, and mild reductions in blood pressure may be theoretically beneficial in many patients.

CONTRAINDICATIONS

Suggested contraindications to thrombolytic therapy, developed at an early NIH consensus conference,[14,95] are shown in Table 4. These contraindications are often relative rather than absolute and continue to evolve with greater clinical experience, especially for the short-term, high-dose regimens used in AMI.

DOSAGE AND ADMINISTRATION

For AMI, SK is generally given by short-term, high-dose IV infusion. The approved dose is 1.5 million IU infused over 1 hour. The drug preparation and administration protocol is summarized in Table 5. More rapid infusion (ie, over 30 minutes) has also been used,[66,68] but the risk of hypotension may be higher.

CONCLUSION

Short-term, high-dose IV streptokinase clearly provides effective thrombolysis in AMI, leading to substantial reductions in morbidity and mortality with an acceptable safety profile when used in appropriately selected patients. A summary of its comparative advantages and disadvantages as a thrombolytic agent is given in Table 6.

Table 4. *Absolute and relative contraindications to thrombolytic therapy*

ABSOLUTE:	1. Active internal bleeding
	2. Recent cerebrovascular accident (within 2 months) or other active intracranial process
RELATIVE: **Major**	1. Recent (within 10 days) major surgery, obstetric delivery, organ biopsy, prior puncture of noncompressible blood vessels
	2. Recent serious gastrointestinal bleeding
	3. Recent serious trauma
	4. Severe arterial hypertension (≥ 200 mm Hg systolic or ≥ 100 mm Hg diastolic)
Minor	1. Recent minor trauma including cardiopulmonary resuscitation
	2. High likelihood of left heart thrombus (mitral disease with atrial fibrillation)
	3. Bacterial endocarditis
	4. Hemostatic defects (including those associated with hepatic and renal disease)
	5. Pregnancy
	6. Age > 75 years
	7. Diabetic hemorrhagic retinopathy

Adapted from Sherry et al[95]

Table 5. *Protocol for IV administration of streptokinase*

1. Confirm that inclusion/exclusion criteria for AMI therapy are met.

2. Give aspirin, 162 to 325 mg immediately (chew), then a daily oral dose.

3. Consider optional premedication (ie, diphenhydramine ± hydrocortisone).

4. Add 5 mL of physiologic sterile saline or 5% dextrose to vial of 1.5 million IU of lyophilized SK. Dissolve gently, avoiding shaking and foaming the solution.

5. Further dilute solution to ≥ 45 mL with diluent (saline or dextrose).

6. Administer by infusion pump at constant rate over 60 minutes.

7. The use of heparin has varied, but many patients have received IV heparin to maintain PTT at 1.5 to 2 times upper limit of normal for 1 to 7 days. Therapy usually begins within 1 to 2 hours of infusion; initial rate may be about 1,000 U/hour.

Table 6. *Relative advantages and disadvantages of IV SK compared with other agents*

Advantages of SK:

Well-studied

Inexpensive

Non-fibrin specificity yields added anticoagulant effect*

Low reocclusion risk

Excellent mortality reduction if given with aspirin

Disadvantages of SK:

Allergic/antigenic potential

Hypotension risk

Lower, slower rates of reperfusion (especially if given at > 4 hours)

---

* Formerly viewed as a disadvantage

REFERENCES

1. Tillet WS, Garner RL: The fibrinolytic activity of streptococci. J Exp Med 1933;58:485-502.

2. Christensen LR, MacLeod M: Streptococcal fibrinolysis: a proteolytic reaction due to a serum enzyme activated by streptococcal fibrinolysin. J Gen Physiol 1945;28:363-383; 559-583.

3. Sherry S: Personal reflections on the development of thrombolytic therapy and its application to acute coronary thrombosis. Am Heart J 1981;102(part 2):1134-1139.

4. Sherry S: Streptokinase, in Messerli FH (ed): *Cardiovascular Drug Therapy*. Philadelphia, WB Saunders Co, 1990, pp 1479-1494.

5. Tillet WS, Sherry S: The effect in patients of streptococcal fibrinolysin (streptokinase) and streptococcal desoxyribonuclease on fibrinous, purulent, and sanguinous pleural exudations. J Clin Invest 1949;28:173-190.

6. Fletcher AP, Alkjaersig N, Smyrniotis FE, et al: The treatment of patients suffering from early myocardial infarction with massive and prolonged streptokinase therapy. Trans Assoc Am Physicians 1958;71:287-296.

7. Fletcher AP, Alkjaersig N, Sherry S: The maintenance of a sustained thrombolytic state in man. I. Induction and effects. J Clin Invest 1959;38:1096-1110.

8. Fletcher AP, Sherry S, Alkjaersig N, et al: The maintenance of a sustained thrombolytic state in man. II. Clinical observations on patients with myocardial infarction and other thromboembolic disorders. J Clin Invest 1959;38:1111-1119.

9. Castellino FJ, Sodetz JM, Brockway NJ, et al: Streptokinase. Methods Enzymol 1976; 45:244.

10. Jackson KW, Tang J: Complete amino acid sequence of streptokinase and its homology with serine proteases. Biochemistry 1982;21:6220.

11. McEvoy GK, McQuarrie GM, Dipietro-Heydorn J (eds): *Drug Information 87*. Thrombolytic agents. American Society of Hospital Pharmacy, Bethesda, Md, 1987, pp 700-705.

12. Barlow GH: Pharmacology of fibrinolytic agents. Prog Cardiovasc Dis 1979;21:315-326.

13. Enzymes, choleretics and other digestive agents, in Wade A, Reynolds JEF, Prasad AB (eds): *Martindale: The Extra Pharmacopoeia*. London, Pharmaceutical Press, ed 28, 1982, pp 644-661.

14. Sharma GVRK, Cella G, Parisi AF, et al: Thrombolytic therapy. N Engl J Med 1982;306:1268-1276.

15. Marder VJ: Pharmacology of thrombolytic agents: implications for therapy of coronary artery thrombosis. Circulation 1983;68:I-2.

16. Oliven A, Gidron E: Orally and rectally administered streptokinase. Investigation of its absorption and activity. Pharmacology 1981;22:135-138.

17. Nunn B, Esmail A, Fears R, et al: Pharmacokinetic properties of anisoylated plasminogen streptokinase activator complex and other thrombolytic agents in animals and in humans. Drugs 1987;33(suppl 3):88-92.

18. Staniforth DH, Smith RAG, Hibbs M: Streptokinase and anisoylated streptokinase plasminogen complex. Their action on haemostasis in human volunteers. Eur J Clin Pharmacol 1983;24:751-756.

19. Mentzer RL, Budzynski AZ, Sherry S: High-dose, brief-duration intravenous infusion of streptokinase in acute myocardial infarction: description of effects in circulation. Am J Cardiol 1986;57:1220-1226.

20. Gonias SL, Einarsson M, Pizzo SV: Catabolic pathways for streptokinase, plasmin, and streptokinase activator complex in mice. J Clin Invest 1982;70:412-423.

21. Marder VJ, Sherry S: Thrombolytic therapy: current status. N Engl J Med 1988;318: 1512-1520;1585-1594.

22. Ferres H: Pre-clinical pharmacological evaluation of Eminase (APSAC). Drugs 1987;33 (suppl 3):33-50.

23. Brogden RN, Speight TM, Avery GS: Streptokinase: a review of its clinical pharmacology, mechanism of action and therapeutic uses. Drugs 1973;5:357-445.

24. Hoffman JJML, Fears R, Bonnier JJRM, et al: Significance of antibodies to streptokinase in coronary thrombolytic therapy with streptokinase of APSAC. Fibrinolysis 1988;2:203.

25. Rentrop P, Blanke H, Karsch KR, et al: Acute myocardial infarction: intracoronary application of nitroglycerin and streptokinase in combination with transluminal recanalization. Clin Cardiol 1979;2:354-359.

26. Rentrop P, Blanke H, Karsch KR, et al: Selective intracoronary thrombolysis in acute myocardial infarction and unstable angina pectoris. Circulation 1981;63:307-317.

27. Ganz W, Buchbinder N, Marcus H, et al: Intracoronary thrombolysis in evolving myocardial infarction. Am Heart J 1981;101:4-14.

28. Mathey DG, Kuck K-H, Tilsner V, et al: Nonsurgical coronary artery recanalization in acute transmural myocardial infarction. Circulation 1981;63:489-499.

29. Reduto LA, Smalling RW, Freund BC, et al: Intracoronary infusion of streptokinase in patients with acute myocardial infarction: effects of reperfusion on left ventricular performance. Am J Cardiol 1981;48:403-409.

30. Merx W, Dorr R, Rentrop P, et al: Evaluation of the effectiveness of intracoronary streptokinase infusion in myocardial infarction: postprocedure management and hospital course in 204 patients. Am Heart J 1981;102:1181.

31. Markis JE, Malagold M, Parker JA, et al: Myocardial salvage after intracoronary thrombolysis with streptokinase in acute myocardial infarction. N Engl J Med 1982;305:777.

32. Laffel GL, Braunwald E: Thrombolytic therapy: a new strategy for the treatment of acute myocardial infarction. N Engl J Med 1984;311:710-717;770-776.

33. Anderson JL: Principles of thrombolytic therapy: intracoronary administration, in Anderson JL (ed): *Acute Myocardial Infarction: New Management Strategies.* Rockville, MD, Aspen Press, 1987, pp 157-184.

34. Anderson JL, Marshall HW, Bray BE, et al: A randomized trial of intracoronary streptokinase in the treatment of acute myocardial infarction. N Engl J Med 1983;308:1312-1318.

35. Khaja F, Walton JA, Brymer JF, et al: Intracoronary fibrinolytic therapy in acute myocardial infarction. Report of a prospective, randomized trial. N Engl J Med 1983;308:1305-1311.

36. Kennedy JW, Ritchie JL, Davis KB, et al: Western Washington randomized trial of intracoronary streptokinase in acute myocardial infarction. N Engl J Med 1983;309: 1477-1482.

37. Rentrop KP, Feit F, Blanke H, et al: Effects of intracoronary streptokinase and intracoronary nitroglycerin infusion on coronary angiographic patterns and mortality in patients with acute myocardial infarction. N Engl J Med 1984;311:1457-1463.

38. Chesebro JH, Knatterud G, Roberts R, et al: Thrombolysis in myocardial infarction (TIMI) trial, phase I: a comparison between intravenous plasminogen activator and intravenous streptokinase. Circulation 1987;76:142-154.

39. Anderson JL, Rothbard RL, Hackworthy RA, et al, for the APSAC Multicenter Investigators: Multicenter reperfusion trial of intravenous anisoylated plasminogen streptokinase activator complex (APSAC) in acute myocardial infarction: controlled comparison with intracoronary streptokinase. J Am Coll Cardiol 1988;11:1153-1163.

40. Bonnier HJRM, Visser RF, Klomp HC, Hoffmann HJML, and the Dutch Invasive Reperfusion Study Group: Comparison of intravenous anisoylated plasminogen streptokinase activator complex and intracoronary streptokinase in acute myocardial infarction. Am J Cardiol 1988;62:25-30.

41. Anderson JL, McIlvaine PM, Marshall HW, et al: Long-term follow-up after intracoronary streptokinase for myocardial infarction: a randomized, controlled study. Am Heart J 1984;108:1402-1407.

42. Spann JF, Sherry S: Coronary thrombolysis for evolving myocardial infarction. Drugs 1984;28:465-483.

43. Anderson JL: Streptokinase and acylated streptokinase: biochemical properties and clinical effects, in Topol EJ (ed): *Acute Coronary Intervention*. New York, Alan R Liss, Inc, 1988, pp 3-23.

44. Simoons ML, Serruys PW, van den Brand M, et al: Improved survival after early thrombolysis in acute myocardial infarction. Lancet 1985;2:578-582.

45. Yusuf S, Collins R, Peto R, et al: Intravenous and intracoronary fibrinolytic therapy in acute myocardial infarction: overview of results on mortality, reinfarction and side effects from 33 randomized controlled trials. Eur Heart J 1985;6:556-585.

46. Yusuf S, Wittes J, Friedman L: Overview of results of randomized clinical trials in heart disease. I: treatments following myocardial infarction. JAMA 1988;260:2088-2093.

47. Richter IH, Musacchio F, Clifton EE, et al: Experiences with clot-lysing agents in coronary thrombosis. Am J Cardiol 1960;6:534.

48. Boucek RJ, Murphy WP Jr: Segmental perfusion of the coronary arteries with fibrinolysin in man following a myocardial infarction. Am J Cardiol 1960;6:525-533.

49. European Cooperative Study Group for Streptokinase Treatment in Acute Myocardial Infarction: Streptokinase in acute myocardial infarction. N Engl J Med 1979;301:797-802.

50. Stampfer MJ, Goldhaber SZ, Yusuf S, et al: Effect of intravenous streptokinase on acute myocardial infarction: pooled results from randomized trials. N Engl J Med 1982;307:1180-1182.

51. DeWood MA, Spores J, Notske R, et al: Prevalence of total coronary occlusion during the early hours of transmural myocardial infarction. N Engl J Med 1980;303:897-902.

52. Davis MJ, Thomas AC: Plaque fissuring: the cause of acute myocardial infarction, sudden ischaemic death, and crescendo angina. Br Heart J 1985;53:363-373.

53. Schroder R, Biamino G, Leitner ER, et al: Intravenous short-term infusion of streptokinase in acute myocardial infarction. Circulation 1983;67:536-548.

54. Anderson JL: Intravenous thrombolysis and other antithrombotic therapy, in Anderson JL (ed): *Acute Myocardial Infarction: New Management Strategies*. Rockville, MD, Aspen Press, 1987, pp 185-217.

55. Rogers WJ, Mantle JA, Hood WP, et al: Prospective randomized trial of intravenous and intracoronary streptokinase in acute myocardial infarction. Circulation 1983;68:1051-1061.

56. Alderman EL, Jutzy KR, Berte LE, et al: Randomized comparison of intravenous versus intracoronary streptokinase for myocardial infarction. Am J Cardiol 1984;54:14-19.

57. Anderson JL, Marshall HW, Askins JC, et al: A randomized trial of intravenous and intracoronary streptokinase in patients with acute myocardial infarction. Circulation 1984; 70:606-618.

58. Verstraete M, Bernard R, Bory M, et al: Randomized trial of intravenous recombinant tissue-type plasminogen activator versus intravenous streptokinase in acute myocardial infarction. Lancet 1985;1:842-847.

59. Pacouret G, Charbonnier B, for the IRS II Study: Multicentre European randomized trial of anistreplase versus streptokinase in acute myocardial infarction. Circulation 1989;80(suppl II):II-420.

60. Anderson JL, Sorensen SG, Moreno FL, et al, for the TEAM-2 Study Investigators: Multicenter patency trial of intravenous anistreplase compared with streptokinase in acute myocardial infarction. Circulation 1991;83:126-140.

61. PRIMI Trial Study Group: Randomized double-blind trial of recombinant pro-urokinase against streptokinase in acute myocardial infarction. Lancet 1989;1:863-867.

62. Yusuf S, Sleight P, Held P, McMahon S: Routine medical management of acute myocardial infarction. Lessons from overviews of recent randomized controlled trials. Circulation 1990;82(suppl II):II-117-II-134.

63. Serruys PW, Simoons ML, Suryapranta H, et al: Preservation of global and regional left ventricular function after early thrombolysis in acute myocardial infarction. J Am Coll Cardiol 1986;7:729-742.

64. Simoons ML, Serruys PW, van den Brand M, et al: Early thrombolysis in acute myocardial infarction: limitation of infarct size and improved survival. J Am Coll Cardiol 1986; 7:717-728.

65. ISAM Study Group: A prospective trial of intravenous streptokinase in acute myocardial infarction (ISAM). Mortality, morbidity, and infarct size at 21 days. N Engl J Med 1986;14:1465-1471.

66. White HD, Norris RM, Brown MA, et al: Effect of intravenous streptokinase on left ventricular function and early survival after acute myocardial infarction. N Engl J Med 1987;317:850-855.

67. Kennedy JW, Martin GV, Davis KB, et al: The Western Washington intravenous streptokinase in acute myocardial infarction randomized trial. Circulation 1988;77:345-352.

68. White HD, Rivers JT, Maslowski AH, et al: Effect of intravenous streptokinase as compared with that of tissue type plasminogen activator on left ventricular function after first myocardial infarction. N Engl J Med 1989;320:817-821.

69. Gruppo Italiano per lo Studio della Sopravvivenza nell'Infarto Miocardico: GISSI-2: a factorial randomised trial of alteplase versus streptokinase and heparin versus no heparin among 12,490 patients with acute myocardial infarction. Lancet 1990;336:65-70.

70. Gruppo Italiano per lo Studio della Streptochinasi nell' Infarcto Miocardico (GISSI): Effectiveness of intravenous thrombolytic treatment in acute myocardial infarction. Lancet 1986;1:397-401.

71. GISSI Study Group: Long-term effects of intravenous thrombolysis in acute myocardial infarction: final report of the GISSI study. Lancet 1987;2:871-874.

72. ISIS-2 Collaborative Group: Randomized trial of intravenous streptokinase, oral aspirin, both, or neither among 17,187 cases of suspected acute myocardial infarction: ISIS-2. Lancet 1988;2:349-360.

73. The International Study Group: In-hospital mortality and clinical course of 20,891 patients with suspected acute myocardial infarction randomised between alteplase and streptokinase with or without heparin. Lancet 1990;336:71-75.

74. White HW: GISSI-2 and the heparin controversy. Lancet 1990;336:297-298.

75. Rentrop KP, Feit F, Sherman W, et al: Serial angiographic assessment of coronary artery obstruction and collateral flow in acute myocardial infarction. Report from the second Mount Sinai-New York University Reperfusion Trial. Circulation 1989;80:1166-1175.

76. The TIMI Study Group: Comparison of invasive and conservative strategies after treatment with intravenous tissue plasminogen activator in acute myocardial infarction: results of the Thrombolysis in Myocardial Infarction (TIMI) Phase II trial. N Engl J Med 1989;320:618-626.

77. SCATI Group: Randomized, controlled trial of subcutaneous calcium-heparin in acute myocardial infarction. Lancet 1989;2:182-186.

78. Melandri G, Branzi A, Semprini F, et al: Enhanced thrombolytic efficacy and reduction of infarct size by simultaneous infusion of streptokinase and heparin. Br Heart J 1990; 64:118-120.

79. Anderson JL, Battistessa SA, Clayton PD, et al: Coronary bypass surgery early after thrombolytic therapy for acute myocardial infarction. Ann Thorac Surg 1986;41:176-183.

80. The TIMI Research Group: Immediate vs delayed catheterization and angioplasty following thrombolytic therapy for acute myocardial infarction. TIMI II A results. JAMA 1988; 260:2849-2858.

81. de Bono DP for the SWIFT Investigator Group: Should we intervene following thrombolysis? The SWIFT study of intervention versus conservative management after anistreplase thrombolysis. Eur Heart J 1989;10:253 (abstract 1318).

82. Erbel R, Pop T, Henrichs K-J, et al: Percutaneous transluminal coronary angioplasty after thrombolytic therapy: a prospective controlled randomized trial. J Am Coll Cardiol 1986; 8:485-495.

83. Sharma GTRK, Burleson VA, Sasahara AA: Effect of thrombolytic therapy on pulmonary capillary blood volume in patients with pulmonary embolism. N Engl J Med 1980; 303:842-845.

84. Dalen JE, Alpert JS: Natural history of pulmonary embolism, in Sasahara AA, Sonnenblick EH, Lesch M (eds): *Pulmonary Emboli*. New York, Grune & Stratton, 1975, pp 77-88.

85. Goldhaber SZ, Buring JE, Lipnick RJ, et al: Pooled analyses of randomized trials of streptokinase and heparin in phlebographically documented deep venous thrombosis. Am J Med 1984;76:393-397.

86. Immelman EJ, Jeffery PC: The post phlebitic syndrome. Pathophysiology, prevention and management. Clin Chest Med 1984;5:537-550.

87. Rao AK, Pratt C, Berke A, et al: The thrombolysis in myocardial infarction (TIMI) trial, phase II: hemorrhagic manifestations and changes in plasma fibrinogen and fibrinolytic system. J Am Coll Cardiol 1988;11:1-11.

88. Anderson JL, Karagounis L, Allen A, et al: Age and systolic hypertension are risk factors for intracranial hemorrhage after thrombolysis. Circulation 1990;82(suppl 2):II-431.

89. Sane DC, Califf RM, Topol EJ, et al: Bleeding during thrombolytic therapy for acute myocardial infarction: mechanisms and management. Ann Intern Med 1989;111:1010-1022.

90. AIMS Trial Study Group: Long-term effects of intravenous anistreplase in acute myocardial infarction: final report of the AIMS study. Lancet 1990;335:427-431.

91. Green J, Dupe RJ, Smith RAG, et al: Comparison of the hypotensive effects of streptokinase (human)-plasmin activator complex and BRL 26921 (p-anisoylated streptokinase-plasminogen activator complex) in the dog after high dose bolus administration. Thromb Res 1984;36:29-36.

92. Lew AS, Laramee P, Cercek B, et al: The hypotensive effect of intravenous streptokinase in patients with acute myocardial infarction. Circulation 1985;72:1321-1326.

93. Hall GH: Bolus streptokinase after myocardial infarction. Lancet 1987;2:96-97.

94. Köhler M, Hellstern P, Doenecke P, et al: High-dose systemic streptokinase and acylated streptokinase-plasminogen complex (BRL 26921) in acute myocardial infarction: alterations of the fibrinolytic system and clearance of fibrinolytic activity. Haemostasis 1987;17:32-39.

95. Sherry S, Bell WR, Duckert FH: Thrombolytic therapy in thrombosis. A National Institutes of Health consensus development conference. Ann Intern Med 1980;93:141-144.

215

Chapter 11

TISSUE PLASMINOGEN ACTIVATOR IN ACUTE MYOCARDIAL INFARCTION

Michael J. Attubato
Frederick Feit

STRUCTURE AND FUNCTION OF TISSUE PLASMINOGEN ACTIVATOR

Although multiple enzymes and factors are involved in the thrombolytic system, the most important enzyme involved in physiologic fibrinolysis is a direct activator: a tissue-type plasminogen activator (t-PA). Tissue plasminogen activator is a serine protease that converts the inactive proenzyme plasminogen to plasmin, an active fibrinolytic enzyme capable of degrading fibrinogen, fibrin, and clotting factors V, VIII, and XIII. Native t-PA, synthesized primarily by vascular endothelial cells,[1,2] is found in the blood in trace concentrations.[3,4] It is one of two plasminogen activators present in the plasma, the other being urokinase.

Tissue plasminogen activator (Figure 1) is synthesized as a single-chain polypeptide of 527 amino acids with a molecular weight of approximately 70,000.[5] It can be converted into a two-chain form by cleavage of a peptide bond by endogenous proteases, including plasmin. Both the one- and two-chain forms have enzymatic activity and similar plasminogen activating properties.[6] The two-chain form consists of a carboxy terminal light chain with the active serine protease domain and an amino terminal heavy chain which contains the two kringle domains.[7] The kringle domains, which are present in several other serine proteases involved in coagulation and fibrinolysis including plasminogen, prothrombin, and urokinase, contain the lysine binding sites responsible for the high affinity of t-PA for fibrin.[8] Through the formation of a cyclic ternary complex,[9] both plasminogen and t-PA bind to fibrin via their lysine binding sites, markedly enhancing the ability of t-PA to convert plasminogen to plasmin. The Michaelis-Menten constant for plasminogen activation by t-PA is decreased from 65 M to 0.16 M in the presence of fibrin,[9] indicating that t-PA has much greater

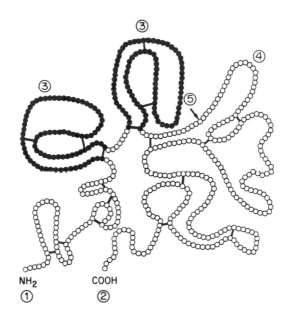

Figure 1. *Tissue plasminogen activator. ① Amino terminal end of heavy ② Carboxy terminal end of light chain ③ Kringle domains ④ Active serine protease domain ⑤ Peptide bond (cleavage at this site generates the double-chain form which consists of a heavy chain and a light chain linked by a single disulfide bond) ⎯ = Disulfide bonds*

affinity for fibrin-bound plasminogen than for free circulating plasminogen. This allows for the preferential activation of plasminogen on the fibrin clot. This fibrin specificity is not absolute, however, and with large pharmacologic doses of t-PA, conversion of plasminogen to plasmin also occurs in the plasma resulting in some systemic fibrinolysis.

The presence of circulating inhibitors of plasmin further limits the extent of systemic fibrinolysis. These inhibitors are present in plasma and inhibit plasmin directly (α_2-antiplasmin)[10] and indirectly by inhibiting the action of t-PA on plasminogen (plasminogen activator inhibitors 1 and 2).[11,12] Plasmin present in the circulating blood is rapidly inhibited by α_2-antiplasmin,[13] providing its lysine binding sites and active proteolytic site are not occupied. When plasmin is bound to fibrin, its lysine binding sites are occupied and inactivation does not occur. As long as free circulating plasmin is inactivated by α_2-antiplasmin, systemic fibrinolysis will not occur. However, when this inhibitor is depleted, fibrinogen and blood coagulation factors V, VIII, and XIII will be degraded by plasmin. Therefore, high infusion rates of t-PA, which raise its plasma concentration to approximately 1000 times the baseline level,[14] cause

218

systemic fibrinolysis to occur, although still to a lesser degree than the systemic fibrinolysis produced by non-fibrin specific thrombolytic agents.

ISOLATION, SYNTHESIS AND INITIAL USE OF TISSUE PLASMINOGEN ACTIVATOR

Plasminogen activators were first identified in 1947 when tissue slices were shown to lyse plasminogen-containing fibrin.[15] In 1980 purified t-PA was isolated, first from human uterine tissue[16] and subsequently from human melanoma cells,[17,18] and produced in sufficient quantities to allow for its further characterization. Human t-PA cDNA was then cloned and expressed in *E. coli*,[5] and ultimately recombinant t-PA (rt-PA) was produced in quantities sufficient for clinical use. The first clinical application of rt-PA was its successful use in two patients with renal vein thrombosis.[19] Tissue plasminogen activator was first administered to patients with AMI in 1983 when Van de Werf et al[20] administered melanoma-derived rt-PA to 7 patients with evolving myocardial infarction and demonstrated coronary thrombolysis within 50 minutes in 6 of them, without depletion of plasminogen, fibrinogen or α_2-antiplasmin. The first multicenter study[21] of recombinant tissue plasminogen activator (rt-PA) confirmed its efficacy in the lysis of coronary artery thrombi, as acute recanalization of a totally occluded infarct-related artery occurred within 90 minutes of therapy in 25 of 33 patients (76%). The initial clinical trials were performed using a predominantly double-chain (95% double-chain) form of rt-PA, while later studies were done with the currently commercially available form of rt-PA, which is 70%-80% single-chain. The same dose of the predominantly single-chain form will result in a 35% lower plasma concentration than the double-chain form.[22]

RATIONALE FOR THROMBOLYTIC THERAPY WITH rt-PA

An occlusive coronary artery thrombus can be demonstrated in 70%-80% of patients with AMI who present within six hours of pain onset and have electrocardiographic evidence of ST-segment elevation.[23,24] Experiments assessing sudden coronary occlusion in anesthetized animals demonstrate myocardial necrosis within 20 minutes in the subendocardial region with extension towards the subepicardium as the occlusion persists.[25,26] Injury is irreversible within three hours and complete within six hours of total occlusion. Recanalization of the occluded artery within this time period can result in the salvage of acutely ischemic but viable myocardium.[27]

The time window for myocardial salvage in patients with AMI may be longer in those patients with preexisting collateral channels[28] and in those with intermittent or incomplete obstruction. Recanalization of an occluded coronary artery may also have benefits other than clinically measurable myocardial salvage, such as prevention of infarct expansion and aneurysm formation[29] or prevention of late arrhythmias.[30] Given the high morbidity and mortality of AMI, large-scale clinical trials were undertaken to assess the potential beneficial effects of rt-PA on coronary artery patency, left ventricular function, and survival and its potential risks including hemorrhagic complications and reinfarction. These large prospective trials have served a pivotal role in defining the subsets of patients with AMI who derive the greatest benefit and those at the greatest risk from the administration of rt-PA. Furthermore, they have clarified the role of adjuvant pharmacologic therapy and other interventions such as percutaneous transluminal coronary angioplasty (PTCA).

EFFECT OF THE INTRAVENOUS ADMINISTRATION OF rt-PA ON CORONARY ARTERY PATENCY

Evaluating the effects of rt-PA on coronary artery thrombosis requires a clear understanding of the definitions of coronary artery recanalization (reperfusion) and patency. Recanalization refers to the restoration of complete antegrade flow in a coronary artery that had been demonstrated to be totally occluded by angiography performed prior to the initiation of treatment. Patency refers to antegrade flow in a vessel following treatment, with or without knowledge of the status of the vessel prior to treatment. Patency rates will generally be higher than reperfusion rates, since arteries which were not totally occluded prior to therapy will be included. Patency rates obtained days following therapy will tend to be even higher due to spontaneous fibrinolysis over time.

The restoration of patency of an occluded coronary artery is the immediate goal of thrombolytic therapy. Angiographic studies following rt-PA have established infarct vessel patency rates of 61%-84% after 60 to 120 minutes of therapy[31-44] (Table 1). Overall, a patency rate of 75% was obtained with the predominantly single-chain form presently in use when treatment was initiated a mean of 3.0 hours after the onset of symptoms of infarction. This compares favorably with patency rates of 60%-80%[45-49] achieved with intracoronary streptokinase and exceeds the angiographically confirmed rates of 10%-62%[50] seen early (90 minutes) after intravenous streptokinase.

Phase I of the Thrombolysis in Myocardial Infarction (TIMI) Trial[32] sponsored by the National Heart, Lung, and Blood Institute was designed to compare the efficacy of rt-PA and streptokinase on coronary artery reperfusion during AMI. Patients aged less than 76 years with at least 30 minutes of ischemic chest pain and 1 mm ST-segment elevation in two contiguous electrocardiographic leads were eligible, if they presented within seven hours of pain onset. Patients were randomly assigned to receive either streptokinase 1.5 million IU intravenously over one hour or 80 mg rt-PA intravenously (predominantly double-chain preparation given as 40 mg over the first hour and 20 mg over each of the next two hours). The primary end point was recanalization, with

Table 1. *Infarct vessel patency 60-120 minutes after treatment with tissue plasminogen activator for acute myocardial infarction*

Trial	Mean time to treatment (hours)	Number of patients	Number patent	Percent patent
		C–2		
TIMI-I Pilot[31]	4.8	47	35	74
TIMI-I[32]	4.8	143	100	70
ECSG (rt-PA/SK)[33]	3.0	61	43	70
ECSG (rt-PA/Placebo)[34]	3.4	62	38	61
ECSG Maintenance[35]	2.5	119	78	66
TAMI-1 Pilot[36]	3.8	38	32	84
Gold et al[37]	—	29	24	83
TOTAL	3.7	499	350	70
		C–1		
Johns et al[38]	—	68	52	76
ECSG (Acute PTCA)[39]	2.6	51	39	76
TIMI-II Pilot[40]	3.0	33	27	82
TIMI-IIA[41]	2.8	193	145	75
Topol et al, Multicenter[42]	3.6	71	49	69
TAMI-1[43]	3.0	386	288	75
TAMI-3[44]	2.8	131	104	79
TOTAL	3.0	933	704	75

C-2 = the predominantly double-chain preparation of rt-PA used in early clinical trials; C-1 = the currently used predominantly single-chain preparation of rt-PA
TIMI = Thrombolysis in Myocardial Infarction Trial; ECSG = European Cooperative Study Group, rt-PA/SK – randomized trial of tissue plasminogen activator vs. streptokinase, rt-PA/Placebo – randomized trial of tissue plasminogen activator vs. placebo; TAMI = Thrombolysis and Angioplasty in Myocardial Infarction

TIMI 2 or 3 flow 90 minutes following initiation of therapy, of a vessel that was totally occluded prior to therapy (Table 2).[32,51] The time from symptom onset to the initiation of therapy was relatively long (4.8 hours) due to the performance of pre-treatment angiography. Successful reperfusion at 90 minutes occurred in 62% of patients with baseline TIMI 0 or 1 flow treated with rt-PA in contrast to only 31% treated with streptokinase (p < 0.001). A patent infarct-related artery with perfusion

Table 2. *Definitions of perfusion in the TIMI trial*

Grade 0 (no perfusion): No antegrade flow beyond the point of occlusion.

Grade 1 (penetration without perfusion): Contrast material passes beyond the area of obstruction but fails to opacify the distal coronary bed.

Grade 2 (partial perfusion): Contrast material passes through the obstruction and opacifies the coronary bed distal to the obstruction, but the rate of entry of contrast into the distal vessel and its clearance are slower than that of nonstenosed vessels.

Grade 3 (complete perfusion): Contrast material promptly enters the coronary bed distal to the obstruction and clears as rapidly as nonstenosed vessels.

grade 2 or 3 at 90 minutes was present in 70% of patients treated with rt-PA and 45% of those treated with streptokinase (p < 0.001). In addition, recanalization rates with rt-PA were higher at 30 minutes (24% vs. 8%) and at 60 minutes (48% vs. 23%) than those with streptokinase therapy. The efficacy of rt-PA was relatively constant whether or not treatment was initiated within four hours of symptom onset, while that of streptokinase decreased dramatically when treatment was initiated after four hours.

The European Cooperative Study Group (ECSG) performed a similar study[33] in which patients were treated with either 1.5 million IU streptokinase intravenously over 90 minutes or 0.75 mg/kg rt-PA intravenously over 90 minutes. Pre-treatment angiography was not performed, thereby decreasing the delay from symptom onset to treatment to approximately three hours. Coronary angiography performed 75-90 minutes after the initiation of therapy revealed a patency rate of 70% in the rt-PA patients and 55% in the streptokinase patients (p = 0.054).

When the data of the TIMI Phase I trial and the ECSG trial are pooled,[52] it is clear that whether or not treatment is administered within three hours of symptom onset, rt-PA results in a higher incidence of infarct vessel patency than does streptokinase 90 minutes following the initiation of therapy (Table 3). These results establish the superiority of rt-PA over streptokinase in achieving rapid recanalization of acutely occluded coronary arteries.

The new predominantly single-chain preparation of rt-PA appears to result in patency rates that are comparable to the double-chain preparation used in TIMI I and the early ECSG trials (Table 1). Patency rates of 75-82% were obtained when angiography was performed 60 to 120 minutes after therapy with the new rt-PA preparation.[38,40-44] Angiography 18-48 hours after rt-PA therapy in Phase II of the TIMI trial[53] (the details of which will be described in the section on elective PTCA) revealed a patent infarct vessel in 85% of cases, with no difference in patency using

Table 3. *Incidence of patency after therapy with tissue plasminogen activator (rt-PA) or streptokinase (SK), according to the time interval from symptom onset to treatment*

	n	Patency rates (%)		P value
		rt-PA	SK	
< 3 hours				
ECSG	64	79	57	0.06
TIMI	34	85	52	0.06
Combined	98	81	55	< 0.01
> 3 hours				
ECSG	58	63	54	0.51
TIMI	255	69	40	< 0.001
Combined	313	67	42	< 0.001

n = number of patients treated with rt-PA or SK
Patency rates were determined 75-90 minutes after the onset of therapy in ECSG and 90 minutes after the onset of therapy in TIMI.
ECSG = European Cooperative Study Group; TIMI = Thrombolysis in Myocardial Infarction Trial
Adapted from Chesebro et al[52]

either 100 mg or 150 mg of this preparation. Other studies in which angiography was delayed for several days after the infarction demonstrated high patency rates ranging from 70% to 81%[54-58] (Table 4).

EFFECTS OF rt-PA ON LEFT VENTRICULAR FUNCTION

Extensive data from prospective, randomized, placebo-controlled trials demonstrate that treatment with rt-PA results in an improvement in left ventricular function.[54-56,59,60] In patients who received rt-PA, ejection fraction increased by an average of 5-6 points compared to the control groups (Table 5). While improvement was greatest in patients with anterior infarction, a benefit was also seen in those with inferior infarction.[54,56,59] Patients who received rt-PA also had a decrease in the prevalence of congestive heart failure[59] and a decrease in end-systolic volume,[60] which has been shown to be an important determinant of survival following myocardial infarction.[61] Although these studies demonstrate that left ventricular function is preserved when

Table 4. *Infarct vessel patency after treatment with tissue plasminogen activator (rt-PA): results with delayed angiography*

Trial	n	Time of angiography	Infarct Vessel Patency (%)		
			rt-PA	Control	SK
TIMI-II[53]	1458	18-48 h	85	—	—
NHF[54]	125	7 d	70	41	—
TPAT[55]	59	9 d	75	56	—
TICO[56]	131	21 d	81	63	—
New Zealand[57]	270	21 d	76	—	75
PAIMS[58]	152	4 d	81	—	74

n = number of patients in whom coronary artery patency was assessed at the specified time; d = day; h = hour; SK = streptokinase
TIMI-II = Thrombolysis in Myocardial Infarction Trial - Phase II; NHF = National Heart Foundation of Australia; TPAT = Tissue Plasminogen Activator: Toronto; TICO = Thrombolysis in Acute Coronary Occlusion; PAIMS = Plasminogen Activator Italian Multicenter Study

Table 5. *Left ventricular function in placebo-controlled trials of tissue plasminogen activator (rt-PA) in acute myocardial infarction*

Trial	n	Mean time to treatment (hours)	Time of eval. (day)	Method	Ejection Fraction (%)		P value
					rt-PA	Placebo	
Johns Hopkins[59]	117	3.2	10	Nuclear	53.2	46.4	< 0.02
NHF[54]	103	3.3	5-7	Cath	57.7	51.7	0.04
ECSG[60]	577	2.9	10-22	Cath	50.7	48.5	*
TPAT[55]	104	3.0	9	Nuclear	53.6	47.8	0.017
TICO[56]	126	1.9	21	Cath	61.0	54.0	0.006

n = number of patients in whom left ventricular function was assessed at the specified time
* = Statistically significant, no p value given
NHF = National Heart Foundation of Australia; ECSG = European Cooperative Study Group; TPAT = Tissue Plasminogen Activator: Toronto; TICO = Thrombolysis in Acute Coronary Occlusion

patients are treated with rt-PA early in the course of an AMI, the improvement by only several ejection fraction points is somewhat disappointing. Because global ejection fraction is dependent on multiple factors including the loading conditions of the ventricle and the presence and degree of hyperkinesis of non-infarct segments, it may not precisely assess the degree of myocardial preservation. End point data are also frequently missing, since patients who expire or are critically ill do not undergo analysis of left ventricular function during the post-intervention period.

Improvement in left ventricular function also results from treatment with intravenous streptokinase,[62-64] and a substantial difference between the two agents regarding this end point has not been demonstrated.[57,58] Thus, although early arterial patency occurs more frequently with rt-PA than streptokinase, no conclusive evidence indicates that this results in greater myocardial preservation.

EFFECTS OF rt-PA ON MORTALITY

Treatment with rt-PA early in the course of AMI results in a marked reduction in mortality, with the greatest benefit seen when therapy is initiated early (Table 6). The Anglo-Scandinavian Study of Early Thrombolysis[65] (ASSET) demonstrated a 26% reduction in mortality within one month in more than 5,000 patients treated with rt-PA. The beneficial effect was similar regardless of whether patients were treated within 3 hours or between 3 and 5 hours from symptom onset. Another smaller study not designed to be a definitive mortality trial,[60] the European Cooperative Study Group, also demonstrated a survival benefit with rt-PA treatment (Table 6). In Phase II of the TIMI trial, a mortality rate of only 4.9% within 42 days was observed in

Table 6. *Mortality rates in placebo-controlled trials of tissue plasminogen activator (rt-PA) in acute myocardial infarction*

Trial	No. of patients	Time to treatment (hours)	Period of follow-up (days)	Mortality (%) rt-PA	Mortality (%) Control	Percent reduction
ASSET[65]	5011	0-5	30	7.2	9.8	26
		< 3		8.1	10.9	26
ECSG[60*]	721	0-5	14	2.8	5.7	51
		< 3		1.1	6.3	82
		0-5	30	5.1	7.9	36
		< 3		3.4	8.2	59

ASSET = Anglo-Scandinavian Study of Early Thrombolysis; ECSG = European Cooperative Study Group
* Not planned with sufficient power to be a definitive mortality trial

patients who were randomized to either invasive or conservative strategies in conjunction with drug treatment.[53] Treatment with intravenous streptokinase also results in a decreased mortality rate following AMI. In the GISSI trial, overall hospital mortality at 21 days was 10.7% in streptokinase recipients compared to 13.0% in control patients, an 18% reduction.[66] In the Second International Study of Infarct Survival (ISIS-2), vascular mortality (deaths attributed to cardiac, cerebral, hemorrhagic, other vascular, or unknown causes) within five weeks of the infarct decreased from 12.0% in the control group to 9.2% in patients who received streptokinase, a 25% reduction.[67]

The International t-PA/SK Mortality Trial (which included GISSI II) assessed in-hospital mortality in 20,891 patients with AMI who were randomly assigned to receive either rt-PA (100 mg over 3 hours) or streptokinase (1.5 million IU over 30-60 minutes).[68] The patients in this study were also randomly assigned to receive either subcutaneous heparin (12,500 units twice daily starting 12 hours after thrombolytic therapy) or no anticoagulation. The in-hospital mortality was 8.9% in the patients who received rt-PA and 8.5% in the patients who received streptokinase, a difference which was not statistically significant. There was also no significant difference in the mortality rate of the patients who received subcutaneous heparin compared to those who did not.

The mortality data from this trial should be interpreted in light of the fact that the early administration of intravenous heparin with rt-PA therapy appears to be necessary to maintain coronary artery patency once recanalization has occurred (see section on adjuvant therapy with heparin), although it might also increase the risk of bleeding.

HEMORRHAGIC COMPLICATIONS

The only significant side effect of rt-PA therapy is bleeding. The initial promise that its relative fibrin specificity would markedly decrease the incidence of bleeding compared to that seen with the other thrombolytic agents has not been fulfilled. The fibrin specificity of rt-PA is not absolute; the extent of systemic fibrinogen degradation is proportional to the dose administered.[22,69] Even if its fibrin specificity was absolute, rt-PA cannot be expected to distinguish between coronary artery thrombi and protective vascular hemostatic plugs, potentially resulting in internal hemorrhage or bleeding at sites of trauma or vascular puncture. Most patients treated with rt-PA also receive concomitant therapy with heparin and aspirin, increasing the likelihood of bleeding.

Absolute and relative contraindications have been adopted for the use of rt-PA. Approximately 15%-20% of patients screened for thrombolytic therapy are excluded on the basis of a contraindication.[65] The absolute contraindications are a bleeding disorder or diathesis, a recent history of cerebrovascular disease, recent head trauma, and refractory severe hypertension. Relative contraindications are recent surgery or trauma, prolonged cardiopulmonary resuscitation, acute hypertension unresponsive to therapy, diabetic hemorrhagic retinopathy, or warfarin therapy. Data are scarce on the actual risk of bleeding in many of these conditions.

Several clinical factors have also been associated with an increased risk of hemorrhagic complications following rt-PA therapy. These include older age, female sex, low body weight, a history of hypertension, and the use of invasive procedures such as coronary artery bypass surgery, PTCA, and intra-aortic balloon counterpulsation.[70]

The risk of bleeding after therapy with rt-PA or streptokinase is similar.[33,71] When acute angiography is performed, the primary bleeding site is the catheterization or other vascular access site in the majority of patients. The incidence of gastrointestinal, genitourinary, retroperitoneal, or intracranial bleeding is low after therapy with either agent. The incidence of bleeding is similar despite the finding from the TIMI I trial that plasma fibrinogen levels decreased by about 25% in patients treated with rt-PA and about 50% in those treated with streptokinase.[71] The percentage of patients whose serum fibrinogen fell below 100 mg/dL was also markedly lower with rt-PA therapy.

In Phase II of the TIMI trial, the incidence of major hemorrhagic events in patients treated with 100 mg of rt-PA was 5.5% and the blood transfusion rate was 4.4%.[72] The patients who underwent routine angiography and PTCA for suitable anatomy 18-48 hours following rt-PA therapy ("invasive strategy") had a slightly higher incidence of major bleeding compared to those assigned to a "conservative strategy" without routine angiography (6.9% vs. 4.1%, p < 0.01).

The most serious complication of rt-PA therapy has been intracranial hemorrhage. Careful patient selection is necessary to minimize its incidence. The overall incidence of stroke after myocardial infarction has not increased with the advent of thrombolytic therapy, due to the decreased incidence of thrombotic and embolic strokes.[73] In fact, the incidence of stroke was been about the same in the ASSET rt-PA and placebo groups.[65]

The risk of intracranial hemorrhage after rt-PA therapy is dose-related. The administration of 150 mg over 6 hours to over 1000 patients in the TIMI studies resulted in intracranial hemorrhage in 1.6% of patients. This led to a protocol change in which the dose was decreased to 100 mg over 6 hours.[74] In over 3000 patients treated with this dose the incidence of intracranial hemorrhage was 0.5% (p < 0.01).[75] Whether the incidence of hemorrhagic stroke can be decreased further is unknown.

Intracranial hemorrhage usually presents in the first several days following therapy, with most cases occurring within the first 24 hours. Any change in the patient's neurologic status should prompt the immediate discontinuation of both rt-PA and anticoagulant therapy. An immediate computerized tomographic scan of the head should be obtained. Further treatment with fresh frozen plasma, protamine, epsilon-aminocaproic acid (a specific plasminogen activator inhibitor) and platelets can be given if needed.

Efforts should be made to minimize the bleeding complications associated with rt-PA. Patient selection is the initial and most important step in decreasing the risk of serious bleeding. Invasive procedures such as immediate angiography and PTCA, intra-aortic balloon counterpulsation, arterial puncture for blood gases, and percutaneous cannulation of the subclavian or internal jugular veins should be avoided if possible. Blood pressure should be well controlled. With proper patient selection and these precautions, the risk of serious bleeding can be minimized.

Other Side Effects

The infusion of rt-PA has been well tolerated with other side effects occurring infrequently. Since rt-PA is a physiologic protein, the occurrence of allergic and pyrogenic reactions and significant hypotension has been low. Antibodies against rt-PA are not detected when serum is tested two weeks after therapy, allowing for its repeated administration.[76]

REOCCLUSION

The importance of thrombolytic therapy lies not only in achieving early coronary artery recanalization to limit myocardial necrosis, but also in maintaining long-term vessel patency. The ruptured atherosclerotic plaque present in most cases of AMI remains a strong stimulus for platelet aggregation and thrombus formation, even after successful thrombolysis has occurred.[77] Early trials with rt-PA reported angiographically documented reocclusion rates of 24%-45%;[31,32,37] however, these studies often used lower doses of rt-PA or heparin and had small numbers of patients. The incidence of angiographically documented reocclusion in recent trials using larger doses of rt-PA and/or heparin with or without angioplasty ranges between 10%-15%.[38,39,41,43]

Several angiographic factors appear to be associated with an increased risk of reocclusion. The presence of a residual thrombus,[78] a post-treatment residual stenosis 75%,[78] TIMI grade 2 (incomplete) perfusion,[79] intermittent patency during acute angiography,[79] and a minimal cross-sectional area mm^2 are each associated with an increased risk of early rethrombosis.[80] Rethrombosis also appears to be inversely related to the degree of systemic fibrinolysis and to the steady-state plasma concentration of rt-PA.[22]

Reocclusion of the infarct related-artery is often not accompanied by a clinical event, due either to improved collateral flow, the lack of sufficient viable myocardium to cause symptoms, or intermittent patency. Most episodes of recurrent ischemia or infarction occur in the first 24 hours after thrombolytic therapy. Early recurrent ischemia occurs in 15%-25% of patients after rt-PA therapy,[39,43,53,55,56,58,59] while reinfarction occurs much less frequently, with an incidence of 0% to 8%.[39,53-58,60]

Because rt-PA has a short plasma half-life, prolonged maintenance infusions of up to six hours have been used in an attempt to prevent early reocclusion.[35,37,38] Results have been variable with benefit shown in studies which maintained higher plasma rt-PA levels for longer periods of time.[37,38] Unfortunately, this has also led to increased bleeding. Other approaches to increasing and maintaining vessel patency have been used. The utility of adjuvant medical therapy and PTCA in preventing recurrent ischemia and enhancing myocardial salvage will be addressed in the next two sections.

ADJUVANT MEDICAL THERAPY

Heparin

While heparin has been administered intravenously to the majority of patients treated with rt-PA, the optimal dosage, duration of infusion and time of initiation of therapy are still controversial. Data from a canine model showed that pretreatment with heparin enhanced thrombolysis by preventing the incorporation of new fibrin into experimentally induced carotid artery thrombi.[81] However, in patients with AMI, infarct-related artery patency rates 90 minutes after the initiation of rt-PA therapy were not significantly increased in patients who received concurrent heparin therapy with rt-PA therapy compared to those who did not.[44] While this study does not support the use of heparin to achieve higher early patency rates, other data indicate that the use of heparin is critical in preventing reocclusion. Two small, prospective, randomized trials indicate that the initiation of intravenous heparin therapy with the rt-PA infusion leads to improved patency rates of the infarct-related artery on day one[82] or day three.[83]

Our standard practice is to administer a 5000 unit bolus of intravenous heparin along with the initial rt-PA bolus, followed by a continuous infusion, except in elderly patients where the heparin therapy is delayed until the conclusion of the rt-PA infusion. Intravenous heparin is continued for three to five days to maintain the partial thromboplastin time at 1.5 to 2 times the control value.

Aspirin

The timing of aspirin therapy in clinical trials of rt-PA has been variable, ranging from administration concurrently with the rt-PA bolus to its not being used at all. The most compelling evidence for the use of early aspirin therapy comes from the ISIS-2 trial where the mortality in patients receiving aspirin concurrent with streptokinase therapy was lower than that in patients receiving streptokinase alone. Aspirin alone also reduced mortality. Whether these effects are due to improved acute patency, decreased reocclusion, or a combination of the two is not known. Recently, it was demonstrated that after therapy with rt-PA and 24 hours of intravenous heparin, aspirin plus dipyridamole are as effective in preventing reocclusion at one week as the continued use of intravenous heparin.[84] Our approach is to administer aspirin therapy at the initiation of the rt-PA therapy and continue it indefinitely.

Beta-Adrenergic Blocking Agents

Several studies have demonstrated the efficacy of β-blockers in reducing mortality following myocardial infarction.[85 88] The intravenous administration of β-blockers increases the degree of myocardial salvage attained with reperfusion in an animal model of AMI, presumably by decreasing the extent of myocardial necrosis.[89] To test the utility of intravenous β-blockade combined with treatment with rt-PA, patients in phase IIB of the TIMI II trial were randomly assigned to either immediate or deferred therapy with metoprolol. Approximately one-half of the patients were eligible for β-blocker randomization (main exclusion criteria were bradycardia, hypotension, a history of asthma, advanced atrioventricular block, significant rales, or current use of β-blockers or calcium channel blockers). Patients were randomly assigned to receive either immediate therapy with intravenous followed by oral metoprolol, or oral metoprolol starting on day 6. Intravenous metoprolol was well tolerated in 90% of patients to whom it was administered.

The primary end point, ejection fraction prior to hospital discharge, did not differ significantly between the two groups. However, intravenous β-blockade did decrease the incidence of recurrent nonfatal myocardial infarction and recurrent ischemia within six days of therapy. At 42 days following therapy, the decreased incidence of recurrent nonfatal infarction persisted. There was no significant difference in total mortality, although the incidence of death in the low-risk group (age < 70 years and an uncomplicated, initial inferior infarction) was decreased. We recommend that when feasible, intravenous β-blockers be administered along with rt-PA, especially in patients with an elevated heart rate or blood pressure.

COMBINATION THROMBOLYTIC THERAPY

Additive effects or synergy between thrombolytic agents which act through different mechanisms has been demonstrated in vitro[90] and in animals.[91,92] Since the degree of systemic fibrinolysis occurring with the fibrin specific agents is dependent on the dose administered, the presence of synergism could theoretically allow for the use of smaller doses of each agent, resulting in effective thrombolysis with a decrease in hemorrhagic complications. The combined infusion of low doses of rt-PA and single-chain urokinase-type plasminogen activator (scu-PA), a naturally occurring fibrin specific agent, is effective and safe.[93,94]

The administration of non-fibrin specific thrombolytic agents in conjunction with rt-PA may be beneficial by increasing the degree of systemic fibrinolysis. When rt-PA and urokinase were administered together, there was no synergistic effect on reperfusion rates.[95] Low-dose therapy with a combination of both agents resulted in a very low patency rate (approximately 40%), while the use of larger doses gave similar patency rates to those obtained with rt-PA therapy alone. However, the reocclusion rate after therapy with the combination was low, particularly in patients undergoing salvage PTCA for failed thrombolysis where the rate of reocclusion after rt-PA therapy alone was higher.[96] Combined thrombolytic therapy with half dose (50 mg) rt-PA and streptokinase leads to a high rate of infarct vessel patency at 90 minutes[97] and may also reduce the rate of reocclusion after salvage PTCA by producing a systemic fibrinolytic state.[98] These combination therapies may result in lower rates of reocclusion and possibly hemorrhage, but further study is necessary to define such advantages.

THE ROLE OF CORONARY ANGIOGRAPHY AND PTCA

PTCA is an effective modality for the primary recanalization of occluded infarct-related arteries.[99,100] In conjunction with rt-PA therapy, PTCA has been used both to establish infarct vessel patency and to decrease the high-grade residual stenosis remaining in most patients after successful thrombolysis. By increasing the luminal diameter, it was postulated that PTCA would improve coronary blood flow (and therefore myocardial function) and decrease the incidence of reocclusion. The role and timing of coronary angiography and PTCA as adjunctive therapy to rt-PA have been studied extensively.

Acute PTCA

The major clinical trials which evaluated emergency catheterization and PTCA during or immediately following rt-PA therapy differed in design and purpose, but significant conclusions can be derived from their findings. These studies, which were conducted by the Thrombolysis and Angioplasty in Myocardial Infarction (TAMI) group,[43] the ECSG group,[39] and the TIMI group,[41] demonstrated no advantage for a strategy of routine immediate angiography with PTCA compared with a conservative approach without immediate angiography (Table 7). Immediate PTCA did not decrease the incidence of coronary reocclusion, recurrent ischemia, or reinfarction, nor did it result in improvement in left ventricular function or early survival. The strategy of immediate angiography and PTCA was also associated with a higher incidence of bleeding complications, blood transfusions, and emergency bypass surgery when compared with either a noninvasive approach,[39] or delayed PTCA at 18-48 hours[41] or 7-10 days.[43]

Table 7. *Clinical outcomes and ventricular function after acute PTCA following therapy with rt-PA*

ECSG[39]

	Immediate Angiography/PTCA n=183	Noninvasive n=184
Reocclusion	11%	13%
Reinfarction	7%	10%
Mortality	7%	10%
LVEF	51%	51%
Blood Transfusion	10%	4%

TIMI IIA[41]

	2 hour Angiography/PTCA n=195	18-48 hour Angiography/PTCA n=194	P value
CABG after PTCA	6.7%	1.5%	0.02
Reocclusion	15%	17%	NS
Reinfarction	6.7%	4.1%	0.27
Mortality	7.2%	5.7%	0.54
LVEF	50.3%	49.0%	0.37
Blood Transfusion	20.0%	7.2%	< 0.001

TAMI[43]

	Immediate Angiography/PTCA n=99	Elective PTCA at 7-10 days n=98	P value
Emergency CABG	7%	2%	0.17
Reocclusion	11%	13%	0.67
Mortality	4%	1%	0.37
LVEF	53.2%	56.4%	0.08

One recently published study of thrombolytic therapy in AMI showed a significant increase in life-threatening complications during catheterization compared with a corresponding observation period in a non-catheterized control group.[101] Thus, the risks of intervention which include excessive bleeding and need for transfusion may be partly responsible for the lack of benefit in left ventricular function or survival.

While these studies demonstrate that routine acute coronary angiography and PTCA are not advantageous to the entire group of patients after rt-PA therapy and specifically to those with a patent vessel and no evidence of ongoing ischemia, perhaps certain subsets of patients would benefit from acute PTCA. The greatest potential benefit of early angiography would be to identify those patients with persistent total or near-total occlusion of the infarct-related artery. These patients would have vessel patency restored by successful PTCA (salvage PTCA), possibly salvaging myocardium and reducing mortality. While the mortality has been high in patients undergoing salvage PTCA it is notable that in patients with successful salvage PTCA the mortality is lower than in those where sustained patency is not obtained.[96]

Other patients who might benefit from early coronary angiography following rt-PA therapy are those with: 1) persistent ischemic pain after several hours of therapy; 2) hemodynamic instability, where achieving early infarct vessel patency may be critical to survival; 3) clinical signs of early reocclusion during or immediately after the rt-PA infusion; and 4) high-risk anatomy such as left main coronary artery disease requiring urgent surgery. Little data are available on these subsets of patients.

Noninvasive methods to assess the patency of the infarct related artery have been limited by low sensitivity and specificity. The triad of complete, rapid resolution of chest pain, ST-segment normalization, and the appearance of reperfusion arrhythmias is usually associated with a patent vessel, but occurs infrequently.[102] Because these clinical signs of reperfusion are not sufficiently accurate to predict vessel patency, determining which patients may derive the greatest benefit from acute intervention may not be possible.

Elective PTCA

The use of routine elective coronary angiography prior to hospital discharge, with prophylactic PTCA for suitable coronary anatomy, may reduce the incidence of recurrent ischemia, reocclusion, and reinfarction, and reduce mortality. This strategy has several advantages over immediate PTCA including: 1) the procedure is performed in an elective setting rather than during the acute infarction; 2) the incidence of hemorrhagic complications is lower since the effects of rt-PA have abated and plasma fibrinogen levels have increased; and 3) there may be less residual thrombus and a more "stable" atherosclerotic plaque due to healing of a ruptured plaque.

Phase II of the TIMI trial compared two treatment strategies after rt-PA therapy for AMI.[53] Following the administration of 100-150 mg of rt-PA, patients were randomly assigned to routine coronary angiography at 18 to 48 hours with prophylactic PTCA for suitable anatomy ("invasive strategy") or to conventional care where angiography and PTCA were performed only for recurrent spontaneous or exercise-induced ischemia ("conservative strategy"). The primary end point was survival free of recurrent myocardial infarction at 42 days. In the patients assigned to the invasive strategy, PTCA was performed in 53.7%. The principal reasons for not attempting the procedure were: 1) no lesion in the infarct-related artery of greater than 60% severity;

2) total occlusion of the infarct vessel; or 3) infarct-related artery unsuitable for PTCA. A high percentage (93.3%) of the PTCA procedures were successful, with a low incidence of emergency coronary artery bypass surgery (2.4%) or death (0.5%) within 24 hours of the procedure. PTCA at 18-48 hours following rt-PA therapy appears to be feasible in the majority of patients and is associated with a low risk.[53,103]

Overall results in the TIMI phase II trial were excellent, with a 42-day mortality of only 4.9%. The clinical outcome was not improved by the invasive strategy; there was no significant difference in the incidence of death and nonfatal reinfarction between the two groups. Left ventricular ejection fraction at hospital discharge and at six weeks following therapy was also the same in both groups. The only advantages observed with the invasive strategy were a decreased incidence of exercise-induced myocardial ischemia at hospital discharge and a slightly greater rise in ejection fraction from rest to exercise at both hospital discharge and six weeks following treatment.

These results indicate that after therapy with rt-PA, coronary angiography can be reserved for those patients with recurrent spontaneous myocardial ischemia or provokable ischemia on a pre-discharge exercise stress test. Of the patients assigned to the conservative strategy, 32.7% underwent coronary angiography within 14 days of study entry and 13.3% underwent PTCA. The mortality rate with this approach (4.7%) was quite low as was the incidence of nonfatal reinfarction, 5.4%. These findings have major implications for the use of thrombolytic therapy with rt-PA for AMI, especially in the community hospital setting. In conjunction with the results of the trials assessing acute PTCA, it is clear that rt-PA can be administered effectively in both tertiary care and community hospitals, whether or not on-site cardiac catheterization facilities are available.

PATIENT SELECTION

Thrombolytic therapy is the treatment of choice for patients 75 years of age or younger presenting within six hours of the onset of symptoms of myocardial infarction with ST-segment elevation who do not have an excessive risk of hemorrhage. The utility of thrombolytic therapy in certain other subsets of patients with AMI has not been established.

Treatment in the Elderly

The risk-benefit ratio of thrombolytic therapy in the elderly has not been established. The mortality in patients older than 65-75 years treated conventionally is approximately four times as great as that in a younger population. Thrombolytic therapy with SK or rt-PA decreases mortality by up to 34% in this group[65-67] (Table 8). Despite the

Table 8. *Mortality rates by age with rt-PA or SK*

ASSET[65]		Mortality (%)		
Age (yrs)	n	rt-PA		% Reduction
≤ 55	748	3.8		14
56-65	963	6.5		18
66-75	827	10.8		34
GISSI[66]		Mortality (%)		
Age (yrs)	n	SK	Control	% Reduction
≤ 65	7608	5.7	7.7	26
65-75	2886	16.6	18.1	8
> 75	1215	28.9	33.1	13
ISIS-2[67]		Mortality (%)		
Age (yrs)	n	SK	Control	% Reduction
< 60	7720	4.2	5.8	28
60-69	6056	10.6	14.4	26
≥ 70	3411	18.2	21.6	16

n = number of patients
ISIS-2 = Second International Study of Infarct Survival; GISSI = Italian Group for the Study of Streptokinase in Myocardial Infarction; ASSET − Anglo-Scandinavian Study of Early Thrombolysis

apparent mortality reduction by intravenous thrombolytic therapy, rt-PA has not been used routinely in patients over the age of 75, due to the increased risk of hemorrhagic complications.[104] An analysis of data from the TIMI group revealed higher rates of hemorrhagic complications, transfusions, and mortality in patients greater than 65 years of age treated with rt-PA.[105] Elderly females are at the highest risk for hemorrhagic complications.[70]

A randomized, multicenter, placebo-controlled trial of rt-PA in patients over the age of 75 assessing **T**hrombolytic **T**herapy in an **O**lder **P**atient **P**opulation (TTOPP) has recently been completed.[106] Patients without other contraindications to thrombolytic therapy received either a weight-adjusted three-hour infusion of rt-PA to a maximum of 100 mg or a placebo in a double-blind fashion. Preliminary data from this small trial in which 69 patients were enrolled indicated that patients in the rt-PA group had a higher mean left ventricular ejection fraction at hospital discharge than those who received placebo (50.5% vs. 41.5%, respectively; p = 0.05). Patients in the placebo group were also significantly more likely to undergo PTCA or coronary artery bypass surgery prior to hospital discharge than those in the rt-PA group. There were favorable trends in the rt-PA group with regard to mortality, the development of severe heart failure, and the incidence of ventricular arrhythmias, although these differences did not reach statistical significance.

Currently, most investigators believe than an arbitrary upper age limit for the administration of thrombolytic therapy is no longer appropriate. The risk-benefit ratio of thrombolytic therapy in the elderly should therefore be evaluated on a case by case basis.

Late Treatment

Many patients presenting to an emergency room with AMI who would otherwise be eligible for thrombolytic therapy do not receive it because they are seen more than 5-6 hours following symptom onset.[65] Patient delay and ambulance transport time are the primary reasons for such delays. The ISIS-2 trial demonstrated improved survival with intravenous streptokinase when therapy was initiated as late as 12-24 hours after the onset of symptoms. This may be due to the fact that myocardial salvage has been shown to occur up to at least 12 hours after symptom onset in patients treated with intracoronary streptokinase and nitroglycerin in whom there was collateral flow to an occluded coronary artery.[28]

However, late reperfusion may improve survival independent of myocardial salvage. In anesthetized rats, reperfusion 24 hours following ligation of a coronary artery decreased infarct expansion and subsequent aneurysm formation without reducing infarct size.[29] The long-term benefits of a patent vessel have also been demonstrated in clinical reperfusion trials. In the Western Washington Intracoronary Streptokinase Trial,[107] a 2.5% one-year mortality was observed in patients with complete perfusion of the infarct related artery, compared with 16.6% mortality in those with partial or no reperfusion, despite the fact that there was no demonstrable difference in global left ventricular function. A decreased mortality rate at 6 and 12 months was also shown in patients with a patent vessel 90 minutes following therapy with rt-PA in the TIMI I trial,[108] again with no demonstrable difference in left ventricular function.[109] In addition, patients with spontaneous late reperfusion occasionally show improvement in ejection fraction even though patency is not achieved until several days post infarction.[76]

The TAMI group has recently completed a randomized, placebo-controlled trial of thrombolytic therapy with rt-PA for patients presenting 6 to 24 hours after the onset of symptoms of myocardial infarction.[110] Although treatment with rt-PA resulted in a significantly higher incidence of early infarct-related artery patency, there was no difference between the two groups in left ventricular ejection fraction determined by contrast ventriculography at six months.

Whether the time window for thrombolytic therapy should be increased from the present limit of 4-6 hours following symptom onset is unknown. Certainly in patients with persistent ischemic pain, which may be a marker of residual viable myocardium, late thrombolytic therapy should be strongly considered.

Inferior Wall Myocardial Infarction

Because inferior wall myocardial infarction usually causes less left ventricular necrosis than anterior wall myocardial infarction, demonstrating myocardial salvage or mortality reduction is more difficult. The use of rt-PA in inferior infarction does result in improved myocardial function compared to control groups, though to a lesser degree than seen with anterior infarction[54,56,59] (Table 9). The greatest benefit is evident when treatment is initiated early.[56] Mortality data on rt-PA therapy in patients with inferior infarction are not available.

We recommend that most patients with inferior infarction who present within six hours of the onset of symptoms should be treated with thrombolytic therapy. Precordial ST-segment depression in inferior wall myocardial infarction is associated with higher CPK release, lower left ventricular ejection fraction and higher mortality than inferior infarction in the absence of precordial ST depression.[111] The finding of precordial ST-segment depression can therefore be of use in the risk stratification of patients presenting with inferior wall myocardial infarction. In those patients in whom this electrocardiographic finding is not present, there should be a lower threshold for withholding thrombolytic therapy when relative contraindications are present.

Table 9. *Left ventricular function in placebo-controlled trials of rt-PA in inferior wall myocardial infarction*

| Trial | n | Time to treatment (hours) | Ejection Fraction (%) | | P value |
			rt-PA	Placebo	
Johns Hopkins[59]	80	3.2	58.8	54.0	0.06
NHF[54]	61	3.3	62.1	57.4	0.10
TICO[56]	69	1.9	66	59	0.017

n = number of patients in whom left ventricular function was assessed
NHF = National Heart Foundation of Australia; TICO = Thrombolysis in Acute Coronary Occlusion

Patients With Isolated ST-Segment Depression on Screening Electrocardiogram

The effectiveness of thrombolytic therapy in patients with suspected myocardial infarction presenting with isolated ST-segment depression is not known, since most trials have required ST-segment elevation for inclusion. In the GISSI and ISIS-2 trials, in which patients with isolated ST-segment depression were eligible, no significant reduction in mortality was achieved with the administration of intravenous streptokinase. Notably, mortality rates in both the treatment and control groups were quite high. The Second Mt. Sinai-NYU Reperfusion Trial provided detailed angiographic and clinical data on these patients.[112] Forty-one of the 393 (11%) patients entered into this trial had new ST-segment depression as their only electrocardiographic inclusion criterion. Myocardial infarction was confirmed by serum CK determination in 92% of these patients, demonstrating the high specificity of isolated ST depression for AMI in patients with more than 30 minutes of chest pain. Patients with isolated ST-segment depression were significantly more likely to have right coronary or left circumflex coronary artery infarct vessels than those with ST-segment elevation. The most common angiographic finding in patients with isolated ST-segment depression was a totally occluded infarct vessel which was collateralized. The incidence of subtotal occlusion of the infarct vessel prior to thrombolytic therapy was low. Although the utility of thrombolytic therapy remains controversial, patients presenting with a history strongly suggestive of myocardial infarction with new ST-segment depression should be considered for treatment.

DOSAGE AND ADMINISTRATION OF rt-PA

The ideal regimen for administering rt-PA has not been established. The conventional dose is a total of 100 mg, given as 60 mg over the first hour and 20 mg over each of the next two hours. While doses in this range result in infarct vessel patency in 75% of cases, with reocclusion rates of 10%-15%, more rapid reperfusion with higher patency rates can be obtained with increased infusion rates. The total dose and duration of the infusion are also important in maintaining patency once it has been achieved. As the dose and duration of therapy are increased in an effort to prevent reocclusion, the risk of hemorrhagic complications rises. The identification of the regimen which maximizes the efficacy of rt-PA with an acceptable risk of hemorrhagic complications is still under investigation.

The initial bolus and first hour dose are important determinants of the speed and efficacy of thrombolysis. The value of achieving a rapid high peak plasma rt-PA level is evident when large first hour doses are administered. The **P**re-hospital **A**dministration of **T**-PA **S**tudy (PATS) evaluated a regimen of rt-PA administration for use in the pre-hospital setting.[113] A 20 mg bolus of rt-PA was administered followed by a delayed infusion 30 minutes later (60 mg over one hour and 20 mg over the subsequent hour) to simulate initial thrombolytic therapy in the field followed by ambulance transport and subsequent thrombolytic therapy in the hospital. The patency rate in 60 patients, determined by coronary angiography performed 90 minutes following the initial bolus, was 92%. In another study, the administration of 100 mg of rt-PA over 90 minutes (15 mg bolus, 50 mg over 30 minutes, 35 mg over 60 minutes) resulted in 60 and 90 minute patency rates of 78% and 92% respectively.[114] When compared with the conventional regimen in a randomized study, this regimen resulted in improved infarct vessel patency at 60 minutes following the initial bolus (76% vs. 63%, p = 0.03), but no significant difference in patency at 90 minutes (81% vs. 77%, p = 0.21).[115] A single 50 mg bolus of rt-PA will also result in high early patency, 75% at 60 minutes.[116]

Weight-adjusted dosing may be the safest, most efficacious method to administer rt-PA.[117] A dose of 1 mg/kg in the first hour, with 10% given as a bolus, results in greater overall patency with more rapid reperfusion and less major bleeding than a fixed dose regimen. Recently, the results of a randomized trial demonstrated that a weight-adjusted high dose infusion of rt-PA (total dose 2 mg/kg to a maximum of 150 mg over 3 hours, with 1.2 mg/kg to a maximum of 100 mg over the first hour) resulted in a higher patency rate of the infarct-related artery at 90 minutes than a weight-adjusted standard dose (total dose 1.25 mg/kg to a maximum of 125 mg over 3 hours, with a 0.75 mg/kg to a maximum of 75 mg over the first hour).[118] The TAMI investigators have examined several accelerated weight-adjusted rt-PA regimens and found patency rates of the infarct-related artery at 90 minutes varied from 64% to 82%, including a rate of 73% for the PATS regimen.[119] These high dose front-loaded rt-PA regimens appear to result in more rapid and frequent early patency of the infarct-related artery, but their safety profile requires further investigation.

ADMINISTRATION OF rt-PA IN THE COMMUNITY HOSPITAL

Most patients with AMI present initially to a community hospital. Treatment should be initiated as soon as the diagnosis and eligibility have been established, rather than delaying therapy until transfer to a hospital with facilities for PTCA takes place. The TAMI investigators have shown that this results in improved ventricular function by shortening the time to initiation of therapy.[120] The safety profile of rt-PA in the community hospital is no different than in tertiary referral centers.[121]

Once thrombolytic therapy has been initiated, the question of transfer to a hospital with PTCA facilities arises. Because acute angiography does not lead to an improved clinical outcome, emergent transfer is not necessary in most cases. Routine cardiac catheterization and prophylactic PTCA during hospitalization offer no advantage over a conservative strategy in which angiography is performed only for recurrent spontaneous or exercise-induced ischemia. Therefore, the main indication for transfer to a hospital with on-site PTCA facilities is recurrent ischemia. Transfer should also be considered in those cases in which other signs of instability have been observed or the patient appears to be in a high-risk subset. The effectiveness of the conservative strategy depends on the ability to perform coronary angiography promptly when indications arise. A comparison of the results at hospitals with (tertiary care) and without (community) PTCA facilities confirms that such a conservative strategy is applicable to community hospitals.[121] In phase IIB of the TIMI trial, 21% of the patients were treated at hospitals without PTCA facilities. A comparison of patients presenting to tertiary and community hospitals assigned to the conservative strategy is shown in Table 10. While baseline characteristics were similar in the two groups, coronary angiography was performed significantly more frequently in patients presenting at tertiary hospitals. Despite the greater use of coronary angiography, PTCA, and CABG (coronary artery bypass grafting) on patients from tertiary hospitals, there was no difference in mortality, recurrent myocardial infarction, left ventricular ejection fraction, or the incidence of a positive exercise stress test between the two sites. It can be concluded that therapy with rt-PA is feasible in hospitals without cardiac catheterization and PTCA facilities.

CONCLUSION AND FUTURE DIRECTIONS

Therapy with rt-PA for patients presenting early in the course of AMI results in coronary artery recanalization, myocardial salvage, and reduced mortality. Although thrombolytic therapy represents a breakthrough in the treatment of myocardial infarction,

Table 10. *Comparison of patients at tertiary and community hospitals in the conservative strategy arm of TIMI IIB (all events assessed within 42 days)*

	Tertiary	Community	P value
Coronary angiography performed	46.8%	30.1%	< 0.001
PTCA	17.6%	10.8%	0.004
CABG	11.3%	7.2%	0.04
Blood transfusion	14.2%	7.2%	0.01
Mortality	4.0%	4.6%	NS
Recurrent nonfatal MI	6.1%	4.9%	NS
Left ventricular EF	50.5%	51.1%	NS
Positive exercise stress	18.9%	22.0%	NS

TIMI IIB = Thrombolysis in Myocardial Infarction Trial – Phase IIB; Tertiary Hospital = on-site angioplasty available; Community = transfer to tertiary for coronary angiography/angioplasty; PTCA = percutaneous transluminal coronary angioplasty; CABG = coronary artery bypass grafting; EF = ejection fraction as determined by radionuclide angiography major limitations still exist. Perhaps the most important is that fewer than half of the patients presenting to the hospital with an AMI are eligible for thrombolytic therapy when the current exclusion criteria are applied. Further public education, the elimination of delays involved in patient transport and evaluation, and improved patient selection are necessary to alleviate this problem.

The optimal regimen of rt-PA which will safely maximize the rate of and time to recanalization and possibly allow for its pre-hospital administration is currently being investigated, as are the proper use and timing of adjunctive therapy. Newer agents including potent inhibitors of platelet function[122,123] and antithrombins[124] may prove useful as adjuvant therapy. Finally, a rapid noninvasive method to detect vessel patency would allow the use of emergency coronary angiography and PTCA in those patients with persistent coronary artery occlusion.

REFERENCES

1. Levin EG: Latent tissue plasminogen activator produced by human endothelial cells in culture: Evidence for an enzyme-inhibitor complex. Proc Natl Acad Sci USA 1983;80: 6804-6808.

2. Rijken DC, Wijngaards G, Welbergen J: Relationship between tissue plasminogen activator and the activators in blood and vascular wall. Thromb Res 1980;18:815-830.

3. Bergsdorf N, Nilsson T, Wallen P: An enzyme linked immunosorbent assay for determination of tissue plasminogen activator applied to patients with thromboembolic disease. Thromb Haemost 1983;50:740-744.

4. Rijken DC, Juhan-Vague I, DeCock F, Collen D: Measurement of human tissue-type plasminogen activator by a two-site immunoradiometric assay. J Lab Clin Med 1983; 101:274-284.

5. Pennica D, Holmes WE, Kohr WJ, et al: Cloning and expression of human tissue-type plasminogen activator cDNA in *E. coli*. Nature 1983;301:214-221.

6. Rijken DC, Hoylaerts M, Collen D: Fibrinolytic properties of one-chain and two-chain human extrinsic (tissue-type) plasminogen activator. J Biol Chem 1982;257:2920-2925.

7. Rijken DC, Groeneveld E: Isolation and functional characterization of the heavy and light chains of human tissue-type plasminogen activator. J Biol Chem 1986;261:3098-3102.

8. Ichinose A, Takio K, Fujikawa K: Localization of the binding site of tissue-type plasminogen activator to fibrin. J Clin Invest 1986;78:163-169.

9. Hoylaerts M, Rijken DC, Lijnen HR, Collen D: Kinetics of the activation of plasminogen by human tissue plasminogen activator: Role of fibrin. J Biol Chem 1982;257:2912-2919.

10. Moroi M, Aoki N: Isolation and characterization of alpha$_2$-plasmin inhibitor from human plasma: A novel proteinase inhibitor which inhibits activator-induced clot lysis. J Biol Chem 1976;251:5956-5965.

11. Erickson LA, Ginsberg MH, Loskutoff DJ: Detection and partial characterization of an inhibitor of plasminogen activator in human platelets. J Clin Invest 1984;74:1465-1472.

12. Wohlwend A, Belin D, Vassali J-D: Plasminogen activator-specific inhibitors produced by human monocytes/macrophages. J Exptl Med 1987;165:320-339.

13. Rijken DC, Juhan-Vague I, Collen D: Complexes between tissue-type plasminogen activator and proteinase inhibitors in human plasma, identified with an immunoradiometric assay. J Lab Clin Med 1983;101:285-294.

14. Collen D, Bounameaux H, De Cock F, et al: Analysis of coagulation and fibrinolysis during intravenous infusion of recombinant human tissue-type plasminogen activator in patients with acute myocardial infarction. Circulation 1986;73:511-517.

15. Astrup T, Permin PM: Fibrinolysis in animal organism. Nature 1947;159:681-682.

16. Rijken DC, Wijngaards G, Zaal-De Jong M, Welbergen J: Purification and partial characterization of plasminogen activator from human uterine tissue. Biochim Biophys Acta 1979;580:140-153.

17. Rijken DC, Collen D: Purification and characterization of the plasminogen activator secreted by human melanoma cells in culture. J Biol Chem 1981;256:7035-7041.

18. Collen D, Rijken DC, Van Damme J, Billiau A: Purification of human tissue-type plasminogen activator in centigram quantities from human melanoma cell culture fluid and its conditioning for use in vivo. Thromb Haemost 1982;48:294-296.

19. Weimar W, Stibbe J, van Seyen AJ, et al: Specific lysis of an iliofemoral thrombus by administration of extrinsic (tissue-type) plasminogen activator. Lancet 1981;2:1018-1020.

20. Van de Werf F, Ludbrook PA, Bergmann SR, et al: Coronary thrombolysis with tissue-type plasminogen activator in patients with evolving myocardial infarction. N Engl J Med 1984;310:609-613.

21. Collen D, Topol EJ, Tiefenbrunn AJ, et al: Coronary thrombolysis with recombinant human tissue-type plasminogen: A prospective, randomized, placebo-controlled trial. Circulation 1984;6:1012-1017.

22. Garabedian HD, Gold HK, Leinbach RC, et al: Comparative properties of two clinical preparations of recombinant human tissue-type plasminogen activator in patients with acute myocardial infarction. J Am Coll Cardiol 1987;9:599-607.

23. DeWood MA, Spores J, Notske R, et al: Prevalence of total coronary occlusion during the early hours of transmural myocardial infarction. N Engl J Med 1980;303:897-902.

24. Rentrop KP, Feit F, Blanke H, et al: Effects of intracoronary streptokinase and intracoronary nitroglycerin infusion on coronary angiographic patterns and mortality in patients with acute myocardial infarction. N Engl J Med 1984;311:1457-1463.

25. Reimer KA, Lowe JE, Rasmussen MM, Jennings RB: The wavefront phenomenon of ischemic cell death. 1. Myocardial infarct size vs duration of coronary occlusion in dogs. Circulation 1977;56:786-794.

26. Reimer KA, Jennings RB: The wavefront phenomenon of myocardial ischemic cell death. II. Transmural progression of necrosis within the framework of ischemic bed size (myocardium at risk) and collateral flow. Lab Invest 1979;40:633-644.

27. Kloner RA, Ellis SG, Lange R, et al: Studies of experimental coronary artery reperfusion. Effects on infarct size, myocardial function, biochemistry, ultrastructure and microvascular damage. Circulation 1983;68:(suppl I):I-8-I-15.

28. Rentrop KP, Feit F, Sherman W, et al: Late thrombolytic therapy preserves left ventricular function in patients with collateralized total coronary occlusion: Primary end point findings of the Second Mt. Sinai-N.Y.U. Reperfusion trial. J Am Coll Cardiol 1989;14:58-64.

29. Hochman JS, Choo H: Limitation of myocardial infarct expansion by reperfusion independent of myocardial salvage. Circulation 1987;75:299-306.

30. Sager PT, Perlmutter RA, Rosenfeld LE, et al: Electrophysiologic effects of thrombolytic therapy in patients with a transmural anterior myocardial infarction complicated by left ventricular aneurysm formation. J Am Coll Cardiol 1988;12:19-24.

31. Williams DO, Borer J, Braunwald E, et al: Intravenous recombinant tissue-type plasminogen activator in patients with acute myocardial infarction: A report from the NHLBI Thrombolysis in Myocardial Infarction trial. Circulation 1986;73:338-346.

32. Chesebro JH, Knatterud G, Roberts R, et al: Thrombolysis in Myocardial Infarction (TIMI) trial, phase I: A comparison between intravenous tissue plasminogen activator and intravenous streptokinase. Circulation 1987;76:142-154.

33. Verstraete M, Bernard R, Bory R, et al: Randomised trial of intravenous recombinant tissue-type plasminogen activator versus intravenous streptokinase in acute myocardial infarction: Report from the European Cooperative Study Group for recombinant tissue-type plasminogen activator. Lancet 1985;1:842-847.

34. Verstraete M, Bleifeld W, Brower RW, et al: Double-blind randomised trial of intravenous tissue-type plasminogen activator versus placebo in acute myocardial infarction. Lancet 1985;2:965-969.

35. Verstraete M, Arnold AER, Brower RW, et al: Acute coronary thrombolysis with recombinant human tissue-type plasminogen activator: Initial patency and influence of maintained infusion on reocclusion rate. Am J Cardiol 1987;60:231-237.

36. Topol EJ, O'Neill WW, Langburd AB, et al: A randomized, placebo-controlled trial of intravenous recombinant tissue-type plasminogen activator and emergency coronary angioplasty in patients with acute myocardial infarction. Circulation 1987;75:420-428.

37. Gold HK, Leinbach RC, Garabedian HD, et al: Acute coronary reocclusion after thrombolysis with recombinant human tissue-type plasminogen activator: Prevention by a maintenance infusion. Circulation 1986;73:347-352.

38. Johns JA, Gold HK, Leinbach RC, et al: Prevention of coronary artery reocclusion and reduction in late coronary artery stenosis after thrombolytic therapy in patients with acute myocardial infarction: A randomized study of maintenance infusion of recombinant human tissue-type plasminogen activator. Circulation 1988;78:546-556.

39. Simoons ML, Arnold AER, Betriu A, et al: Thrombolysis with tissue plasminogen activator in acute myocardial infarction: No additional benefit from immediate percutaneous coronary angioplasty. Lancet 1988;1:197-203.

40. Passamani E, Hodges M, Herman M, et al: The Thrombolysis in Myocardial Infarction (TIMI) phase II pilot study: Tissue plasminogen activator followed by percutaneous transluminal coronary angioplasty. J Am Coll Cardiol 1987;10:51B-64B.

41. TIMI Study Group: Immediate vs delayed catheterization and angioplasty following thrombolytic therapy for acute myocardial infarction: TIMI IIA results. JAMA 1988; 260:2849-2858.

42. Topol EJ, Morris DC, Smalling RW, et al: A multicenter, randomized, placebo-controlled trial of a new form of intravenous recombinant tissue-type plasminogen activator (Activase) in acute myocardial infarction. J Am Coll Cardiol 1987;9:1205-1213.

43. Topol EJ, Califf RM, George BS, et al: A randomized trial of immediate versus delayed elective angioplasty after intravenous tissue plasminogen activator in acute myocardial infarction. N Engl J Med 1987;317:581-588.

44. Topol EJ, George BS, Kereiakes DJ, et al: A randomized controlled trial of intravenous tissue plasminogen activator and early intravenous heparin in acute myocardial infarction. Circulation 1989;79:281-286.

45. Khaja F, Walton JA, Brymer JF, et al: Intracoronary fibrinolytic therapy in acute myocardial infarction: Report of a prospective randomized trial. N Engl J Med 1983;308:1305-1311.

46. Anderson JL, Marshall HW, Bray BE, et al: A randomized trial of intracoronary streptokinase in the treatment of acute myocardial infarction. N Engl J Med 1983;308:1312-1318.

47. Rentrop KP, Blanke H, Karsch KR: Selective intracoronary thrombolysis in acute myocardial infarction and unstable angina pectoris. Circulation 1981;63:307-317.

48. Leiboff RH, Katz RJ, Wasserman AG, et al: A randomized, angiographically controlled trial of intracoronary streptokinase in acute myocardial infarction. Am J Cardiol 1984; 53:404-407.

49. Kennedy JW, Ritchie JL, Davis KB, Fritz JK: Western Washington randomized trial of intracoronary streptokinase in acute myocardial infarction. N Engl J Med 1983;309:1477-1482.

50. Rentrop KP: Thrombolytic therapy in patients with acute myocardial infarction. Circulation 1985;71:627-631.

51. TIMI Study Group: The Thrombolysis in Myocardial Infarction (TIMI) Trial: Phase I findings. N Engl J Med 1985;312:932-936.

52. Chesebro JH, Knatterud G, Braunwald E: Thrombolytic therapy (letter). N Engl J Med 1988;319:1544-1545.

53. TIMI Study Group: Comparison of invasive and conservative strategies after treatment with intravenous tissue plasminogen activator in acute myocardial infarction: Results of the Thrombolysis in Myocardial Infarction (TIMI) Phase II Trial. N Engl J Med 1989; 320:618-627.

54. National Heart Foundation of Australia Coronary Thrombolysis Group: Coronary thrombolysis and myocardial salvage by tissue plasminogen activator given up to 4 hours after onset of myocardial infarction. Lancet 1988;1:203-208.

55. Armstrong PW, Baigrie RS, Daly PA, et al: Tissue plasminogen activator: Toronto (TPAT) placebo-controlled randomized trial in acute myocardial infarction. J Am Coll Cardiol 1989;13:1469-1476.

56. O'Rourke M, Baron D, Keogh A, et al: Limitation of myocardial infarction by early infusion of recombinant tissue-type plasminogen activator. Circulation 1988;77:1311-1315.

57. White HD, Rivers JT, Maslowski AH, et al: Effect of intravenous streptokinase as compared with that of tissue plasminogen activator on left ventricular function after first myocardial infarction. N Engl J Med 1989;320:817-821.

58. Magnani B and the PAIMS Investigators: Plasminogen Activator Italian Multicenter Study (PAIMS): Comparison of intravenous recombinant single-chain human tissue-type plasminogen activator (rt-PA) with intravenous streptokinase in acute myocardial infarction. J Am Coll Cardiol 1989;13:19-26.

59. Guerci AD, Gerstenblith G, Brinker JA, et al: A randomized trial of intravenous tissue plasminogen activator for acute myocardial infarction with subsequent randomization to elective coronary angioplasty. N Engl J Med 1987;317:1613-1618.

60. Van de Werf F, Arnold AER: Intravenous tissue plasminogen activator and size of infarct, left ventricular function, and survival in acute myocardial infarction. Br Med J 1988;297:1374-1379.

61. White HD, Norris RM, Brown MA, et al: Left ventricular end-systolic volume as the major determinant of survival after recovery from myocardial infarction. Circulation 1987;76:44-51.

62. Schroder R, Neuhaus K-L, Leizorovicz A, et al: A prospective placebo-controlled double-blind multicenter trial of intravenous streptokinase in acute myocardial infarction (ISAM): Long-term mortality and morbidity. J Am Coll Cardiol 1989;9:197-203.

63. Kennedy JW, Martin GV, Davis KB, et al: The Western Washington intravenous streptokinase in acute myocardial infarction randomized trial. Circulation 1988;77:345-52.

64. White HD, Norris RM, Brown MA, et al: Effect of intravenous streptokinase on left ventricular function and early survival after acute myocardial infarction. N Engl J Med 1987;317:850-855.

65. Wilcox RG, von der Lippe G, Olsson CG, et al: Trial of tissue plasminogen activator for mortality reduction in acute myocardial infarction: Anglo-Scandinavian study of early thrombolysis (ASSET). Lancet 1988;2:525-530.

66. Gruppo Italiano per lo studio della streptochinasi nell'infarto miocardico (GISSI): Effectiveness of intravenous thrombolytic treatment in acute myocardial infarction. Lancet 1986;1:397-402.

67. ISIS-2 (Second International Study of Infarct Survival) Collaborative Group: Randomised trial of intravenous streptokinase, oral aspirin, both, or neither among 17,187 cases of suspected acute myocardial infarction: ISIS-2. Lancet 1988;2:349-360.

68. The International Study Group: In-hospital mortality and clinical course of 20,891 patients with suspected acute myocardial infarction randomised between alteplase and streptokinase with or without heparin. Lancet 1990;336:71-75.

69. Mueller HS, Rao AK, Forman SA, and the TIMI Investigators: Thrombolysis in Myocardial Infarction (TIMI): Comparative studies of coronary reperfusion and systemic fibrinogenolysis with two forms of recombinant tissue-type plasminogen activator. J Am Coll Cardiol 1987;10:479-490.

70. Califf RM, Topol EJ, George BS, et al: Hemorrhagic complications associated with the use of intravenous tissue plasminogen activator in treatment of acute myocardial infarction. Am J Med 1988;85:353-359.

71. Rao AK, Pratt C, Berke A, et al: Thrombolysis in Myocardial Infarction (TIMI) Trial-Phase I: Hemorrhagic manifestations and changes in plasma fibrinogen and the fibrinolytic system in patients treated with recombinant tissue plasminogen activator and streptokinase. J Am Coll Cardiol 1988;11:1-11.

72. Bovill E, Stump D, Tracy R, et al: Dose response relationship of rt-PA infusion to induction of systemic fibrin(ogen)olysis in the NHLBI Thrombolysis in Myocardial Infarction (TIMI-II) trial. J Am coll Cardiol 1989;13:198A.

73. Thompson PL, Robinson JS: Stroke after acute myocardial infarction: Relation to infarct size. Br Med J 1978;2:457-459.

74. Braunwald E, Knatterud GL, Passamani ER, Robertson TL: Announcement of protocol change in Thrombolysis in Myocardial Infarction trial (letter). J Am Coll Cardiol 1987; 9:467.

75. Braunwald E, Knatterud GL, Passamani E, et al: Update from the Thrombolysis in Myocardial Infarction trial (letter). J Am Coll Cardiol 1987;10:970.

76. Jang I-K, Vanhaecke J, De Geest H, et al: Coronary thrombolysis with recombinant tissue-type plasminogen activator: Patency rate and regional wall motion after 3 months. J Am Coll Cardiol 1988;8:1455-1460.

77. Fuster V, Stein B, Badimon L, Chesebro JH: Antithrombotic therapy after myocardial reperfusion in acute myocardial infarction. J Am Coll Cardiol 1988;12:78A-84A.

78. Gash AK, Spann JF, Sherry S, et al: Factors influencing reocclusion after coronary thrombolysis for acute myocardial infarction. Am J Cardiol 1986;57:175-177.

79. Grines CL, Topol EJ, Bates ER, et al: Infarct vessel status after intravenous tissue plasminogen activator and acute coronary angioplasty: Prediction of clinical outcome. Am Heart J 1988;115:1-7.

80. Harrison DG, Ferguson DW, Collins SM, et al: Rethrombosis after reperfusion with streptokinase: Importance of geometry of residual lesions. Circulation 1984;69:991-999.

81. Cercek B, Lew AS, Hod H, et al: Enhancement of thrombolysis with tissue-type plasminogen activator by pretreatment with heparin. Circulation 1986;74:583-587.

82. Hsia J, Hamilton WP, Kleiman N, et al: A comparison between heparin and low-dose aspirin as adjunctive therapy with tissue plasminogen activator for acute myocardial infarction. N Engl J Med 1990;323:1433-1437.

83. Bleich SD, Nichols TC, Schumacher RR, et al: Effect of heparin on coronary arterial patency after thrombolysis with tissue plasminogen activator (t-PA) in acute myocardial infarction. Am J Cardiol 1990;66:1412-1417.

84. National Heart Foundation of Australia Coronary Thrombolysis Group: A randomized comparison of oral aspirin/dipyridamole versus intravenous heparin after rt-PA for acute myocardial infarction. Circulation 1989;80(suppl II):II-114.

85. ISIS-1 (First International Study of Infarct Survival) Collaborative Group: Randomised trial of intravenous atenolol among 16,027 cases of suspected myocardial infarction: ISIS-1. Lancet 1986;2:57-66.

86. Hjalmarson A, Herlitz J,Malek I, et al: Effect on mortality of metoprolol in acute myocardial infarction: A double-blind randomised trial. Lancet 1981;2:823-827.

87. The Norwegian Multicenter Study Group: Timolol-induced reduction in mortality and reinfarction in patients surviving acute myocardial infarction. N Engl J Med 1981;304:801-807.

88. Beta-Blocker Heart Attack Trial Research Group: A randomized trial of propranolol in patients with acute myocardial infarction: I. Mortality results. JAMA 1982;247:1707-1714.

89. Hammerman H, Kloner RA, Briggs LL, Braunwald E: Enhancement of salvage of reperfused myocardium by early beta-adrenergic blockade (timolol). J Am Coll Cardiol 1984;3:1438-1443.

90. Gurewich V, Pannell R: A comparative study of the efficacy and specificity of tissue plasminogen activator and pro-urokinase: Demonstration of synergism and of different thresholds of non-selectivity. Thromb Res 1986;44:217-228.

91. Collen D, Stassen J-M, Stump DC, Verstraete M: Synergism of thrombolytic agents in vivo. Circulation 1986;74:838-842.

92. Ziskind AA, Gold HK, Yasuda T, et al: Coronary thrombolysis in dogs with synergistic combinations of human tissue-type plasminogen activator (t-PA) and single chain urokinase-type plasminogen activator (scu-PA). Clin Res 1987;35:337A.

93. Collen D, Stump DC, Van de Werf F: Coronary thrombolysis in patients with acute myocardial infarction by intravenous infusion of synergic thrombolytic agents. Am Heart J 1986;112:1083-1084.

94. Collen D, Van de Werf F: Coronary arterial thrombolysis with low-dose synergistic combinations of recombinant tissue-type plasminogen activator (rt-PA) and recombinant single-chain urokinase-type plasminogen activator (rscu-PA) for acute myocardial infarction. Am J Cardiol 1987;60:431-434.

95. Topol EJ, Califf RM, George BS, et al: Coronary arterial thrombolysis with combined infusion of recombinant tissue-type plasminogen activator and urokinase in patients with acute myocardial infarction. Circulation 1988;77:1100-1107.

96. Califf RM, Topol EJ, George BS, et al: Characteristics and outcome of patients in whom reperfusion with intravenous tissue-type plasminogen activator fails: Results of the Thrombolysis and Angioplasty in Myocardial Infarction (TAMI) I trial. Circulation 1988;77:1090-1099.

97. Grines CL, Nissen SE, Booth DC: A prospective randomized trial comparing combination half dose tPA with streptokinase to full dose tPA in acute myocardial infarction: preliminary report. J Am Coll Cardiol 1990;15:4A.

98. Grines CL, Nissen SE, Booth DC, et al: A new thrombolytic regimen for acute myocardial infarction using combination half dose tissue-type plasminogen activator with full dose streptokinase: A pilot study. J Am Coll Cardiol 1989;14:573-580.

99. O'Neill W, Timmis GC, Bourdillon PD, et al: A prospective randomized clinical trial of intracoronary streptokinase versus coronary angioplasty for acute myocardial infarction. N Engl J Med 1986;314:812-818.

100. Hartzler GO, Rutherford BD, McConahay DR, et al: Percutaneous transluminal coronary angioplasty with and without thrombolytic therapy for treatment of acute myocardial infarction. Am Heart J 1983;106:965-973.

101. Rentrop KP, Feit F, Sherman W, Thornton JC: Serial angiographic assessment of coronary artery obstruction and collateral flow in acute myocardial infarction: Report from the Second Mt. Sinai-New York University Reperfusion trial. Circulation 1989;80:1166-1175.

102. Califf RM, O'Neill W, Stack RS, et al: Failure of simple clinical measurements to predict perfusion status after intravenous thrombolysis. Ann Intern Med 1988;108:658-662.

103. Williams DO, Ruocco NA, Forman S, and the TIMI Investigators: Coronary angioplasty after recombinant tissue-type plasminogen activator in acute myocardial infarction: A report from the Thrombolysis in Myocardial Infarction (TIMI) trial. J Am Coll Cardiol 1987;10:45B-50B.

104. Lew AS, Hod H, Cercek B, et al: Mortality and morbidity rates of patients older and younger than 75 years with acute myocardial infarction treated with intravenous streptokinase. Am J Cardiol 1987;59:1-5.

105. Chaitman BR, Thompson B, Wittry MD, et al: The use of tissue-type plasminogen activator for acute myocardial infarction in the elderly: Results from Thrombolysis in Myocardial Infarction phase I, open label studies and the Thrombolysis in Myocardial Infarction phase II pilot study. J Am Coll Cardiol 1989;14:1159-1165.

106. Feit F, Breed J, Anderson JL, Attubato MJ, et al: A randomized, placebo-controlled trial of tissue plasminogen activator in elderly patients with acute myocardial infarction. Circulation 1990;82(suppl III):III-666.

107. Kennedy JW, Ritchie JL, Davis KB, et al: The Western Washington randomized trial of intracoronary streptokinase in acute myocardial infarction: A 12 month follow-up report. N Engl J Med 1985;312:1073-1078.

108. Dalen JE, Gore JM, Braunwald E, et al: Six- and twelve-month follow-up of the phase I Thrombolysis in Myocardial Infarction (TIMI) trial. Am J Cardiol 1988;62:179-185.

109. Sheehan FH, Braunwald E, Canner P, et al: The effect of intravenous thrombolytic therapy on left ventricular function: A report on tissue-type plasminogen activator and streptokinase from the Thrombolysis in Myocardial Infarction (TIMI Phase I) trial. Circulation 1987;75:817-829.

110. Topol EJ, Ellis SG, Wall TC, et al: A randomized, controlled trial of late (6-24 hour) reperfusion for acute myocardial infarction. Circulation 1990;82(suppl III):III-539.

111. Bates ER, Clemmensen PM, Gorman LE, Aronson LG: Precordial ST segment depression predicts a worse prognosis in inferior infarction despite reperfusion therapy. Circulation 1988;78(suppl II):II-211.

112. Feit F, Rey M, Sherman W, et al: Second Mt. Sinai-N.Y.U. Reperfusion trial: Incidence and significance of isolated ST depression at screening. Circulation 1988;78(suppl II): II-212.

113. McKendall GR, Attubato MJ, Drew TM, et al: Improved infarct artery patency using a new modified regimen of tPA: Results of the Pre-hospital Administration of tPA (PATS) Pilot Trial. J Am Coll Cardiol 1990;15:3A.

114. Neuhaus K-L, Feuerer W, Jeep-Tebbe S, et al: Improved thrombolysis with a modified dose regimen of recombinant tissue-type plasminogen activator. J Am Coll Cardiol 1989;14:1566-1569.

115. Carney R, Brandt T, Daley P, et al: Increased efficacy of rt-PA by more rapid administration: The RAAMI Trial. Circulation 1990;82(suppl III):III-538.

116. Tebbe U, Tanswell P, Seifried E, et al: Single-bolus injection of recombinant tissue-type plasminogen activator in acute myocardial infarction. Am J Cardiol 1989;64:448-453.

117. Topol EJ, George BS, Kereiakes DJ, et al: Comparison of two dose regimens of intravenous tissue plasminogen activator for acute myocardial infarction. Am J Cardiol 1988; 61:723-728.

118. Smalling RW, Schumacher R, Morris D, et al: Improved infarct-related arterial patency after high dose, weight-adjusted, rapid infusion of tissue-type plasminogen activator in myocardial infarction: results of a multicenter randomized trial of two dosage regimens. J Am Coll Cardiol 1990;15:915-921.

119. Wall TC, Topol EJ, George BS, et al: The TAMI-7 trial of accelerated plasminogen activator dose regimens for coronary thrombolysis. Circulation 1990;82(suppl III):III-538.

120. Topol EJ, Bates ER, Walton JA, et al: Community hospital administration of intravenous tissue plasminogen activator in acute myocardial infarction: Improved timing, thrombolytic efficacy and ventricular function. J Am Coll Cardiol 1987;10:1173-1177.

121. Feit F, Mueller HS, Ross R, et al: Coronary angiography and angioplasty in the conservative arm of TIMI IIB: A comparison of primary and satellite hospitals. Circulation 1989;80(suppl II):II-626.

122. Shebuski RJ, Ramjit DR, Lumma PK, et al: Prevention of canine coronary artery thrombosis with echistatin, a potent inhibitor of platelet aggregation from the venom of the viper, Echis carinatus. Circulation 1989;80(suppl II):II-645.

123. Gold HK, Gimple L, Yasuda T, et al: Phase I human trial of the potent anti-platelet agent 7E3-F(ab')$_2$, a monoclonal antibody to the GPIIb/IIIa receptor. Circulation 1989;80(suppl II):II-267.

124. Jang I-K, Gold HK, Ziskind AA, et al: Prevention of arterial thrombosis by short-term thrombin inhibition. Circulation 1989;80(suppl II):II-23.

Chapter 12

CLINICAL APPLICATIONS OF UROKINASE
The First Tissue Plasminogen Activating Thrombolytic Agent

William R. Bell, Jr.*

INTRODUCTION

Recognition of the existence of proteolytic activity in human urine was first reported in 1861.[1] Nearly 25 years later, proteolytic activity with some degree of specificity for fibrin was identified in human urine.[2] Many additional proteolytic enzymes were discovered in human urine before 1900.[3,4] Several years elapsed before the proteolytic enzyme capable of fibrin degradation could be isolated and purified from human urine.[5,6] Many studies indicated that proteolytic activity resulted when the substance found in human urine acted upon plasminogen to promote and induce the formation of plasmin. This substance was designated urokinase (UK) by Sobel in 1952.[7] Considerable controversy concerning the cellular production site of urokinase then ensued.

It has now been established that the renal parenchymal cell is the cellular production site for UK, the first known tissue plasminogen activator. Urokinase currently employed in the North American continent is prepared from renal parenchymal cells grown in tissue culture.[8-10] The molecular species of UK purified from human urine is of a different form and higher in molecular weight (55,000 daltons) than the UK obtained from tissue culture (33,000 daltons). Clinically the therapeutic efficacy of these two molecular species is very similar. Recently, molecular engineering techniques have allowed the expression of UK in *E. coli* and in mammalian cell lines in tissue culture;[11-14] in the future, these techniques may become the source of therapeutic quantities of UK. In contrast to streptokinase, UK is a trypsin-type serine protease that is not normally found in the circulation. It is composed of two polypeptide chains

---

* Hubert E. and Ann E. Rogers Scholar in Academic Medicine

251

connected by a single disulfide bridge and totals 410 amino acid residues. The UK that has been employed therapeutically occurs in two molecular forms: a relatively high molecular weight form of 54,000 daltons and a lower molecular weight form of 33,000 daltons. The latter is almost certainly a proteolytic degradative product of the higher molecular weight form.[15] The complete primary structure of human UK has been identified, with 253 amino acids in the heavy chain and 157 amino acids in the light chain (Figure 1).[16-18] A single bolus of this agent given intravenously in man is cleared with a half-life of 14 ± 6 minutes.[19] Like streptokinase, most of urokinase is degraded to inert metabolites by the liver.[20] A number of circulating proteases in the blood inhibit to some degree the activity of UK, including α_2 antiplasmin, α_2 macro-

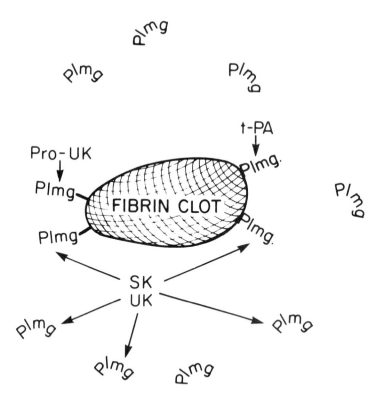

Figure 1. *Amino acid sequence of streptokinase. Reproduced from Bell WR, Sasahara AA (eds):* Review of Thrombolytic Therapy and Thromboembolic Disease. Glenview, IL, Physicians & Scientists Publishing Co., 1989, p 6, with permission.

globulin, α_1 antitrypsin, antithrombin III, and a new fast-acting inhibitor (official name pending).[21-23]

Urokinase converts inert plasminogen to proteolytically active plasmin by directly inducing an enzymatic clip at a 560 arginine-valine 561 site (the identical site attacked by streptokinase). This reaction occurs without any additional cofactors.

Therapeutic utilization of the plasminogen-plasmin proteolytic enzyme system was first made possible as a result of a discovery by Tillet in 1933.[24] Tillet discovered that β-hemolytic streptococci elaborated a substance, designated streptokinase (SK), that was capable of activating the fibrinolytic system. Now, less than 60 years later, molecular biologic techniques have allowed the expression of a cloned human tissue plasminogen activator (t-PA) in mammalian cell culture.[25] A large number of studies have demonstrated that these agents induce the lysis of thrombi and emboli in arteries and veins throughout the human body. Numerous studies[26-34] have clearly demonstrated that these agents, as the result of inducing lysis of thrombi and emboli, promptly return cardiopulmonary, peripheral venous, arterial and coronary arterial hemodynamics back toward normal. By inducing lysis of endogenously formed thrombi, these agents prevent end organ damage and avoid the development of such problems as pulmonary hypertension, renal failure, mesenteric infarction, soft tissue necrosis, peripheral venous hypertension, and the sequelae of the post-phlebitic syndrome.

The clinical indications for which thrombolytic therapy has been approved by the Center for Drugs and Biologics of the Food and Drug Administration in the United States include:

1) Pulmonary thromboemboli
2) Deep vein thrombosis
3) Arterial thromboembolic disease
4) External arteriovenous-shunts (thrombosis in)
5) Indwelling arterial or venous catheters (intraluminal thrombosis or catheter-associated thrombosis)
6) Acute myocardial infarction (AMI)

Pulmonary Thromboemboli

Pulmonary embolism (PE) affects approximately 500,000 people each year in the United States alone, although some data suggest that the actual incidence of PE may be higher.[35] In approximately 30% of untreated patients and 8-10% of treated patients, the PE is fatal.[35]

Embolic obstruction of pulmonary arterial blood flow prevents perfusion of lung areas still undergoing ventilation, producing a ventilation-perfusion mismatch. Clinically, symptoms include dyspnea, tachycardia, fever, cough, chest pain, and syncope. Often, clinical evidence of deep venous thrombosis can be found concurrently. Arterial hypoxemia is a common finding and is especially pronounced in massive PE. In acute PE, pulmonary hypertension occurs infrequently due to the large vascular reserve of the lungs and the development of collateral circulation, but it may be significant in massive PE. The fibrinolytic system attempts to address the effect of emboli by dissolving the clot to whatever extent possible. The residual is then organized and recanalized. Over time, patients may have recurrence of dyspnea and persistent pulmonary hypertension due to incomplete removal of the arterial obstruction by these mechanisms.[35,36]

Traditionally, acute PE has been treated with supportive measures and a combination of heparin and warfarin. Anticoagulants only prevent further thrombus formation or extension of existing thrombi. They do not lyse thrombi or emboli. In extreme cases, surgical intervention may be required to remove a massive obstruction caused by emboli.

Pulmonary thromboembolism remains the most common cause of death of all diseases of the thorax. In many institutions it remains the most common cause of all in-hospital deaths. The need for better treatment of this problem is obvious. A number of investigators have studied the role of thrombolytic therapy in patients with pulmonary emboli.[26-34] Some of these studies compared the efficacy of heparin to that of thrombolytic therapy in this condition. Results of these studies indicate that those patients with massive pulmonary emboli (two or more lobar arteries obstructed with emboli or the equivalent), massive pulmonary emboli and shock, or sub-massive pulmonary emboli superimposed on chronic cardiopulmonary disease where even minimal amounts of embolic material induce cardiopulmonary decompensation, should receive thrombolytic therapy as the initial treatment of choice. Patients in these categories require prompt resolution of the obstruction in the pulmonary arterial system. With the use of thrombolytic agents, there is prompt return of cardiopulmonary hemodynamics back to normal. Rapid resolution of embolic material avoids the subsequent problems of pulmonary hypertension, pulmonary failure and cardiac failure.

In patients with smaller amounts of embolic material with minimal intravascular obstruction and without significant hemodynamic decompensation, heparin treatment may be acceptable. In these patients, no data demonstrate that thrombolytic therapy is superior to heparin alone. However, if thromboembolic material can be safely dissolved from the pulmonary arterial vasculature, it may be prudent to employ thrombolytic therapy to achieve this goal.

In our experience in treating more than 700 patients and in most published reports, the usual duration of thrombolytic therapy for most patients with pulmonary emboli is 24-48 hours. The technique for administration of the thrombolytic agents is continuous infusion by an automated pump in a forearm vein. Since approximately 30% of the cardiac output goes to the lungs, it is not necessary to infuse the thrombolytic agent directly into the pulmonary artery. Although such direct delivery into the pulmonary artery is possible, local infusion of thrombolytic therapy becomes systemic immediately because of the high blood flow in this circuit. The overall success rate for thrombolytic therapy of pulmonary embolism is 65-85% of patients treated with forearm vein infusion.

Thrombolytic therapy with UK has been compared with anticoagulation to determine if the former may have benefits over traditional therapy in managing both the short-term and long-term consequences of PE. The Urokinase Pulmonary Embolism Trial (UPET), sponsored by the National Heart and Lung Institute, was a modified double-blinded, randomized trial in which UK was compared to heparin in the treatment of acute, massive, and sub-massive PE as demonstrated by lung scan and angiography.[26] Urokinase was administered at an IV loading dose of 2,000 U/lb and was followed by an infusion of 2,000 U/lb/hr for 12 hours (n = 82). Heparin was administered at an IV loading dose of 75 U/lb and was followed by an infusion of 10 U/lb/hr for 12 hours (n = 78). Both regimens were followed by heparinization for a minimum of 5 days and then warfarin anticoagulation.

The group treated with UK showed significantly greater improvement in both angiogram and lung scan (performed before and after therapy) rating scores after treatment (24 hours after initiation of therapy). Similarly, hemodynamic measurements including total pulmonary resistance, mean pulmonary artery pressure, right atrial systolic and diastolic pressures, and right atrial mean pressure were improved to a significantly greater extent in the UK group. At day seven post-therapy, the lung scan improvement was similar in the two groups. Improvement in lung scan persisted at the 3-, 6-, and 12-month evaluations. Additionally, comparison of the overall clinical improvement between the groups showed no difference in the rate of dyspnea resolution obtained at 24 hours. Analysis of those classified as having massive PE did show faster resolution of dyspnea with UK therapy. The mortality rates observed in the two treatment groups were comparable at the 14-day (7/78 heparin vs. 6/82 UK) and one-year (10/70 heparin vs. 11/69 UK) follow-up periods.

The most common clinical adverse event was bleeding, which occurred in 37/82 (45%) UK and 21/78 (27%) heparin recipients. Most of the bleeding episodes with UK occurred during the first 24 hours of therapy (29/37) and were attributed in most cases (21/29) to cut-down procedures required to perform the aggressive angiographic and hemodynamic monitoring required in the study. The mean fibrinogen concentration decreased from 514 mg/dL before UK therapy to 264 mg/dL after UK therapy. This decrease in fibrinogen concentration was not believed to be a causative factor in the bleeding episodes observed during UK therapy. Bleeding episodes related to heparin were evenly distributed throughout the 14-day adverse event monitoring period.

In this study, UK produced a significantly more rapid overall improvement, as demonstrated by angiography, lung scan, and hemodynamic measurements, than did heparin therapy. In the massive PE subgroup, improvement in dyspnea 24 hours after the initiation of therapy was greater with UK than with heparin.

As a follow-up to the overall UPET study, Sharma et al[29] followed patients treated with heparin (n = 21) and UK (n = 19) for one year to determine the influence of therapy on long-term pulmonary function. The pulmonary capillary blood volume was abnormally low before therapy in both treatment groups. At the 14-day and one-year follow-up visits, this measurement remained abnormally low in those who were treated with heparin, but it was normal in those who were treated with UK (p < 0.001). Similarly, pulmonary diffusing capacity was only 69% and 72% of the predicted values at the 14-day and one-year evaluation in the heparin group, respectively. In the UK group, these values were 85% and 93% of predicted at the 14-day and one-year follow-up visits, respectively (p < 0.001). These data show that thrombolytic therapy produced a greater short-term and long-term resolution in pulmonary perfusion and diffusion studies than did heparin therapy.

The **U**rokinase-**S**treptokinase **P**ulmonary **E**mbolism **T**rial (USPET) sponsored by the National Heart and Lung Institute enlisted 11 centers in the United States to study patients with angiographically proven, acute, symptomatic pulmonary embolism.[27] The purpose of the study was to determine if 24 hours of UK therapy was more effective than 12 hours of UK. Secondly, it was designed to determine if any differences existed between UK and SK with regard to efficacy in PE.

The Urokinase Pulmonary Embolism Trial demonstrated that thrombolytic therapy with UK produced significantly greater angiographic and hemodynamic improvement than heparin. Hence, a heparin group was not included in the USPET. Since the study designs were similar, the heparin group of the UPET was used for certain comparisons in the USPET. In the USPET, therapy with UK consisted of an IV loading dose of 2,000 U/lb, followed by an infusion of 2,000 U/lb/hr for either 12 hours (UK12) or 24 hours (UK24). Therapy with SK consisted of an IV loading dose of 250,000 IU, followed by an infusion of 100,000 IU/hr for 24 hours (SK24). Heparin was given for a minimum of five days following termination of thrombolytic therapy. This was followed by warfarin anticoagulation to complete a minimum of 14 days of total therapy.

A total of 166 patients met the entry criteria. Fifty-nine received UK12, 53 received UK24, and 54 received SK24. The PE was characterized as massive in 33/59 UK12 patients, 31/53 UK24 patients, and 31/54 SK24 patients. Analysis of angiograms performed 24 hours after the initiation of therapy showed that all three treatments produced equal angiographic improvement. Comparison of the UK12 arm in USPET with UK12 in UPET showed the improvement to be equal in the two studies, confirming both the UPET results and the validity of the interpretive criteria used in both studies. Thus, it can be stated that UK12, UK24, and SK24 therapy produced significantly greater angiographic improvement than did heparin therapy.

Complete hemodynamic measurements were available in about 50% of cases after 24 hours, and 89% of patients had at least eight cardiac and pulmonary artery pressure measurements performed. There were no differences among the three treatment groups in the amount of hemodynamic improvement produced by therapy. The mean pre-therapy perfusion defect detected by lung scan was about 33% (approximately two-thirds of one lung). The amount of resolution from baseline determined at 24 hours, 3 months, and 6 months from initiation of therapy was not different, although the amount of improvement in the UK24 group at 24 hours was greater than that in the SK24 group. These data, analyzing overall results of therapy, demonstrate that UK12, UK24, and SK24 are equal in their ability to produce angiographic, hemodynamic, and lung scan improvement.

The effect of thrombolytic therapy on patient survival at two weeks and six months post-therapy did not differ among the three treatment groups. At two weeks, the mortality rates were 7%, 9% and 9% for the UK12, UK24, and SK24 groups, respectively. At six months, these had increased to 10%, 15% and 15% for UK12, UK24, and SK24, respectively. These data indicate that UK12, UK24, and SK24 therapy produced equal overall angiographic, hemodynamic, lung scan, and survival results. In the group with massive PE, UK therapy produced significantly greater 24-hour resolution in lung scan and pulmonary artery pressure measurements.

There was no difference between the UK groups with regard to plasminogen and fibrinogen concentrations or in euglobulin lysis time. The effect of SK on these same studies was significantly greater than that produced by UK.[27,37] Although all three groups had evidence of systemic fibrinolysis, SK therapy was associated with greater abnormalities in coagulation studies than UK.

Clinical adverse events observed within 24 hours of the termination of thrombolytic therapy were not different among the three groups in the number of bleeding episodes during therapy. The monitoring of coagulation studies revealed a greater impact of SK on plasma proteins than was observed with UK. These differences were not reflected in a greater occurrence of clinical adverse events.

Recombinant tissue plasminogen activator (rt-PA) has been evaluated in an open, non-comparative clinical trial for the treatment of angiographically-proven, acute symptomatic PE.[38] Entrance and evaluation criteria were similar to those used in the UPET and USPET.[26,27] The dose of rt-PA was 50 mg given IV over 2 hours. If the repeat angiogram at that time showed clot lysis, no further doses of rt-PA were given. If no clot lysis had occurred, an additional 40 mg was given over 4 hours. Most patients received heparin post-rt-PA administration.

Thirty-six cases were evaluated; 14/36 received one dose, and 22/36 received two doses of rt-PA. There was a statistically significant improvement in angiograms after therapy with rt-PA (p < 0.001). Complete hemodynamic measurements were made before and after therapy. Therapy with rt-PA produced a significant improvement in mean pulmonary artery pressure (22 mg Hg pre-treatment vs. 18 mg Hg post-treatment, p = 0.003).

Complications of therapy included groin hematoma in 5 cases, which prevented administration of the full intended dose of rt-PA. Other bleeding complications included hematuria (n = 2), periodontal oozing (n = 3), and superficial oozing from venous or arterial puncture sites (n = 18). Major hemorrhagic episodes occurred in 2 cases, both of which required surgical intervention. Thus, a total of 30 bleeding events occurred in the 36 cases studied. The measurement of coagulation proteins showed a decrease in mean fibrinogen concentration from 360 mg/dL to 253 mg/dl with two-hour therapy, and to 223 mg/dL with six-hour therapy (p < 0.001). The fibrinogen concentration never fell below 100 mg/dL in patients whose initial value was > 100 mg/dL. Mean fibrin degradation products increased from 10 mg/mL to 96 mg/mL with two-hour therapy and to 87 mg/mL with six-hour therapy (p < 0.0001).

In this study 83% of patients treated with rt-PA showed a moderate-to-marked angiographic improvement when the one-dose and two-dose groups were combined. The authors contrast this with a 4% moderate-to-marked improvement with heparin and a 42% improvement with UK12 in UPET (although the actual values stated in UPET were 9% for heparin and 53% for UK12). Despite this stated difference, it should be noted that the average improvement in actual angiogram rating scores was similar (49% with rt-PA vs. 45% with UK12). The authors also point out that the rate of severe bleeding complications was 6% with rt-PA and 12% and 27% for UK in the USPET and UPET, respectively. Nevertheless, the overall rate of bleeding complications with rt-PA (30/36, 83%) was higher than those with UK12 (31/59, 53%) and UK24 (37/53, 70%) in USPET and with UK12 (21/78, 45%) in UPET.

Although similar criteria were used to evaluate cases treated with rt-PA and UK in separate studies, the results are subject to conflicting interpretations. Therefore, comparison of data from the preliminary study of rt-PA therapy of PE with those obtained for UK in UPET and USPET must be made with caution. Further direct comparative clinical studies of rt-PA and UK are required to assess the comparative efficacy and safety of these agents.

In a follow-up study[39] comparing rt-PA with UK in treatment of pulmonary emboli, 45 patients were studied. The total dose of rt-PA was given in 120 minutes, while the UK was given by continuous infusion over 24 hours. At 2 hours considerably more lysis occurred in the group receiving the rt-PA. At 24 hours perfusion lung scans revealed equal resolution in both UK- and rt-PA-treated groups.

Four additional studies[40-43] in patients with pulmonary emboli confirmed the excellent success rate in dissolution of emboli. In one study of 133 patients,[40] forearm vein infusion of UK was compared with intrapulmonary artery UK infusion. Equal rates of resolution were observed in the two treatment groups. In another study considerably greater efficacy of UK as compared with heparin was clearly observed.[41]

Deep Vein Thrombosis

Deep venous thrombosis (DVT) in the peripheral venous system is characterized by swelling, tenderness, heat, and pain in the affected area. Pulmonary embolism, however, may be the presenting sign.[44-54] The major source of pulmonary emboli in man is probably the deep venous system of the lower extremities. Veins of the pelvis, abdomen, upper extremities, neck, thorax, and the right side of the heart also give rise to thrombi from which pulmonary emboli may derive. Traditional therapy of DVT has revolved around symptomatic treatment combined with the use of heparin and warfarin. Unfortunately, these agents are only effective in preventing further thrombus extension; they do not augment the patient's thrombolytic system in dissolving the existing obstruction. Complete clot lysis occurs in < 10% of cases treated with anticoagulation therapy alone.[36,55] In patients in whom anticoagulant therapy is ineffective, the clot undergoes organization and subsequent recanalization, which leads to permanent damage in the affected venous valves. This damage produces venous hypertension. If severe, it is manifested clinically as the post-phlebitic syndrome, characterized by chronic edema, pain, pigmentation, cellulitis, and non-healing ulcers in the affected limb.[36,54-59]

Many studies have demonstrated that thrombolytic therapy is indicated in patients with proximal deep vein thrombosis.[44-52] In this situation thrombus formation extends into the thigh or even more proximally above the inguinal ligament or even into the inferior vena cava. Thrombolytic therapy is also indicated in patients with upper extremity thrombosis, abdominal venous thrombosis, pelvic venous thrombosis and in certain patients with intra-cardiac thrombus formation.

Patients in these categories, particularly the group with proximal venous thrombosis of the lower extremities with extensive thrombus formation, are more likely to experience pulmonary embolism and to develop post-phlebitic syndrome with pain, venous engorgement, edema, dermal breakdown, necrosis, and cellulitis. When thrombi in these venous compartments undergo resolution, the problems of the post-phlebitic syndrome and its sequelae can be avoided.[53]

From the available data, the optimal treatment of deep vein thrombosis is the use of the same doses of thrombolytic agents as are used in patients with pulmonary emboli. The mean lysis time for most patients with lower extremity venous thrombosis is between 34-36 hours of continuous infusion. Thus, at present the optimal duration of therapy is 48-72 hours. Rarely, excellent resolution in the lower extremities may occur after only 12 hours of therapy. In several patients in whom only moderate improvement occurred after 48-72 hours of continuous infusion, we have continued therapy for up to five days with excellent resolution.

Although no study has been conducted, it may be reasonable to administer the thrombolytic agent in standard doses into a vein in the ankle or foot of the involved extremity in patients with extensive venous thrombosis and massive edema of the leg. Such an approach may allow better contact of the thrombolytic agent with the thrombus. The overall success rate in the treatment of proximal venous thrombosis varies from 46-85%. This degree of variability is most likely due to the fact that in some patients the thrombus may be of very long duration and not susceptible to fibrinolysis.

Studies comparing thrombolytic therapy to anticoagulant therapy have shown that thrombolytic therapy produces significantly better clinical and venographic/phlebographic responses when therapy is given within 3-7 days of the onset of the venous obstruction.[36-38,54,55,57-61] Patients who receive thrombolytic therapy can expect clot lysis to occur 50-77% of the time. In comparison, clot lysis occurs in only 5-30% of patients treated with heparin and warfarin.[36-38,54,55,57-60]

Evaluation of UK in open non-comparative trials confirmed that complete clot lysis occurred in 14/30 patients and partial clot lysis occurred in 7/30 patients when UK was given within 6 days of the onset of disease.[62,63] When therapy was given for clots that were 1-6 weeks in duration, the rate of complete lysis decreased to 11/67, but partial lysis still occurred in 39/67 cases.

Following the open trials, UK was compared to SK in prospective randomized trials.[64,65] Initially, 33 patients with acute iliofemoral thrombosis were treated with either UK or SK.[64] Symptoms were present a mean of 3.0-4.1 days. All patients had a positive phlebogram before undergoing therapy. Patients were randomized to receive UK in an intravenous (IV) loading dose of 4,400 IU/kg, followed by an IV infusion of either 2,200 IU/kg/hr (group I, n = 11) or 1,100 IU/kg/hr (group II, n = 11) 12 hours/day for 3 days, or SK with an IV loading dose of 250,000 IU, followed by an infusion of 100,000 u/hr continuously for 3 days (group III, n = 11). Patients in the UK-treated groups received heparin during the 12 hours of each day when thrombolytic therapy was not given. Patients were evaluated with phlebograms on day 3.

At the end of therapy, 5/10 patients in group I, 7/11 patients in group II, and 6/10 patients in group III had improved. The remaining patients in each group had either no change or worsening occlusions. Two patients (1 each from groups I and III) could not be evaluated. Based on these results, 10, 9, and 5 patients in groups I, II, and III, respectively, received a second 3-day course of therapy. Of these, 7, 8, and 4 patients in groups I, II, and III, respectively, were able to be evaluated on day 6. The response rate in these cases was 4/7 in group I, 5/8 in group II, and 4/4 in group III.

These results indicate that in cases of acute thrombi in iliofemoral veins, UK and SK are equally effective in producing clot lysis. These regimens differed in terms of their effects on coagulation proteins and in their propensity to produce adverse clinical events. For example, in the SK group all patients had a fibrinogen concentration of < 100 mg/dL on all days of therapy. In contrast, all patients in the UK groups had a concentration of > 100 mg/dL on all days of therapy. Clinically, hematuria developed in 3 patients in group I, 2 patients in group II, and in 7 patients in group III. Additionally, one patient each in groups I and III developed bleeding at an IV puncture site.

One SK recipient developed a "shock-like" syndrome that required discontinuation of therapy. Fever (38.5°-40° C) developed in all SK recipients but in only one UK recipient. In summary, a total of 20 adverse events occurred in 11 SK recipients, as compared to 7 adverse events in 22 UK recipients.

In a second prospective, randomized trial, 40 patients with deep venous thrombosis were assigned to receive UK in an IV loading dose of 4,000 U/kg followed by 4,000 U/kg/hr, or SK 250,000 IU IV followed by 100,000 IU/hr.[65] The duration of initial therapy averaged 5 days for each agent. A second treatment course was administered if indicated. Both groups received heparin concurrently in a dose of 18 U/kg/hr. All patients had positive phlebograms before therapy.

Substantial clot lysis occurred in 76% of UK and 79% of SK recipients, indicating that the two regimens were equally effective in lysing clots. Once again, the incidence of adverse events differed between the two groups. Fever and bleeding accounted for most of the increased incidence of adverse events in the SK recipients. All UK recipients completed therapy, while 42% of SK recipients had therapy discontinued due to an adverse event. These data suggest that while UK and SK appear to be equally effective in lysing venous thrombi, SK therapy is associated with more complications.

Sharma et al[66] reviewed their experience with UK and SK in the treatment of DVT in those patients with documented DVTs at the time they were entered into the prospective, randomized Urokinase-Streptokinase Pulmonary Embolism Trial (USPET).[26] In this study, patients were randomized to receive one of three regimens: 1) UK at a loading dose of 200 U/lb, followed by an IV infusion of 2,000 U/lb/hr for 12 hours (group I, n = 6) or 24 hours (group II, n = 5); 2) SK at an IV loading dose of 250,000 IU followed by an infusion of 100,000 IU/hr for 24 hours (group III, n = 5); or 3) heparin 1,000-2,000 U/hr for 7 days to maintain the partial thromboplastin time at two times normal (group IV, n = 16). All patients had positive electrical impedance phlebography before therapy.

After 24 hours of therapy, 3/6 patients in group I, 4/5 patients in group II, 4/5 patients in group III, and 1/16 patients in group IV had negative phlebograms. Repeat evaluations on day 7 yielded only one additional patient in group I and 3 patients in group IV with a negative test result. In summary, UK and SK appeared to be equally effective in lysing thrombi, and both agents were more effective than heparin.

A comparison of the effects of UK and SK on coagulation values has been reported.[27] At 18 hours the mean fibrinogen concentration decreased to < 200 mg/dL in the SK group, although it exceeded this value at all other time points in the 24-hour sample period. Mean fibrinogen concentrations were > 300 mg/dL at all sample points in both UK groups. Mean fibrin degradation products exceeded 400 mg/dL at all time points (peaking at approximately 600 mg/dL at 12 hours) in the SK group, while this value was < 200 mg/dL in the 12-hour UK group and < 400 mg/dL in the 24-hour UK group at all times. Mean plasminogen concentrations were < 1 u/mL in both the UK and SK groups, although values in the UK groups exceeded those in the SK group by about two-fold. Thus, patients in the SK group showed a trend toward more systemic manifestations of a lytic state than those in the UK groups.

A decrease in hematocrit value of > 5% occurred in 3/16 heparin, 2/5 SK and 5/11 UK recipients. Only one patient (in the UK group) required a transfusion. These events were due to bleeding at the IV cut-down site in 8 cases; in 2 other cases the cause was unknown. Thus, despite the differences in laboratory coagulation measurements in UK and SK recipients, there was no significant difference between these two regimens with regard to clinical bleeding.

Graor et al[67] recently analyzed the outcomes of 60 patients who were assigned to receive either UK (n = 30) or SK (n = 30) for the treatment of DVT. All patients had venographically proven acute venous thrombosis (duration ≤ 7 days) in thigh or pelvic veins. SK was given at an IV loading dose of 250,000 IU followed by a 100,000 IU/hr infusion for a mean duration of 58 hours (range 48-106). UK was given at an IV loading dose of 4,400 U/kg followed by an infusion of 4,400 U/kg/hr for a mean of 26 hours (range 24-48). UK and SK were equally effective in lysing clots. Complete clot lysis occurred in 24/30 (80%) SK-treated patients and in 25/30 (83%) UK-treated patients. Partial lysis was observed in 4/30 (13%) patients in each group. Clot lysis was not achieved in 1 UK patient and in 2 SK recipients. The effect of each agent on fibrinogen concentration was also studied. In the SK group, 19/30 (63%) patients had a fibrinogen concentration < 100 mg/dL during therapy, while only 9/30 (30%) UK recipients had this finding (p = 0.01). In the SK group, fibrinogen decreased an average of 83% from the baseline reading, as compared to 61% in the UK group.

Minor adverse clinical events (e.g., fever, vomiting, nausea, urticaria) occurred in 16/30 (53%) SK and 0/30 UK recipients. Major complications such as hemorrhage occurred in 5/30 (17%) patients who received SK. These 5 patients required therapy in the form of blood transfusion, fresh frozen plasma, surgery, or chest tube insertion. Only 1/30 UK-treated patients suffered a hemorrhagic episode; this was treated with 2 units of fresh frozen plasma. The difference in the number of bleeding complications between the two treatment groups was significant (p = 0.019).

Based on this analysis, these authors concluded that when such factors as differences in the duration of thrombolytic infusion required, length of hospital stay, and complications due to adverse events were taken into account, the cost of UK therapy was only $11.40 more per patient than that of SK therapy (based on a cost of $140.00 per 250,000 U for UK and $18.45 per 250,000 IU for SK). This was due to the increased cost for major interventions to control hemorrhage in the SK group. In this regard, an average of $641 was spent on each SK case for complications, while only $2.50 was spent per UK case. The mean length of stay was 8 days for SK-treated patients and 4.3 days for UK-treated patients.

Thus, although the results of studies of DVT therapy indicate that SK and UK are equal in efficacy, the majority of patients treated with UK suffered significantly fewer major and minor complications, with the decrease in cost for treatment of adverse events nearly offsetting the difference in cost between the two thrombolytic agents. More recent studies have again confirmed the high success rate of thrombolysis with UK in the venous circulation.[68-71] It is clear from these studies that UK is efficacious in the upper extremities as well as in the lower extremities.[71]

The treatment of DVT with recombinant tissue plasminogen activator (rt-PA) has been evaluated in an open study with 20 patients.[72] Patients received heparin plus either rt-PA or placebo. rt-PA was administered intravenously in a dose of 0.5 mg/kg for 4 hours. Patients received a second course of therapy (rt-PA 0.5 mg/kg or placebo) over a 1-hour period if the venogram was not improved at 72 hours post-initial therapy.

In the heparin plus rt-PA group, 2/10 patients achieved complete clot lysis, 3/10 patients had partial lysis, and 5/10 patients had no lysis of their clots. In the heparin plus placebo group, only 1/10 patients had partial clot lysis, and 9/10 had no improvement. It was not specified if these were the results at the end of the first or second course of therapy. Patients who received rt-PA were noted to have a 40% decrease in plasminogen, a 50% decrease in fibrinogen, reduction of α_2 -antiplasmin to undetectable levels, and a four-fold increase in fibrin degradation products compared to baseline.

Thus, in this preliminary report, rt-PA plus heparin was substantially more active than heparin plus placebo in the dissolution of clots in the deep venous system. Although the rates for complete and partial clot lysis appear to be somewhat lower than those reported for UK and SK,[33,34,44-46] any conclusions concerning the efficacy and safety of rt-PA in the treatment of DVT must await studies comparing this agent directly with UK and/or SK.

Arterial Thromboembolic Disease

Peripheral arterial thromboembolic disease is one of the most disabling diseases of elderly people. Although surgical techniques are sometimes useful in the treatment of thrombo-occlusive disease of the large and some of the proximal medium-size arteries, these techniques are not useful in distal medium-size vessels, small arteries and the microvascular circulation. Frequently, surgical techniques, because of distortion of or injury to vascular endothelium, may induce thrombus formation. The advent of thrombolytic therapy provides an alternative approach to the reconstitution of arterial blood flow.

Thrombolytic therapy is indicated whenever acute thrombo-occlusive disease occurs any place in the arterial system, with the exception of those vessels directly supplying the central nervous system. Most frequently, thrombolytic therapy is employed for thrombo-occlusive disease involving the superficial and deep arteries of the lower extremities, the renal and mesenteric arteries, the arteries of the upper extremities and in particular, the hands and fingers, and the aorta.[73,74] Recently, thrombolytic therapy has been employed successfully to induce the dissolution of intra-cardiac thrombus formation.[75] Fibrinolytic agents have also been used successfully to restore patency to arterial bypass grafts, predominantly in the aorta and lower extremities.

When treating thrombo-occlusive disease on the arterial side of the circulatory system, two techniques are currently utilized. One technique is systemic infusion of the thrombolytic agent, employing the standard dose (SK 250,000 IU loading dose followed by 100,000 IU/hr sustaining dose, or UK 4,000 U/kg loading dose followed by 4,000 U/kg/hr sustaining dose) delivered into a forearm vein. The second technique is the local infusion method. With this technique an angiocatheter is passed into the proximal portion of the involved vessel and placed adjacent to or directly into the substance of the thrombus. With the catheter in place, infusion of the thrombolytic agent is initiated. No loading doses are administered. A continuous infusion of SK at 7,500 IU/hr or UK at 15,000 U/hr is given. Utilizing this technique, McNamara and Fischer[76] have had excellent success using UK at 4,000 U/minute.

With the local perfusion technique, because of a relatively lower degree of systemic fibrinolytic activity (at least for the first 8-10 hours), there is occasionally a tendency for thrombus formation to occur on the catheter employed to deliver the thrombolytic agent. To avoid this problem either a double lumen catheter or a two-catheter technique is employed. Into the second lumen or the second catheter heparin at a concentration of 0.25 units/mL is infused at a "keep open" rate, concomitantly with the infusion of the thrombolytic agent. In this way thrombus formation on the infusion catheter is avoided.

A successful result with thrombolytic therapy in the arterial circulation can frequently be appreciated early (2-3 hours) in the course of treatment. Usually the first sign appreciated by the patient is a decrease in the intensity of pain. Promptly thereafter the temperature in the involved area increases. If these signs are observed, it is important to continue the infusion and pursue complete reconstitution of blood flow. If success is achieved with thrombolytic therapy, complex surgical procedures can be avoided. If no signs of success are observed in the early hours of treatment, the thrombolytic agent can be discontinued, and within less than one hour the patient can safely be taken to the operating theater for surgery. Thus, with respect to time, thrombolytic therapy can be judiciously used without additional risk to the jeopardized tissue distal to the site of arterial thrombus or embolus. Even in the most ideal situation, several hours are required to arrange for the surgical procedure. This time can be used to try thrombolytic therapy. If successful, surgery is avoided; if it fails, surgery can still be performed without an excessive delay.

If surgery is performed initially and fails because of reformation of thrombus material despite heparin anticoagulation, the clinician must decide whether to initiate thrombolytic therapy. However, in this setting, following 2-3 surgical attempts, some degree of oozing at the arterial site(s) of surgical intervention is common. The administration of thrombolytic therapy immediately following arterial surgery is usually very risky. Thus, it is reasonable to try thrombolytic therapy before rather than imme-diately following surgery on the arterial vascular compartment.

The overall success of thrombolytic therapy in the treatment of thrombo-occlusive disease of the arterial network is 55-70%. Employing the local perfusion technique the frequency of success is higher than with the systemic infusion technique.

Acute arterial obstruction may result from thrombosis or emboli.[54] When collat-eral vessels cannot supply blood to the affected areas, the patient experiences pain, pallor, coldness, and numbness in the affected areas. Eventually, ischemia and gan-grene may develop if therapeutic interventions to restore blood supply are not undertaken. When indicated, these interventions have included embolectomy and angioplasty along with the judicious use of anticoagulants. In spite of aggressive treatment, however, mortality rates of 12-34% and amputation rates of 5-45% have been reported.[77,78]

Thrombolytic therapy has been evaluated as a possible intervention in arterial occlusion and peripheral arterial graft occlusion. In these cases, thrombolytic therapy has generally been administered in relatively low doses directly into the thrombus or embolus via a catheter. Presumably, this provides therapy to the affected site without activating the systemic fibrinolytic system to as great an extent as would full-dose intravenous therapy. This may lead to fewer bleeding complications.

The results obtained with streptokinase (SK) have been compared to those ob-tained with heparin therapy. In 17 patients the limb salvage rate was 75% with SK, which far exceeded the 33% rate observed with heparin.[57] In open studies with SK, clot lysis was achieved in > 70% of the cases of acute arterial thrombosis when the clot was present for < 3 days.[56] In another open study involving 600 patients with femoral or iliac artery obstruction, the figure was 75% when the obstruction was present for < 2 weeks.[57] In some cases, after thrombolytic therapy had dissolved the obstructing clot, angioplasty was performed if residual stenosis was present at the site of obstruction (e.g., an atherosclerotic plaque).

A retrospective study compared UK and SK therapy of arterial occlusion in 33 symptomatic patients with positive arteriograms who had 37 acute episodes of arterial occlusion.[79] The median duration of occlusion was 24 hours (range 3 hours to 3 weeks). Occlusions involved the lower extremities (n = 33), upper extremities (n = 3) and a visceral artery (n = 1). Twenty-two of these patients had a known history of peripheral vascular disease and 18 had undergone previous femoral-popliteal or fem-oral-tibial bypass grafting.

Patients received an intra-arterial (IA) infusion of SK 5,000 IU/hr (n = 25) for an average of 44 hours, or UK 40,000 U/hr (up to 60,000 U/hr) for an average of 46 hours (n = 12). All treatment courses lasted a minimum of 12 hours. Heparin was co-adminis-tered at a rate of 200-500 U/hr to prevent thrombosis of the infusion catheter.

In the SK group, 11/22 (50%) of the evaluable episodes were associated with both clinical and angiographic improvement, while in the UK group, 10/10 (100%) improved (p < 0.005). One patient who responded to UK therapy had failed to respond to 24 hours of SK therapy. Of the 21 totally successful courses with UK and SK, 5 patients required angioplasty and 4 patients required surgery to repair anatomic abnormalities.

The two treatment regimens also differed in their effects on coagulation studies and in their tendency to produce adverse events. Mean coagulation protein determinations were markedly abnormal in the SK group. In the UK group, only a minimal elevation of prothrombin time was noted, and only one UK patient had a significant abnormality in coagulation studies. These differences were reflected in the fact that 12/25 (48%) SK courses were associated with a bleeding episode that was believed to be due to abnormalities in the coagulation profile. These included 7 major (bleeding that required surgical repair or transfusion) and 5 minor (oozing at access site, groin hematoma) bleeding episodes. Additionally, two more cases had new cerebrovascular accidents thought to be due to emboli. Only 3/12 (25%) UK courses were associated with a bleeding episode, but 2 of these were believed to be due to procedures performed concurrently. A total of 22 adverse events occurred in 25 SK treatment courses as compared to 6 adverse events in 12 UK treatment courses. Thus, in this study, UK was shown to be more effective than SK in the treatment of arterial occlusions and was also associated with fewer adverse events.

Gardiner et al[78] retrospectively analyzed 44 cases of angiographically proven thrombosis of femoral-popliteal bypass grafts that were treated with UK (n = 22) between 1984-1985 or SK (n = 22) between 1979-1984. The age of the obstruction was < 7 days in 30 cases and > 7 days in 14 cases. Patients received a UK loading dose of 30,000-60,000 U followed by an IA infusion of 4,000 U/min for 2 hours, 2,000 U/min for 2 hours, and 1,000 U/min until therapy was completed (mean 26 hours in responders). In the SK group, loading doses of 25,000-250,000 IU were followed by IA infusion of 5,000-15,000 IU/hr for a mean of 47 hours (in responders). Prior to initiating therapy, a guidewire was passed through the clot 1-2 times.

Overall, UK completely lysed the thrombus in 17/22 cases (77%), while this was accomplished in only 9/22 (41%) SK cases (p < 0.05). None of the 18 patients who failed UK or SK therapy had a successful thrombectomy, and 10 eventually required amputation.

The number of adverse events recorded during therapy was also different for the two treatment groups. In the UK group, 5/22 (23%) patients had an adverse event. These included embolus (2), hematoma (1), acute renal insufficiency and congestive heart failure (1), and angina plus pulmonary embolism (1). In the SK group, 11/22 (50%) patients had an adverse event. These included hematoma (7), embolus (1), renal failure (1), hypotension plus myocardial infarction (1), and leaking aortic aneurysm (1). Four patients in the SK group had therapy terminated due to bleeding complications. In this study, UK was not only more effective than SK in lysing occluded arterial grafts but was also associated with fewer adverse events.

266

McNamara and Fischer[76] compared their experience with intra-arterial UK for angiographically proven peripheral arterial or arterial graft occlusion to historical controls who received SK. Controls were obtained by reviewing six studies in the medical literature. There were 93 UK treatment courses in 85 patients. In the current study, occlusion was present for < 10 days in 72 cases and > 10 days in 21 cases. Seventy-one cases were thrombotic in origin, while 22 involved obstruction due to embolism. In this series, UK was given in an IA dose of 4,000 U/min for 4 hours, decreasing to 1,000-2,000 U/min for 14-18 hours. Heparin 1,000 U/hr was co-administered with UK in 86/93 courses. The treatment was completed in 84/93 courses. In the other nine courses, therapy was discontinued due to adverse events (n = 6) or the need for surgical intervention (n = 3). No patient who completed therapy required an amputation. Canalization was achieved in 84/93 (90%) patients. Complete clot lysis was achieved in 70/93 (75%) cases (including failures with SK), while 75/93 (81%) cases resulted in clinical improvement that was sufficient to obviate the need for surgical intervention. In the 64 cases of thrombotic obstruction that were evaluable, 50 eventually required angioplasty for residual stenosis. These results are substantially better than those observed in controls who received SK administered either IA or IV in doses up to 100,000 IU/hr. In these patients, complete clot lysis was observed in 70/155 (45%) cases, despite longer mean durations of SK infusion (41 hours).

The mean time to initial clot opening was 3.3 hours in UK patients with 73% (61/84) and occurred within two hours of the initiation of treatment. Interestingly, all patients who had initial clot opening within 2 hours ultimately had complete clot lysis as compared to only 39% who achieved initial opening after 2 hours of therapy. An additional predictor of response was the ability to pass a guidewire through the clot prior to initiation of therapy. In 62 cases in which this was attempted, passage was obtained in 52; none of these patients went on to fail therapy. In contrast, all 10 patients in whom the guidewire could not pass also failed to respond to therapy.

Evaluation of coagulation factors revealed mean fibrinogen levels of 265 mg/dL at the 4,000 U/min UK dose and 208 mg/dL at the 1,000 U/min dose (normal 170-410 mg/dL). A total of 32 adverse events were noted during 15/93 UK infusions. All cases of bleeding were at a vascular puncture site. One patient with moderate bleeding was also thrombocytopenic, and another with severe bleeding had been therapeutically anticoagulated with warfarin. In one case of severe bleeding, the fibrinogen level was 60 mg/dL. This was the only case in which the fibrinogen was < 100 mg/dL. Streptokinase controls had a frequency of severe bleeding of 13% as compared to 4% for UK therapy, despite the use of relatively high UK doses. Pericatheter thrombosis occurred in 2/7 cases (29%) in which heparin was not co-administered but in only 3/86 (4%) cases in which heparin was administered concurrently. These data are similar to those reported for SK controls, who had a 35% thrombosis rate without heparin and a 12% rate with concurrent heparin administration. Distal clot migration led to increasing ischemia in two cases, one of which required surgery. Therapy was discontinued due to an adverse event in only 5 cases.

As in previous studies, these comparative data indicate that in the treatment of peripheral arterial or arterial graft occlusion, the use of relatively high-dose UK produces a two-fold greater rate of clot lysis than SK therapy while causing about one-third the number of severe bleeding complications.

McNamara and Bomberger[80] subsequently updated this experience to include their first 100 cases of UK therapy for arterial occlusion and to assess the results by site of occlusion. Consistent with their previous report, complete clot lysis occurred in 77/100 treatment courses. Six-month follow-up data revealed that 86% of supra-inguinal sites remained open as compared to 38% of infra-inguinal sites. Native arterial occlusions responded better than arterial graft occlusions (71% versus 41% at a six-month follow-up, respectively). A final predictor of outcome was residual stenosis; only 8% of arteries with residual stenosis after therapy remained open as compared to 85% of those without residual stenosis.

During the past two years, several studies have reconfirmed the excellent rate of resolution of thromboembolic disease in the arterial circulation.[70,81-96] Several of these studies[82-90] demonstrate a success rate of 80-85% in patients treated with UK. A novel approach in the administration of UK has been employed in patients with thrombotic occlusions of hemodialysis grafts, arterial bypass grafts, and native peripheral arteries.[95] This procedure involved the use of a small pulse of highly concentrated UK forcefully sprayed into the thrombus. This resulted in complete resolution in 46 of the 47 patients treated. Clearly, further attention needs to be directed to this technique.

Recombinant tissue plasminogen activator (rt-PA) has recently been evaluated in 18 patients with thrombosed peripheral arteries (n = 12) or peripheral arterial grafts (n = 6).[97] The mean duration of occlusion was 6.8 days (range 1-21). The dose of rt-PA was 0.1 mg/kg/hr given as an intra-arterial infusion for a mean of 202 minutes (range 60-390). The mean total dose was 29.2 mg (range 9-58). Heparin was not given concurrently. In 15/18 (83%) cases, both clinical and angiographic improvement were noted. Following rt-PA therapy 2 patients required angioplasty, and 5 required surgical intervention for residual abnormalities. Of 3 non-responders, 2 were believed to have anatomic abnormalities that prevented the optimal delivery of thrombolytic therapy. The fibrinogen concentration fell below 100 mg/dL in 3/18 (17%) patients and decreased an average of 40% from baseline. Plasminogen and α_2-antiplasmin decreased an average of 47% and 93% from baseline, respectively. Adverse events included groin hematomas in three cases. One patient had a cerebrovascular hemorrhage 48 hours post-rt-PA therapy, but he was receiving heparin at the time.

Although no direct comparisons are available for rt-PA versus UK or SK, these preliminary data suggest that rt-PA is of equal efficacy to these agents in the treatment of acute arterial thrombosis and graft occlusion. These data suggest a safety and laboratory profile similar to those seen with UK and SK.

External A-V Shunts and Indwelling Catheters

When the lumen of external A-V shunts and indwelling venous and arterial catheters becomes obliterated by thrombus formation, function diminishes and concern over possible thrombus extension arises. In the past, treatment of this problem required removal of the shunt or catheter (Hickman, Broviac, Infusaport, etc.) and implantation of a new device at a different location. Currently, thrombolytic therapy is indicated to promptly restore patency and function to these devices. This is accomplished by instillation of 5-10 mL (depending on the size of the device) containing 5,000 U of UK. After incubation of the thrombolytic solution for 1-3 hours, the contents of the catheter can usually be aspirated and patency restored. This may have to be repeated for complete clearance. When this is achieved, the need for removal and reimplantation at a different site is completely avoided. Recently completed studies[98-100] indicate that patency can be restored in greater than 90% of such devices obstructed by thrombus formation. If the obstruction results from crystalline precipitation, kinking of the device tubing, or movement of the device beyond the blood vessel wall, thrombolytic agents are not indicated and are not helpful.

Although the indwelling catheter may remain patent, thrombus formation may occur near the location of the catheter tip. In this situation thrombolytic therapy is indicated to dissolve the thrombus and to prevent growth and propagation that might obstruct not only the catheter but also adjacent vessels. An acceptable way to deal with this problem is to employ the local perfusion technique using the indwelling catheter to infuse the thrombolytic agent in low doses. In most instances this approach results in resolution of the thrombus and allows continued safe use of the indwelling catheter.

Additional studies employing various regimens of UK in the treatment of thrombi obstructing indwelling catheters and A-V shunts demonstrate 90% success in restoring patency.[101-104]

Acute Myocardial Infarction

Acute myocardial infarction is a major cause of hospitalization in the United States. Approximately 1.5 million persons sustain myocardial infarctions each year in this country, and of these about 550,000 die. Acute myocardial infarction is responsible for 36% of all deaths in males between the ages of 28 and 64 years. Many studies[105-137] strongly indicate this will be reduced by treatment with thrombolytic therapy.

The cause of cardiac ischemia resulting in the clinical and electrocardiographic evidence of AMI has been disputed for many years. Recent angiographic and surgical data support the presence of occlusive coronary artery thrombi as the cause of obstruction to coronary blood flow in 87% of AMI cases examined within four hours of the onset of symptoms.[135] Intraluminal thrombus formation is the final event in a series of vascular and endothelial disturbances that result in complete cessation of blood flow.

Studies in laboratory animals and later in patients undergoing coronary artery bypass surgery within six hours of the onset of symptoms showed that less permanent myocardial damage occurred when the thrombosed artery recanalized early after the development of symptoms. Several clinical trials with the thrombolytic agent SK showed that intervention within the first 3-6 hours after the onset of symptoms significantly reduced the early mortality of MI compared with standard therapy.[131,138-141] The myocardial salvage produced by removal of thrombotic obstruction also led to preservation of myocardial contractility and left ventricular function. The initial approach to the treatment of AMI with thrombolytic therapy was to deliver the thrombolytic agent directly into the coronary arteries by catheter cannulation of the coronary ostia of the occluded vessel(s). Following the initial successful studies of Rentrop et al,[105,106] successful reconstitution of coronary blood flow with thrombolytic therapy has been achieved in 57-96% of patients treated in a large number of studies.[107-134] Most of these studies were performed using intracoronary SK at a dose of 20,000 IU loading and 2,000 IU/min for 90 minutes; a small number of studies used intracoronary UK at a dose of 6,000 IU/min for 90 minutes.

Within the past several years numerous studies have been carried out with systemic infusion of thrombolytic therapy in the treatment of myocardial infarction. With this technique, successful reperfusion of the coronary arteries occurs nearly as often as with direct intracoronary infusion. Using systemic infusion techniques, an amazing number of different doses, schedules, and durations have been employed. No single best regimen has been identified.

Intracoronary Thrombolytic Therapy of Acute Myocardial Infarction

One of the early studies compared therapy with UK to SK in a randomized, double-blinded study of 80 patients suffering an AMI.[134,142] Patients had symptoms for < 12 hours (mean 5.3 hr), electrocardiographic evidence of AMI, and angiographic evidence of coronary artery obstruction. Patients received intracoronary (IC) UK (n = 45) at a rate of 6,000 U/min or IC SK (n = 35) at a rate of 2,000 IU/minute. Angiograms were repeated every 15 minutes until maximal coronary opening occurred. No infusion lasted longer than two hours.

The results of therapy were similar for the two treatment groups. The occluded artery was opened in 27/45 (60%) UK and 20/35 (57%) SK patients (p = 0.8). Time to first opening of the obstruction occurred at 35 ± 21 minutes in the UK group and 45 ± 27 minutes in the SK group (p = 0.17). The only difference between the two groups was in the total duration of therapy, which was 81 ± 34 minutes in the UK group and 97 ± 29 minutes in the SK group (p < 0.05).

Monitoring of laboratory measurements and clinical adverse events revealed significant differences in the two treatments. Fibrinogen concentration decreased to < 100 mg/dL in 2/34 (6%) UK and 19/29 (66%) SK recipients in whom these measurements were performed before and after therapy (p < 0.001). This translated into an incidence of hemorrhage of 11% (5/45) in UK-treated patients and 29% (10/35) in SK recipients (p < 0.05). Of these, 7/10 SK and 1/5 UK bleeding episodes were considered major and required transfusion, surgical intervention, drainage, or discontinuation of therapy. The fibrinogen concentration was < 100 mg/dL during 8/9 bleeding episodes with SK therapy and 1/5 episodes with UK therapy. Additionally, 4/5 SK recipients who had coronary bypass surgery within 20 hours of thrombolytic therapy had bleeding complications.

In this study, UK and SK were equally effective in opening obstructed coronary arteries. A significantly lower number of complications occurred with UK therapy. Despite the use of local IC infusion, SK produced a significantly greater abnormality in coagulation protein concentrations, which may have contributed to the increased incidence of bleeding events with this agent.

INTRAVENOUS THERAPY FOR MYOCARDIAL INFARCTION

Urokinase therapy by the intravenous (IV) route has been evaluated in open noncomparative studies of the treatment of AMI.[143,144] A total of 35 patients with angiographic evidence of obstructed coronary arteries, electrocardiographic evidence of MI, and symptoms of MI for < 3 hours duration were treated with IV UK.[143] Patients received either 200,000 U IV bolus followed by an IV infusion of 1,200,000 U over 1.5 hours (n = 21; group I) or an IV bolus dose of 500,000 U without subsequent infusion (n = 14; group II). Angiography performed 48 hours after the onset of therapy showed that 14/21 (66%) group I and 13/14 (93%) group II patients had their obstructed coronary arteries opened. The mean time to peak CPK-MB concentrations was 12 hours for those who were reperfused and 20 hours in those without reperfusion. No adverse events were reported.

Mathey et al[144] administered a single IV bolus of 2,000,000 U of UK (n = 50) to patients with symptoms of MI < 3 hours and electrocardiographic evidence of MI. Heparin 200 u/kg/12 hours was also given to prevent thrombosis of angiography catheters. The dose of UK was given an average of 1.8 hours after the onset of symptoms. Initial coronary angiography was not performed until after UK was given and occurred a mean of 1.1 ± 0.6 hours after the dose. At this time, coronary arteries were open in 30/50 (60%) patients. Because of the study design, it is not known if any of these arteries were patent before UK was administered. Follow-up at three weeks was available in 24 patients with open coronary arteries after therapy. Of these, 23/24 (96%) still had patent coronary arteries. Ventriculograms could be analyzed in 32 acutely ill patients and in 36 patients at follow-up (both studies were available in 25 patients). In those with patent coronary arteries following UK administration, the left ventricular ejection fraction (LVEF) was 55%. This was unchanged at follow-up (53%). Wall motion was depressed (–2.2 SD/Chord) initially but improved (–1.5 SD/Chord) at follow-up. Wall motion was significantly better in those who were reperfused with UK (–1.2 SD/Chord) within 2 hours of the onset of symptoms than those in whom reperfusion never occurred (–2.5 SD/Chord) (p = 0.05).

The effects of IV bolus UK therapy on coagulation proteins revealed significant abnormalities when measured two hours after the dose of UK. At 24 hours, however, these values were within the normal range. Despite these abnormalities in coagulation proteins, no clinical adverse events were reported. There was a significant difference in the mean maximal level of creatinine kinase between those who responded to UK therapy (802 u/L) versus those who did not respond (1,848 u/L in patients in whom angioplasty or IC SK ultimately opened the artery, p < 0.05; 1,973 u/L in those whose coronary arteries did not reopen, p < 0.005).

These two studies of IV UK in AMI show that 60-92% of obstructed coronary arteries could be reperfused with either bolus or infusion UK therapy. When administered within two hours of this event, successful UK therapy produced significant improvement in left ventricular wall motion as compared to unsuccessful therapy. Despite abnormalities in coagulation values, no adverse bleeding events occurred in either study. Although the optimal dose of any available thrombolytic agent in the treatment of acute coronary thrombosis has not be absolutely established, for UK it is probably somewhere between 1.5 and 3.0 million units given over 60-90 minutes. Studies comparing rt-PA to SK in the treatment of AMI have been carried out, and are summarized in Chapters 10 and 11.[137-140]

During the past three years there has been a progressive increase in the number of studies employing UK thrombolysis in patients with AMI, unstable angina, and related problems.[145-167] These studies suggest that the frequency of reperfusion patency with UK is about as high as seen with SK, rt-PA, or acylated streptokinase plasminogen activator complex (APSAC). In one large study comparing UK with rt-PA, although the overall reperfusion success was equal in the two treatment groups, there were two subgroups categorized on the basis of the degree of coronary artery obstruction and duration of symptoms in which UK opened the arteries faster and with statistically greater frequency than did rt-PA.[156] In this study, angiography performed at the completion of the infusion revealed a patent infarct-related artery in 69.4% of 121 patients receiving rt-PA versus 66% of 117 patients given urokinase (p = not significant). In those patients treated within 3 hours of symptom onset, a patent infarct-related artery was identified in 63.9% of 72 patients receiving rt-PA versus 70 patients receiving urokinase (p = not significant). There were five cardiac deaths in each treatment group and one fatal intracranial hemorrhage in the rt-PA treatment group. The rate of reinfarction was the same in each group and there was no improvement in left ventricular function after treatment. Reocclusion following treatment was less in patients receiving urokinase.

The results of UK in opening reoccluded coronary bypass grafts in those who failed to respond to rt-PA have been particularly impressive.[168-170] In these reports, the authors have demonstrated the prolonged (17-70 hours) infusion of urokinase 50,000-100,000 U/hr given through a wire imbedded directly into the thrombus in the coronary artery results in a high rate of patency. These patients presented with coronary thrombosis of 2-8 weeks in duration. This technique was successful in native coronary vessels as well as occluded vein bypass grafts. Most recently, several studies have employed combinations of thrombolytic agents.[151,152,159,162,167] These studies have attempted to identify synergy: two agents yielding greater efficacy and fewer complications than a single agent. In some studies, an attempt has been made to reduce the dose of agents employed in combination. In general, no striking differences have been observed with combination therapy, although a trend toward a better outcome than with single-agent therapy has been seen.

Miscellaneous Uses

Both UK and SK have been used for several thrombotic diseases in which their use has not yet been officially approved by the Center for Drugs and Biologics of the Food and Drug Administration. Successful therapy with fibrinolytic agents has been reported in a variety of unusual or threatening clinical states including thrombosis of cardiac valves,[139,171,172] renal artery thrombosis,[173] renal vein thrombosis,[174-176] retinal artery and vein thrombosis, central nervous system vascular thrombosis,[177,178] paroxysmal nocturnal hemoglobinuria with abdominal venous thrombosis,[179] priapism,[180] Budd-Chiari syndrome[179,181,182] and for clots or fibrosis in body cavities such as occur after pleural exudates,[183-185] and cardiac chamber thrombosis.[75,186-189] Since fibrinolytic therapy can produce dramatic results, especially in the most seriously or acutely ill patients, it is reasonable to consider this therapeutic possibility for patients with all types of thrombotic disorders.

Recently, the diuretic amiloride has been found to inhibit the activity of UK in the conversion of plasminogen to plasmin.[190] Thus, amiloride should be discontinued in any patient treated with UK.[190]

Urokinase in the Pediatric Population

During the past decade, experience has accumulated on the use of UK thrombolysis in premature infants, infants and children.[191-196] The results of these studies clearly indicate that this agent can safely be employed in the younger age group, and success is fairly impressive.

273

PRACTICAL USE OF UROKINASE

Pulmonary Emboli

Urokinase is given in a forearm vein infusion in the following manner:

1. Loading dose
   4,000 U/Kg in 50 or 100 mL D5W or NSS over 30-45 minutes
2. Sustaining dose
   4,000 U/Kg/hr in 500 or 1,000 mL
3. Duration of infusion
   It is thought that the optimal duration of infusion is 24-36 hours. It is seldom that 48 hours of therapy are required.

Deep Vein Thrombosis*

1. Loading dose
   4,000 U/Kg IV in 50 or 100 mL over 30-45 minutes
2. Sustaining dose
   4,000 U/Kg/hr IV
3. Duration of infusion
   Most patients require 48 hours of treatment and very seldom is an additional 24 hours required. Some patients experience excellent resolution in 12 hours or less.

Arterial Thrombosis

This condition is most frequently and most successfully treated when the infusion of urokinase is given adjacent to or directly into the substance of the thrombus.

1. Loading dose — usually not given
2. Sustaining infusion dose
   4,000 U/min for 1-2 hours
   followed by
   2,000 U/min for 1-2 hours
   followed by
   1,000 U/min until successful opening is achieved
3. Duration of infusion
   Most infusions are given for 6-12 hours, rarely for 18-24 hours

---

* See footnote on following page.

274

Indwelling Infusion Catheters

If the obstruction is confined to the lumen of the infusion catheter:
1. UK given in 5-10 mL volume containing 5,000 U directly into the catheter and allowed to incubate 1-2 hours. At this time, attempts are made to aspirate the obstructing thrombus. This may have to be repeated 2-3 times.

If the obstruction extends from the catheter tip into distal veins, the dose of UK and technique is that as described under venous thrombosis. In this situation, every attempt is made to infuse the UK directly into the involved venous network.

Acute Myocardial Infarction

Intra-coronary Route (IC)

1. After cannulation of the obstructed infarct-related artery, UK is given directly in a dose of 6,000 U for 90-120 minutes.

Intravenous Route*

1. The UK is infused in a forearm vein in one of the following ways:
   a) 3,000,000 U given in 45-60 minutes
   b) 1,500,000 U given in 5 minutes followed by an additional 1,500,000 U given over 45-60 minutes

At the completion of all the various infusions of UK, the patient within 15-30 minutes is started on a continuous infusion of heparin at approximately 1,000 U/hr. A loading bolus dose is usually not given. The patient may then be switched to warfarin. The duration of heparin and warfarin is decided by the patients' physician.

SUMMARY

Since urokinase became commercially available in January of 1979, a large number of studies has confirmed the clinical utility of this agent. It is evident from the reported data that UK is capable of activating the plasminogen-plasmin proteolytic enzyme system, thereby inducing resolution of thrombi and emboli on both the arterial and venous side of the circulation. The frequency of successful resolution of thrombi/emboli with this agent is excellent and not statistically different from that observed with

---

* Not FDA approved for this condition, but the use of UK in these situations is widespread and has been reported in several publications.

SK, rt-PA, or APSAC. In comparative studies with rt-PA in the treatment of AMI in certain subcategories of patients, the time required to open the coronary arteries was shorter with UK than with rt-PA, and the frequency of coronary vessel patency was greater with UK in contrast to rt-PA. In the treatment of pulmonary emboli, deep vein thrombosis, and arterial thromboembolic occlusive disease, the success rate has been excellent but not significantly better than that seen with SK. In the category of restoration of patency of indwelling catheters of all types, greater than 90% success has been observed with UK. In the treatment of peripheral vascular disease, particularly peripheral thrombo/embolic arterial occlusive disease, studies have shown UK to be associated with a greater degree of success and fewer complications than other thrombolytic agents. For this reason, virtually all interventional radiologists are now routinely employing urokinase therapy.

From all available published data, the frequency of complications associated with thrombolytic therapy is lowest when UK is employed. This is particularly evident with respect to hemorrhage. The frequency of intracranial hemorrhage associated with urokinase is lower than that observed with any other thrombolytic agent. Associated fever seldom occurs. In addition, urokinase administration does not lead to the formation of antibodies against the drug.

REFERENCES

1. von Brucke E: Die verdauende substanz im urin. SB Akad Wiss (Vienna) 1861;43:601-615.

2. Sahli W: Uber das vorkommen non pepsin und trypsin in mornalen menschlichen harn. Pflugers Arch ges Physiol 1886;38:35-93.

3. Gehrig F: Uber fermente in harn. Pflugers Arch ges Physiol 1886;38:35-93.

4. Grutzner P: Uber fermente in harn. Dtsch Med Wschr 1891;17:10-13.

5. MacFarlane RG, Pilling J: Fibrinolytic activity of normal urine. Nature 1947;159:779.

6. Williams JRB: The fibrinolytic activity of the urine. Br J Exptl Pathol 1951;32:530-537.

7. Sobel GW, Mohler SR, Jones NW, et al: Urokinase: An activator of plasma pro-fibrinolysin extracted from urine. Am J Physiol 1952;171:768-769.

8. Bernik MB, Kwaan MC: Plasminogen activator activity in cultures from human tissues. An immunological and histochemical study. J Clin Invest 1969;48:1740-1753.

9. Bernik MB: Increased plasminogen activator (urokinase) in tissue cultures after fibrin deposition. J Clin Invest 1973;52:823-834.

10. Bernik MB, White WF, Oller EP, et al: Immunologic identity of plasminogen activator in human urine, heart, blood vessels and tissue culture. J Lab Clin Med 1974;84:456-558.

11. Ratzkin B, Lee SG, Schrenk WJ, et al: Expression in Escherichia coli of biologically active enzyme by a DNA sequence coding for the human, plasminogen activator urokinase. Proc Natl Acad Sci USA 1981;78:3313-3317.

12. Hung PP: The cloning, isolation and characterization of a biologically active human enzyme, urokinase, in E. coli. Adv Exptl Med Biol 1984;172:281-293.

13. Kalyan NK, Hung PP, Levner MH, et al: Site-specific DNA splicing: a general procedure for the creation of a restriction site at a predetermined position in a DNA sequence. Gene 1986;42:331-337.

14. Cheng SM, Lee SG, Kalyan NK: Isolation of a human cDNA of urokinase and its expression in COS-1 cells. Gene 1988;69:357-363.

15. White WF, Barlow GH, Mozen MN, et al: The isolation and characterization of plasminogen activators (urokinase) from human urine. Biochemistry 1966;5:2160-2169.

16. Steffens GJ, Gunzler WA, Otting F, et al: The complete amino acid sequence of low molecular mass urokinase from human urine. Z Physiol Chem 1982;363:1043-1058.

17. Gunzler WA, Steffens GJ, Otting F, et al: The primary structure of high molecular mass urokinase from human urine: the complete amino acid sequence of the A chain. Z Physiol Chem 1982;363:1155-1165.

18. Gunzler WA, Steffens GJ, Otting F, et al: Structural relationship between human high and low molecular mass urokinase. Z Physiol Chem 1982;363:133-141.

19. Fletcher AP, Alkjaersig N, Sherry S, et al: The development of urokinase as a thrombolytic agent. Maintenance of a sustained thrombolytic state in man by its intravenous infusion. J Lab Clin Med 1965;65:713-731.

20. Collen D, DeCock F, Lijnen HR: Biological and thrombolytic properties of proto-enzyme and active forms of urokinase. II. Turnover of natural and recombinant urokinase in rabbits and squirrel monkeys. Thromb Haemostas 1984;52:24-26.

21. Ogston D, Bennett B, Herbert J, et al: The inhibition of urokinase by alpha 2-macroglobulin. Clin Sci 1973;44:73-79.

22. Clemmensen I, Christensen U: Inhibition of urokinase by complex formation with human alpha 1-antitrypsin. Biophys Acta 1978;249:591-599.

23. Podor TJ, Schleef RR, Loskutoff DJ: A competitive radioimmunoassay (RIA) for a fast acting inhibitor of plasminogen activator (PA). Thromb Haemostas 1985;54:218.

24. Tillet WS, Garner RL: The fibrinolytic activity of hemolytic streptococci. J Exp Med 1933;58:485-502.

25. Pennica D, Holmes WE, Kohr WJ, et al: Cloning and expression of human tissue-type plasminogen activator cDNA in *E. coli*. Nature 1983;301:214-221.

26. Urokinase Pulmonary Embolism Trial Study Group. A Urokinase Pulmonary Embolism Trial. A national cooperative study. Circulation 1973;47(suppl 2):1-108.

27. Urokinase-Streptokinase Pulmonary Embolism Trial Study Group: Urokinase-Streptokinase Pulmonary Embolism Trial. Phase II Results. A national cooperative study. JAMA 1974;229:1606-1613.

28. Dalen JE, Alpert JS: Natural history of pulmonary embolism, in Sasahara AA, Sonenblick EH, Lesch M (eds): *Pulmonary Emboli*. New York, Grune & Stratton, pp 77-88, 1975.

29. Sharma GVRK, Burleson VA, Sasahara AA: Effect of thrombolytic therapy on pulmonary capillary blood volume in patients with pulmonary embolism. N Engl J Med 1980;303:842-845.

30. Robertson BR: On thrombosis, thrombolysis and fibrinolysis. Acta Chir Scand 1971;421(suppl):551.

31. Miller II GA, Hall RJC, Paneth MM: Pulmonary embolectomy, heparin and streptokinase; their place in the treatment of acute massive pulmonary embolism. Am Heart J 1977;93:568-574.

32. Ly B, Arnesen H, Eie H, et al: A controlled trial of streptokinase and heparin in the treatment of major pulmonary embolism. Acta Med Scand 1978;203:465-470.

33. Bell WR, Simon TL: Current status of pulmonary thromboembolic disease: pathophysiology, diagnosis, prevention and treatment. Am Heart J 1982;103:239-262.

34. Bell WR: Pulmonary embolism: progress and problems. Am J Med 1982;72:181-183.

35. Bell WR, Bartholomew JR: Pulmonary thromboembolic disease. Curr Prob Cardiol 1985;10:1-70.

36. Sherry S, Gustafson E: The current and future use of thrombolytic therapy. Ann Rev Pharmacol Toxicol 1985;25:413-431.

37. Bell WR: Thrombolytic therapy: A comparison between urokinase and streptokinase-from a national cooperative study. Semin Thromb Hemostas 1975;2:1-13.

38. Goldhaber SZ, Vaughan DE, Markis JE, et al: Acute pulmonary embolism treated with tissue plasminogen activator. Lancet 1986;2:886-888.

39. Goldhaber SZ, Kessler CM, Heit J, et al: Randomized controlled trial of recombinant tissue plasminogen activator versus urokinase in the treatment of acute pulmonary embolism. Lancet 1988;2:293-298.

40. The UKEP Study Research Group: The UKEP study: multicentre clinical trial on two local regimens of urokinase in massive pulmonary embolism. Eur Heart J 1987;8:2-10.

41. Berger T, Schafer H, von Gemmeren D, et al: Local fibrinolytic therapy in acute pulmonary embolism. Ann Radiol 1987;30:151-155.

42. Marini C, DiRicco G, Rossi G, et al: Fibrinolytic effects of urokinase and heparin in acute pulmonary embolism: a randomized clinical trial. Respiration 1988;54:162-173.

43. Rosenthal D, Evans D, Borrero E, et al: Massive pulmonary embolism: Triple-armed therapy. J Vasc Surg 1989;9:261-270.

44. Browse NL, Thomas ML, Pim HP: Streptokinase and deep vein thrombosis. Br Med J 1968;3:717-720.

45. Kakkar VV, Flauc C, Howe CT, et al: Treatment of deep vein thrombosis. A trial of heparin, streptokinase, and arvin. Br Med J 1969;1:806-810.

46. Robertson BR, Nilsson IM, Nylauder G: Thrombolytic effect of streptokinase as evaluated by phlebography of deep venous thrombi of the leg. Acta Chir Scand 1970;136:173-180.

47. Tsapogas MJ, Peabody RA, Wu KT, et al: Controlled study of thrombolytic therapy in deep vein thrombosis. Surgery 1973;74:973-984.

48. Duckert F, Muller G, Nyman D, et al: Treatment of deep vein thrombosis with streptokinase. Br Med J 1975;1:479-481.

49. Porter JM, Seaman AJ, Common HH, et al: Comparison of heparin and streptokinase in the treatment of venous thrombosis. Am Surg 1975;41:511-519.

50. Marder VJ, Soulen RL, Atichartakarn V: Quantitative venographic assessment of deep vein thrombosis in the evaluation of streptokinase and heparin therapy. J Lab Clin Med 1977;89:1018-1029.

51. Arnesen H, Heilo A, Jakobsen E, et al: A prospective study of streptokinase and heparin in the treatment of venous thrombosis. Acta Med Scand 1978;203:457-463.

52. Elliott MS, Immelman EJ, Jeffrey P, et al: A comparative randomized trial of heparin versus streptokinase in the treatment of acute proximal venous thrombosis: an interim report of a prospective trial. Br J Surg 1979;66:838-843.

53. O'Donnel TF, Browse NL, Burnand KG, et al: The socioeconomic effects of an ileofemoral thrombosis. J Surg Res 1977;22:483-488.

54. Strandness DE: Vascular diseases of the extremities, in Isselbacher KJ, Adams RD, Braunwald E, Petersdorf RG, Wilson JD (eds): *Harrison's Principles of Internal Medicine.* New York, McGraw-Hill, 1980, pp 1181-1188.

55. Klatte EC, Becker GJ, Holden RE, et al: Fibrinolytic therapy. Radiology 1986;159:619-624.

56. Marder VJ: The use of thrombolytic agents: choice of patient, drug administration, laboratory monitoring. Ann Intern Med 1979;90:802-808.

57. Rutkowski DM, Burkle WS: Advances in thrombolytic therapy. Drug Intell Clin Pharm 1982;16:115-121.

58. Porter JM, Taylor LM: Current status of thrombolytic therapy. J Vasc Surg 1985;2:239-249.

59. Kwaan HC: Thrombolytic therapy with urokinase and streptokinase. Med Chall 1978;10:25-38.

60. Vogelsang GB, Bell WR: Treatment of pulmonary embolism and deep vein thrombosis with thrombolytic therapy. Clin Chest Med 1984;5:487-494.

61. Stambaugh RL, Alexander MR: Therapeutic use of thrombolytic agents. Am J Hosp Pharm 1981;38:817-824.

62. Tesi M, Carini A, Mirchioni R, et al: Thrombolytic therapy with urokinase in deep vein thrombosis. Int Angiol (Italy) 1984;3:373-376.

63. Trubestein G, Brecht T, Ludwig M, et al: Experience with urokinase therapy in the treatment of fresh and older deep-vein thromboses, in Trebestein G (ed): *Urokinase Therapy*. New York, FK Schattauer Verlag, 1981, pp 67-89.

64. van de Loo JCW, Kriessmann A, Trubestein G, et al: Controlled multicenter pilot study of urokinase-heparin and streptokinase in deep venous thrombosis. Thromb Haemostas 1983;50:660-663.

65. Zimmermann R, Epping J, Rasche H, et al: Urokinase and streptokinase treatment of deep vein thrombosis. Results of a randomized study. Haemostasis 1986;16(suppl 5):9.

66. Sharma GVRK, O'Connell DJ, Belko JS, et al: Thrombolytic therapy in deep vein thrombosis, in Paoletti R, Sherry S (eds): *Thrombosis and Urokinase*. New York, Academic Press, 1977, pp 181-189.

67. Graor RA, Young JR, Risius B, et al: Comparison of cost-effectiveness of streptokinase and urokinase in the treatment of deep vein thrombosis. Ann Vasc Surg 1987;1:524-528.

68. Scheffler P, Leipnitz G, Braun B, et al: Thrombus formation in deep venous thrombosis. A clinical approach to diagnosis and control of lysis efficacy. Int Angiol 1988;7:207-213.

69. Pilla T, Comerota AJ: Basic data related to thrombolytic therapy for venous thrombosis. Ann Vasc Surg 1989;3:81-85.

70. Sniderman KW, Kalman PG, Oderny A, et al: Low-dose fibrinolytic therapy for recent lower extremity thromboembolism. J Can Assoc Radiol 1989;40:98-103.

71. Meister FL, McLauglin TF, Tenney RD, et al: Urokinase. A cost-effective alternative treatment of superior vena cava thrombosis and obstruction. Arch Intern Med 1989; 149:1209-1210.

72. Turpie AGG, Jay RM, Carter CJ, et al: A randomized trial of recombinant tissue plasminogen activator for the treatment of proximal deep vein thrombosis. Circulation 1985;72:111-193.

73. Marder VJ, Bell WR: Fibrinolytic therapy in hemostasis and thrombosis, in Colman RW, Hirsh J, Marder VJ, Salzman EW (eds): *Hemostasis and Thrombosis: Basic Principles and Clinical Practice*. Philadelphia, JB Lippincott Co., 1982, pp 1037-1057.

74. Hess H, Ingrisch H, Mietaschk A, et al: Local low-dose thrombolytic therapy of peripheral arterial occlusions. N Engl J Med 1982;307:1627-1630.

75. Kremer P, Feibig R, Tilsner V, et al: Lysis of ventricular thrombi with urokinase. Circulation 1985;72:112-118.

76. McNamara TO, Fischer JR: Thrombolysis of peripheral arterial and graft occlusions. Am J Radiol 1985;144:769-775.

77. Persson AV, Thompson JE, Patman RD: Acute arterial occlusions. Vasc Surg 1977; 11:359-363.

78. Gardiner GA, Koltun W, Kandarpa K, et al: Thrombolysis of occluded femoral-popliteal grafts. Am J Roentgenol 1986;147:621-626.

79. Belkin M, Belkin B, Buckman CA, et al: Intra-arterial fibrinolytic therapy - efficacy of streptokinase versus urokinase. Arch Surg 1986;121:769-773.

80. McNamara TO, Bomberger RA: Factors affecting initial and 6 month patency rates after intraarterial thrombolysis with high dose urokinase. Am J Surg 1986;152:709-712.

81. Andrews JC, Griggs TJ, Ensminger WD, et al: Local thrombolytic therapy for hepatic artery thrombosis following chemotherapy infusion catheter placement. Invest Radiol 1987;22:467-471.

82. McNamara TO: Role of thrombolysis in peripheral arterial occlusion. Am J Med 1987; 83:6-10.

83. Pernes JM, de Almeida Augusto M, Vitoux JF, et al: Local thrombolysis in peripheral arteries and bypass grafts. J Vasc Surg 1987;6:372-378.

84. Traughber PD, Cook PS, Micklos TJ, et al: Intraarterial fibrinolytic therapy for popliteal and tibial artery obstruction: comparison of streptokinase and urokinase. Am J Radiol 1987;149:453-456.

85. van Breda A, Katzen BT, Deutsch AS: Urokinase versus streptokinase in local thrombolysis. Radiology 1987;165:109-111.

86. Koltun WA, Gardiner GA, Harrington DP, et al: Thrombolysis in the treatment of peripheral arterial vascular occlusions. Arch Surg 1987;122:901-905.

87. Hess H, Mietaschk A, Bruckl R: Peripheral arterial occlusions: A 6-year experience with local low-dose thrombolytic therapy. Radiology 1987;163:753-758.

88. Comerata AJ, Rubin RN, Tyson RR, et al: Intra-arterial thrombolytic therapy in peripheral vascular disease. Surg Gyn Obstet 1987;165:1-8.

89. Price C, Jacocks MA, Tytle T: Thrombolytic therapy in acute arterial thrombosis. Am J Surg 1988;156:488-491.

90. Lupatelli L, Barzi F, Corneli P, et al: Selective thrombolysis with low-dose urokinase in chronic arteriosclerotic obstructions. Cardiovasc Intern Radiol 1988;11:123-126.

91. Abu-Nama T, Ayyash K, Wafaii IK, et al: Jellyfish sting resulting in severe hard ischaemia successfully treated with intra-arterial urokinase. Br J Acc Surg 1988;19:294-296.

92. Parent FN, Bernhard VM, Pabst TS, et al: Fibrinolytic treatment of residual thrombus after catheter embolectomy for severe lower limb ischemia. J Vasc Surg 1989;9:153-160.

93. Durham JD, Geller SC, Abbott WM, et al: Regional infusion of urokinase into occluded lower-extremity bypass grafts: long-term clinical results. Radiology 1989;172:83-87.

94. Italian Cooperative Group (Bologna): Endoarterial treatment of acute ischemia of the limbs with urokinase. Int Angiol 1989;8:53-56.

95. Bookstein JJ, Fellmeth B, Roberts A, et al: Pulsed-spray pharmacomechanical thrombolysis: preliminary clinical results. Am J Roentgenol 1989;152:1097-1100.

96. Goffette P, Kurdziel JC, Dondelinger RD: Local urokinase infusion for total occlusion of the lower abdominal aorta. Report of two cases and a review of the literature. Eur J Radiol 1989;9:121-124.

97. Graor RA, Risius B, Young JR, et al: Peripheral artery and bypass graft thrombolysis with recombinant human tissue-type plasminogen activator. J Vasc Surg 1986;3:115-124.

98. Hurtubise MR, Bottino JC, Lawson M, et al: Restoring patency of occluded central venous catheters. Arch Surg 1980:115:212-213.

99. Glynn MFX, et al: Therapy for thrombotic occlusion of long-term intravenous alimentation catheters. J Parenter Enteral Nutr 1980;4:387-390

100. Lawson M, Bottino JC, Hurtubise MR, et al: The use of urokinase to restore the patency of occluded central venous catheters. Am J IV Ther Clin Nutr 1982;9:29-30,32.

101. Fraschini G, Jadega J, Lawson M, et al: Local infusion of urokinase for the lysis of thrombosis associated with permanent central venous catheters in cancer patients. J Clin Oncol 1987;5:672-678.

102. Bjeletich J: Declotting central venous catheters with urokinase in the home by nurse clinicians. NITA 1987;10:428-430.

103. Suarez CR, Ow EP, Lambert GH, et al: Urokinase therapy for a central venous catheter thrombosis. Am J Hematol 1989;31:269-272.

104. Stokes DC, Rao BN, Mirro J Jr, et al: Early detection and simplified management of obstructed Hickman and Broviac catheters. J Pediatr Surg 1989;24:257-262.

105. Rentrop KP, Blanke H, Karsch KR, et al: Acute myocardial infarction: intracoronary application of nitroglycerin and streptokinase. Clin Cardiol 1979;2:354-363.

106. Rentrop P, Blanke H, Kostering H, et al: Intrakoronare streptokinase applikation bei akutem infarkt and instabiler angina pectoris. Dtsch Med Wschr 1980;105:221-228.

107. Rentrop P, Blanke H, Karsch KR, et al: Selective intracoronary thrombolysis in acute myocardial infarction and unstable angin pectoris. Circulation 1981;63:307-317.

108. Ganz W, Buchbinder N, Marcus H, et al: Intracoronary thrombolysis in evolving myocardial infarction. Am Heart J 1981;101:4-13.

109. Mathey DG, Kuck KH, Tilsner V, et al: Nonsurgical coronary artery recanalization in acute transmural myocardial infarction. Circulation 1981;63:489-497.

110. Reduto LA, Smalling RW, Freund GC, et al: Intracoronary infusion of streptokinase in patients with acute myocardial infarction: effects of reperfusion on left ventricular performance. Am J Cardiol 1981;48:403-409.

111. Gold HK, Leinbach RC, Buckley MJ, et al: Intracoronary streptokinase in evolving infarction. Hosp Pract 1981;16:105-119.

112. Markis JE, Malagold M, Parker JA, et al: Myocardial salvage after intracoronary thrombolysis with streptokinase in acute myocardial infarction: assessment by intracoronary thallium-201. N Engl J Med 1981;305:777-782.

113. Lee G, Amsterdam EA, Low R, et al: Efficacy of percutaneous transluminal coronary recanalization utilizing streptokinase thrombolysis in patients with acute myocardial infarction. Am Heart J 1981;102:1159-1167.

114. Cowley MJ, Hastillo A, Vetrovec GW, et al: Effects of intracoronary streptokinase in acute myocardial infarction. Am Heart J 1981;102:1149-1158.

115. Reduto LA, Freund GC, Gaeta JM, et al: Coronary artery reperfusion in acute myocardial infarction: beneficial effects of intracoronary streptokinase on left ventricular salvage and performance. Am Heart J 1981;102:1168-1177.

116. Kaziwara N, Kanmatsuse S, Yagi H, et al: Urokinase in acute myocardial infarction. Shindan to chiryo (diagnosis and treatment) 1981;69:420-428.

117. Schuler G, Schwarz F, Hofmann M, et al: Thrombolysis in acute myocardial infarction using intracoronary streptokinase: assessment by thallium-201 scintigraphy. Circulation 1982;66:658-664.

118. Meyer J, Merx W, Schmitz H, et al: Percutaneous transluminal angioplasty immediately after intracoronary streptolysis of transmural myocardial infarction. Circulation 1982; 66:905-916.

119. Spann JF, Sherry S, Caraballo BA, et al: High dose brief intravenous streptokinase early in acute myocardial infarction. Am Heart J 1982;104:939-945.

120. Mathey DG, Schofer J, Kuck KH, et al: Transmural haemorrhagic myocardial infarction after intracoronary streptokinase. Br Heart J 1982;48:546-551.

121. Cowley MJ, Gold HK: Use of intracoronary streptokinase in acute myocardial infarction. Mod Concepts Cardiovasc Dis 1982;51:97-102.

122. Goldberg S, Urban PL, Greenspon A, et al: Combination therapy for evolving myocardial infarction: intracoronary thrombolysis and percutaneous transluminal angioplasty. Am J Med 1982;72:994-997.

123. Stampfer MJ, Goldhaber SZ, Yusuf S, et al: Effect of intravenous streptokinase on acute myocardial infarction. N Engl J Med 1982;307:1180-1182.

124. Cowley NJ, Hastillo A, Vetrovec GW, et al: Fibrinolytic effects of intracoronary streptokinase administration in patients with acute myocardial infarction and coronary insufficiency. Circulation 1983;67:1031-1038.

125. Anderson JL, Marshall HW, Bray BE, et al: A randomized trial of intracoronary streptokinase in the treatment of acute myocardial infarction. N Engl J Med 1983;308:1312-1318.

126. Khaja F, Walton JA, Brymer JF, et al: Intracoronary fibrinolytic therapy in acute myocardial infarction. N Engl J Med 1983;308:1305-1311.

127. Kennedy JW, Ritchie JL, David KB, et al: Western Washington randomized trial of intracoronary streptokinase in acute myocardial infarction. N Engl J Med 1983;309:1477-1482.

128. Rogers WJ, Mantle JA, Hood, et al: Prospective randomized trial of intravenous and intracoronary streptokinase in acute myocardial infarction. Circulation 1983;68:1051-1061.

129. Schroeder R, Biamino G, Leitner ER, et al: Intravenous short-term infusion of streptokinase in acute myocardial infarction. Circulation 1983;67:536-548.

130. Alderman EL, Jutzy KR, Berte LE, et al: Randomized comparison of intravenous versus intracoronary streptokinase for myocardial infarction. Am J Cardiol 1984;54:14-19.

131. Laffel GL, Braunwald E: Thrombolytic therapy: a new strategy for the treatment of acute myocardial infarction. N Engl J Med 1984;311:710-717, 770-776.

132. Furberg CD: Clinical value of intracoronary streptokinase. Am J Cardiol 1984;53:626-627.

133. Leiboff Rh, Katz JR, Wasserman AG, et al: A randomized, angiographically controlled trial of intracoronary streptokinase in acute myocardial infarction. Am J Cardiol 1984; 53:404-407.

134. Tennant SN, Dixon J, Venable TC, et al: Intracoronary thrombolysis in patients with acute myocardial infarction comparison of efficacy of urokinase and streptokinase. Circulation 1984;69:756-760.

135. DeWood MA, Spores J, Notske MD, et al: Prevalence of total coronary occlusion during the early hours of transmural myocardial infarction. N Engl J Med 1980;303:897-902.

136. The TIMI Study Group. The thrombolysis in myocardial infarction (TIMI) trial. N Engl J Med 1985;312:932-936.

137. Verstraete M, Bernard R, Borey M, et al: Randomized trial of intravenous recombinant tissue-type plasminogen activator versus intravenous streptokinase in acute myocardial infarction. Lancet 1985;1:842-847.

138. Kennedy JW: Streptokinase for the treatment of acute myocardial infarction: A brief review of randomized trials. J Am Coll Cardiol 1987;10:28B-32B.

139. Inberg MV, Havia T, Arstila M: Thrombolytic treatment for thrombolytic complication of valve prosthesis after tricuspid valve replacement. Scand J Thorac Cardiovasc Surg 1977;11:195-198.

140. Braunwald E, Alpert JS, Ross RS: Acute myocardial infarction, in Isselbacher KJ, Adams RD, Braunwald E, Petersdorf RG, Wilson JD (eds): *Harrison's Principles of Internal Medicine*. New York, pp 1125-1136, 1980.

141. Spann JF, Sherry S: Coronary thrombosis for evolving myocardial infarction. Drugs 1984;28:465-483.

142. Kubler W, Doorey A: Reduction of infarct size, an attractive concept. Br Heart J 1985; 53:5-8.

143. Cernigliaro C, Sansa M, Campi A, et al: Efficacy of intracoronary and intravenous urokinase in acute myocardial infarction. J Ital Cardiol 1984;14:927-930.

144. Mathey DG, Schofer J, Sheehan H, et al: Intravenous urokinase in acute myocardial infarction. Am J Cardiol 1985;55:878-882.

145. Topol EJ: Clinical use of streptokinase and urokinase therapy for acute myocardial infarction. Heart Lung 1987;16:760-774.

146. Matsuda M, Fujiwara H, Onodera T, et al: Quantitative analysis of infarct size, contraction band necrosis and coagulation necrosis in human autopsied hearts with acute myocardial infarction after treatment with selective intracoronary thrombolysis. Circulation 1987;76:981-989.

147. Katari R, Ishikawa K, Kanamasa K, et al: Improved prognosis after coronary thrombolysis with urokinase in acute myocardial infarction. Jpn Heart J 1987;28:863-872.

148. Ohyagi A, Hirose K, Watanabe Y, et al: Dose of urokinase for intra-coronary thrombolysis in patients with acute myocardial infarction. Clin Cardiol 1987;10:453-456.

149. Kambara H, Kammatsuse K, Nobuyoshi M, et al: Randomized double-blind trial of intracoronary urokinase for acute myocardial infarction: multicenter study. Jpn Circ J 1987;51:1072-1076.

150. Cernigliaro C, Sansa M, Campi A, et al: Clinical experience with urokinase in intracoronary thrombolysis. Clin Cardiol 1987;10:222-230.

151. Gurewich V: Experiences with pro-urokinase and potentiation of its fibrinolytic effect by urokinase and by tissue plasminogen activator. J Am Coll Cardiol 1987;10:16B-21B.

152. Collen D, Van de Werf F: Coronary arterial thrombolysis with low-dose synergistic combinations of recombinant tissue-type plasminogen activator (rt-PA) and recombinant single-chain urokinase-type plasminogen activator (rscu-PA) for acute myocardial infarction. Am J Cardiol 1987;60:431-434.

153. Mathey DG, Schofer J, Sheehan FH: Coronary thrombolysis with intravenous urokinase in patients with acute myocardial infarction. Am J Med 1987;83:26-30.

284

154. Motomiya, T, Tokuyasu Y, Watanabe K, et al: Intracoronary urokinase in acute myocardial infarction: prevalence of total coronary occlusion during the early hours, effects on myocardial infarct size and left ventricular function, and outcome of residual coronary stenosis. Jpn Circ J 1988;52:702-708.

155. Gotoh K, Minamino T, Katoh O, et al: The role of intracoronary thrombus in unstable angina: angiographic assessment and thrombolytic therapy during ongoing anginal attacks. Circulation 1988;77:526-534.

156. Neuhaus KL, Tebbe U, Gottwik M, et al: Intravenous recombinant tissue plasminogen activator (rt-PA) and urokinase in acute myocardial infarction: results of the German Activator Urokinase Study (GAUS). J Am Coll Cardiol 1988;12:581-587.

157. Nakagawa S, Hanada Y, Kowaya Y, et al: Angiographic features in the infarct-related artery after intracoronary urokinase followed by prolonged anticoagulation. Circulation 1988;78:1335-1344.

158. Kambara H, Kawai C, Kajiwara N, et al: Randomized, double-blinded multicenter study. Comparison of intracoronary single-chain urokinase-type plasminogen activator, pro-urokinase (GE-0943), and intracoronary urokinase in patients with acute myocardial infarction. Circulation 1988;78:899-905.

159. Topol EJ, Califf RM, George BS, et al: Coronary arterial thrombolysis with combined infusion of recombinant tissue-type plasminogen activator and urokinase in patients with acute myocardial infarction. Circulation 1988;77:1100-1107.

160. Ishikawa K, Oda A, Kanamasa K, et al: Effects of coronary thrombolysis on left ventricular ejection fraction in patients with acute myocardial infarction. Jpn Circ J 1988;52:1141-1148.

161. Brunelli C, Spallarossa P, Ghigliotti G, et al: Peaking time of creatine-kinase MB in patients treated with urokinase or conventionally during acute myocardial infarction. Cardiologia 1988;33:669-674.

162. Kasper W, Meinertz T, Hohnloser S, et al: Coronary thrombolysis in man with pro-urokinase: improved efficacy with low dose urokinase. Klin Wochenschr 1988;66:109-114.

163. Diefenbach C, Erbel R, Pop T, et al: Recombinant single-chain urokinase-type plasminogen activator during acute myocardial infarction. Am J Cardiol 1988;61:966-970.

164. Ogassawara K, Aizawa T, Nakamura F: Angina preceding myocardial infarction and residual coronary narrowing after intracoronary thrombolysis. Am Heart J 1989;117:804-808.

165. Schreiber TL, Macina G, McNulty A, et al: Urokinase plus heparin versus aspirin in unstable angina and non-Q wave myocardial infarction. Am J Cardiol 1989;64:840-844.

166. Marx M, Armstrong WP, Wach JP, et al: Short duration, high-dose urokinase infusion for recanalization of occluded saphenous aorta coronary bypass grafts. Am J Roentgenol 1989;153:167-171.

167. Gulba DC, Fischer K, Barthels M, et al: Low dose urokinase preactivated natural pro-urokinase for thrombolysis in acute myocardial infarction. Am J Cardiol 1989;63:1025-1031.

168. McKeever L, Hartmann J, Bufalino V, et al: Prolonged selective urokinase infusion in totally occluded coronary arteries and bypass grafts. Cath Cardiovasc Diag 1988;15:247-251.

169. Hartmann J, McKeever L, Teran J, et al: Prolonged infusion of urokinase for recanalization of chronically occluded aortocoronary bypass grafts. Am J Cardiol 1988;61:189-191.

170. McKeever LS, Hartmann JR, Bufalino VJ, et al: Acute myocardial infarction complicating recanalization of aortocoronary bypass grafts with urokinase therapy. Am J Cardiol 1989;64:683-685.

171. Luluaga IT, Carrera D, Oliveria J, et al: Successful thrombolytic therapy after acute tricuspid-valve obstruction. Lancet 1971;1:1067-1068.

172. Sugawa M, Ohkubo S, Nakamura M, et al: Successful fibrinolytic treatment for recurrent thrombosis on aortic valve prosthesis. Jpn J Med 1988;27:200-202.

173. Jones FE, Black PJ, Cameron JS, et al: Local infusion of urokinase and heparin into renal arteries in impending renal cortical necrosis. Br Med J 1975;4:547-549.

174. Rowe JM, Rasmussen RL, Mader SL, et al: Successful thrombolytic therapy in two patients with renal vein thrombosis. Am J Med 1984;77:1111-1114.

175. Burrow CR, Walker WG, Bell WR, et al: Streptokinase salvage of renal function after renal vein thrombosis. Ann Intern Med 1984;100:237-238.

176. Vogelzang RL, Moel DI, Cohn RA, et al: Acute renal vein thrombosis: Successful treatment with intra-arterial urokinase. Radiol 1988;169:681-682.

177. Hacke W, Zeumer H, Ferhert A, et al: Intra-arterial thrombolytic therapy improves outcome in patients with acute vertebrobasilar occlusive disease. Stroke 1988;19:1216-1222.

178. Poeck K: Intra-arterial thrombolytic therapy in acute stroke. Acta Neurol Belg 1988;88:35-45.

179. Sholar PM, Bell WR: The use of thrombolytic therapy to resolve inferior vena cava thrombosis in PNH. Ann Intern Med 1985;103:539-541.

180. King LM, McCune DP, Harris JJ, et al: Fibrinolysin therapy for thrombosis of priapism. J Urol 1964;92:692-695.

181. Warren RL, Schlant RC, Wenger NK: Treatment of Budd-Chiari syndrome with streptokinase. Gastroenterology 1973;64:200.

182. Yankes JR, Uglietta JP, Grant J, et al: Percutaneous trans-hepatic recanalization and thrombolysis of the superior mesenteric vein. Am J Radiol 1988;151:289-290.

183. Bergh NP, Ekroth R, Larsson S, et al: Intrapleural streptokinase in the treatment of haemothorax and empyema. Scand J Thorac Cardiovasc Surg 1977;11:265-268.

184. Yoshimato T, Ohwada K, Takahashi K, et al: Magnetic urokinase: targeting of urokinase to fibrin clot. Biochem Biophys Res Commun 1988;152:739-743.

185. Moulton JS, Moore PT, Mencini RA: Treatment of loculated pleural effusions with transcatheter intracavitary urokinase. Am J Roentgenol 1989;153:941-945.

186. Keren A, Medina A, Gottlieb S, et al: Lysis of mobile left ventricular thrombi during acute myocardial infarction with urokinase. Am J Cardiol 1987;60:1180-1181.

187. Goldhaber SZ, Nagel JS, Theard M, et al: Treatment of right atrial thrombus with urokinase. Am Heart J 1988;115:894-897.

188. Paulson EK, Miller FJ: Embolization of cardiac mural thrombosis; complication of intra-arterial fibrinolysis. Radiol 1988;168:95-96.

189. Perez JE, Eisenberg PR: Lysis of venous, pulmonary, prosthetic valvular, arterial and ventricular clots. Cardiol Clin 1987;5:113-124.

190. Vassalli JD, Belin D: Amiloride selectively inhibits the urokinase-type plasminogen activator. FEBS 1987;214:187-191.

191. Kellam B, Fraze D, Kamarek KS: Clot lysis for thrombosed central venous catheters in pediatric patients. J Perinatol 1987;7:242-244.

192. Griffin MP, Casta A: Successful urokinase therapy for superior vena cava syndrome in a premature infant. Am J Dis Child 1988;142:1267-1268.

193. Wilson CM, Merritt RJ, Thomas DW: Successful treatment of superior vena cava syndrome with urokinase in an infant. J Parenter Enteral Nutr 1988;12:81-83.

194. Strife JL, Ball WS Jr, Towbin R, et al: Arterial occlusions in neonates: use of fibrinolytic therapy. Radiol 1988;166:395-400.

195. Goldberg RE, Cohen AM, Bryan PJ, et al: Neonatal aortic thrombosis treated with intra-arterial urokinase therapy. J Can Assoc Radiol 1989;40:55-56.

196. Bagnall HA, Gomperts E, Atkinson JB: Continuous infusion of low-dose urokinase in the treatment of central venous catheter thrombosis in infants and children. Pediatrics 1989;83:963-966.

Chapter 13

PRO-UROKINASE
An Experimental Thrombolytic

Victor Gurewich

INTRODUCTION

Pro-urokinase (pro-UK), a novel single chain form of urokinase (UK), was first isolated from urine and partially characterized by Husain et al.[1-3] Subsequently, it was purified from the culture fluid of human epidermoid cancer cells and identified as a proenzyme, precursor form of two-chain UK.[4] This proenzyme property of single chain UK is of special pharmacological importance and sets pro-UK apart from other plasminogen activators. Pro-urokinase is the only activator which is inert in plasma and does not form inhibitor complexes.

In the presence of a fibrin clot, pro-UK becomes active and induces focal plasminogen activation. Surprisingly, the fibrin-dependent mechanisms by which pro-UK induces plasminogen activation, in contrast to the mechanisms of tissue plasminogen activator (t-PA), are independent of fibrin-binding.[5] At the physiological pH of blood, little binding to fibrin appears to take place, but pro-UK has nevertheless been shown in vitro and in vivo to be at least as fibrin-specific as t-PA.[6,7]

The mechanism for this fibrin-specificity has not been firmly established but appears to be related to at least three elements: 1) the pro-enzyme property of pro-UK; 2) a conformational change in plasminogen which is induced when the latter binds to fibrin; and 3) plasma inhibitors which help confine the proteolytic activity to the clot surface.

Pro-urokinase is activated to urokinase by plasmin with a resultant 250-fold increase in its plasminogen-activating activity.[8,9] Therefore, pro-UK and plasminogen are mutually activated, and this provides a positive feedback which greatly amplifies plasmin generation on the clot surface.[10-12] Since pro-UK has only a low intrinsic activity, the main active principle of pro-UK is UK. However, unlike UK, pro-UK gets to the clot intact without being partially dissipated by the formation of inhibitor complexes and without inducing non-specific plasminogen activation. In a sense, the pro-UK form can be seen as serving a transport function, like an invisible catheter, for getting UK to a fibrin clot without impairing hemostasis.

FIBRIN-SPECIFIC THROMBOLYSIS

Pharmacological thrombolysis with streptokinase (SK), UK, anistreplase (anisoylated plasminogen-streptokinase activator complex or APSAC), or rt-PA, in contrast to physiological fibrinolysis, is invariably accompanied by systemic plasmin generation which may compromise both the safety and the efficacy of the therapy. These potential adverse effects are related to the multiple substrates of plasmin.

Plasmin is an enzyme with broad specificity; systemic plasminogen activation induces a number of proteolytic reactions. These include degradation of certain clotting factors (I, V, VIII, XII), proteolysis of certain constituents of platelets and basement membrane, and activation of the complement pathway through activation of C1, C3, and C5.

The most obvious clinical consequence of plasminemia is compromised hemostasis, not only as a result of clotting factor depletion, but also because of the generation of fibrinogen degradation products which interfere with platelet aggregation and fibrin polymerization and may enhance vascular permeability. The resulting bleeding diathesis is believed to be largely responsible for the high incidence of hemorrhagic myocardial infarction associated with thrombolytic therapy but not with reperfusion induced by angioplasty.[13] On the other hand, the generation of fibrinogen degradation products may be viewed as advantageous to the extent that they reduce the risk of rethrombosis. Paradoxically, plasmin also induces platelet aggregation and the platelet release reaction.[14] This phenomenon may contribute to certain clot promoting effects of SK and UK observed in experimental studies.[15,16] It is not known whether a pro-thrombotic effect due to free plasmin is involved in the mechanism of rethrombosis which occurs in up to 24% of rt-PA-treated patients.[17]

The activation of certain complement zymogens by plasmin results in the release of anaphylotoxins which are present in high concentrations in the blood of patients undergoing thrombolytic therapy with SK or rt-PA.[18] Since anaphylotoxins induce tissue necrosis, their release during therapeutic thrombolysis may compromise myocardial salvage.

Finally, systemic plasmin generation results in a major depletion of circulating plasminogen, the substrate required for fibrinolysis. It was shown experimentally by Chesterman et al almost 20 years ago that reduction of the plasminogen concentration in the ambient fluid compromises clot lysis.[19] Maintenance of the reservoir of plasminogen may therefore be necessary if optimal thrombolysis is to be achieved.

These potentially deleterious effects of non-specific plasminogen activation have long made fibrin specificity an attractive therapeutic objective which has yet to be achieved. The endogenous plasminogen activators t-PA and pro-UK are each capable of selectively activating fibrin-bound plasminogen. Unfortunately, at the high doses required for effective coronary thrombolysis by monotherapy with either rt-PA or pro-UK, non-specific activation of plasma plasminogen is unavoidable. At lower, fibrin-specific doses, each activator is relatively ineffective in coronary thrombolysis.

THE FIBRINOLYTIC PROPERTIES OF PRO-UK

Since pro-UK was first isolated because of its selective binding to fibrin/Celite,[1-3] it was assumed that pro-UK had a fibrin clot affinity similar to that of t-PA. This assumption proved to be incorrect.[20] Certain properties of fibrin/Celite and of freshly voided urine were found to be required for binding, which occurred predominantly at an acid pH.[21] By contrast, in a plasma milieu, little or no binding of pro-UK to a fibrin clot occurred. Nevertheless, pro-UK was shown to induce fibrin specific clot lysis in plasma both in vitro and in vivo.[22,23] This phenomenon may be due in part to a conformational change in plasminogen which takes place when it binds to fibrin.[20] Alternatively, it has been proposed that dissociation of a pro-UK/inhibitor complex in plasma is triggered by fibrin.[24] However, pro-UK fails to form complexes with known inhibitors, and no alternative inhibitor has yet been identified. Regardless of the mechanism, all investigators agree that pro-UK is inert and stable in plasma for extended periods, and in contrast to UK, does not form sodium dodecyl sulfate (SDS)-stable inhibitor complexes.[20] As a result, the fibrinolytic properties of pro-UK when incubated for several days in plasma remain uncompromised,[22] and plasma plasminogen remains intact.[25]

The potential importance of this zymogenic property of pro-UK can be appreciated when contrasted to the enzymatic property of other activators. For example, t-PA is inactivated by several plasma inhibitors which include PAI-1, C1-esterase inhibitor, α_2-antiplasmin, and α_2-macroglobulin. Therefore, when rt-PA is infused peripherally, binding by inhibitors results in loss of some of the rt-PA activity by the time it reaches the clot. As a result, consumption of important plasma defenses against plasmin also takes place, and non-specific proteolysis is facilitated. In physiological fibrinolysis, t-PA is released locally from the vessel wall at the site of a thrombus. The high fibrin affinity of t-PA then allows it to initiate fibrinolysis efficiently and to evade inhibition. In contrast to t-PA, pro-UK can be infused peripherally without consuming inhibitors and circulates to a clot intact. However, since it does not bind to a clot, it is ill-suited for bolus therapy. The clinical value of this property of pro-UK, which allows it to be infused for protracted periods without compromising hemostasis, has yet to be exploited since only patients with acute myocardial infarction (AMI), in whom the rate of thrombolysis is critical, have thus far been treated with pro-UK.

291

Another difference between pro-UK and t-PA relates to the separate mechanisms by which they induce activation of fibrin-bound plasminogen. To appreciate the importance of this difference, a brief explanation of the fibrin-binding of plasminogen is required. Lysine binding sites on plasminogen bind to two types of lysine residues in fibrin. One type is situated internally and is therefore present on intact fibrin. The other is formed only after plasmin degradation of fibrin has been initiated, resulting in specific breaks in the α, β and γ chains of fibrin. As a result, new lysine residues (called carboxyterminal lysines) are exposed at the carboxyterminal ends of each of these chains.

Pro-UK activates predominantly the plasminogen bound to the carboxyterminal lysines which are present in fibrin only after limited digestion by plasmin. When plasminogen binds to any lysine residues in fibrin, it undergoes a conformational change.[26] The selective activation of plasminogen by pro-UK may be mediated by a particular conformational change which is induced only when plasminogen binds to carboxyterminal lysines.[27] Tissue plasminogen activator, on the other hand, appears to activate predominantly plasminogen bound to the internal lysine residues,[28,29] which are present on intact fibrin. As a result, t-PA is more effective in initiating lysis, priming the clot for pro-UK, which can then bring the lytic process efficiently to completion.[30]

These complementary mechanisms of action may explain the synergy in fibrinolysis found when t-PA and pro-UK are combined.[27] These complementary mechanisms also explain why rt-PA and pro-UK are *relatively* ineffective when given alone, since neither efficiently activates the alternate plasminogen. A schema that illustrates non-specific plasminogen activation by SK and UK, and fibrin-dependent plasminogen activation by pro-UK and t-PA, is shown in Figure 1.

Since pro-UK appears to preferentially activate plasminogen available only on partially degraded fibrin, the lytic effect of pro-UK should be potentiated not only by t-PA but also by other activators. That has indeed turned out to be the case. For example, pro-UK-induced clot lysis in vitro[31] or in patients with AMI[32] is potentiated by a small, sub-therapeutic bolus of UK. Similarly, a bolus of heparin potentiates the thrombolytic effect of pro-UK. This potentiation appears to be predominantly an in vivo phenomenon. Since heparin has been shown to release t-PA from the vessel wall,[33] we have postulated that the potentiating effect of heparin on pro-UK induced thrombolysis is in fact mediated by t-PA. No combination therapy with SK has yet been tested, but SK should also potentiate thrombolysis by pro-UK.

Finally, when t-PA and pro-UK are given sequentially in animals, a synergistic thrombolytic effect is found only when t-PA is given first, but not when the sequence is reversed.[34] This observation in animals provides strong support for the sequential mechanisms of action of t-PA and pro-UK, and for the importance of priming a thrombus with another thrombolytic agent in order to provide the optimal substrate for pro-UK.

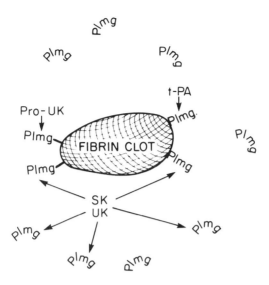

Figure 1. *Model illustrating non-specific plasminogen activation by SK or UK which activate both free and fibrin-bound plasminogen. By contrast, t-PA and pro-UK selectively activate fibrin-bound plasminogen and therefore are capable of inducing fibrin-specific clot lysis.*

MONOTHERAPY WITH PRO-UK

Only a limited number of clinical trials involving small numbers of patients have been completed at the time of this writing. The findings obtained are consistent with the basic mechanism of action summarized above. At a dose ranging from 36-69 mg infused over 90 minutes, clot lysis was quite specific (fibrinogen fell only 10%), but reperfusion of the infarct-related artery at one hour was only 51%.[35] That is, lysis of an unprimed thrombus appears to be relatively slow or incomplete, but a high degree of fibrin selectivity can be maintained. When a priming dose of UK (2-2.5 mg) was given first, efficacy was improved[32] and a reperfusion rate of 81% (9/11) at 90 minutes was reported with only 48 mg of pro-UK.[36]

The largest clinical trial published to date involved 401 patients randomly allocated to receive either recombinant pro-UK (80 mg) or SK (1.5 million IU) each infused over 60 minutes.[37] Angiographically demonstrated patency rates at 60 and 90 minutes were 71.8% and 71.2%, respectively, for recombinant pro-UK, and 48.0% and 63.9% for SK. At 60 minutes, but not 90 minutes, the difference was highly significant (p < 0.001) in favor of rec-pro-UK, and bleeding complications were also significantly (p < 0.01) less in this group.[37] However, at this dose of pro-UK, specificity was lost and plasminemia with extensive fibrinogen degradation occurred. Since pro-UK is very sensitive to activation by plasmin, it is likely that most of the pro-UK was converted to UK, so that much of the therapeutic advantage of pro-UK over UK was probably lost. The overall results with pro-UK are therefore similar to those reported for rt-PA monotherapy. That is, rapid coronary thrombolysis requires high doses at which fibrin specificity is lost. At fibrin selective doses, pro-UK, like rt-PA, induced coronary reperfusion in only about 50% of patients. This clinical experience is consistent with the mechanisms of action of t-PA and pro-UK which are illustrated in Figure 2a and Figure 2b.

These limitations of monotherapy with rt-PA or pro-UK in AMI make both of these new activators look deceptively similar to the old non-specific activators (SK and UK). Nevertheless, there are a number of other clinical indications for which monotherapy with pro-UK appears to have great potential.

The clinical indications proposed for pro-UK monotherapy are listed in Table 1 and include conditions requiring more prolonged therapy than the 30-90 minutes currently employed for AMI. For example, the mass of thrombus present in deep venous thrombosis or pulmonary embolism requires a more protracted course of treatment. The natural history of unstable angina or transient ischemic attacks dictates a course of treatment of several days; a long duration of therapy is not as safe with the other activators, not only because of their propensity to induce bleeding but also because they consume plasminogen, an effect of treatment which eventually under-

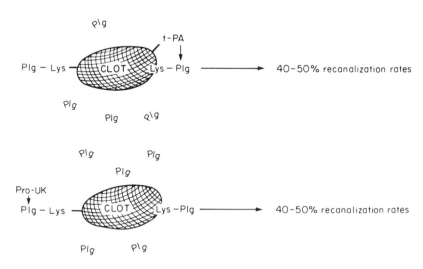

Figure 2a. *Model illustrating why clot lysis by t-PA (above) and pro-UK (below) is suboptimal at fibrin-specific doses. The t-PA activates plasminogen available on intact fibrin (bound to an internal lysine residue) whereas pro-UK activates plasminogen bound to new sites created on partially degraded fibrin (carboxyterminal lysines). Since neither activator appears to activate all available fibrin-bound plasminogen, the rates of lysis are suboptimal, explaining the relatively low recanalization rates (40-50%) obtained with fibrin-specific doses of t-PA or pro-UK.*

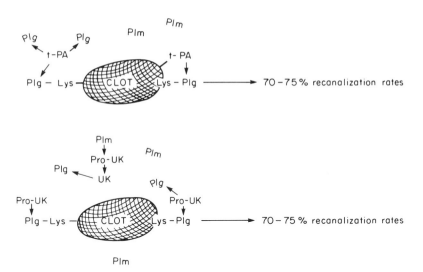

Figure 2b. *Model illustrating the effect of monotherapy at high doses of t-PA (above) or pro-UK (below). At a dose at which non-specific plasminogen activation takes place, t-PA activates the alternate plasminogen (on the left) thereby improving the recanalization rate but losing specificity. Similarly, pro-UK at these doses also activates the alternate plasminogen (on the right) thereby improving the recanalization rate. Generation of free plasmin (plm) is apt to convert most of the pro-UK to UK as shown.*

Table 1. *Clinical indications for which the zymogenic properties of pro-UK make it the plasminogen activator of choice*

1. **Deep vein thrombosis and pulmonary embolism** – in which the thrombus mass may necessitate prolonged (12-24 h) treatment

2. **Unstable angina** – prolonged (days) treatment desirable

3. **Transient ischemic attacks** – prolonged treatment desirable

4. **Prevention of rethrombosis following PTCA or after acute lytic therapy** – use of relatively low-dose infusions for hours to days

5. **Completion of coronary thrombolysis** – follow-up to ensure that all fibrin deposits have been lysed

6. **Prevention of cardiovascular disease** – for this a pro-UK modified to give it a long half-life will need to be developed

mines its efficacy. Rethrombosis following angioplasty or thrombolytic therapy in peripheral artery or coronary artery disease remains a major problem. The use of pro-UK at a relatively low infusion rate for this indication has not been tested but is a rational clinical application of its zymogenic property. Experience with coronary thrombolysis indicates that the residual stenosis in the infarct-related artery present at the end of the infusion undergoes significant further reduction when evaluated a few days after treatment as compared to initial (90 minutes) assessments. This observation indicates that fibrinolysis had not been completed by the end of the short infusion currently employed, and that a longer infusion may be needed to remove all of the lysable fibrin. This may have the additional benefit of reducing the incidence of rethrombosis.

Finally, it has been well-established that patients with cardiovascular disease tend to have impaired fibrinolytic activity that may be an important risk factor for coronary thrombosis. Since pro-UK is a plasminogen activator found normally in the blood, giving a pharmacological boost to the physiological level of pro-UK may be a safe and effective way of correcting this risk factor. The short half-life of pharmacological pro-UK would, of course, have to be considerably modified to make this idea practical.

THE FIBRINOLYTIC EFFICACY OF COMBINATION THERAPY WITH rt-PA AND PRO-UK

As shown in Figure 2c, when rt-PA and pro-UK are combined, effective thrombolysis can be achieved without sacrificing specificity. This result is related not only to the selective activation of all available fibrin-bound plasminogen but also to the preserva-

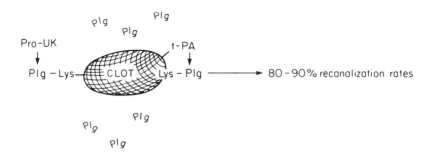

Figure 2c. *Model illustrating the effect of combination therapy with t-PA and pro-UK. The combination is capable of activating all available fibrin-bound plasminogen without sacrificing fibrin-specificity. Since the reservoir of plasma plasminogen is thereby spared, optimal lysis rates and recanalization rates may be achievable. The preliminary clinical experience supports this expectation.*

tion of the reservoir of plasminogen in plasma. In vitro studies,[25,27,30] experimental studies in animal models[38] and pilot clinical trials,[39-41] have all demonstrated a synergistic effect. Fractional combinations of rt-PA and pro-UK, corresponding to about 22% and 72% of the total monotherapy dose, have been reported to produce patency rates that are somewhat higher than those generally reported for high-dose monotherapy.[39,40] Pilot clinical trials of synergistic combinations are continuing in order to establish the optimal combination of rt-PA and pro-UK, including the optimal method of administration of rt-PA; ie, by bolus or infusion.

Since rt-PA has a strong clot affinity but is rapidly inactivated in the circulation by inhibitors, bolus therapy might have significant advantages. For example, bolus therapy should minimize non-specific effects without compromising efficacy. Pro-urokinase, in contrast, is a true circulating plasminogen activator. Therefore, a bolus or boluses of rt-PA followed by an infusion of pro-UK constitutes a therapeutic approach modeled after the natural design of how these activators are believed to function in physiologic fibrinolysis.

The potential advantages of combination therapy are three-fold. First, by avoiding a systemic lytic effect, the toxic effects of plasmin may be prevented. Second, specificity permits conservation of the plasminogen reservoir in plasma which is important for optimal fibrinolysis.[19] Third, the lower dose requirements should reduce the cost of treatment. Clinical exploitation of the special properties of pro-UK is still in its infancy. Their rational utilization should make thrombolytic therapy more specific, more effective, and enable its duration to be extended to meet a number of important clinical needs.

CONCLUSION

Pro-urokinase, the relatively inactive precursor of classical high molecular weight (55 kDa) urokinase, is a plasminogen activator with unique thrombolytic properties. Although only limited clinical trials have been performed to date, its properties have been thoroughly investigated over the past 10 years. It is known that pro-UK is inert in plasma in the absence of a clot, and therefore has the potential to be infused for indefinite periods without untoward effects. For this reason, monotherapy with pro-UK has a number of potential clinical indications other than AMI for which other activators are less suitable. Since pro-urokinase induces fibrin-specific clot lysis by a mechanism which is different from that of t-PA, the combination of the two activators has a synergistic fibrinolytic effect in experimental studies. Utilization of the complementary properties of t-PA and pro-UK may be the best way to induce rapid thrombolysis without sacrificing fibrin-specificity, a hypothesis which should undergo clinical testing in the future.

REFERENCES

1. Husain SS, Lipinski B, Gurewich V: Isolation of plasminogen activators useful as thera-peutic and diagnostic agents (single-chain, high fibrin affinity urokinase). US Patent No. 4 381 346 (filed 1979; issued 1983).

2. Husain SS, Gurewich V, Lipinski B: Purification of a new high MW single chain form of urokinase (UK) from urine. Thromb Haemost 1981;47:11 (abstract).

3. Husain SS, Gurewich V: Purification and partial characterization of a single chain, high molecular weight form of urokinase from human urine. Arch Biochem Biophys 1983; 220:31-38.

4. Wun T, Ossowski L, Reich E: A proenzyme form of urokinase. J Biol Chem 1982;257: 7262.

5. Gurewich V, Pannell R: The fibrin specificity of single chain-urokinase (sc-UK) induced proteolysis is not dependent on fibrin binding. Thromb Haemost 1986;50:386.

6. Gurewich V, Pannell R, Louie S, Kelley P, Suddith RL, Greenlee R: Effective and fibrin-specific clot lysis by a zymogen precursor form of urokinase (pro-urokinase). A study in vitro and in two animal species. J Clin Invest 1984;73:1731-1739.

7. Van de Werf F, Nobuhara M, Collen D: Coronary thrombolysis with human single chain urokinase-type plasminogen activator (pro-urokinase) in patients with acute myocardial infarction. Ann Int Med 1986;104:345-348.

8. Pannell R, Gurewich V: The activation of plasminogen by single-chain urokinase or by two-chain urokinase - A demonstration that single chain urokinase has a low catalytic activity (pro-urokinase). Blood 1987;69:22-26.

9. Petersen LC, Lund LR, Dano K, Nielsen LS, Skriver L: One-chain urokinase type plas-minogen activator from human sarcoma cells is a proenzyme with little or no intrinsic activity. J Biol Chem 1988;263:11189-11195.

10. Gurewich V, Characterization and thrombolytic properties of pro-urokinase, in Verstraete M, Collen D (eds): *Thrombolysis: Biological and Therapeutic Properties of New Throm-bolytic Agents.* London, Churchill Livingstone, 1985, pp 92-110.

11. Gurewich V, Pannell R, Broeze RJ, Mao J-I: Characterization of the intrinsic fibrinolytic properties of pro-urokinase through a study of plasmin resistant mutant forms produced by site specific mutagenesis of lysine-158. J Clin Invest 1988;82:1956-1962.

12. Lijnen HR, Van Hoef B, DeCock F, Collen D: The mechanism of plasminogen activation and fibrin dissolution by single chain urokinase-type plasminogen activator in a plasma milieu in vitro. Blood 1989;73:1864-1872.

13. Waller BF, Rothbaum DA, Pinkerton CA, Cowley MJ, Linnemeier TJ, Orr C, Irons M, Helmuth RA, Wills ER, Anst C: Status of myocardium and infarct-related coronary artery in 19 necropsy patients with acute recanalization using pharmacologic (streptokinase, r-tissue plasminogen activator) or combined types of reperfusion therapy. J Am Coll Cardiol 1987;9:785-801.

14. Niewiarowski S, Senyi AF, Gillies P: Plasmin-induced platelet aggregation and platelet release reaction. Effects on hemostasis. J Clin Invest 1973;52:1647-1659.

15. Godal HC, Hale I: Studies of the clot promoting effect of large concentrations of strepto-kinase. Scand J Clin Lab 1963;15:375-379.

16. Hirsh J, Buchanan M, Glynn MF, Mustard JF: Effect of activation of the fibrinolytic mechanism on experimental platelet rich thrombi in rabbits. J Lab Clin Med 1968;72: 245-255.

17. Chesebro JH, Knotterud G, Roberts R, Borer J, Cohen GS, Dalen JR, Dodge HT, Francis CK, Hillis D, Ludbrook P: Thrombolysis in myocardial infarction (TIMI) trial phase I: A comparison between intravenous tissue plasminogen activator and intravenous streptokinase: Clinical findings through hospital discharge. Circulation 1987;76:142-154.

18. Bennett WR, Yawn DH, Migliove PJ, Young JB, Pratt CM, Raizner AE, Roberts R, Bolli R: Activation of the complement system by recombinant tissue plasminogen activator. J Am Coll Cardiol 1987;10:627-633.

19. Chesterman CN, Allington MJ, Sharp AA: Relationship of plasminogen activator to fibrin. Nature 1972;238:15-17.

20. Pannell R, Gurewich V: Pro-urokinase - A study of its stability in plasma and a mechanism for its selective fibrinolytic effect. Blood 1986;67:1215-1223.

21. Pannell R, Angles-Cano E, Gurewich V: The pH dependence of the binding of pro-urokinase to fibrin/Celite. Thromb Haemostas 1991;64(4).

22. Gurewich V, Pannell R, Louie S, Kelley P, Suddith RL, Greenlee R: Effective and fibrin-specific clot lysis by a zymogen precursor form of urokinase (pro-urokinase). A study in vitro and in two animal species. J Clin Invest 1984;73:1731-1739.

23. Van de Werf F, Nobuhara M, Collen D: Coronary thrombolysis with human single chain urokinase-type plasminogen activator (pro-urokinase) in patients with acute myocardial infarction. Ann Int Med 1986;104:345-348.

24. Lijnen HR, Zammarron C, Blaber M, Winkler ME, Collen D: Activation of plasminogen by pro-urokinase. I Mechanism. J Biol Chem 1986;261:1253-1258.

25. Gurewich V, Pannell R: A comparative study of the efficacy and specificity of tissue plasminogen activator and pro-urokinase: Demonstration of synergism and of different thresholds of non-selectivity. Thromb Res 1986;44:217-228.

26. Violand BN, Sodetz JM, Castellino FJ: The effect of epsilon aminocaproic acid on the gross conformation of plasminogen and plasmin. Arch Biochem Biophys 1975;170:300.

27. Pannell R, Black J, Gurewich V: The complementary modes of action of tissue plasminogen activator (t-PA) and pro-urokinase (pro-UK) by which their synergistic effect on clot lysis may be explained. J Clin Invest 1988;81:853-859.

28. Nieuwenhuizen W, Vermond A, Voskuilen M, Traas DW, Verheijen JH: Identification of a site in fibrin(ogen) which is involved in the acceleration of plasminogen activation by tissue-type plasminogen activator. Biochim Biophys Acta 1983;748:86-92.

29. Nieuwenhuizen W, Voskuilen M, Vermond A, Veeneman G, Boom JV: Lysine residue A-157 of fibrinogen plays a crucial role in the acceleration of the plasminogen activation by tissue plasminogen activator (t-PA). Fibrinolysis 1986;1(suppl 1):Abstract 9.

30. Gurewich V: The sequential, complementary and synergistic activation of fibrin-bound plasminogen by tissue plasminogen activator and pro-urokinase. Fibrinolysis 1989;3:59-66.

31. Gurewich V: Experiences with pro-urokinase and potentiation of its fibrinolytic effect by urokinase and by tissue plasminogen activator. J Am Coll Cardiol 1987;10:16B-21B.

32. Bode C, Schoenermark S, Schuller G, Zimmerman R, Schwarz F, Kuebler W: Efficacy of intravenous prourokinase and a combination of prourokinase and urokinase in acute myocardial infarction. Am J Cardiol 1988;61:971-974.

33. Fareed J, Walenga J, Hoppensteadt D, Messmore HL: Studies on the pro-fibrinolytic action of heparin and its fractions. Semin Thromb Haemostas 1985;11:199-207.

34. Collen D, Stassen JM, DeCock F: Synergistic effect on thrombolysis of sequential infusion of tissue-type plasminogen activator (t-PA) single-chain urokinase-type plasminogen activator (scu-PA) and urokinase in the rabbit jugular vein thrombosis model. Thromb Haemostas 1987;58:943-946.

35. Loscalzo J, Wharton TP, Kirshenbaum JM, Levine HJ, Flaherty JT, Topol EJ, Ramaswamy K, Kosowsky BD, Salem DN, Ganz P, Brinker JA, Gurewich V, Muller JE, and the Prourokinase for Myocardial Infarction Study Group: Clot selective coronary thrombolysis with prourokinase. Circulation 1989;79:776-782.

36. Kasper W, Meinertz T, Hohnloser S, Engler H, Hasler C, Rossler W, Wolfe H, Welzel D, Just H, Gurewich V: Coronary thrombolysis in man with prourokinase: Improved efficacy with low dose urokinase. Klin Wochenschr 1988;66:109-114.

37. PRIMI Trial Study Group: Randomized double blind trial of recombinant pro-urokinase against streptokinase in acute myocardial infarction. Lancet 1989;1:863-867.

38. Spriggs DJ, Stassen JM, Hashimoto Y, Collen D: Thrombolytic properties of human tissue-type plasminogen activator, single chain urokinase-type plasminogen activator, and synergistic combinations in venous thrombosis models in dogs and rabbits. Blood 1989;73:1207-1212.

39. Collen D, Stassen JM, Stump DC, Verstraete M: In vivo synergism of thrombolytic agents. Circulation 1986;74:838-842.

40. Bode C, Schoenermark S, Schaler S, Banman H, Richardt G, Dietz R, Gurewich V, Kubler W: Intravenous thrombolytic therapy with a combination single-chain urokinase-type plasminogen activator and recombinant tissue-type plasminogen activator in acute myocardial infarction. Clin Res 1989;37:247A.

41. Collen D, Van de Werf F: Coronary arterial thrombolysis with low dose synergistic combinations of recombinant tissue type plasminogen activator and recombinant single chain urokinase type plasminogen activator for acute myocardial infarction. Am J Cardiol 1987;60:431-434.

MECHANICAL INTERVENTIONS

Section IV

Chapter 14

THE ROLE OF CORONARY ANGIOPLASTY IN ACUTE MYOCARDIAL INFARCTION

Jeffrey J. Popma
Eric J. Topol

"Every tool carries with it the spirit by which it has been created."
– Werner Heisenberg 1901-1976

INTRODUCTION

The timely use of intravenous thrombolytics soon after the onset of symptoms of acute myocardial infarction (AMI) has been shown to reduce myocardial infarct size,[1,2] improve both regional[1] and global left ventricular function,[1-4] and enhance survival.[3,5-8] Depending upon the specific thrombolytic agent or combination of agents employed, however, antegrade coronary flow is reestablished in a disappointing 35-75% of infarct-related vessels 90-150 minutes following initiation of therapy;[4,9-13] in those infarct-related arteries that achieve reperfusion, a high-grade coronary stenosis frequently persists,[4,9-13] providing a potential substrate for recurrent ischemic events and reinfarction.[5,14,15] Furthermore, the instability of the recanalized vessel coupled with the flow-limiting characteristics of the residual atheroma may impede recovery of left ventricular function.[16-18]

By modifying the obstructive geometry of the residual coronary stenosis and removing the nidus for recurrent thrombosis, coronary angioplasty may potentially benefit patients with AMI, either directly, in lieu of thrombolysis,[18-21] or electively, following thrombolysis to alleviate spontaneous or provoked ischemia.[22] Despite numerous clinical investigations aimed at determining the optimal timing and patient profile suitable for mechanical revascularization following myocardial infarction, the role of coronary angioplasty in this group of patients remains controversial. Its profound socioeconomic impact makes imperative a judicious strategy for the triage of patients with AMI to cardiac catheterization and coronary angioplasty; the community

303

physician managing patients in the early stages of myocardial infarction is the pivotal decision maker in this process. Therefore, based upon currently available data, the utility, indications, and guidelines for the timely application of coronary angioplasty in patients with myocardial infarction will be discussed.

THE DEVELOPMENT OF CORONARY ANGIOPLASTY IN ACUTE MYOCARDIAL INFARCTION

Pathologic investigation in the late 1970s led to revised speculations concerning the mechanisms responsible for the conversion of stable to acute coronary syndromes.[23-26] Post-mortem studies in patients with myocardial infarction suggested that the stimulus for this conversion was endothelial injury, such as plaque rupture, hemorrhage, or ulceration, and exposure of the subintimal collagen, elastin, and smooth muscle cells to circulating platelets. These potent stimuli for platelet aggregation and activation were felt to culminate in the release of a variety of thrombogenic and vasoregulatory mediators; in the absence of effective intrinsic thrombolysis, an acute coronary thrombus resulted, and transmural coronary flow ceased.[27] Angiographic confirmation of these findings was obtained by DeWood and colleagues[28] who demonstrated that when coronary arteriography was performed within 4 hours of the onset of symptoms of myocardial infarction, a coronary thrombus was visualized in nearly 90% of patients. Previous experimental models of coronary occlusion had suggested that myocardial necrosis occurred progressively from endocardium to epicardium over the first six hours following coronary ligation.[29,30] When reperfusion occurred earlier than six hours, myocardial salvage was possible.[29,30] Furthermore, the degree of myocardial salvage was inversely proportional to the duration of coronary occlusion.[29,30] These landmark findings became the impetus for the development of aggressive pharmacologic and mechanical strategies aimed at restoring myocardial perfusion in patients soon after the onset of symptoms of AMI.

In 1979 Rentrop and colleagues[31] reported one of the earliest series of patients with AMI in whom successful coronary recanalization was performed by means of a transluminal catheter technique. Using a standard guidewire, the coronary thrombus was mechanically dislodged and coronary perfusion restored. Despite the rather rudimentary equipment available and the small sample size, a late improvement in regional wall motion and global left ventricular function was noted in patients in whom mechanical revascularization was achieved. Significantly, these improvements occurred despite the fact that a high-grade residual stenosis remained in all patients following coronary reperfusion.

In the late 1970s the technique of coronary angioplasty was introduced by Gruentzig et al,[32] but despite the encouraging results of early mechanical reperfusion,[31] coronary angioplasty was not performed in patients with AMI until several

304

years later (Figure 1). This was due, in part, to the fact that in the early 1980s infarct-vessel recanalization was primarily achieved by the administration of intra-coronary streptokinase; when intracoronary streptokinase was administered early fol-lowing the onset of symptoms of AMI, improvements in both left ventricular function and survival were noted.[33-35] With the expanding use of cardiac catheterization in AMI, obtaining angiographic visualization of the infarct-related artery soon after thrombolysis, it became increasingly apparent that despite effective thrombus disso-lution in up to 75% of cases, a significant obstructive stenosis persisted at the site of vessel occlusion.[18-20,33,34]

In an effort to alleviate the underlying coronary stenosis and nidus for further ischemic events, Meyer and colleagues[36] performed coronary angioplasty following intracoronary streptokinase in 21 patients within 4 ± 1 hours of the onset of symptoms of myocardial infarction. Coronary angioplasty was successful in markedly reducing the severity of the obstructive lesion in over 80% of patients and compared with

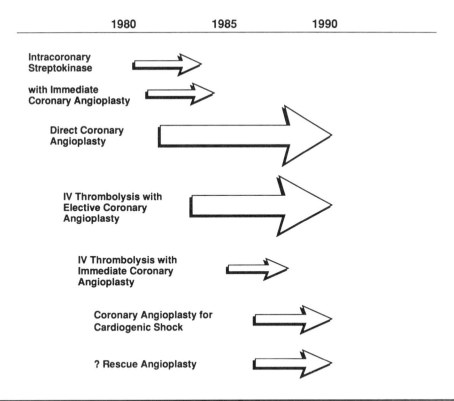

Figure 1. *Evolution of strategies for reducing mortality associated with myocar-dial infarction. The arrows indicate the time frame for the utilization of these varying strategies and the size of the arrows indicates the degree of their impact on mortality.*

patients receiving intracoronary streptokinase alone, appeared to improve prognosis. Over the next several years this combined approach of intracoronary thrombolysis and coronary angioplasty was advocated[19,20] and, in pooled experience of nearly 500 patients summarized by Topol,[37] resulted in a overall angiographic success rate of 82% with a relatively low incidence of abrupt closure and an acceptable requirement for emergency coronary bypass grafting. Furthermore, the pooled in-hospital mortality rate compared favorably with that of patients not receiving such therapy.[37]

Despite the beneficial effects on left ventricular function and survival, several factors prevented the widespread utilization of the combination of intracoronary streptokinase and coronary angioplasty in patients with AMI. First, the time lag needed for the administration of intracoronary streptokinase approached 1-2 hours for most cardiac catheterization labs,[19,20] and the expense involved in maintaining 24 hour on-call catheterization facilities was prohibitive.[38] Second, the newer fibrin-specific intravenous thrombolytic agents were shown to achieve similar recanalization rates as those obtained with intracoronary streptokinase,[9] allowing the initiation of thrombolysis in the community hospital.[38] Finally, a randomized trial comparing intracoronary streptokinase with coronary angioplasty demonstrated that the latter approach was associated with a substantial improvement in left ventricular function, a lower incidence of recurrent ischemic events, and a reduction of the residual stenosis of the infarct-related vessel.[18] Thus, by the mid 1980s the interventional approach to the patient with AMI had evolved from the use of immediate coronary arteriography and coronary reperfusion using intracoronary thrombolytics, to the addition of coronary angioplasty when significant residual stenoses persisted and finally, to the use of intravenous thrombolytics with subsequent triage to immediate, delayed, or elective coronary angioplasty.

PATHOLOGIC CHANGES FOLLOWING CORONARY ANGIOPLASTY

Twenty-five years ago Dotter and Judkins introduced the technique of transluminal dilatation of arterial obstructions due to atherosclerosis.[39] Using a Teflon guiding catheter to dilate peripheral arterial obstructions, they proposed that mechanical forces applied to the interior of the vessel compressed and remodelled the fibroatheroma. By reducing the volume of the luminal obstruction, it was felt that favorable hemodynamic effects within the arterial wall were achieved.[39] It was not until the late 1970s, however, that using techniques derived from cardiac catheterization, coronary angioplasty was introduced.[32] By positioning an expandable balloon catheter across a coronary obstruction, sequential balloon inflations were possible; the coronary artery was stretched, the atheromatous plaque disrupted, and the cross-sectional area of the artery improved (Figure 2). Subsequent histologic examination following

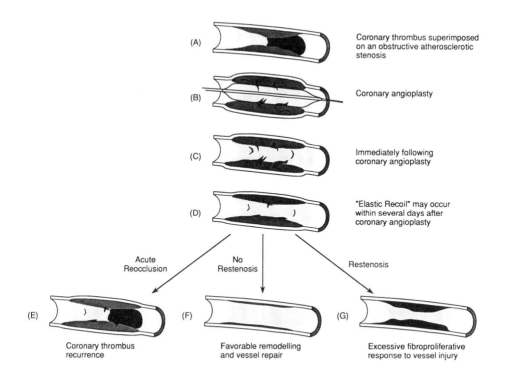

(A) Coronary thrombus superimposed on an obstructive atherosclerotic stenosis

(B) Coronary angioplasty

(C) Immediately following coronary angioplasty

(D) "Elastic Recoil" may occur within several days after coronary angioplasty

Acute Reocclusion   No Restenosis   Restenosis

(E) Coronary thrombus recurrence

(F) Favorable remodelling and vessel repair

(G) Excessive fibroproliferative response to vessel injury

Figure 2. *With acute myocardial infarction, coronary flow is obstructed by an occlusive coronary thrombus superimposed upon a fixed atheromatous lesion (A). Coronary angioplasty is performed (B), and the arterial dimensions are improved as a result of splitting and tearing the fibroatheroma and stretching the vessel wall (C). Early "elastic recoil" of the vessel wall may diminish part of the initial improvement in vessel dimensions (D). In the days to months following coronary angioplasty, reocclusion (E), restenosis (F), or a favorable angiographic outcome may be obtained (G).*

human angioplasty has demonstrated varying degrees of endothelial disruption, neointimal fracture, and medial dissection.[40-42] Furthermore, the compliant components of the vessel wall, such as the media and adventitia, are stretched to conform to the maximal dimension of the inflated balloon.[40] The intimal flaps and intraluminal haziness typically seen angiographically are correlated with intimal-medial splits, localized dissection, and thrombus formation.[40]

In the setting of AMI, an occlusive coronary thrombus is generally present and in most circumstances is easily crossed by a coronary guidewire, allowing transluminal passage of the balloon dilatation catheter. Similar to findings with coronary angioplasty in patients with stable coronary syndromes, coronary angioplasty in the setting of

AMI results in varying degrees of intimal hemorrhage and plaque disruption.[43-45] However, when coronary angioplasty is performed in association with thrombolytic therapy, hemorrhagic myocardial infarction is typically demonstrated histologically,[43] similar to patients undergoing thrombolysis alone.[46] Conversely, in patients undergoing direct coronary angioplasty in lieu of thrombolytic therapy, the incidence of intraplaque hemorrhage and hemorrhagic infarction appears to be substantially lower.[43] While the clinical significance of a hemorrhagic infarction has not been clearly defined,[43] its presence may delay the usual infarct healing process and impede recovery of left ventricular function.[47]

Several interactive biologic processes of vessel repair are initiated at the site of vessel injury immediately following coronary angioplasty (Figure 3). Depending upon the extent of the response to vessel injury, varying degrees of platelet aggregation, vasoconstriction and thrombosis may result. Marked platelet deposition occurs at the site of endothelial injury, with the degree of platelet aggregation correlating with the depth of vascular damage. Upon exposure to subintimal elements, platelets are activated and their granular contents, including thromboxane A_2, serotonin, thrombin

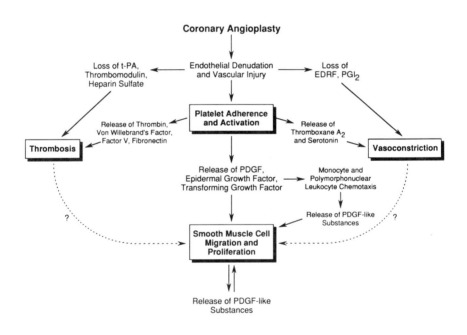

Figure 3. *Interactive biologic processes responsible for vessel repair that are initiated with endothelial denudation and vascular injury following coronary angioplasty in patients with acute myocardial infarction. Abbreviations: t-PA, tissue plasminogen activator; EDRF, endothelial derived growth factor; PGI_2, prostacyclin; PDGF, platelet derived growth factor. (Reproduced with permission, Popma JJ, Topol EJ: Factors influencing restenosis following coronary angioplasty. Am J Med 1990;88:1-16N.)*

and fibrinogen are released.[48] The polymerization of fibrin stabilizes the platelet mass, and hemostasis is achieved.[48] In addition to providing an important nidus for platelet adhesion, injury to the endothelium following balloon angioplasty results in loss of the normal production of heparin sulfate, tissue plasminogen activator (t-PA), thrombomodulin, and prostacyclin (PGI_2), each of which plays an important counter-regulatory role to the thrombotic response seen with vessel injury.[48,49] As a result, the capacity for plasmin generation, fibrinolysis, and thrombus dissolution is diminished following coronary angioplasty. Further, varying degrees of coronary vasoconstriction may result from endothelial denudation and loss of the ability to produce endothelial dependent relaxant factor and degrade humoral substances such as serotonin and thromboxane A_2.[49,50] Using quantitative techniques, sequential angiograms obtained up to 30 minutes following coronary angioplasty have demonstrated progressive coronary vasoconstriction in both the dilated segment and in the segment distal to the coronary stenosis.[50] The high risk characteristics of the infarct-related artery which typically result in intraluminal fibrin, spontaneous intimal disruption, and avid platelet aggregation may increase the tendency for vasoconstriction and acute vessel closure in patients with AMI; these features may be exacerbated by coronary angioplasty. The intense aggregative features of the infarct-related artery also result in the release of mitogenic factors which stimulate a fibroproliferative response, including smooth muscle cell proliferation. When myointimal proliferation is sufficient to encroach upon the arterial lumen, restenosis results. The 25-40% risk of restenosis in patients with AMI undergoing coronary angioplasty, however, appears to be similar to the risk of restenosis in those with stable coronary syndromes.[21,51,52]

CURRENT CLINICAL GUIDELINES FOR THE USE OF CORONARY ANGIOPLASTY IN PATIENTS WITH MYOCARDIAL INFARCTION

The value of various strategies of coronary arteriography and angioplasty in patients with AMI has been traditionally assessed by clinical and angiographic outcome measurements such as mortality, immediate and predischarge infarct vessel patency and resting left ventricular function. Despite their objectivity, these "hard" clinical endpoints may not address which strategy maximizes such functional indices as exercise capacity or quality of life. For example, cerebral hemorrhage that develops as a result of thrombolysis may lead to complete disability despite infarct vessel patency and preserved left ventricular function. The future development of symptomatic congestive heart failure or limitation of excrcise capacity may not be reliably predicted by resting left ventricular ejection fraction obtained prior to hospital discharge. Moreover, early identification of "low risk" anatomy by coronary arteriography may provide psychological reassurance to the patient and physician and lead to early hospital discharge and return to work.[53] Thus, each strategy of mechanical coronary revascularization following myocardial infarction varies with respect to advantages, disadvantages, appropriate timing and concomitant use of thrombolytic therapy (Table 1); the application of these strategies must be highly individualized and be based upon the balance of *relative* risks and potential long-term benefits.

DIRECT OR PRIMARY CORONARY ANGIOPLASTY

In the minority of community hospitals where cardiac catheterization facilities are immediately available or readily accessed, direct coronary angioplasty soon after the onset of symptoms of AMI may confer several potential but unproven advantages over conventional thrombolytic therapy.[21,51,52,54-57] First, the "ceiling" of infarct vessel recanalization using currently available thrombolytic regimens is approximately 75%.[4,9-13] Based on clinical studies in which more than 50 patients were enrolled, successful primary recanalization using direct coronary angioplasty has been achieved in nearly 90% of patients with AMI[21,51,54,55] (Table 2); these favorable recanalization rates have been noted in the elderly,[57] in patients with multivessel disease,[58] and in those who would otherwise be candidates for thrombolytic therapy.[59] Second, a significant residual coronary stenosis is generally present in patients who achieve successful thrombolysis using conventional thrombolytic therapy.[4,9-12] Direct mechanical restoration of antegrade flow using coronary angioplasty significantly reduces the residual coronary stenosis and may promote enhanced recovery of left ventricular function.[16,17] Third, by avoiding systemic fibrinolysis, direct coronary angioplasty may reduce the occurrence of bleeding complications and intraplaque and intramyocardial hemorrhage that accompany standard thrombolytic therapy.[43] Finally, compared with intracoronary streptokinase, direct coronary angioplasty has been associated with an improvement in global and regional left ventricular function and infarct vessel caliber and a reduction in recurrent ischemic events.[18] Inducible myocardial ischemia was present more frequently in patients receiving intracoronary streptokinase than in those undergoing direct coronary angioplasty.[60]

Despite these potential advantages, when coronary arteriography is performed prior to hospital discharge following successful primary coronary revascularization, reocclusion occurs in 8-23% of patients (Table 2), limiting the long-term benefit of establishing initial coronary patency. Thus, the 7-21 day patency rate may be similar to that obtained with conventional thrombolysis.[2,3] Preliminary data comparing direct coronary angioplasty with fibrin-specific thrombolytic therapy using rt-PA suggest similar initial recanalization rates but significantly lower residual stenoses in those undergoing direct coronary angioplasty.[61] However, resting left ventricular ejection fraction 6 weeks after infarction was similar in the two groups.[61] Extremely low post-hospital mortality rates have been noted in patients undergoing direct coronary angioplasty;[21,51,54] whether direct coronary angioplasty confers a survival advantage over conventional thrombolysis is not known.

Table 1. *Strategies for coronary angioplasty in patients with acute myocardial infarction*

Strategy	Timing	Advantages	Disadvantages	Indications
Direct	0-6 hours	Avoidance of thrombolysis Improved immediate patency and reduction of residual stenoses ? Improved global and regional wall motion	Cost of 24-hour on-call Reocclusion in 8-23%	Contraindication to thrombolytics Cath lab immediately available Uncertain diagnosis
Immediate	0-2 hours	Reduced residual stenosis	Increased mortality rate Increased emergency CABG Increased bleeding No improvement of LV function	Cardiogenic shock Ongoing myocardial ischemia Reocclusion
Rescue	0-2 hours	Potentially improved myocardial salvage ? Improved global and regional LV function Less recurrent ischemia	May be detrimental in RCA 24-hour on-call facilities	Cardiogenic shock Ongoing myocardial ischemia
Deferred	1-7 days	May improve exercise LVEF	No improvement in resting LVEF compared with elective approach	? Anterior infarction ? Patients unable to exercise
Elective	>7 days	Reserved for patients with documented ischemia	No benefits of patent artery High-risk anatomy may be missed	Spontaneous or exercise-induced ischemia

LV = left ventricular; LVEF = left ventricular ejection fraction; CABG = coronary bypass surgery; RCA = right coronary artery

Table 2. Direct coronary angioplasty in patients with acute myocardial infarction

Study	No. pts.	Time to thrombo (hr)	Successful (%)	Improvement in LV function (%)	Reocclusion (%)	In-hospital mortality (%)	CABG (%)	Restenosis rate (%)	12-month survival after discharge (%)
O'Neill et al[18]	29	4.1 ± 1.4	82		8	6.8	0		
Rothbaum et al[21]	151	3.1	87	+12	5	9	4	40	98
Miller et al[51]	127*	3.3 ± 1.8	92	+8.2	8	8.6	7.9	36	99
Prida et al[52]	29	6.5	86		23	4	0	25	
O'Keefe et al[54]	614		94	+6.0	9	8			95
Kimura et al[55]	58		88		14				
Topol et al[56]	29		83	+7.7	−2	6.3			
Owens et al[57]	45†		82		8	16.0	8		

* Includes 18 patients with full-dose and 46 patients with partial dose intracoronary streptokinase or urokinase at time of coronary angioplasty, and 8 patients with cardiogenic shock
† All patients 70 years of age
CABG = coronary bypass surgery; improvements in left ventricular ejection fraction expressed as an increase in ejection fraction from time of randomization to discharge
Thrombo = thrombolysis

The strategy of direct coronary angioplasty is further limited by the relative paucity (< 20%) of community hospitals in which facilities for coronary angioplasty are presently available; in those community hospitals with such facilities, a strategy of direct coronary angioplasty would require 24-hour on-call facilities, experienced operators, and a commitment to use coronary angioplasty as a first-line approach.[21,38,54] Thus, judicious triage and transfer of the subset of patients who may be candidates for direct coronary angioplasty is indicated. Myocardial reperfusion may be deemed important in patients who have contraindications to thrombolytic therapy, such as those with an extensive anterior infarction and prior stroke or recent surgery. The time delay required for inter-hospital transfer at a time when the patient may be somewhat unstable may be justified by a high success rate of direct coronary angioplasty for recanalization in patients with symptoms of more than 3 hours duration.[21] In patients in whom the diagnosis of AMI is uncertain, because of an atypical history or lack of diagnostic electrocardiographic features, cardiac catheterization and coronary angioplasty when appropriate may be preferable to empiric thrombolytic therapy. Finally, in those community hospitals with on-call catheterization facilities where direct coronary angioplasty can be performed within 30-40 minutes of the onset of symptoms, recanalization may be achieved sooner than with intravenous thrombolytic therapy.[61]

IMMEDIATE ANGIOPLASTY AS AN ADJUNCT TO THROMBOLYTIC THERAPY

In the mid-1980s the strategy of coronary angioplasty performed soon after pharmacologic coronary reperfusion was advocated as a valuable adjunct to conventional thrombolysis; it was felt that by alleviating the residual coronary stenosis, potential reductions in recurrent ischemic events and improvement in left ventricular function could be achieved. To ascertain the optimum timing of coronary angioplasty, three large clinical trials were conducted utilizing immediate and delayed strategies of coronary angioplasty following thrombolysis.[10-12] In the first of these trials, Thrombolysis and Angioplasty in Acute Myocardial Infarction (TAMI-1), 288 patients received 150 mg of intravenous rt-PA 3.0 ± 1.1 hours after the onset of symptoms of AMI.[10] Ninety-minute coronary arteriography was performed in all patients, and those with complex multivessel disease, left main coronary stenoses, cardiogenic shock, and failed thrombolysis were excluded. Patients with antegrade infarct-related artery flow but significant residual coronary stenoses were randomized to immediate coronary angioplasty (n = 99) or repeat coronary arteriography and coronary angioplasty at 7 days (n = 98)[10] (Table 3). While coronary angioplasty was performed with a high rate of success in both groups, no significant differences were noted in global or regional left ventricular function or reocclusion rate at 7 days[10] (Figure 4). Compared with the delayed strategy of coronary angioplasty, however, immediate angio-

Table 3. Comparison of immediate and delayed coronary angioplasty following thrombolysis in patients with acute myocardial infarction

	Immediate PTCA			Delayed PTCA		Arteriography Only
	TAMI[10] (60-90 min)	TIMI IIA[11] (120 min)	ECSG[12] (60 min)	TAMI[10] (7-10 d)	TIMI IIA[11] (18-48 hr)	ECSG[12] (10-22 d)
Number of patients	99	195	183	98	194	184
PTCA success rate (%)	85	84	61	94	93	
Late left ventricular function (% EF)	53 ± 11	50	51	56 ± 0	49	51
In-hospital mortality (%)	4	7	7	1	6	3
Complication rate						
Bleeding (%)	20	41		7	23	
Recurrent ischemia (%)	5	7	30	16	4	15
Reocclusion (%)	11		12	13		11
CABG						
Emergency	7	7		2	2	
In-hospital	8	16	2	13	8	1

TAMI = Thrombolysis and Angioplasty in Myocardial Infarction; TIMI = Thrombolysis In Myocardial Infarction; ECSG = European Cooperative Study Group; PTCA = coronary angioplasty; EF = ejection fraction; CABG = coronary bypass surgery

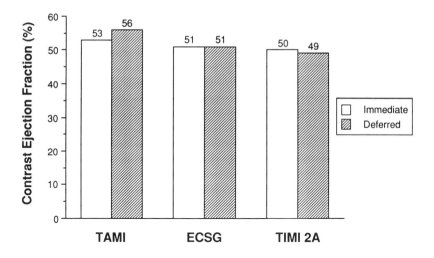

Figure 4. *Left ventricular function in the Immediate Coronary Angioplasty Trials. No differences were seen in predischarge ejection fraction for the immediate (solid blocks) and deferred (striped blocks) strategies. TAMI = Thrombolysis and Angioplasty in Myocardial Infarction Study Group; ECSG = European Cooperative Study Group; TIMI 2A = Thrombolysis in Myocardial Infarction Study Group. (Reprinted with permission, Topol EJ, Ann Intern Med 1988;109:1970.)*

plasty was associated with a higher emergency coronary bypass surgery rate[10] and, as a consequence of immediate cardiac catheterization, bleeding complications and transfusion requirements were substantial in both groups.[10] Interestingly, thrombus resolution occurred over the ensuing 7 days in 15% of patients, thus obviating the need for delayed coronary angioplasty.[10] The authors concluded that immediate coronary angioplasty following thrombolysis offered no clear advantage and possibly increased risk compared with the strategy of delayed coronary angioplasty following myocardial infarction.

Despite differences in study methodology, the findings of both the European Cooperative Study Group (ECSG) and the Thrombolysis In Myocardial Infarction (TIMI) Phase 2A trials were remarkably concordant with the results of the TAMI-1 trial. In the TIMI IIA trial, 389 patients were given 100-150 mg rt-PA within 2.9 ± 0.1 hours of the onset of symptoms of myocardial infarction; 195 and 194 patients were randomized to immediate and 18- to 48-hour coronary angioplasty, respectively. Of these, 141 (72%) and 107 (55%) in the immediate and delayed strategies, respectively, were found to have residual coronary stenoses suitable for mechanical revascularization.[11] While no significant differences were found in the primary end-point, left ventricular function, bleeding complications and the requirement for emergency coronary bypass surgery was higher in the immediate coronary angioplasty group.[11] In the European Cooperative Study, 367 patients received 150 mg of t-PA, aspirin and heparin within 2.6 hours of the onset of symptoms of myocardial infarction. Of these, 183 were randomized to immediate coronary arteriography and coronary angioplasty, and 184 were assigned to a non-invasive strategy of delayed catheterization 10-22 days following myocardial infarction. Surprisingly, no significant differences in left ventricular function were demonstrated between the invasive and non-invasive strategies. Furthermore, mortality rate, bleeding rate, and recurrent ischemia rate were all higher in the invasive study group.[12] In aggregate, these important findings suggest that the strategy of immediate coronary angioplasty in combination with thrombolytic therapy is associated with a lower safety profile and similar indices of left ventricular function when compared with a strategy of delayed coronary angioplasty.[11-13,62]

Now that an effective form of thrombolysis is available in most community hospitals, initial efforts to reestablish coronary perfusion in patients with myocardial infarction should be attempted using pharmacologic methods. Although immediate coronary angioplasty has not been shown to enhance left ventricular function or survival in patients with otherwise uncomplicated myocardial infarction, certain high-risk subsets of patients with hemodynamic compromise, failure of pharmacologic thrombolysis or those with persisting or recurrent myocardial ischemia may benefit from early intervention using coronary angioplasty. Identification and triage of these high-risk patients to a facility equipped for immediate coronary arteriography and angioplasty may have profound effects on both early and late mortality and long-term left ventricular function.

Myocardial Infarction Associated with Cardiogenic Shock

Hypotension associated with elevated left ventricular filling pressures develops in up to 12% of patients with AMI, and with standard medical therapy, portends an in-hospital mortality ranging from 70-87%[5,63-65] (Table 4). This extraordinarily high-risk subgroup of patients may potentially benefit from an aggressive attempt at restoring myocardial perfusion early in the course of myocardial infarction. Although efforts to improve mortality using streptokinase in patients with cardiogenic shock have been somewhat disappointing,[5] results obtained from the TIMI IIB trial suggest that the six-week survival may be as high as 51% when rt-PA is administered soon after the onset of symptoms of myocardial infarction.[66] Patients in the TIMI IIB trial randomized to early arteriography and coronary angioplasty did not appear to have substantially improved survival; others, however, have noted markedly improved survival with early mechanical revascularization[64,65,67-69] (Table 4). In the retrospective analysis of 59 patients with cardiogenic shock by Lee et al,[64] the 30-day survival was significantly improved in patients undergoing emergency coronary angioplasty, often in combination with thrombolytic therapy, over conventionally treated patients (50%

Table 4. *Mortality associated with various treatment strategies for cardiogenic shock*

Authors	Number of patients	Mortality Overall (%)	Successful (%)	Unsuccessful (%)
Conventional Therapy				
Mirowski et al[63]	149	87		
GISSI[5]	134	70		
Lee et al[64]	59	84		
Gacioch and Topol[65]	16	81		
Thrombolysis				
Streptokinase				
GISSI[5]	146	70		
Kennedy et al[34]	45	67	42	84
rt-PA				
Garrahy et al[66]	188	49		
Coronary Angioplasty				
Lee et al[64]	24	50	23	82
Brown et al[67]	28	57	41	81
Gacioch and Topol[65]	25	58	22	100
Shani et al[68]	9	33		
Heuser et al[69]	10	30		

rt-PA = tissue plasminogen activator

vs. 17%; $p = 0.006$). In those patients with successful angioplasty, the survival was 77%.[64]

Based on these encouraging findings, patients who develop hemodynamic compromise at the time of, or soon after the administration of intravenous thrombolytics should be considered for early referral to a facility capable of intraaortic balloon counterpulsation and emergency cardiac catheterization in an effort to reestablish coronary perfusion either with balloon angioplasty or surgical revascularization. Whether more aggressive interventions such as left ventricular assistance and percutaneous cardiopulmonary bypass support will aid further in the stabilization of this high-risk subgroup of patients is currently under study.

Rescue or Salvage Coronary
Angioplasty When Thrombolysis Fails

Patients who achieve successful recanalization of the infarct-related artery using standard thrombolytic therapy appear to have an improved prognosis compared with those in whom thrombolysis fails.[70-72] In the Western Washington trial the 12 month mortality among patients with myocardial infarction was reduced following administration of intracoronary streptokinase, but the improvement in survival was limited to those patients who achieved successful coronary artery recanalization.[71] Using intravenous rt-PA, a doubling of the in-hospital mortality rate was noted in patients with unsuccessful thrombolysis.[70] Cigarroa et al[72] retrospectively reviewed the long-term survival of 179 patients with single vessel coronary artery disease and AMI. During their 10-year follow-up period, the incidence of long-term morbidity and mortality was greatly reduced with residual anterograde perfusion in the infarct-related artery.[72] Since the "ceiling" of infarct-vessel recanalization using presently available agents is only 60-75%,[4,9-13] 25-40% of patients are thrombolytic failures. These patients are at the highest risk for cardiac death.[70-72]

While coronary angioplasty has been advocated to restore infarct-related artery perfusion when pharmacologic methods fail, several features of "rescue" or salvage coronary angioplasty have prevented its widespread use in patients with myocardial infarction. First, the ability to detect which patients have failed thrombolysis using noninvasive methods would be useful in identifying those who may be candidates for immediate coronary arteriography and "rescue angioplasty". Unfortunately, usual clinical and electrocardiographic criteria are poor predictors for accurately determining whether reperfusion has occurred.[73,74] Califf et al[74] compared commonly used markers of coronary reperfusion with infarct-related vessel patency at 90-minute coronary arteriography in 386 patients with AMI receiving rt-PA. Of those patients who developed complete resolution of ST-segment elevation following initiation of therapy, 96% achieved successful reperfusion; this finding, however, was present in only 6% of all patients. Similarly, when chest pain completely resolved following initiation of therapy, reperfusion occurred in 84% of patients, but this finding was present in only 29% of patients.[74] New methods for predicting reperfusion including rapid creatine kinase isoforms assay[75,76] and continuous ST-segment with or without QRS vector monitoring[77] are currently under investigation. Thus, in the absence of sensitive signs of coronary reperfusion, the strategy of rescue coronary angioplasty would require immediate coronary arteriography in all patients with AMI and would therefore be limited to those facilities with 24-hour access to cardiac catheterization facilities.

Second, despite a high successful recanalization rate in most series of patients, depending upon the thrombolytic agent or combination employed, the reocclusion rate may be substantial (Table 5).[13,78-83] For example, when rt-PA is used as mono-

Table 5. Rescue coronary angioplasty after failed thrombolysis in patients with myocardial infarction

Author	Number	Agent	Success rate (%)	Reocclusion (%)	Improvement in EF (%)	In-Hospital Mortality Overall (%)	Successful (%)	Unsuccessful (%)
Fibrin Selective								
Califf et al[78]	86	rt-PA	73	29	NC	12.0	6	44
Baim et al [79]	77	rt-PA	92	26		5.4		
Fibrin Non-Selective								
Fung et al[80]	13	SK	92	16	+10	7.6		
O'Conner et al[81]	90	SK	89	14	−1	17.0		
Holmes et al[82]	34	SK	71			3		
Combination								
Grines et al[83]	10	rt-PA+SK	90		+5			
Topol et al[13]	27	rt-PA+UK	95	4	+5	0		

EF = ejection fraction; rt-PA = tissue plasminogen activator; SK = streptokinase; UK = urokinase; NC = no change therapy, seven-day reocclusion occurs in as many as 26-29% of patients undergoing successful rescue coronary angioplasty.[78,79] Using a longer-acting and fibrin-nonselective agent such as streptokinase, lower reocclusion rates following rescue angioplasty have been noted.[80,81] Using a combination of rt-PA and urokinase, Topol et al[13] have demonstrated an extremely low reocclusion rate and low in-hospital mortality rate following rescue coronary angioplasty. A trial of early administration of urokinase, rt-PA or the combination with subsequent randomization to immediate coronary arteriography with rescue coronary angioplasty or to a delayed strategy of coronary arteriography has recently been reported as part of TAMI-5.[84] While infarct-related vessel patency rates were similar in all groups, the strategy of immediate coronary arteriography with rescue coronary angioplasty was associated with improved regional left ventricular function and a lower clinical event rate.[84] Furthermore, controlling for multivessel disease and prior myocardial infarction, the strategy of rescue coronary angioplasty was associated with improved global left ventricular function.[84] Rescue angioplasty should be used with caution, however, in patients with failed thrombolysis of the right coronary artery; rescue coronary angioplasty in this setting may be associated with an increased incidence of hypotension, bradycardia and mortality despite the low anticipated event rate associated with uncomplicated inferior infarction.[85] The mechanism for the sudden deterioration may be due to an exaggerated Bezold-Jarisch reflex, distal showering of thrombi into the microcirculation, or other factors.

From the foregoing discussion it is apparent that the role of rescue coronary angioplasty in the absence of ongoing myocardial ischemia is, at present, uncertain. Nevertheless, rescue coronary angioplasty may be especially beneficial in certain subsets of patients, such as those with anterior infarction or those with hemodynamic compromise.[86]

Recurrent Ischemia and Reocclusion Following Thrombolysis

In patients receiving thrombolytic therapy, most deaths occur during the first three days of hospitalization.[11] These deaths may occur as a consequence of myocardial rupture, hemodynamic compromise imparted by the extent of myocardial necrosis, or from rhythm disturbances arising in electrically unstable peri-infarction tissue. Recurrent ischemia resulting from coronary reocclusion in the zone of, or at some distance from the prior myocardial infarction, may also occur. It is essential that patients with evidence of persisting or recurrent myocardial ischemia following initially successful thrombolysis be transferred to a facility where immediate coronary arteriography can be performed. Unfortunately, no clinical or angiographic variable has been found to predict the development of reocclusion.[87-89] Recurrent ischemic events may occur in 12-20% of patients following thrombolytic therapy,[88] usually within the first 72 hours. When patients with evidence of recurrent or persistent myocardial ischemia undergo cardiac catheterization, only 50-60% actually demonstrate recurrent thrombosis; the remaining patients manifest ischemia with a patent infarct vessel.[87]

The management of the patient with recurrent ischemia following thrombolytic therapy should initially include a repeated dosage of a thrombolytic agent, either rt-PA not to exceed a total of 135 mg or 1.5 mg/kg in the first 4-6 hours or a non-fibrin selective agent such as urokinase 1.5 million units intravenously. If more than 12 hours have passed since the last dosage of a thrombolytic agent, then 1 mg/kg rt-PA up to 90 mg maximum can be given. While such therapy is being administered, the patient should be transferred to a facility that can perform immediate coronary arteriography and coronary angioplasty. The aggressive response to such events is appropriate and necessary to prevent reinfarction and improve survival.[90] If reocclusion has occurred, coronary angioplasty should be performed unless the infarct vessel anatomy is unsuitable, whereupon emergency coronary bypass surgery should be considered.

ELECTIVE OR DEFERRED CORONARY ANGIOPLASTY

Two strategies of coronary angioplasty are possible in the late-hospital phase following myocardial infarction. Using a deferred strategy, coronary angioplasty is performed in patients when residual coronary stenoses persist prior to hospital discharge; this approach has the advantage of improving the obstructive geometry, potentially improving left ventricular function, and impacting on long-term survival. Using an elective strategy, coronary angioplasty is performed only with the demonstration of spontaneous or provokable myocardial ischemia following myocardial infarction. This approach has the advantage that patients who do not demonstrate myocardial ischemia prior to hospital discharge are not subjected to the expense and risk of coronary angioplasty. The preferred approach has been controversial and the subject of several clinical trials.[4,22]

In the Johns Hopkins trial, 85 patients who received rt-PA or placebo were randomly assigned to receive either deferred or elective angioplasty.[4] Although the mean improvement in left ventricular ejection fraction was similar in the two groups, patients in the deferred coronary angioplasty group demonstrated a greater augmentation of ejection fraction with maximal exercise compared with patients with an elective approach (8.1% vs. 1.2%).[4] Furthermore, recurrent ischemia and reinfarction occurred less frequently in the deferred angioplasty group.

In the TIMI IIB trial, 3,262 patients were given intravenous rt-PA within four hours of the onset of symptoms of AMI and randomized to one of two clinical strategies. The "invasive" limb consisted of cardiac catheterization and coronary angioplasty with suitable coronary anatomy within 18-48 hours following thrombolytic therapy. In the "conservative" arm, cardiac catheterization and coronary angioplasty were performed only if spontaneous or provoked ischemia was present. In this study, angioplasty was performed in 60% of patients in the invasive arm and in 17% of patients in the conservative arm. There were no significant differences between the two groups with respect to resting left ventricular ejection fraction at hospital discharge, rate of reinfarction, or death at six weeks. Similar results were found when the period of follow-up was extended to 12 months.[91]

Preliminary results from the SWIFT trial[92] (**S**hould **We** **I**ntervene **F**ollowing **T**hrombolysis?) support the findings of TIMI IIB. Following administration of anisoylated plasminogen streptokinase activator complex (APSAC), 800 patients were randomized to a strategy of delayed cardiac catheterization and coronary angioplasty at 48 72 hours (n = 397) or to a conservative strategy of cardiac catheterization and coronary angioplasty only for recurrent or provoked ischemia (n = 403). Despite the fact that coronary revascularization was performed in 58% of patients in the invasive group compared with 25% in the conservative group, 3-month left ventricular ejection fraction, reinfarction and mortality rates were similar in the two groups.

Data derived from these trials demonstrate the lack of efficacy of deferred coronary angioplasty and underscore the need for objective evidence of jeopardized myocardium before exposing patients to the risk of coronary angioplasty. The overall conclusion of these trials must, however, be viewed in the context of the study design. In TIMI IIB, patients with failed reperfusion at the time of an 18-48 hour angiogram in the invasive arm only underwent coronary angioplasty for persistent myocardial ischemia. The benefit of a "patent" artery on long term prognosis may not have been fully realized. In the TIMI IIB trial, 5.4% of patients in the "invasive" approach experienced myocardial infarction within 24 hours of the procedure. In many cases, aspirin, which is known to reduce the incidence of acute vessel closure and myocardial infarction following coronary angioplasty, was not given or was given in small (80 mg) doses. Finally, standard thallium-201 or other radionuclide methods of detecting residual myocardial ischemia using submaximal exercise testing prior to hospital discharge may have limited sensitivity in detecting regional coronary stenoses.[93] Moreover, the presence of a "fixed" defect by thallium-201 imaging may actually represent viable myocardium;[94] thus, patients with a "negative" exercise tolerance test may have substantial residual myocardium at risk.[95] The strategy of elective coronary angioplasty following myocardial infarction mandates that patients be aggressively stratified for their risk of recurrent ischemic events using presently available clinical and exercise information. Moderate- and high-risk patients should be referred for coronary arteriography, and when appropriate, coronary revascularization.

Should Coronary Arteriography Be Routinely Performed Following Thrombolysis?

The role of routine coronary arteriography following myocardial infarction remains controversial. Critical to the use of coronary arteriography following thrombolysis is the "uncoupling" of coronary arteriography from coronary angioplasty. Coronary arteriography can identify important prognostic subgroups. For example, patients with minimal lesion syndrome represent approximately 15% of patients who receive thrombolytic therapy for ST-segment elevation consistent with myocardial infarction[10,22] (Figure 5). Further treatment in this subgroup of patients would include antiplatelet agents aimed at preventing recurrent coronary thrombosis. Other subsets of patients identified by early coronary arteriography are those with left main stem disease and those with multiple vessel coronary disease, comprising 35% of patients following myocardial infarction. Surgical revascularization is clearly of benefit in the former group, and the latter group represents patients with a three-fold higher in-hospital mortality rate.[96] Finally, the largest subgroup of patients, those with single vessel coronary artery disease, are best managed by performing a functional test, with coronary angioplasty reserved for those with demonstrable residual coronary ischemia. Thus, the decision to refer a patient for coronary arteriography following myocardial infarction must be individualized and based on both patient and physician preference. Candidates for coronary arteriography in the absence of spontaneous or provokable myocardial ischemia would include young patients, those with evidence of diminished left ventricular function, and those who are unable to perform adequate exercise stress testing prior to hospital discharge.

CONCLUSION

State-of-the-art management of the patient with acute transmural myocardial infarction in the community hospital should begin with early administration of intravenous

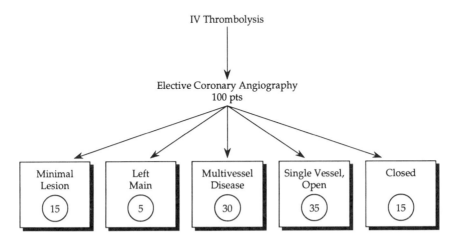

Figure 5. *Anticipated coronary angiographic subgroups after intravenous thrombolytic therapy of 100 patients undergoing the procedure electively at some point prior to hospital discharge (reproduced with permission from Topol[87]).*

thrombolytic agents and close observation for the development of persistent or recurrent ischemia. Direct coronary angioplasty will continue to have a role as primary therapy in those community hospitals with immediate access to cardiac catheterization facilities and operators skilled in acute intervention. In addition, patients should be considered for direct coronary angioplasty when contraindications to thrombolysis are present or the diagnosis of myocardial infarction is uncertain due to inconsistent clinical or electrocardiographic data.

Immediate coronary angioplasty of a recanalized vessel is currently not indicated unless hemodynamic compromise or clear-cut ongoing myocardial ischemia is present. The role of rescue coronary angioplasty is uncertain at the present time and may be detrimental in patients with uncomplicated inferior myocardial infarction and right coronary artery occlusion. Deferred coronary angioplasty in the setting of a negative functional test appears to confer little advantage over an elective approach for demonstrated spontaneous or provokable ischemia. Elective coronary angioplasty in cases of myocardial ischemia following thrombolysis is easily applied and has been associated with an overall favorable 6-week and 12-month survival. Over the next few years, further refinements in angiography and new percutaneous transcoronary devices will become available to patients with evolving or recurrent myocardial infarction.

REFERENCES

1. The I.S.A.M. Study Group: A prospective trial of intravenous streptokinase in acute myocardial infarction (I.S.A.M): Mortality, morbidity, and infarct size at 21 days. N Engl J Med 1986;314:1465-1471.

2. National Heart Foundation of Australia Coronary Thrombolysis Group: Coronary thrombolysis and myocardial salvage by tissue plasminogen activator given up to 4 hours after onset of myocardial infarction. Lancet 1988;1:203-208.

3. White HD, Norris RM, Brown MA, et al: Effect of intravenous streptokinase on left ventricular function and early survival after acute myocardial infarction. N Engl J Med 1987;317:850-855.

4. Guerci AD, Gerstenblith G, Brinker JA, et al: A randomized trial of intravenous tissue plasminogen activator for acute myocardial infarction with subsequent randomization to elective coronary angioplasty. N Engl J Med 1987;317:1613-1618.

5. Gruppo Italiano per lo studio della streptochinasi nell'infarto miocardico (GISSI): Effectiveness of intravenous thrombolytic treatment in acute myocardial infarction. Lancet 1986;1:397-402.

6. Gruppo Italiano per lo studio della streptochinasi nell'infarto miocardico (GISSI): Long-term effects of intravenous thrombolysis in acute myocardial infarction: Final report of the GISSI study. Lancet 1987;2:871-874.

7. ISIS Steering Committee: Intravenous streptokinase given within 0-4 hours of onset of myocardial infarction reduced mortality in ISIS-2 [Letter]. Lancet 1987;1:502.

8. ISIS-2 (Second International Study of Infarct Survival) Collaborative Group: Randomised trial of intravenous streptokinase, oral aspirin, both, or neither among 17,187 cases of suspected acute myocardial infarction: ISIS-2. Lancet 1988;2:349-360.

9. The TIMI Study Group: The Thrombolysis in Myocardial Infarction (TIMI) Trial. Phase I Findings. N Engl J Med 1985;312:932-936.

10. Topol EJ, Califf RM, George BS, et al: A randomized trial of immediate versus delayed elective angioplasty after intravenous tissue plasminogen activator in acute myocardial infarction. N Engl J Med 1987;317:581-588.

11. The TIMI Research Group: Immediate vs delayed catheterization and angioplasty following thrombolytic therapy for acute myocardial infarction: TIMI IIA Results. JAMA 1988; 260:2849-2858.

12. Simoons ML, Arnold AER, Betriu A, et al: Thrombolysis with tissue plasminogen activator in acute myocardial infarction: No additional benefit from immediate percutaneous coronary angioplasty. Lancet 1988;1:197-203.

13. Topol EJ, Califf RM, George BS, et al: Coronary arterial thrombolysis with combined infusion of recombinant tissue-type plasminogen activator and urokinase in patients with acute myocardial infarction. Circulation 1988;77:1100-1107.

14. Harrison DG, Ferguson DW, Collins SM, et al: Rethrombosis after reperfusion with streptokinase: Importance of geometry of residual lesions. Circulation 1984;69:991-999.

15. Gash AK, Spann JF, Sherry S, et al: Factors influencing reocclusion after coronary thrombolysis for acute myocardial infarction. Am J Cardiol 1986;57:175-177.

16. Sheehan FH, Mathey DG, Schofer J, et al: Factors that determine recovery of left ventricular function after thrombolysis in patients with acute myocardial infarction. Circulation 1985;71:1121-1128.

17. Topol EJ, Weiss JL, Brinker JA, et al: Regional wall motion improvement after coronary thrombolysis with recombinant tissue plasminogen activator: Importance of coronary angioplasty. J Am Coll Cardiol 1985;6:426-433.

18. O'Neill W, Timmis GC, Bourdillon P, et al: A prospective randomized clinical trial of intracoronary streptokinase versus coronary angioplasty for acute myocardial infarction. N Engl J Med 1986;314:812-818.

19. Hartzler GO, Rutherford BD, McConahay DR, et al: Percutaneous transluminal coronary angioplasty with and without thrombolytic therapy for treatment of acute myocardial infarction. Am Heart J 1983;106:965-973.

20. Holmes DR Jr, Smith HC, Vlietstra RE, et al: Percutaneous transluminal coronary angioplasty, alone or in combination with streptokinase therapy, during acute myocardial infarction. Mayo Clin Proc 1985;60:449-456.

21. Rothbaum DA, Linnemeier TJ, Landin RJ, et al: Emergency percutaneous transluminal coronary angioplasty in acute myocardial infarction: A 3 year experience. J Am Coll Cardiol 1987;10:264-272.

22. The TIMI Study Group: Comparison of invasive and conservative strategies after treatment with intravenous tissue plasminogen activator in acute myocardial infarction: Results of the Thrombolysis in Myocardial Infarction (TIMI) Phase II Trial. N Engl J Med 1989;320:618-627.

23. Buja LM, Willerson JT: Clinicopathologic correlates of acute ischemic heart disease syndromes. Am J Cardiol 1981;47:343-356.

24. Davies MJ, Woolf N, Robertson WB: Pathology of acute myocardial infarction with particular reference to occlusive coronary thrombi. Br Heart J 1976;38:659-664.

25. Horie T, Sekiguchi M, Hirosawa K: Coronary thrombosis in pathogenesis of acute myocardial infarction. Histopathological study of coronary arteries in 108 necropsied cases using serial sections. Br Heart J 1978;40:153-161.

26. Ridolfi RL, Hutchins GM: The relationship between coronary artery lesions and myocardial infarcts: Ulceration of atherosclerotic plaques precipitating coronary thrombosis. Am Heart J 1977;93:468-486.

27. Oliva PB: Pathophysiology of acute myocardial infarction, 1981. Ann Intern Med 1981; 94:236-250.

28. DeWood MA, Spores J, Notske R, et al: Prevalence of total coronary occlusion during the early hours of transmural myocardial infarction. N Engl J Med 1980;303:897-902.

29. Reimer KA, Lowe JE, Rasmussen MM, et al: The wavefront phenomenon of ischemic cell death. 1. Myocardial infarct size vs duration of coronary occlusion in dogs. Circulation 1977;56:786-794.

30. Reimer KA, Jennings RB: The "wavefront phenomenon" of myocardial ischemic cell death. II. Transmural progression of necrosis within the framework of ischemic bed size (myocardium at risk) and collateral flow. Lab Invest 1979;40:633-44.

31. Rentrop KP, Blanke H, Karsch KR, et al: Initial experience with transluminal recanalization of the recently occluded infarct-related coronary artery in acute myocardial infarction- comparison with conventionally treated patients. Clin Cardiol 1979;2:92-105.

32. Gruentzig AR, Senning A, Siegenthaler WE: Nonoperative dilatation of coronary artery stenosis: Percutaneous transluminal coronary angioplasty. N Engl J Med 1979;301:61-68.

33. Kennedy JW, Ritchie JL, Davis KB, et al: Western Washington randomized trial of intracoronary streptokinase in acute myocardial infarction. New Engl J Med 1983; 309: 1477-1482.

34. Kennedy JW, Gensini GG, Timmis GC, et al: Acute myocardial infarction treated with intracoronary streptokinase: A report of the Society for Cardiac Angiography. Am J Cardiol 1985;55:871-877.

35. Anderson JL, Marshall HW, Bray BE, et al: A randomized trial of intracoronary streptokinase in the treatment of acute myocardial infarction. N Engl J Med 1983;308:1312-1318.

36. Meyer J, Merx W, Schmitz H, et al: Percutaneous transluminal coronary angioplasty immediately after intracoronary streptolysis of transmural myocardial infarction. Circulation 1982;66:905-913.

37. Topol EJ: Coronary angioplasty for acute myocardial infarction. Ann Int Med 1988;109: 970-980.

38. Topol EJ, Bates ER, Walton JA, et al: Community hospital administration of intravenous tissue plasminogen activator in acute myocardial infarction: Improved timing, thrombolytic efficacy and ventricular function. J Am Coll Cardiol 1987;10:1173-1177.

39. Dotter CT, Judkins MP: Transluminal treatment of arteriosclerotic obstruction: Description of a new technic and a preliminary report of its application. Circulation 1964;30: 654-670.

40. Waller BF: "Crackers, breakers, stretchers, drillers, scrapers, shavers, burners, welders, and melters" — The future treatment of atherosclerotic coronary artery disease? A clinical-morphologic assessment. J Am Coll Cardiol 1989;13:969-987.

41. Block PC, Myler RK, Stertzer S, et al: Morphology after transluminal angioplasty in human beings. N Engl J Med. 1981;305:382-385.

42. Austin GE, Ratliff NB, Hollman J, et al: Intimal proliferation of smooth muscle cells as an explanation for recurrent coronary artery stenosis after percutaneous transluminal coronary angioplasty. J Am Coll Cardiol 1985;6:369-375.

43. Waller BF, Rothbaum DA, Pickerton CA, et al: Status of the myocardium and infarct-related coronary artery in 19 necropsy patients with acute recanalization using pharmacologic (streptokinase, r-tissue plasminogen activator), mechanical (percutaneous transluminal coronary angioplasty) or combined types of reperfusion therapy. J Am Coll Cardiol 1987;9:785-801.

44. Colavita PG, Ideker RE, Reimer KA, et al: The spectrum of pathology associated with percutaneous transluminal coronary angioplasty during acute myocardial infarction. J Am Coll Cardiol 1986;8:855-860.

45. Duber C, Jungbluth A, Rumpelt HJ, et al: Morphology of the coronary arteries after combined thrombolysis and percutaneous transluminal coronary angioplasty for acute myocardial infarction. Am J Cardiol 1986;58:698-703.

46. Mattfeldt T, Schwarz F, Schuler G, et al: Necropsy evaluation in seven patients with evolving acute myocardial infarction treated with thrombolytic therapy. Am J Cardiol 1984;54:530-534.

47. Mathey DG, Schofer J, Kuck K-H, et al: Transmural, hemorrhagic myocardial infarction after intracoronary streptokinase. Clinical, angiographic, and necropsy findings. Br Heart J 1982;48:546-551.

48. Fuster V, Badimon L, Cohen M, et al: Insights into the pathogenesis of acute ischemic syndromes. Circulation 1988;77:1213-1220.

49. Brum JM, Sufan Q, Lane G, et al: Increased vasoconstrictor activity of proximal coronary arteries with endothelial damage in intact dogs. Circulation 1984;70:1066-1073.

50. Fischell TA, Derby G, Tse TM, et al: Coronary artery vasoconstriction routinely occurs after percutaneous transluminal coronary angioplasty: A quantitative arteriographic analysis. Circulation 1988;78:1323-1334.

51. Miller PF, Brodie BR, Weintraub RA, et al: Emergency coronary angioplasty for acute myocardial infarction: Results from a community hospital. Arch Int Med 1987;147:1565-1570.

52. Prida XE, Holland JP, Feldman RL, et al: Percutaneous transluminal coronary angioplasty in evolving acute myocardial infarction. Am J Cardiol 1986;57:1069-1074.

53. Topol EJ, Burek K, O'Neill WW, et al: A randomized controlled trial of hospital discharge three days after myocardial infarction in the era of reperfusion. N Engl J Med 1988;318:1083-1088.

54. O'Keefe JH, Rutherford DR, Ligon RW, et al: Direct PTCA for acute infarction in 614 consecutive patients from 11/1980 to 3/1989 (abstract). Circulation 1989;80(suppl-II):II-479.

55. Kimura T, Nosaka H, Ueno K, et al: Role of coronary angioplasty in acute myocardial infarction (abstract). Circulation 1986;74(suppl-II):II-22.

56. Topol EJ, O'Neill WW, Lai P, et al: Sequential intravenous thrombolysis and coronary angioplasty vs. direct PTCA therapy for acute myocardial infarction (abstract). J Am Coll Cardiol 1986;7:18A.

57. Owens SD, Robuck OW, Beauchamp GD: Direct coronary angioplasty in elderly patients with acute myocardial infarction (abstract). Circulation 1989;80(suppl-II):II-624.

58. Kahn JK, Rutherford BD, McConahay DR, et al: Primary angioplasty of acute myocardial infarction in patients with multivessel coronary artery disease (abstract). Circulation 1989;80(suppl-II):II-625.

59. Brodie BR, Weintraub RA, Stuckey TD, et al: Direct angioplasty for acute myocardial infarction: Results in candidates and non-candidates for thrombolytic therapy (abstract). Circulation 1989;80(suppl-II):II-624.

60. Fung AY, Lai P, Juni JE, et al: Prevention of subsequent exercise-induced periinfarct ischemia by emergency coronary angioplasty in acute myocardial infarction: Comparison with intracoronary streptokinase. J Am Coll Cardiol 1986;8:496-503.

61. DeWood MA, Fisher MJ: Direct PTCA versus intravenous r-tPA in acute myocardial infarction: Preliminary results from a prospective randomized trial (abstract). Circulation 1989;80(suppl-II):II-418.

62. Holland K, Topol EJ, Walton JA Jr., et al: Emergency coronary angioplasty therapy for elderly patients with acute myocardial infarction; cautionary results (abstract). J Am Coll Cardiol 1987;9:232A.

63. Mirowski M, Israel W, Antonopoulos AG, et al: Treatment of myocardial infarction in a community hospital coronary care unit. Arch Intern Med 1978;138:210-215.

64. Lee L, Bates ER, Pitt B, et al: Percutaneous transluminal coronary angioplasty improves survival in acute myocardial infarction complicated by cardiogenic shock. Circulation 1988;78:1345-1351.

328

65. Gacioch GM, Topol EJ: Frontiers in cardiogenic shock management: Integration of angioplasty and new support devices (abstract). Circulation 1989;80 (suppl-II):II-624.

66. Garrahy PJ, Henzlova MJ, Forman S, et al: Has thrombolytic therapy improved survival from cardiogenic shock? Thrombolysis in Myocardial Infarction (TIMI II) results (abstract). Circulation 1989;80(suppl-II):II-623.

67. Brown TM Jr., Iannone LA, Gordon DF, et al: Percutaneous myocardial perfusion (PMR) reduces mortality in acute myocardial infarction (MI) complicated by cardiogenic shock (abstract). Circulation 1985;72(suppl-III):III-309.

68. Shani J, Rivera M, Greengart A, et al: Percutaneous transluminal coronary angioplasty in cardiogenic shock (abstract). J Am Coll Cardiol 1986;7:149A.

69. Heuser RR, Maddoux GL, Goss JE, et al: Coronary angioplasty in the treatment of cardiogenic shock: The therapy of choice (abstract). J Am Coll Cardiol 1986;7:219A.

70. Dalen JE for the TIMI Investigators: Intravenous thrombolytic therapy in acute myocardial infarction-six month followup: The NHLBI Thrombolysis In Myocardial Infarction (TIMI) Trial (abstract). J Am Coll Cardiol 1987;9:60A.

71. Kennedy JW, Ritchie JL, Davis KB, et al: The Western Washington randomized trial of intracoronary streptokinase in acute myocardial infarction: A 12-month follow-up report. N Engl J Med 1985;312:1073-1078.

72. Cigarroa RG, Lange RA, Hillis LD: Prognosis after acute myocardial infarction in patients with and without residual anterograde coronary blood flow. Am J Cardiol 1989; 64:155-160.

73. Kircher RJ, Topol EJ, O'Neill WW, et al: Prediction of infarct coronary artery recanalization after intravenous thrombolytic therapy. Am J Cardiol 1987;59:513-515.

74. Califf RM, O'Neill W, Stack RS, et al: Failure of simple clinical measurements to predict perfusion status after intravenous thrombolysis. Ann Int Med 1988;108:658-662.

75. Puleo PR, Perryman B, Bresser MA, et al: Creatine kinase isoform analysis in the detection and assessment of thrombolysis in man. Circulation 1987;75:1162-1169.

76. van der Laarse A, van der Wall EE, van den Pol RC, et al: Rapid enzyme release from acutely infarcted myocardium after early thrombolytic therapy: Washout or reperfusion damage? Am Heart J 1988;115:711-716.

77. Hogg KJ, Hornung RS, Howie CA, et al: Electrocardiographic prediction of coronary artery patency after thrombolytic treatment in acute myocardial infarction: Use of the ST segment as a non-invasive marker. Br Heart J 1988;60:275-280.

78. Califf RM, Topol EJ, George BS, et al: Characteristic and outcome of patients in whom reperfusion with intravenous tissue-type plasminogen activator fails: Results of the Thrombolysis and Angioplasty in Myocardial Infarction (TAMI) I trial. Circulation 1988; 77:1090-1099.

79. Baim DS, Diver DJ, Knatterud GL and the TIMI II-A Investigators: PTCA "Salvage" for thrombolytic failures-implication from TIMI II-A (abstract). Circulation 1988;78(suppl-II): II-112.

80. Fung AY, Lai P, Topol EJ, et al: Value of percutaneous transluminal coronary angioplasty after unsuccessful intravenous streptokinase therapy in acute myocardial infarction. Am J Cardiol 1986;58:686-691.

81. O'Conner CM, Mark DB, Hinohara T, et al: Rescue coronary angioplasty after failure of intravenous streptokinase in acute myocardial infarction: In-hospital and long-term outcomes. J Inv Cardiol 1989;1:85-95.

82. Holmes DR, Gersh BJ, Bailey KR, et al: "Rescue" percutaneous transluminal coronary angioplasty after failed thrombolytic therapy- 4 year follow-up. J Am Coll Cardiol 1989; 13:193A.

83. Grines CL, Nissen SE, Booth DC, et al: Efficacy, safety and cost effectiveness of a new thrombolytic regimen for acute myocardial infarction using half dose tPA with full dose streptokinase (abstract). Circulation 1988;78(suppl-II):II-304.

84. Topol EJ, Califf RM, George BS, et al: Can emergency coronary angioplasty and rescue angioplasty improve infarct vessel patency after thrombolysis?: The TAMI-5 trial preliminary results (abstract). Circulation 1989;80(suppl-II):II-48.

85. Gacioch GM, Topol EJ: Sudden paradoxical clinical deterioration during angioplasty of the occluded right coronary artery in acute myocardial infarction. J Am Coll Cardiol 1989;14:1202-1209.

86. Ellis SG, O'Neill WW, Gallison L, et al: Triage to immediate catheterization and angioplasty with acute myocardial infarction — Implications from survival analyses of 452 patients undergoing angioplasty (abstract). Circulation 1988;78(suppl-II):II-112.

87. Topol EJ: Mechanical Interventions for acute myocardial infarction, in Topol EJ (ed.), *Textbook of Interventional Cardiology*, Philadelphia, WB Saunders, 1990, pp 269-299.

88. Dote K, Sato H, Tateishi H, et al: Post-hospital re-infarction after reperfusion therapy with or without emergency coronary angioplasty (PTCA) (abstract). Circulation 1989;80 (suppl-II):II-46.

89. Ellis SG, Topol EJ, George BS, et al: Recurrent ischemia without warning: Analysis of risk factors for in-hospital ischemic events following successful thrombolysis with intravenous tissue plasminogen activator. Circulation 1989;80:1159-1165.

90. Ohman EM, Nelson C, Kong Y-H, et al: Characteristics and clinical consequences of reinfarction: Benefits of aggressive reperfusion (abstract). Circulation 1989;80(suppl-II):II-479.

91. Williams DO, Braunwald E, Knatterud G, et al: The Thrombolysis in Myocardial Infarction (TIMI) Trial: Outcome at one year of patients randomized to either invasive or conservative management (abstract). Circulation 1989;(suppl-II):II-519.

92. de Bono DP, Pocock SJ for the SWIFT Investigators Group: The SWIFT study of intervention versus conservative management after anistreplase thrombolysis (abstract). Circulation 1989;80(suppl-II):II-418.

93. Iskandrian AS, Heo J, Kong B, et al: Effect of exercise level on the ability of thallium-201 tomographic imaging in detecting coronary artery disease: Analysis of 461 patients. J Am Coll Cardiol 1989;14:1477-1486.

94. Liu P, Kiess MC, Okada RD, et al: The persistent defect on exercise thallium imaging and its fate after myocardial revascularization: Does it represent scar or ischemia? Am Heart J 1985:110:996-1001.

95. Sutton JM, Topol EJ: The paradox of a tight residual stenosis and a negative exercise SPECT thallium test after thrombolysis for evolving myocardial infarction (abstract). Circulation 1989;80(suppl-II):II-521

96. Topol EJ, Ellis SG, George BS, et al: The pivotal role of multivessel coronary artery disease and the remote zone in the reperfusion era. J Am Coll Cardiol 1989;13:92A.

OTHER POST-INFARCTION
MEDICAL AND DIAGNOSTIC CARE

Section V

Chapter 15

MANAGEMENT OF EARLY AND LATE ARRHYTHMIAS IN ACUTE MYOCARDIAL INFARCTION

D. George Wyse

INTRODUCTION

The occurrence of a variety of arrhythmias in acute myocardial infarction (AMI) was a major impetus to the formation of coronary care units beginning over 30 years ago. However, in spite of the fact that disturbances of cardiac rhythm are commonly found in association with AMI, are potential contributing factors in the morbidity of AMI, and are often noted as part of terminal events when death occurs, death from a primary disturbance of the cardiac rhythm in the hospital phase of AMI is distinctly unusual in modern times.[1] Low mortality directly attributable to cardiac arrhythmias alone in the hospital phase of AMI is probably at least partially related to increased knowledge of cardiac rhythm management and to development of better management tools.

Table 1 lists the sequential steps to be followed in the management of arrhythmias. This framework is also applicable to the management of cardiac rhythm problems in patients with AMI. Although reviewing this list in each clinical situation may be laborious and may seem somewhat contrived, with practice it becomes a routine that is quickly done and ensures that key management points are not missed. Learning to do this automatically is akin to learning a systematic approach to ECG interpretation, which is difficult at first but eventually becomes routine.

EARLY ARRHYTHMIA MANAGEMENT

There is no clear consensus about a precise definition of "early" and "late" with respect to the cardiac rhythm disturbances of AMI. In this chapter the term "early" will be applied to those arrhythmias occurring within the first six days of coronary occlusion and/or the onset of pain.

Table 1. *Basic steps of arrhythmia management*

Characterize the rhythm disturbance

Stabilize the patient

Identify and correct reversible causes

Characterize and optimally treat the underlying heart disease

Characterize and treat underlying disease of other major organs

Withdraw antiarrhythmic drug therapy

Quantify arrhythmia in the drug-free state

Decide whether or not further treatment is needed

Set goals for antiarrhythmic therapy

Select and administer antiarrhythmic therapy

Evaluate therapy against preset goals

Reevaluate goals if necessary

Plan long-term follow-up

Supraventricular Arrhythmias

The most common supraventricular arrhythmias encountered in the setting of an AMI are atrial flutter and fibrillation which are noted in approximately 15-20% of patients.[2] Diagnosis is usually straightforward, but in the setting of aberrant conduction it may be difficult. Frequently the episodes are transient and do not require specific therapy. When episodes are sustained, and particularly when they have hemodynamic consequences and/or aggravate ischemic chest pain, specific treatment will be needed. Rarely is atrial flutter/fibrillation an acute emergency. However, when it contributes to severe pain, pulmonary edema or shock, it may require transthoracic cardioversion.

Atrial flutter and fibrillation are more common in the setting of certain other problems associated with myocardial infarction such as heart failure, particularly with co-existent mitral regurgitation, pericarditis, or atrial infarction. Therapy of this rhythm problem thus begins with optimal treatment of any other problems that are present. When sustained atrial flutter/fibrillation occurs in the setting of a small and uncomplicated AMI, other factors known to be associated with these rhythm disturbances outside the setting of AMI should be sought. These include mitral valve disease, hypertension, hyperthyroidism, and others.[3] Management of the atrial flutter/fibrillation will then include correction of any of these factors that are reversible.

After the rhythm has been accurately characterized, emergent treatment (ie, electrical cardioversion) has been administered when necessary, and any potential reversible factors have been identified and corrected, consideration can be given to specific therapy. Specific treatment has two goals: heart rate control and conversion/maintenance. These two goals may sometimes be achieved concurrently, but heart rate control should usually take precedence because it is such an important determinant of myocardial oxygen demand. Only in situations in which atrial transport function provided by atrioventricular synchrony is vital will conversion to sinus rhythm take precedence over rate control.

Rate control by drugs is aimed at retarding atrioventricular nodal conduction. Early administration of intravenous β-adrenergic receptor blocking agents has several salutary effects in the early phase of an AMI.[4] Beta-blockers should be considered among the best agents to control the heart rate in atrial flutter/fibrillation in this setting when there are no contraindications to their use. Two or three doses of 5 mg of intravenous metoprolol or three to four doses of 2 mg of intravenous propranolol given 5 minutes apart with careful clinical monitoring of the patient and the ECG will give rapid and satisfactory β-adrenergic receptor blockade. Alternatively, and especially when adverse effects of β-adrenergic receptor blocking agents are of concern, an infusion of the very short acting agent esmolol may be used. The effects of esmolol quickly dissipate as soon as the infusion is stopped.[5] Oral therapy can be instituted immediately after intravenous dosing and should be given frequently (eg, every six hours) in small doses, using those β-adrenergic receptor blocking agents with shorter half-lives. This approach will permit more rapid dissipation of the effects of β-adrenergic receptor blocking agents should their withdrawal become necessary.

Diltiazem is the only calcium channel blocker shown to have any potential benefit in AMI[6,7] (although recent evidence suggests verapamil may also have benefit[8]), and this fact, coupled with a propensity for calcium channel blockers to cause marked hypotension in some patients, suggests that these agents be relegated to second or third choice for heart rate control of atrial flutter/fibrillation in AMI. When they are used, consideration should be given to the administration of intravenous calcium to offset the potential for serious hypotension.[9]

When β-adrenergic receptor blocking agents cannot be used, and particularly when there is no urgency, digoxin may be readily substituted or even added when rate control has not been satisfactory with other agents. The average person will require a loading dose of 1.25 to 1.5 mg of digoxin given intravenously or orally to be fully digitalized. How rapidly this loading dose should be administered is determined by the clinical circumstances. The positive inotropic effect of digoxin and, when given quickly,[10] its propensity to increase afterload are theoretical points against its use in the setting of an AMI. These effects in the absence of other changes will increase myocardial oxygen demand. Practically, however, the control of heart rate and/or decreased wall tension with restoration of sinus rhythm will more than offset the relatively weak effects of digoxin on inotropy and afterload. The initial portion of the total 1.25 to 1.5 mg intravenous loading dose of digoxin should be 0.5 mg given over at least 15 minutes. The remainder may be given intravenously or orally in 0.125 to 0.25 mg portions every 4 to 6 hours. When more rapid loading is needed, 0.125 mg can be given intravenously every hour until the target heart rate or total loading dose is achieved. The usual oral or intravenous maintenance dose of 0.125 mg to 0.25 mg once a day is started on the day following administration of the loading dose.

The tendency of atrial flutter/fibrillation to terminate spontaneously is well known,[11] and this seems to occur often in the setting of AMI. The drugs discussed so far, which have their major effects on the atrioventricular node, probably do not produce reversion to sinus rhythm, since the atrioventricular node plays little or no role in atrial flutter/fibrillation (other than to conduct the wave of depolarization to the ventricles). Thus, when reversion to sinus rhythm occurs after the use of one of these drugs, it is often more likely a spontaneous event.[11] On the other hand, Class 1A antiarrhythmics, which are often used to restore sinus rhythm, can increase atrioventricular nodal conduction.[12] This is another important reason to control heart rate first and restore sinus rhythm second in most circumstances.

After heart rate is controlled but atrial flutter/fibrillation persists, conversion to sinus rhythm may be attempted, usually with drug therapy. Oral therapy with a standard Class 1A antiarrhythmic drug such as quinidine, procainamide, or disopyramide may be started without any loading dose. The choice of agent requires a clinical assessment of previous antiarrhythmic drug use, underlying heart disease — particularly left ventricular function — and status of other major organ systems, especially the liver and kidneys. All three of these agents can be myocardial depressants in patients with poor ventricular function, with disopyramide having a greater depressant effect than quinidine or procainamide. If quinidine is selected and digoxin has been used, the digoxin-quinidine interaction must be taken into account, usually by halving the maintenance dosage of digoxin.

When the intravenous route is required, procainamide is probably the agent of choice. The loading dose of 10-15 mg/kg is given in 100 mg boluses over 3-5 minutes repeated every 5 minutes, or continuous infusion over 45-60 minutes, with careful monitoring of the blood pressure and the ECG. When the distinction between atrial flutter/fibrillation with aberrancy and ventricular tachycardia cannot be made with certainty, procainamide is the most suitable agent since it is effective therapy for either problem. The Class 1B antiarrhythmic agents — lidocaine, mexiletine, and tocainide — are generally not useful in atrial flutter/fibrillation.

The Class 1C antiarrhythmic drugs propafenone, encainide, and flecainide are all useful for atrial flutter/fibrillation in other settings,[13-16] but their use in the setting of an AMI has not yet been fully evaluated. Propafenone and flecainide in particular can cause significant myocardial depression.[17,18] Proarrhythmia remains a significant concern with these drugs, and the results of the **C**ardiac **A**rrhythmia **S**uppression **T**rial (CAST) should temper their use in this situation.[19] One theoretical advantage of these agents is their ability to provide heart rate control and conversion to sinus rhythm as single agents. This is because these drugs can directly act to slow atrioventricular conduction, and in the case of propafenone, this effect may be enhanced by its β-adrenoceptor blocking properties.[20] The use of these agents as single-drug therapy for atrial flutter/fibrillation is not recommended, however, because they can promote 1:1 conduction of a slowed atrial rhythm with a widened QRS which can be mistaken for *ventricular* flutter.[21]

The Class 3 antiarrhythmic drugs, sotalol and amiodarone, may also be used for management of atrial flutter/fibrillation in an AMI. Both of these drugs can be used as single agents for both rate control and medical conversion to sinus rhythm. Sotalol has considerable β-adrenergic receptor blocking properties which tend to reach a maximum at lower dosages while its Class 3 effects continue to increase as the dosage is increased.[22] Sotalol also has myocardial depressant effects and can provoke heart failure in some patients.[23,24] The usual dosage of sotalol is 160 to 480 mg per day given as two or three divided oral doses.

The use of amiodarone in North America is usually reserved for cases of failure of or intolerance to other antiarrhythmic drugs. Its pharmacokinetic profile (eg, long half-life) and the fear of serious and/or frequent adverse effects of amiodarone inhibit its use. Intravenous amiodarone is not generally used for atrial flutter/fibrillation. An oral loading period of 2 or 3 weeks is common, and several weeks may be needed before the full effects of amiodarone are seen, although rate control through slowed atrioventricular conduction occurs much earlier.[25] An average loading dose for atrial flutter/fibrillation during the first 2 or 3 weeks is 400 to 800 mg per day, usually in divided doses. The maintenance dose for atrial flutter/fibrillation is 200 mg per day for 5 or 7 days per week. These doses are lower than those generally used for chronic life-threatening ventricular arrhythmias, but careful and prolonged surveillance for the multitude of adverse effects of amiodarone[26] must still be maintained. Bradycardia can be a problem during the loading phase. The longer term adverse effects of amiodarone are outlined below.

Initiation of therapy with amiodarone must never be undertaken without careful consideration of the potential consequences. If referral to a specialized arrhythmia center is contemplated, the drug should not be started without consultation with that center. The very long half-life of amiodarone means that washout is lengthy, and once a patient is loaded with the drug, evaluation of other therapy is not possible in the short-term. Furthermore, starting this drug initiates a commitment by the physician for regular and careful evaluation for adverse effects for the rest of the patient's life. All patients on prolonged therapy with amiodarone require sun screen protection and most require a regular laxative. Prior to or at initiation of therapy patients require a thorough neurological evaluation, chest x-ray and pulmonary function tests, thyroid function tests, and liver enzyme measurement. These evaluations must be repeated at regular intervals as long as the patient is on the drug. All patients will get cornea microdeposits but these do not usually interfere with vision. However, some patients complain of light sensitivity and scotomata. As indicated above, most patients on chronic amiodarone therapy experience photosensitivity and constipation. Skin rashes occur and rarely can be a serious Stevens-Johnson type reaction. Long-term therapy can lead to delayed problems such as pulmonary fibrosis, although alveolitis can occur earlier. Other delayed problems include hepatitis, peripheral neuropathy, hypothyroidism, or paradoxically, hyperthyroidism, which sometimes presents as a puzzling myositis.[26]

Several other management considerations for atrial flutter/fibrillation in the setting of AMI should be mentioned. Atrial flutter, but not atrial fibrillation, is often amenable to pace-termination. Although pace-termination is not usually a primary mode of therapy, it represents an alternative to medical or electrical cardioversion, particularly when a pacing catheter is already in place in the right atrium or central venous access is already available. The transesophageal route may also be used.[27] Pace-termination is more rapid than medical conversion and does not require the general anesthesia of transthoracic cardioversion.

Atrial fibrillation (but probably not atrial flutter) is a risk factor for thromboembolic complications at any time,[3] and probably adds to the risk of thromboembolism already present in all patients with AMI. Atrial fibrillation for more than brief, unsustained episodes should prompt consideration of more vigorous anticoagulant therapy including full anticoagulation with intravenous heparin and/or oral warfarin if these therapies are not already in use. Coexistence of other risk factors for thromboembolism, including obesity, congestive heart failure and mitral regurgitation in the presence of atrial fibrillation mandates full anticoagulation, unless a strong contraindication exists.

Other supraventricular arrhythmias can, of course, occur in the setting of AMI. For the most part, however, these do not usually require therapy, or their therapy is similar to that applied in other situations. Management of these arrhythmias will not be discussed here.

Bradycardia

Bradycardia is frequently encountered in AMI.[2,28] The sinus node artery in man originates more frequently from the right coronary artery and when it originates from the left, it is usually from the circumflex branch.[28] Thus, sinus bradycardia is more frequently a problem with inferior/posterior infarctions.

In most instances, specific therapy for these arrhythmias is not necessary since they are usually transient. A stable and reliable secondary pacemaker with an adequate rate emerges, usually from the atrioventricular junction. However, when sinus brady-cardia is marked and/or seriously disrupts atrioventricular synchrony, specific therapy may be needed.[29] Although rate is not usually an important determinant of cardiac output over a wide range in normal healthy hearts unless the rate becomes very low, in AMI a decline in cardiac output may be seen with heart rates considered acceptable in other circumstances — 55-60 beats per minute. When atrioventricular synchrony is lost, particularly in association with a right ventricular infarction, the decrease in cardiac output can be profound.[29]

The first step in managing sinus bradycardia is to determine whether any poten-tially reversible causes are present, such as β-adrenergic receptor blocking agents. Other drugs are also capable of causing sinus bradycardia and/or sinus arrest, including α-methyldopa and, although it is not widely recognized, lidocaine.[30] Drug-induced sinus bradycardia/arrest is easily reversed by discontinuation of the offending agent. Sometimes small doses (0.3 to 0.6 mg) of intravenous atropine are administered as temporary therapy for transient bradycardia in AMI. When no obvious reversible cause of bradycardia is apparent, temporary pacing may be necessary. Temporary atrial pacing may be particularly helpful when persistent sinus bradycardia produces hemodynamic compromise in inferior infarction with concomitant right ventricular infarction.[29] In this case, decreased heart rate and atrial transport both diminish cardiac output, and therefore atrial pacing is more beneficial than ventricular pacing. When atrioventricular conduction is impaired, as it often is under these circumstances, tem-porary dual chamber pacing may be needed.

Beta-adrenergic receptor stimulating agents may also be used as temporary ther-apy for hemodynamically significant sinus bradycardia, but in many cases the addi-tional inotropic effects of such agents are unwanted because they cause a dramatic increase in myocardial oxygen demand. On the other hand, in the setting of inferior/posterior infarction with right ventricular infarction, heart rate and atrioventricular synchrony in themselves may be insufficient for an adequate hemodynamic response, and the positive inotropic effects of β-adrenergic receptor agonists such as dobutamine and dopamine may be needed in addition to pacing.

Heart Block

Atrioventricular (AV) block of varying degrees is extremely common in inferior/posterior myocardial infarction. The anatomic explanation for this phenomenon is that the major blood supply to the atrioventricular node is provided by the dominant coronary artery; ie, the artery giving rise to the posterior descending coronary artery. In approx-imately 90% of humans this is the right coronary artery.[28] Although AV block is extremely common in inferior/posterior infarction and may even progress to third degree or complete AV block, it does not always require cardiac pacing. One reason pacing is usually not needed, or is needed only temporarily, is that the conduction problem is usually transient. Transient AV block in this circumstance is often due to ischemia rather than infarction, perhaps as a consequence of the rich dual blood supply of the AV node region and/or a high rate of spontaneous reperfusion. More importantly, however, a stable secondary pacemaker with an adequate rate will usually emerge from the AV junction. Drug therapy (eg, digoxin, β-adrenergic receptor blocking agents, calcium channel blockers) which impairs AV nodal conduction should be discontinued if marked first, second, or third degree AV block develops. Extreme hypokalemia or hyperkalemia is another reversible cause of atrioventricular block.

Bundle branch blocks and fascicular blocks are also found in AMI, and they may portend complete heart block requiring pacemaker therapy. These conduction problems occur most frequently with anterior myocardial infarctions and determining whether the conduction problem is new or chronic may be difficult. Whether these conduction disturbances are chronic or new is important in decisions concerning temporary pacing. In cases of high risk bundle branch and fascicular blocks in anterior myocardial infarction, complete heart block may ensue precipitously, and the escape rhythm that results is inadequate and unreliable. Potentially fatal hemodynamic collapse from asystole may be the consequence of complete heart block under these circumstances.

When Type 2 second degree AV block occurs in the setting of new bifascicular block, complete heart block often follows and may occur suddenly and unpredictably. Much effort has been made to distinguish "high risk" patients who might benefit from prophylactic insertion of a temporary pacemaker. However, considerable disagreement remains, and the need for prophylactic temporary pacing in AMI should be individualized, although published guidelines exist.[31-33] "Low," "intermediate," and "high" risk conduction characteristics, in which temporary prophylactic pacing may be considered, are outlined in Table 2. These divisions are somewhat arbitrary and should be regarded as analogous to the categorization of indications for permanent pacemakers.[31] That is, low risk means general agreement that prophylactic temporary pacing is not indicated; intermediate risk means a divergence of opinion concerning whether or not prophylactic temporary pacing is indicated; and high risk means general agreement that prophylactic temporary pacing is indicated.

Complete heart block in patients who have left bundle branch block and undergo right heart catheterization with a flow-directed (Swan-Ganz) catheter may result from temporary catheter-induced right bundle branch block. Therefore, it may be prudent to place a temporary pacemaker before inserting a flow-directed right heart catheter, or alternatively, to use a technique which allows rapid institution of temporary pacing if complete heart block develops. Temporary pacing in AMI may need to be continued beyond the six-day period arbitrarily set as the "early" phase of AMI. Discontinuation of temporary pacing and institution of permanent pacing will be discussed below.

Table 2. *Conduction characteristics of patients at "low," "intermediate," and "high" risk for development of complete heart block in acute myocardial infarction*

Low Risk (Temporary Cardiac Pacemaker Not Indicated)

First Degree AV Block with Pre-existing LBBB or Isolated RBBB

First Degree AV Block with New RBBB

Normal PR Interval with Pre-existing Alternating LBBB and RBBB

Normal PR Interval with New LBBB or Isolated RBBB

Intermediate Risk (Temporary Cardiac Pacemaker Optional)

New RBBB + LAH with normal PR Interval

LBBB or RBBB + Hemiblock and Prolonged HV Interval

First Degree AV Block and New LBBB

High Risk (Temporary Cardiac Pacemaker Indicated)

New Alternating LBBB and RBBB, Regardless of PR Interval

New RBBB + Alternating LAH and LPH, Regardless of PR Interval

New RBBB + LPH, Regardless of PR Interval

New RBBB + LAH with First Degree AV Block

AV = Atrioventricular
HV Interval = Time from bundle of His depolarization to QRS; ie, Infranodal Conduction Time
LAH = Left Anterior Hemiblock
LBBB = Left Bundle Branch Block
LPH = Left Posterior Hemiblock
RBBB = Right Bundle Branch Block
Adapted from references 29-31

Ventricular Arrhythmias

The management of ventricular arrhythmias during the acute phase of myocardial infarction has been one of the most controversial issues in arrhythmia management over the last two decades. Even now, not all aspects of this controversy have been settled. When Coronary Care Units were first instituted, treatment of ventricular arrhythmias was aimed at prevention of sustained ventricular tachycardia and ventricular fibrillation and improvement of hospital survival. More recently, animal studies have suggested that lesser ventricular arrhythmias may impact on infarct size,[34] and ventricular premature depolarizations have been shown to activate the sympathetic nervous system in man,[35] perhaps increasing the propensity for more serious and life-threatening arrhythmias.

Even the prognostic significance of early ventricular fibrillation in patients with AMI is controversial. It is commonly stated that early ventricular fibrillation has no long term consequences or significance.[36] As shown in Figure 1, however, hospital mortality is increased in patients who have early ventricular fibrillation.[37,38] Whether the increase in hospital mortality is due to the ventricular fibrillation directly or to an association between early ventricular fibrillation and greater infarct size is not clear.[39]

There is also a consensus that for patients who survive and leave hospital after a myocardial infarction, the one-year survival of those with early ventricular fibrillation is equal to those without this problem.[37,38,40] However, careful review of the data in the study with longest follow-up suggests that those patients who sustained early ventricular fibrillation have a decreased survival at four years.[37]

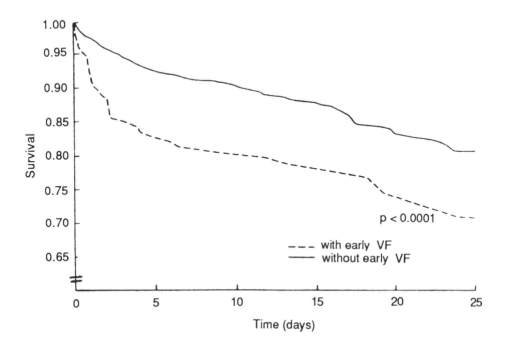

Figure 1. *Relationship between occurrence of early ventricular fibrillation (VF) and in-hospital survival following acute myocardial infarction. From Nicod et al,[38] with permission.*

The incidence of ventricular fibrillation is greatest in the very earliest phase of an AMI and declines very rapidly thereafter.[2,41] The exact incidence in the first hour is unknown, partly because some of these patients do not survive to reach the hospital (Figure 2). The incidence of primary ventricular fibrillation then falls very sharply and after 4 to 6 hours, when the majority of patients have reached the hospital, it reaches a stable and low level of probably less than 1% for the remainder of the hospital course. It remains at this level until 24-36 hours following the infarct. After that, ventricular fibrillation in the absence of heart failure, continued ischemia, hemodynamic compromise, failure of another major organ system, or drug or electrolyte abnormalities is unusual during the remainder of the hospital course. The overall incidence of primary ventricular fibrillation in the 1974 study of hospitalized patients by Lie et al[41]

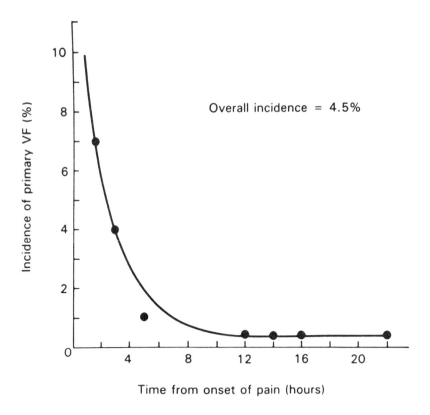

Figure 2. *Relationship between onset of chest pain and incidence of primary ventricular fibrillation (VF) in acute myocardial infarction.*
Source: Wyse, DG: Initiation of the treatment of ventricular tachyarrhythmias, in Mexiletine: A Significant Advance in Arrhythmia Therapy *(MEDICINE Publishing Foundation Symposium Series, 15), Toronto, MES Medical Education Services, 1985 pp 1-13, with permission.*

was 4.5%. The impact of early intervention and reperfusion on the incidence of early ventricular fibrillation in AMI is not known with certainty but has probably not been large. The overall incidence of primary ventricular fibrillation in the hospital phase of GISSI was approximately 3%, and no difference in incidence was observed between those given thrombolytic therapy and the control group.[42]

Many authorities have advocated universal early preventive therapy for ventricular fibrillation. The lack of any reliable indicator to predict which patients are at greatest risk for primary ventricular fibrillation favors this prophylactic strategy. In the past, complex ventricular premature beats were thought to indicate a high risk of impending ventricular fibrillation. However, about half the patients with early ventricular fibrillation during an AMI have no previously detected complex ventricular premature beats, or detection of such beats occurs too late to intervene effectively.[43-45] Nevertheless, many have continued to advocate a more selective prophylactic strategy, and the arguments in favor of such a position are also compelling. First, antiarrhythmic drug therapy has its own inherent risks, and these risks accrue to all patients treated, whether or not they have an AMI.[1] Studies have shown that when antiarrhythmic drug therapy is initiated (appropriately) very early, up to two-thirds of the patients treated will be subsequently shown not to have an AMI.[46] These patients have virtually no risk of ventricular fibrillation and yet are exposed to the measurable risk of potentially serious adverse effects of antiarrhythmic drug therapy.[1,30,46] Analysis of the available data[47] suggests that while the universal prophylactic strategy may decrease the incidence of early ventricular fibrillation, it may actually increase the hospital mortality of AMI (Figures 3 and 4). Thus, the pooled data suggest the value of a cautious rather than an aggressive treatment of early ventricular arrhythmias of AMI.

For the present, the data do not clearly favor either the universal prophylactic or the selective strategy, and treatment must be individualized.[1] The prophylactic strategy appears to be most suitable when the diagnosis of AMI is certain, the duration of pain is less than four hours, and the availability of cardiac monitoring and resuscitation are uncertain. Conversely, when the diagnosis of AMI is uncertain, the duration of pain is greater than four hours, and the availability of monitoring and resuscitation are certain, a selective strategy would be more appropriate. When therapy is started, it should be discontinued as early as possible, preferably within 12 hours, since the toxicity of lidocaine (the drug most commonly used) increases with prolonged infusion.[30]

Lidocaine is the drug of choice, and its pharmacokinetics determine its most appropriate use.[48] A loading infusion of 150 to 250 mg is given as 3-4 divided doses each separated by 8-10 minutes. The maintenance infusion should be 2-3 mg per minute and should be reduced or discontinued after 12 hours. Beta-adrenergic receptor blocking agents also have antiarrhythmic properties in AMI. Part of the benefit

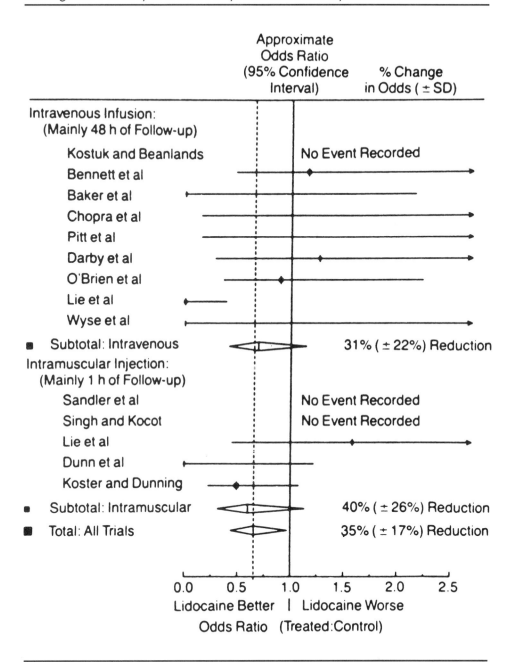

Figure 3. *Meta-analysis of odds ratios for ventricular fibrillation with prophylactic lidocaine versus placebo in 14 randomized trials of therapy for 48 hours after acute myocardial infarction. From MacMahon et al,[47] with permission. JAMA 1988;260:1910-1916. Copyright 1988, American Medical Association.*

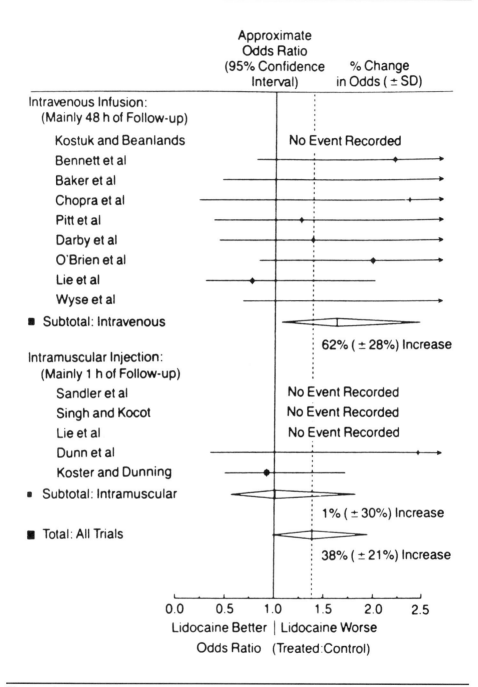

Figure 4. *Meta-analysis of odds ratio for mortality with prophylactic lidocaine versus placebo in 14 randomized trials of therapy for 48 hours after acute myocardial infarction. From MacMahon et al,[47] with permission. JAMA 1988;260:1910-1916. Copyright 1988, American Medical Association.*

from early use of these agents may be attributable to reduction of ventricular arrhythmias (Figure 5).[49]

Once a patient has experienced sustained ventricular tachycardia or fibrillation during the early phase of an AMI, a more aggressive therapy may be needed, especially when sustained ventricular tachycardia and/or fibrillation have occurred in spite of lidocaine prophylaxis. The first step after failure of adequate doses of lidocaine is usually intravenous administration of a Class 1A antiarrhythmic drug such as procainamide while administration of lidocaine continues. Other general measures include optimal therapy of any potential reversible causes such as heart failure, continued

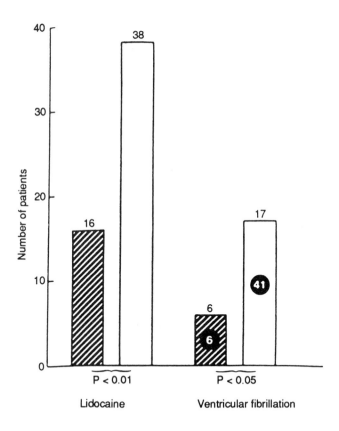

Figure 5. *Number of patients requiring lidocaine treatment and number of patients having ventricular fibrillation among those randomized to early treatment with metoprolol (hatched bars) or placebo (open bars) during acute myocardial infarction. Numbers in circles are episodes of ventricular fibrillation, ie more than one per patient in placebo group. From Ryden et al,[49] with permission.*

ischemia and electrolyte abnormalities. Administration of potassium and magnesium may be helpful. Often small doses of an intravenous β-adrenergic receptor blocking agent may help to stabilize a difficult ventricular rhythm. Second-line antiarrhythmic agents such as bretylium and amiodarone may be required but should be used only by those experienced with these agents. Cardiac pacing and temporary transvenous cardio verters/defibrillators are available in centers specializing in such problems and may bridge the gap from this very unstable phase to more long-term management. In the absence of severe and uncorrectable cardiac pump failure, it is unusual to lose a patient from cardiac rhythm problems, although this clearly does happen occasionally even in the best of centers.

Torsade de pointes ventricular tachycardia can easily be mistaken for ventricular fibrillation. However, its recognition is important since its management is quite different. The characteristics of torsade de pointes ventricular tachycardia[50,51] are a polymorphic ventricular tachycardia, self-terminating episodes, long QT interval and T-U abnormality, short-long-short RR interval initiation sequence, and the appropriate clinical milieu (bradycardia, hypokalemia, use of Class 1A antiarrhythmic drugs). These characteristics should be looked for very carefully whenever an episode of "self-terminating ventricular fibrillation" or a salvo of polymorphic ventricular tachycardia occurs. The treatment of torsade de pointes is markedly different from the treatment of the ventricular tachycardia more commonly seen in the setting of an AMI and usually includes withholding drugs which prolong repolarization (Class 1A and Class 3 antiarrhythmic drugs), administration of potassium and magnesium (magnesium should be given even if serum levels are normal), increasing the heart rate (usually via pacing), and possibly addition of a Class 1B antiarrhythmic drug such as lidocaine.

A common ventricular arrhythmia in the setting of an AMI is accelerated ventricular rhythm. This arrhythmia is benign and does not require therapy. In fact, occasionally it is a more hemodynamically stable rhythm than the underlying rhythm (eg, sinus bradycardia), and suppression of the accelerated ventricular rhythm may actually worsen the patient's status. For this reason, a clear definition of ventricular tachycardia is important, recognizing that all definitions are arbitrary. The elements of ventricular tachycardia in addition to its ventricular origin are the number of successive beats and the RR interval. A useful functional definition of ventricular tachycardia is a rhythm of ventricular origin consisting of 5 or more successive beats with an average RR interval ≤ 600 msec (ie, 100 beats per minute). Three successive beats are called triplets and four successive beats are called salvoes or runs of ventricular premature depolarizations. Sustained ventricular tachycardia is that lasting 30 seconds or longer or requiring termination by cardioversion in less than 30 seconds to avoid hemodynamic collapse. The definition of accelerated ventricular rhythm is a rhythm of ventricular origin of 5 or more successive beats with an average RR interval of 601 to 1000 msec (ie, 60 to 99 beats per minute). "Slow" couplets, triplets or runs with RR intervals of 601 to 1000 msec are thus related to accelerated ventricular rhythm and not to ventricular tachycardia.

LATE ARRHYTHMIA MANAGEMENT

Supraventricular Arrhythmias

Long-term therapy of atrial flutter/fibrillation is probably not needed in most cases. In many cases, patients with atrial flutter/fibrillation in AMI are placed on digoxin and then remain on the drug indefinitely for reasons that are long forgotten. Withdrawal of drug therapy for atrial flutter/fibrillation may be appropriate in some patients prior to hospital discharge. In other cases, particularly those with a previous history of hypertension, chronic left atrial enlargement, mitral regurgitation, poor left ventricular function, or heart failure, atrial flutter/fibrillation therapy will be needed permanently. In most patients, a trial withdrawal of drug therapy for atrial flutter/fibrillation should be done 6 to 12 weeks after myocardial infarction.

Bradycardia and Heart Block

The need for temporary pacing early in the course of AMI does not by itself constitute an indication for permanent pacing.[31-33] Permanent pacing is seldom needed for sinus bradycardia occurring in AMI since this is almost always a transient problem unless underlying Sick Sinus Syndrome is present. Symptomatic sinus bradycardia is the usual indication for permanent pacing and the guidelines of the American College of Cardiology/American Heart Association for sinus node dysfunction should be followed.[31] In the case of heart block, however, the extent of myocardial injury and the character of intraventricular conduction after AMI will determine the need for permanent pacing. The criteria for permanent pacing in heart block after AMI do not depend on the presence of symptoms.

Patients with persistent advanced AV block or complete heart block following AMI require a permanent pacemaker.[31-33] Some cardiologists also recommend permanent pacemakers for patients with persistent first degree AV block with a new bundle-branch block or for those with bundle branch block (old or new) who have transient advanced AV block.[31-33] Transient advanced AV block in the setting of complete right bundle branch block and left anterior hemiblock (old or new) is felt by many to constitute an indication for permanent pacing.[31-33]

Ventricular Arrhythmias

Considerable controversy surrounds the long-term management of ventricular arrhythmias occurring in the late phase of AMI. A number of large, multicenter clinical trials currently underway or about to begin will probably clarify this area substantially within the next 5 to 10 years.

Most arrhythmia specialists regard ventricular fibrillation or sustained, hemodynamically significant ventricular tachycardia occurring more than six days after myocardial infarction as indicating a high risk for further recurrences of these arrhythmias. Most would recommend an aggressive management strategy in the absence of an identifiable reversible cause. Such a strategy would include optimal therapy of congestive heart failure and of ischemic heart disease including revascularization if indicated. Only after this has been accomplished should attention focus on the finalization of rhythm control. At this point, any antiarrhythmic drug therapy that was instituted earlier should be discontinued, and arrhythmia quantification should be undertaken in the drug-free state. Arrhythmia quantification should include 24-hour ambulatory ECG monitoring, treadmill exercise testing, and invasive electrophysiological testing. Measurement of late potentials via the signal-averaged ECG has recently been shown to be an important prognostic indicator of the risk of sudden arrhythmic death in the post-AMI patient and can be done, if available.[52-54]

When withdrawal of antiarrhythmic drug therapy results in no significant spontaneous arrhythmias on the ambulatory ECG and if none is induced on exercise testing or with invasive electrophysiologic testing, an important clinical decision must be made. Such patients may have a low risk of sudden arrhythmic death or recurrence of sustained ventricular arrhythmias,[55,56] perhaps because of therapy applied for ischemia or heart failure. However, these patients may simply fail to possess a suitable surrogate endpoint to guide antiarrhythmic therapy.[55,56] The first decision to be made is which of these two possibilities is correct. Factors such as age, residual left ventricular function, and the presence or absence of late potentials may be helpful. If a decision is made to treat, very few therapeutic choices are available because of the absence of surrogate endpoints to guide therapy. One choice is empiric antiarrhythmic drug therapy; that is, selecting the best possible drug and using whatever means possible to optimize therapy, such as monitoring plasma drug levels. Many experts use empiric amiodarone in this situation. The other choice is an automatic implantable cardioverter/defibrillator. Which of these two choices is best is unknown, but some trials recently begun or in the planning stages may eventually provide an answer. The use of catheter fulguration and arrhythmia surgery in these clinical circumstances must be considered investigational at this time.

When the drug-free arrhythmia quantification reveals frequent and complex ventricular ectopy on the ambulatory ECG and/or treadmill exercise test but no inducible ventricular arrhythmias on invasive electrophysiologic testing, a similarly important clinical decision point is reached. These findings may indicate a low risk of sudden arrhythmic death or recurrence of sustained ventricular arrhythmias or may merely indicate the lack of a suitable electrophysiologic testing endpoint to guide antiarrhythmic drug therapy.[55,56] Most arrhythmia specialists favor the latter interpretation and use the combination of ambulatory ECG testing and treadmill exercise testing to guide antiarrhythmic drug therapy. A parallel situation can occur in which there are no significant arrhythmias on ambulatory ECG and/or treadmill exercise testing in the drug-free state (a clinical circumstance which mandates invasive electrophysiologic testing in a patient with previous ventricular fibrillation or sustained ventricular tachycardia), but ventricular fibrillation or sustained ventricular tachycardia are reliably reproduced by invasive electrophysiologic testing. In this circumstance, antiarrhythmic drug therapy should be guided by the results of invasive electrophysiologic testing.

Finally, the drug-free assessment may reveal frequent and complex ventricular ectopy on ambulatory ECG monitoring and/or treadmill exercise testing and reliably reproducible induction of ventricular fibrillation or sustained ventricular tachycardia during invasive electrophysiologic testing. Present evidence suggests that antiarrhythmic drug therapy selected by invasive electrophysiologic testing is superior to that selected by ambulatory ECG monitoring and/or treadmill exercise testing for long term control of ventricular arrhythmias (Figure 6).[57] A large multicenter trial is currently underway which makes a similar comparison to that shown in Figure 6, although with a different protocol and less stringent endpoints for therapy.[58] Further information on this point may soon be available.

The point at which attempts to guide antiarrhythmic drug therapy by either invasive or noninvasive means should be abandoned in favor of empiric amiodarone therapy, an automatic implantable cardioverter/defibrillator, catheter fulguration, or arrhythmia surgery is not known with certainty at present. The unknown factors which require further assessment include efficacy and reliability and cost-benefit analysis. It is known that "suitable" drug therapy can be found during initial assessment for virtually all patients when noninvasive techniques are used but for only about 40-50% of patients when invasive techniques are used.[57] Furthermore, recent evidence suggests that after four unsuccessful antiarrhythmic drug trials using the invasive techniques, virtually no chance exists of finding a "suitable" drug therapy by this technique, and the cumulative risk of procedural complications begins to rise after two or three such tests.[59]

The greatest controversy in the entire area of arrhythmia management in the late phase after AMI centers on what is the most appropriate treatment for those patients who have frequent ventricular premature beats but who have not had ventricular fibrillation or sustained ventricular tachycardia (after the first six days following their myocardial infarction). Earlier studies of antiarrhythmic drug therapy in the post-AMI are summarized in Figure 7, but all such studies have serious deficiencies.[60] The β-adrenergic receptor blocking agents in myocardial infarction trials have shown that these drugs reduce not only total deaths but also sudden cardiac deaths.[61] Beta-adrenergic receptor blocking agents seem to have significant antiarrhythmic efficacy in both the early (see above) and late phases after an AMI, and these effects have been

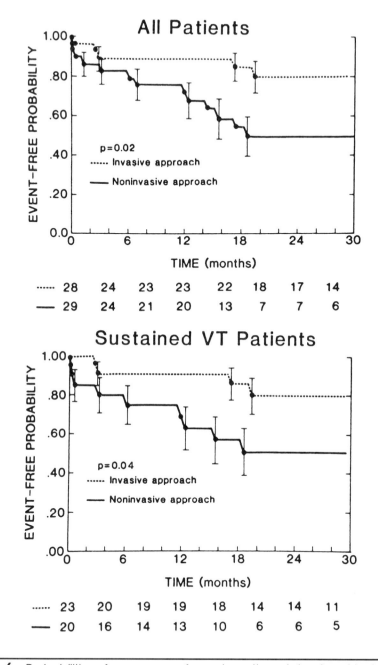

Figure 6. *Probabilities of recurrence of symptomatic sustained ventricular tachyarrhythmia (VT) among patients randomized to the invasive or noninvasive approaches From Mitchel et al,[57] with permission.*

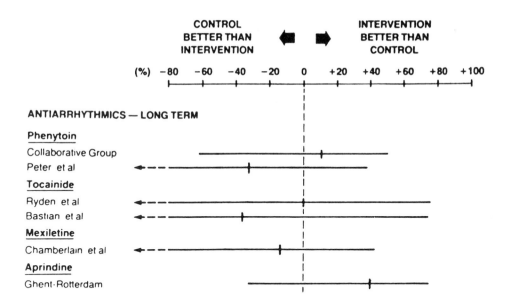

Figure 7. *Meta-analysis of percent difference in total mortality with 95% confidence interval with antiarrhythmic drug (intervention) versus placebo (control) in six randomized trials of long-term therapy following acute myocardial infarction. From Furberg,[60] with permission.*

demonstrated in large trials without any attempt to use spontaneous arrhythmia suppression as a guide to therapy or to select patients with frequent ventricular ectopy. However, the fact that frequent and complex ventricular premature beats are an independent prognostic factor for poor outcome is now well-recognized.[62] A criticism often leveled at the earlier studies of antiarrhythmic drugs in this situation is the failure to select patients who had frequent and complex ventricular premature beats on their ambulatory ECGs.

Some patients are symptomatic because of their frequent and complex ventricular ectopy, and particularly when the ventricular ectopy includes unsustained ventricular tachycardia and the symptoms include presyncope and syncope, most arrhythmia specialists recommend therapy. However, therapy in this instance is for relief of symptoms, and no evidence suggests that suppression of these arrhythmias will improve survival. The recent Cardiac Arrhythmia Suppression Trial (CAST) suggested that therapy may actually decrease survival in some patient subsets. It is important to stress, however, that patients with symptoms such as syncope and presyncope from unsustained ventricular tachycardia were not included in CAST.[19] The CAST results are therefore not applicable to patients with syncope and presyncope from ventricular arrhythmias, although caution should be exercised until a survival benefit has been shown in such patients.

Unless there is an important contraindication to its use, a β-adrenergic receptor blocking agent should be the initial drug used to relieve symptomatic ventricular arrhythmias in the post-AMI patient because of the proven efficacy of this group of drugs in reducing sudden death.[61] However, β-adrenergic receptor blocking agents are not particularly effective in eliminating or reducing complex ventricular ectopy,[63] and addition of another drug may be necessary. There are no data to suggest what that drug should be. However, several trials currently underway may clarify this issue over the next few years. The CAST results suggest the danger of using flecainide and encainide and possible other Class 1C agents in such patients. The continuation of CAST will provide further data on moricizine, a Class 1A agent. Other Class 1A agents have not been rigorously investigated, and trials of Class 1B agents are inconclusive.[60] Trials to assess the Class 3 agent, amiodarone, are soon to begin, and Class 4 agents (calcium channel blockers) have no consistent long-term benefit in patients with recent myocardial infarction.[7,8,64,65]

The CAST, which enrolled patients with asymptomatic or mildly symptomatic but frequent ventricular ectopy after a myocardial infarction, has recently produced results which will have profound effects, not only on the way in which such patients are managed, but also on the way antiarrhythmic drugs are evaluated.[19,66] A common supposition that has guided clinical thinking about arrhythmia pathophysiology in recent years has been that a fortuitous and unpredictable confluence of "triggers," "substrate," and "modulating factors" are necessary to produce an arrhythmia such as ventricular fibrillation or sustained ventricular tachycardia.[67] Elimination or marked reduction of triggers such as ventricular premature depolarizations has been thought to reduce the likelihood of ventricular fibrillation or sustained ventricular tachycardia, provided there is no counter-balancing change in the substrate or modulating factors. CAST was designed to test this "Suppression Hypothesis." Patients selected after screening entered an open-label drug titration phase in which antiarrhythmic drugs were given in sequence, and ambulatory ECG monitoring was used to assess suppression of ventricular ectopy. Three drugs — encainide, flecainide, and moricizine — were used, and the selection of these drugs was based on the Cardiac Arrhythmia Pilot Study (CAPS).[68] In CAST, patients who demonstrate suppression are then randomized to double-blind therapy with effective drug or matching placebo; patients who demonstrate partial suppression are then randomized to double-blind therapy with best drug or matching placebo; and patients who demonstrate no suppression, drug intolerance, or other problems precluding randomization are followed without antiarrhythmic drug therapy.

The recently published interim report of CAST deals only with results in the first group who were randomized to flecainide, encainide, or their matching placebos.[19] As can be seen in Figures 8 and 9, use of flecainide and encainide in those patients demonstrating suppression of ventricular ectopy was associated with increased total and arrhythmic death, and this finding was consistent across all subgroups.[19] CAST continues with the single drug, moricizine, and is enrolling even higher risk patients by lowering the ceiling on left ventricular ejection fraction from 0.55 to 0.40.

At present, antiarrhythmic drug therapy for asymptomatic or mildly symptomatic lower risk patients (ie, those with left ventricular ejection fractions > 0.40) is not prudent, and antiarrhythmic drug therapy for the asymptomatic or mildly symptomatic higher risk group (ie, those with left ventricular ejection fractions ≤ 0.40) is unproven, and in the case of encainide and flecainide, is harmful.

NEWER THERAPIES

New drugs for the management of arrhythmias are under development. The CAST results will clearly affect how such drugs are evaluated, but the final resolution of

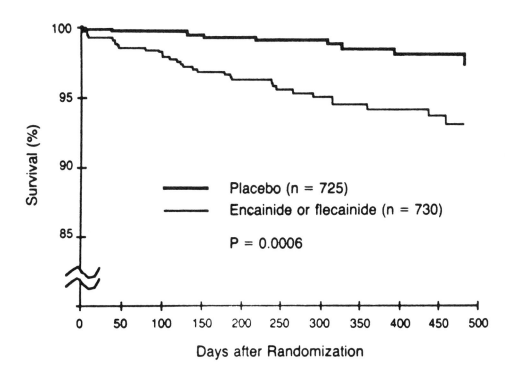

Figure 8. *Survival to sudden arrhythmic death or cardiac arrest in patients randomized to encainide/flecainide or placebo after myocardial infarction. From reference 19, with permission.*

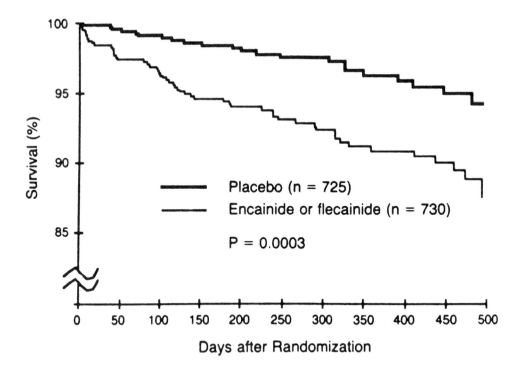

Figure 9. *Survival to death from all causes in patients randomized to encainide/flecainide or placebo after myocardial infarction. From reference 19, with permission.*

antiarrhythmic drug therapy in post-AMI patients will require more information and careful consideration of the data available thus far. Nevertheless, the weaknesses and the dangers of antiarrhythmic drug therapy are now more widely recognized than they have ever been in the past. Drug therapy in the future will require more knowledge of the basic pathogenesis of arrhythmias and of drug effects. Entirely novel approaches may be required.[69] It is clear that as new developments occur, more therapeutic options will be added to the list of alternative modalities of therapy including catheter fulguration, implantable electronic devices, and arrhythmia surgery. Presently such techniques are used only in those with the most life-threatening and drug-resistant arrhythmias.

REFERENCES

1. Wyse DG, Kellen J, Rademaker AW: Prophylactic versus selective lidocaine for early ventricular arrhythmias of myocardial infarction. J Am Coll Cardiol 1988;12:507-513.

2. O'Doherty M, Tayler DI, Quinn E, Vincent R, Chamberlain DA: Five hundred patients with myocardial infarction monitored within one hour of symptoms. Br Med J 1983;286: 1405-1408.

3. Dunn M, Alexander J, de Silva R, Hildner F: Antithrombotic therapy in atrial fibrillation. Chest 1989;95:118S-127S.

4. The MIAMI Trial Research Group: MIAMI: Metoprolol in acute myocardial infarction. Am J Cardiol 1985;56:1G-57G.

5. Gray RJ, Bateman TM, Czer LSC, Conklin CM, Matloff JM: Esmolol: A new ultrashort-acting beta-adrenergic blocking agent for rapid control of heart rate in postoperative supraventricular tachyarrhythmias. J Am Coll Cardiol 1985;5:1451-1456.

6. Gibson RS, Boden WE, Theroux P, Strauss HD, Pratt CM, Gheorghiade M, Capone RJ, Crawford MH, Schlant RC, Kleiger RE, Young PM, Schechtman K, Perryman MB, Roberts R: The Diltiazem Reinfarction Study Group: Diltiazem and reinfarction in patients with non-Q-wave myocardial infarction. Results of a double-blind, randomized, multicenter trial. New Engl J Med 1986;315:423-429.

7. The Multicenter Diltiazem Postinfarction Trial Research Group: The effect of diltiazem on mortality and reinfarction after myocardial infarction. New Engl J Med 1988;319:385-392.

8. The Danish Study Group on Verapamil in Myocardial Infarction: Effect of verapamil on mortality and major events after acute myocardial infarction (The Danish Verapamil Infarction Trial II - DAVIT II). Am J Cardiol 1990;66:779-785.

9. Haft JI, Habbab MA: Treatment of atrial arrhythmias. Effectiveness of verapamil when preceded by calcium infusion. Arch Intern Med 1986;146:1085-1089.

10. De Mots H, Rahimtoola SH, McAnulty J, Porter G: Effects of ouabain on systemic vascular resistance and myocardial oxygen consumption in patients without heart failure. Am J Cardiol 1978;41:88-93.

11. Falk RH, Knowlton AA, Bernard SA, Gotlieb NE, Battinelli NJ: Digoxin for converting recent-onset atrial fibrillation to sinus rhythm. A randomized, double-blind trial. Ann Int Med 1987;106:503-506.

12. Singh BN, Mandel WJ: Antiarrhythmic drugs: basic concepts of their actions, pharmacokinetic characteristics, and clinical applications, in Mandel WJ, (ed): *Cardiac Arrhythmias: Their Mechanism, Diagnosis and Management.* Philadelphia, JB Lippincott, 1980, pp 558-588.

13. Antman EM, Beamer AD, Cantillon C, McGowan N, Goldman L, Friedman PL: Long-term oral propafenone therapy for suppression of refractory symptomatic atrial fibrillation and atrial flutter. J Am Coll Cardiol 1988;12:1005-1011.

14. Connolly SJ, Hoffert DL: Usefulness of propafenone for recurrent paroxysmal atrial fibrillation. Am J Cardiol 1989;63:817-819.

15. Suttorp MJ, Kingma JH, Lie-A-Huen L, Mast EG: Intravenous flecainide versus verapamil for acute conversion of paroxysmal atrial fibrillation or flutter to sinus rhythm. Am J Cardiol 1989;63:693-696.

16. Pool PE: Treatment of supraventricular arrhythmias with encainide. Am J Cardiol 1986; 58:55C-57C.

17. de Paola AAV, Horowitz LN, Morganroth J, Senior S, Spielman SR, Greenspan AM, Kay HR: Influence of left ventricular dysfunction on flecainide therapy. J Am Coll Cardiol 1987;9:163-168.

18. Baker BJ, Dinh H, Kroskey D, de Soyza NDB, Murphy ML, Franciosa JA: Effect of propafenone on left ventricular ejection fraction. Am J Cardiol 1984;54:20D-22D.

19. The CAST Investigators: Preliminary report: Effect of encainide and flecainide on mortality in a randomized trial of arrhythmia suppression after myocardial infarction. New Engl J Med 1989;321:406-412.

20. Sadoway LA, Roden DM, Woosley RL: Clinical pharmacology of propafenone: Pharmacokinetics, metabolism and concentration-response relations. Am J Cardiol 1984;54:9D-12D.

21. Crijns HJ, van Gelder IC, Lie KI: Supraventricular tachycardia mimicking ventricular tachycardia during flecainide treatment. Am J Cardiol 1988;62:1303-1306.

22. Mitchell LB, Wyse DG, Duff H: The electropharmacology of sotalol in the Wolff-Parkinson-White syndrome. Circulation 1987;76:810-818.

23. Senges J, Hengfelder W, Jauernig R, Czyan E, Brachmann A, Rizos I, Cobbe S, Kubler W: Electrophysiologic testing in assessment of therapy with sotalol for sustained ventricular tachycardia. Circulation 1984;69:577-584.

24. Seipel L, Hoffmeister HM: Hemodynamic effects of antiarrhythmic drugs: negative inotropy versus influence on peripheral circulation. Am J Cardiol 1989;64:37J-40J.

25. Mitchell LB, Wyse DG, Gillis AM, Duff HJ: Electropharmacology of amiodarone therapy initiation: Time courses of onset of electrophysiologic effects and antiarrhythmic effects. Circulation 1989;80:34-42.

26. Mason JW: Amiodarone. N Engl J Med 1987;316:455-466.

27. Gallagher JJ, Smith WM, Kerr CR, Kasell J, Cook L, Reiter M, Sterba R, Harte M: Esophageal pacing: A diagnostic and therapeutic tool. Circulation 1982;65:336-341.

28. Rotman M, Wagner GS, Wallace AG: Bradyarrhythmias in acute myocardial infarction. Circulation 1972;45:703-722.

29. Matangi MF: Temporary physiologic pacing in inferior wall acute myocardial infarction with right ventricular damage. Am J Cardiol 1987;59:1207-1208.

30. Rademaker AW, Kellen J, Tam YK, Wyse DG: Character of adverse effects of prophylactic lidocaine in the coronary care unit. Clin Pharmacol Ther 1986;40:71-80.

31. Frye RL, Collins JJ, De Sanctis RW, Dodge HT, Dreifus LS, Fisch C, Gettes LS, Gillette PC, Parsonnet V, Reeves TJ, Weinberg SL: Guidelines for permanent pacemaker implantation, May 1984. A report of the joint American College of Cardiology/American Heart Association Task Force on Assessment of Cardiovascular Procedures (Subcommittee on Pacemaker Implantation). Circulation 1984;70:331A-339A.

32. Klein RC, Vera Z, Mason DT: Intraventricular conduction defects in acute myocardial infarction: Incidence, prognosis, and therapy. Am Heart J 1984;108:1007-1013.

33. Lamas GA, Muller JE, Turi ZG, Stone PH, Rutherford JD, Jaffe AS, Raabe DS, Rude RE, Mark DB, Califf RM, Gold HK, Robertson T, Passamani ER, Braunwald E, The MILIS Study Group. A simplified method to predict occurrence of complete heart block during acute myocardial infarction. Am J Cardiol 1986;57:1213-1219.

34. Nattel S, Beau S, McCarragher G: Effect of frequent ventricular ectopy on myocardial infarct size in dogs. Cardiovasc Res 1987;21:286-292.

35. Welch WJ, Smith ML, Rea RF, Bauernfeind RA, Eckberg DL: Enhancement of sympathetic nerve activity by single premature ventricular beats in humans. J Am Coll Cardiol 1989;13:69-75.

36. Hurst JW, Logue RB, Walter PF: The clinical recognition and management of coronary atherosclerotic heart disease, in Hurst JW, Logue RB, Schlant RC, Kass Wenger N (eds), *The Heart, Arteries and Veins*, 4th edition. McGraw-Hill, New York, 1978, p 1202.

37. Tofler GH, Stone PH, Muller JE, Rutherford JD, Willich SN, Gustafson NF, Poole WK, Sobel BE, Willerson JT, Robertson T, Passamani E, Braunwald E, The MILIS Study Group: Prognosis after cardiac arrest due to ventricular tachycardia or ventricular fibrillation associated with acute myocardial infarction (The MILIS Study). Am J Cardiol 1987;60:755-761.

38. Nicod P, Gilpin E, Dittrich H, Wright M, Engler R, Rittlemeyer J, Henning H, Ross J Jr: Late clinical outcome in patients with early ventricular fibrillation after myocardial infarction. J Am Coll Cardiol 1988;11:464-470.

39. Herlitz J, Hjalmarson A, Swedberg K, Waagstein F, Holmberg S, Waldenstrom J: Relationship between infarct size and incidence of severe ventricular arrhythmias in a double-blind trial with metoprolol in acute myocardial infarction. Int J Cardiol 1984;6:47-60.

40. Volpi A, Cavalli A, Franzosi MG, Maggioni A, Mauri F, Santoro E, Tognoni G, The GISSI Investigators: One-year prognosis of primary ventricular fibrillation complicating acute myocardial infarction. Am J Cardiol 1989;63:1174-1178.

41. Lie JT, Wellens HJJ, Durrer D: Characteristics and predictability of primary ventricular fibrillation. Eur J Cardiol 1974;1:379-384.

42. Volpi A, Maggioni A, Franzosi MG, Pampallona S, Mauri F, Tognoni G: In-hospital prognosis of patients with acute myocardial infarction complicated by primary ventricular fibrillation. N Engl J Med 1987;317:257-261.

43. Lie JT, Wellens HJJ, Downar E, Durrer D: Observations on patients with primary ventricular fibrillation complicating acute myocardial infarction. Circulation 1975;52:755-759.

44. El-Sherif N, Myerburg RJ, Scherlag BJ, Befeler B, Aranda JM, Castellanos A, Lazzara R: Electrocardiographic antecedents of primary ventricular fibrillation. Value of the R-on-T phenomenon in myocardial infarction. Br Heart J 1976;38:415-422.

45. Campbell RWF, Murray A, Julian DG: Ventricular arrhythmias in the first 12 hours of acute myocardial infarction. Br Heart J 1981;46:351-357.

46. Koster RW, Dunning AJ: Intramuscular lidocaine for prevention of lethal arrhythmias in the prehospitalization phase of acute myocardial infarction. N Engl J Med 1985;313:1105-1110.

47. MacMahon S, Collins R, Peto R, Koster RW, Yusef S: Effects of prophylactic lidocaine in suspected acute myocardial infarction. An overview of results from the randomized, controlled trials. JAMA 1988;260:1910-1916.

48. Salzer LB, Weinrib AB, Marina RJ, Lima JJ: A comparison of methods of lidocaine administration in patients. Clin Pharmacol Ther 1981;29:617-624.

49. Ryden L, Ariniego R, Arnman K, Herlitz J, Hjalmarson A, Holmberg S, Reyes C, Smedgard P, Svedberg K, Vedin A, Waagstein F, Waldenstrom A, Wilhelmsson C, Wedel H, Yamamoto M: A double-blind trial of metoprolol in acute myocardial infarction; effects on ventricular tachycardia. New Eng J Med 1983;308:614-618.

50. Smith WM, Gallagher JJ: "Les torsade des pointes": An unusual ventricular arrhythmia. Ann Int Med 1980;93:578-584.

51. Roden DM, Woosley RL, Primm RK: Incidence and clinical features of the quinidine-associated long QT syndrome: Implications for patient care. Am Heart J 1986;111:l088-l093.

52. Turitto G, Caref EB, Macina G, Fontaine GM, Ursell SN, El-Sherif N: Time course of ventricular arrhythmias and the signal averaged electrocardiogram in the post-infarction period: A prospective study of correlation. Br Heart J 1988;60:17-22.

53. El-Sherif N, Ursell SN, Bekheit S, Fontaine J, Turitto G, Henkin R, Caref EB: Prognostic significance of the signal-averaged ECG depends on the time of recording in the post-infarction period. Am Heart J 1989;118:256-264.

54. Berbari EJ, Lazzara R: An introduction to high-resolution ECG recordings of cardiac late potentials. Arch Int Med 1988;148:1859-1863.

55. McLaren CJ, Gersh BJ, Sugrue DD, Hammill SC, Zinmeister AR, Wood DL, Holmes DR Jr, Osborn MJ: Out-of-hospital cardiac arrest in patients without clinically significant coronary artery disease: Comparison of clinical, electrophysiological and survival characteristics with those in similar patients who have clinically significant coronary artery disease. Br Heart J 1987;58:583-591.

56. Swerdlow CD, Freedman RA, Peterson J, Clay D: Determinants of prognosis in ventricular tachyarrhythmia patients without induced sustained arrhythmias. Am Heart J 1986; 111:433-438.

57. Mitchell LB, Duff H, Manyari D, Wyse DG: A randomized clinical trial of the noninvasive and invasive approaches to drug therapy of ventricular tachycardia. New Eng J Med 1987;317:1681-1687.

58. The ESVEM Investigators: The ESVEM Trial. Electrophysiologic study versus electrocardiographic monitoring for selection of antiarrhythmic therapy of ventricular tachyarrhythmias. Circulation 1989;79:1354-1360.

59. Kavanagh KM, Wyse DG, Duff HJ, Gillis AM, Mitchell LB: Drug selection for therapy of ventricular tachycardia. How may electropharmacologic tests are appropriate? Circulation 1987;76:IV 509.

60. Furberg CD: Effect of antiarrhythmic drugs on mortality after myocardial infarction. Am J Cardiol 1983;52:32C-36C.

61. Beta-Blocker Heart Attack Trial Research Group: A randomized trial of propranolol in patients with acute myocardial infarction. I. Mortality Results. JAMA 1982;247:1707-1714.

62. Bigger JT, Fleiss JL, Kleiger R, Miller JP, Rolnitzky LM, and the Multicenter Post-Infarction Research Group. The relationships among ventricular arrhythmias, left ventricular dysfunction and mortality in the 2 years after myocardial infarction. Circulation 1984; 69:250-258.

63. Koppes GM, Beckman CH, Jones FG: Propranolol therapy for ventricular arrhythmias 2 months after acute myocardial infarction. Am J Cardiol 1980;46:322-328.

64. The Danish Study Group on Verapamil in Myocardial Infarction: Verapamil in acute myocardial infarction. Eur Heart J 1984;5:516-528.

65. Muller JE, Morrison J, Stone PH, Rude RE, Rosner B, Roberts R, Pearle DL, Turi ZG, Schneider JF, Serfas DH, Tate C, Scheiner E, Sobel BE, Hennekens CH, Braunwald E: Nifedipine therapy for patients with threatened and acute myocardial infarction: A randomized, double-blind, placebo-controlled comparison. Circulation 1984;69:740-747.

66. Garratt C, Ward DE, Camm AJ: Lessons from the cardiac arrhythmia suppression trial. Br Med J. 1989;299:805-806.

67. Myerberg RJ, Kessler KM, Bassett AL, Castellanos A: A biological approach to sudden cardiac death: Structure, function and cause. Am J Cardiol 1989;63:1512-1516.

68. The Cardiac Arrhythmia Pilot Study (CAPS) Investigators: Effects of encainide, flecainide, imipramine and moricizine on ventricular arrhythmias during the year after acute myocardial infarction: The CAPS. Am J Cardiol 1988;61:501-509.

69. Duff HJ, Mitchell LB, Kavanagh KM, Manyari DE, Gillis AM, Wyse DG: Amiloride: Antiarrhythmic and electrophysiologic actions in patients with inducible sustained ventricular tachycardia. Circulation 1989;79:1257-1263.

Chapter 16

MEDICAL THERAPY IN THE CONVALESCENT AND RECOVERY PERIODS FOLLOWING AN ACUTE MYOCARDIAL INFARCTION

Sidney Goldstein

INTRODUCTION

During the past three decades many interventions have been tested in patients who have sustained acute myocardial infarctions. This chapter considers some of these therapeutic options for patients who have survived the acute episode and who are in the convalescent or recovery phase of the illness. In these patients therapy is directed toward prevention of recurrent ischemic events including reinfarction and death. Since this therapy is often administered to asymptomatic patients, its effects are difficult to judge. In this setting, therapeutic benefit is measured as events that *do not* happen. On the other hand, these interventions may have risks and side effects which are all too evident, particularly in asymptomatic individuals.

The Coronary Drug Prevention Project was one of the first attempts to alter morbidity and mortality in patients following acute myocardial infarction (AMI) by modifying coronary risk factors.[1] This trial evaluated the role of estrogens, dextrothyroxine, clofibrate, and niacin. One of the estrogen arms of the study was dropped early on, and an aspirin arm was added. Subsequent investigations of a number of different drugs were conducted by both governments and pharmaceutical companies in the United States and Europe. These trials elucidated many aspects of the natural history of coronary artery disease following initial myocardial infarction and defined many of the predictors of subsequent events.

NATURAL HISTORY

Early studies called attention to the accelerated mortality in the first few months after myocardial infarction. Later studies, including the Beta Blocker Heart Attack Trial,[2] the Norwegian Timolol Trial,[3] and the Multicenter Rochester Postinfarction Research Group,[4] described the demographic and physiologic risk factors for subsequent events and the temporal pattern of late mortality. Age, previous history of myocardial infarction, extent of the myocardial infarction, presence of ventricular ectopy, and other factors were shown to affect the natural history of patients following a myocardial infarction.

Risk Stratification

The risk factors for recurrent myocardial infarction derive from two major areas: those factors which the patient brings to the event such as age and previous medical history, and those factors which characterize the event itself such as magnitude of the infarction and presence of associated problems including congestive heart failure and ventricular ectopy. In addition to age and medical history, race has also been thought to affect survival.[5] A number of studies suggest, however, that the increased mortality of black patients with AMI is due to a greater incidence of preexisting cardiovascular disease, especially hypertension.

The size of the myocardial infarction and the residual ejection fraction (Figure 1) clearly have an important effect on subsequent survival.[4] This effect relates both to previous myocardial injury and location of the current infarction. Patients with anterior wall infarctions have a worse prognosis than those with inferior infarctions.[2] The anterior wall is usually supplied by the left anterior descending coronary artery while the inferior surface usually receives its blood supply from the right coronary artery which affects a smaller volume of myocardium. Furthermore, the inferior surface often has a rich collateral network and is therefore usually associated with smaller myocardial infarctions. Occasionally, however, inferior myocardial infarctions may cause right ventricular damage and septal wall involvement leading to a severe degree of both right and left ventricular dysfunction.

The development of ventricular failure both acutely and during the post-infarction phase is, not unexpectedly, associated with an increased mortality. Congestive heart failure is also associated with the other major predictor of recurrent events, ventricular ectopy (Figure 2). Ventricular premature beats are highly predictive of both total and sudden death mortality[6,7] and are intimately related to the extent of left ventricular dysfunction[8] (Figure 3). The presence of either a decreased ejection fraction or of ventricular ectopy causes a doubling of the mortality rate, and when both occur together, the mortality rate is increased almost threefold.[9]

Ventricular ectopy is the most important predictor of sudden cardiac death in the post-infarction period.[6] Approximately half of all deaths following myocardial infarction occur suddenly and are presumably associated with ventricular fibrillation either as a primary event or secondary to recurrent ischemia.[10] Patients with high frequency ventricular ectopy following AMI experience a substantial increase in the incidence of

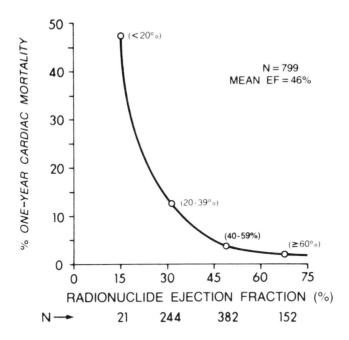

Figure 1. *Cardiac mortality rate in four categories of radionuclide ejection fraction (EF) determined before discharge. N denotes the number of patients in the total population and in each category. Of 811 patients in whom the ejection fraction was recorded, 12 were lost to follow-up during the first year after hospitalization. From reference 4, with permission.*

sudden death. Whether ventricular ectopy acts as an independent risk factor for late mortality in the post-infarction period or simply indicates the extent of left ventricular dysfunction remains to be established.

The severity of myocardial necrosis may also represent a risk factor for recurrent events. Whether the infarction is transmural or non-transmural affects both short and long-term mortality and also predicts the timing and character of recurrent events.[11] With the early use of thrombolytic therapy, blood flow can be restored and myocardial damage may be limited to "incomplete" or non-transmural infarction. Although the mortality rate at the end of one year is the same for transmural and non-transmural infarctions, early recurrent events (recurrent ischemia and early reinfarction) are more common in patients with non-transmural infarcts.

In the early post-infarction period, particularly in patients with non-transmural or incomplete infarctions, progression of infarction appears to be caused primarily by platelet aggregation and thrombogenesis. Therapeutic interventions directed against these processes using agents that alter platelet aggregation have produced substantial

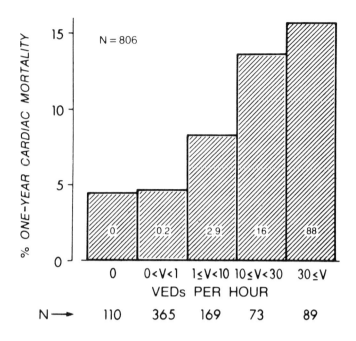

Figure 2. *Cardiac mortality rate in five categories for frequency of ventricular ectopic depolarizations (VEDs) determined by 24-hour Holter recording before discharge. N denotes the number of patients in the total population and in each category. Of 819 patients with Holter recordings, 13 were lost to follow-up during the first year after hospitalization. The numbers within each of the boxes denote the median frequency of ventricular ectopy. From reference 4, with permission.*

improvement in morbidity and mortality.[12,13] Vasomotor reactivity may also be important in this phase, and some calcium-blocking agents have shown beneficial effects in patients with non-transmural or incomplete infarctions.[14]

Medical Therapy

In the last three decades, tremendous interest has centered around secondary prevention following an initial myocardial infarction. Numerous therapeutic interventions have been proposed, including β-adrenergic blocking agents, anticoagulants, antiplatelet agents, calcium blocking agents, and most recently, drugs directed at improving left ventricular function. All of this information will be reviewed in this chapter. The use of antiarrhythmic agents is discussed in Chapter 15.

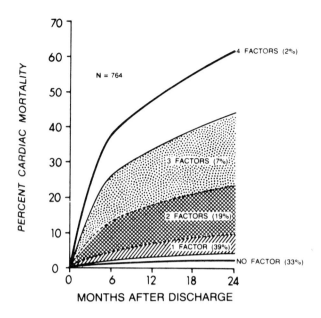

Figure 3. *Mortality curves after discharge and zones of risk, according to number of risk factors.The risk factors were New York Heart Association functional class II through IV before admission, pulmonary rales, occurrence of 10 or more ventricular ectopic depolarizations per hour, and a radionuclide ejection fraction below 0.40. The variation of risk within each zone reflects the spectrum of relative risk for individual factors as well as the range of multiplicative risks for combinations of two and three factors. The numbers in the parentheses denote the percentage of the population with the specified number of factors. See text for details. From reference 4, with permission.*

Beta-Adrenergic Blocking Agents

Observations that β-adrenergic blocking agents can modify myocardial oxygen demands by decreasing blood pressure and heart rate suggested that these agents might be useful in the treatment of patients in the post-infarction period. Early studies by Wilhelmsson et al[15] with alprenolol were followed by two major studies in the United States[2] and Scandinavia[3] which demonstrated that propranolol and timolol were effective in reducing the overall mortality rate in post-infarction patients. In the Beta Blocker Heart Attack Trial, propranolol decreased the post-infarction mortality rate from 9.8% to 7.2%, a 26% decrease over a two-year period (Figure 4). The Timolol

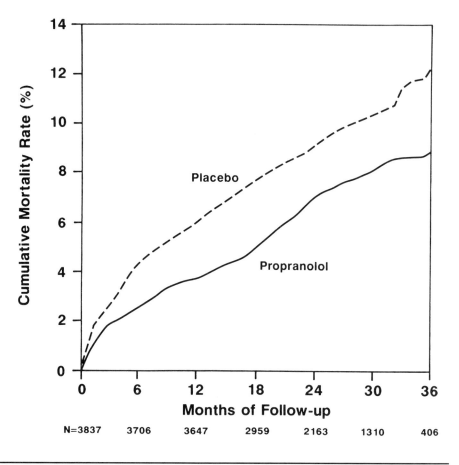

Figure 4. *Life-table cumulative mortality curves for groups receiving propranolol hydrochloride and placebo. N indicates total number of patients followed up through each time point. From reference 2, with permission.*

Trial achieved a 35% reduction in mortality over a one-year follow-up period. Both of these studies have withstood considerable scrutiny in the nearly two decades since their publication. The results seem unassailable: these drugs lead to a decrease in the mortality rate. The success of these agents in the convalescent phase of myocardial infarction led to their investigation and subsequent demonstration of additional bene-fit in the early acute phase of myocardial infarction in the ISIS-1 study.[16]

Despite almost three decades of research, the mechanism by which β-adrenergic blocking agents achieve their effect is not entirely clear. Some studies suggest that the extent of benefit depends on the relative degree of bradycardia achieved by the β-blocker employed.[17] Beta-adrenergic blocking agents also decrease the response to circulating catecholamines, which may explain their ability to decrease ventricular ectopy. Studies by Kloner et al[18] indicate that β-blockers also modify mitochondrial function and preserve myocardial cellular integrity in the setting of ischemia. These agents may also have a mechanical effect on ventricular integrity by decreasing myocardial wall stress and consequently decreasing the risk of cardiac rupture. In the ISIS-1 study,[19] the benefit of β-blockers was expressed primarily as a decrease in the occurrence of cardiac rupture and ventricular fibrillation without an effect on left ventricular function.

Other clinical studies using a variety of indirect measurements indicate that β-blockers limit the extent of myocardial damage when administered in the hyperacute phase.[20] Animal studies have shown that β-adrenergic blocking agents increase the ventricular fibrillation threshold in ischemic and non-ischemic myocardium,[21] thus explaining the observation that these agents decrease ventricular ectopy and ventricular fibrillation in both the hyperacute and late phases of myocardial infarction.[22,23]

Reductions in the occurrence of early morning acute myocardial infarctions and sudden cardiac deaths with β-blocker therapy suggested that these drugs might alter circadian phenomena.[24,25] The circadian increase in early morning blood pressure and pulse rate is known to be associated with increased circulating catecholamine levels, increase in platelet aggregation,[26] and decrease in thrombolytic activity.[27] Beta-adrenergic blocking agents may affect one or all of these phenomena. The effect of β-blockers on platelet aggregation and hemostasis is controversial, however.[28,29] Catecholamine levels themselves are not affected by β-blockers; rather, these agents probably block β-adrenergic receptors in the vascular bed, modulating the circadian increase in blood pressure and pulse rate in this manner. Reduction of symptomatic and asymptomatic myocardial ischemia[30] and of the early morning increase in ventricular ectopy[31] by β-blockers may be mediated through their effect on these cardiac β-adrenergic receptors.

Certain subgroups of patients derive greater benefit in terms of mortality reduction from β-blockers than others. Older patients[32] and those with more extensive left ventricular dysfunction with mild to moderate heart failure and with frequent ventricular arrhythmias appear to have the greatest relative and absolute benefit.[33,34] Those patients who begin β-blocker therapy earlier also derive greater benefit.[35] In a retrospective analysis of patients in the Beta Blocker Heart Attack Trial, those with a history of heart failure achieved the greatest reduction of both total mortality and sudden death mortality rates[33] (Figure 5). In a high risk population studied by Hansteen et al, patients with left ventricular dysfunction and ventricular arrhythmias and ventricular fibrillation experienced a significant decrease in sudden cardiac death if treated with propranolol.[36]

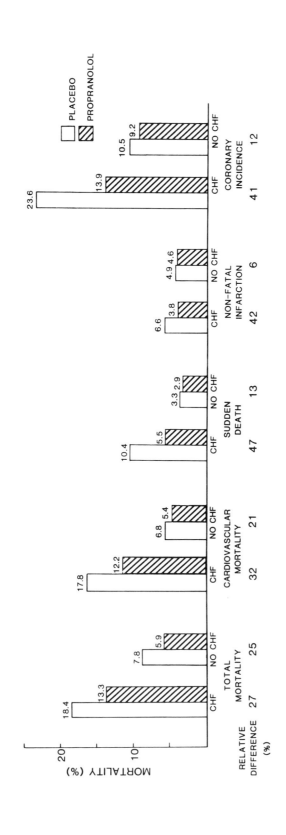

Figure 5. Effect of propranolol on morbidity and mortality related to the presence or absence of congestive heart failure (CHF). From Chadda et al,[33] with permission.

Beta-blocker therapy also lowers the mortality rate in other patients at high risk, particularly cigarette smokers and former smokers.[37] Although some inconsistencies have been described, Jafri et al[37] observed that propranolol had a unique and profound salutary effect on mortality rate in the post-infarction period in both current smokers and former smokers.

The doses of β-blockers used in the clinical trials described above have been variable. In general, the dose of a β-blocker should be adjusted to achieve the desired decrease in heart rate and blood pressure. This usually requires 160 to 240 mg of propranolol, 10 to 20 mg of timolol, and 100 mg daily of either metoprolol or atenolol. Not all β-blockers are beneficial in reducing mortality in the post-infarction period. Those agents which possess sympathomimetic activity, such as oxprenolol[38] and pindolol,[39] are not useful in this setting. Although contraindicated in patients with chronic lung disease, asthma, and severe left ventricular dysfunction, β-blockers are well tolerated by most other patients. In placebo-controlled studies, patients receiving β-blockers report a slightly higher incidence of fatigue, cold extremities, and reduced sexual activity compared with patients receiving placebos.[2]

Calcium Channel Blockers

Although theoretically attractive as agents for secondary prevention following an AMI, calcium channel blockers have failed to demonstrate any improvement in survival in a multitude of studies. Currently available calcium blocking agents, often considered as a homogeneous group of drugs, actually have varying effects on blood pressure, heart rate, AV conduction, vasomotor tone, and myocardial contractility. Nifedipine accelerates heart rate; verapamil produces some bradycardia and delay in atrioventricular conduction; and diltiazem only decreases atrioventricular conduction. In general, however, drugs of this class decrease myocardial oxygen demand by lowering blood pressure and reducing contractility. They also cause a significant degree of coronary arterial dilatation. All of these drugs are thought to stabilize the movement of intracellular calcium in the setting of ischemia, thereby improving myocardial metabolism.

All three currently available calcium channel blockers — nifedipine, verapamil, and diltiazem — have undergone extensive trials for secondary prevention of AMI. None has demonstrated any benefit. Nifedipine has been studied in Europe and in the United States in patients with unstable angina and with AMI.[40,41] When compared with placebo, nifedipine treatment either produced no benefit or an adverse effect. The failure of nifedipine to prevent subsequent ischemic events has been attributed to its acceleration of heart rate and resultant instability of blood pressure. The initial study of verapamil, although demonstrating an overall lack of efficacy, suggested a benefit after 22 days of therapy.[42] A second study[43] was therefore carried out in which 360 mg of verapamil daily was administered beginning on the second week after an AMI. The mortality was 11.1% in the verapamil group and 13.8% in the control group (p = 0.11). When analyzed for the first major event, either death or first reinfarction, patients in the verapamil group had an incidence of 18.0% and the control group 21.6% (p = 0.03). In patients without heart failure, a beneficial effect on mortality was observed in the verapamil group compared to the control group. In contrast, in patients with heart failure, there was no observed benefit. In a recent trial,[44] diltiazem actually had an adverse effect on patients with low ejection fractions and a previous history of heart failure. However, when diltiazem was administered to patients with non-transmural myocardial infarction, a therapeutic benefit was observed.[14] In this placebo-controlled trial, patients who received diltiazem following a non-transmural myocardial infarction had a lower incidence of recurrent angina and reinfarction. Even in this trial, however, a favorable mortality trend was not observed. Although calcium channel blockers are effective as primary or adjunctive therapy for angina pectoris, they are ineffective for routine secondary prevention. It is appropriate to administer calcium channel blockers for post-myocardial infarction angina in conjunction with β-blockers when β-blocker therapy alone has failed, or to patients in whom β-blockers are contraindicated. Routine prophylactic use of calcium channel blockers, however, cannot be recommended at this time, especially in patients with left ventricular dysfunction.

Anticoagulants

The use of anticoagulants has been advocated for almost 40 years. Initially they were used in an attempt to decrease the occurrence of thromboembolism in patients with myocardial infarction in an era when patients were hospitalized at bed rest for almost five weeks.[45] Over the years, however, the evidence for efficacy of anticoagulants has not been persuasive, and their use has not achieved widespread acceptance. However, in 1977 Chalmers et al examined the pooled data of all randomized trials with anticoagulants and concluded that this treatment did reduce mortality rate.[46] Investigators in Norway recently completed a placebo-controlled study of warfarin in 1214 survivors of an AMI and reported a 24% decrease in mortality over a 37-month period.[47] In addition, they observed a 61% decrease in cerebrovascular events.

Anticoagulant therapy has become more appealing with the recognition that thrombosis is an important cause of AMI. Consequently, anticoagulants have been used in combination with thrombolytic therapy for up to three months following an AMI.[48] The specific role of anticoagulant therapy in thrombolytic therapy studies has not been analyzed. Long-term anticoagulation has also been advocated in the treatment of patients with large anterior myocardial infarctions with and without ventricular mural thrombi in order to prevent systemic emboli.[49,50] Neither one of these therapeutic hypotheses has been tested in randomized trials.

372

Antiplatelet Agents

The suggestion that aspirin might have a beneficial effect on survival after a myocardial infarction developed from the coronary drug project in which patients treated with aspirin showed a trend toward improved survival.[51] In the subsequent Aspirin Myocardial Infarction Study,[52] aspirin was administered to patients who had experienced a myocardial infarction within the previous five years. Although no effect on mortality was demonstrated, a significant decrease occurred in the rate of reinfarction in the aspirin-treated patients, a fact that was not fully appreciated at the time.

Recently, interest in aspirin therapy has been stimulated by the emphasis on thrombogenesis as a precipitating event in acute ischemic syndromes. Aspirin has been used in combination with thrombolytic therapy, particularly in the ISIS-2 study which evaluated streptokinase in combination with aspirin.[53] In that study, acute and continued use of aspirin alone decreased the mortality rate by 20%. The combination of aspirin and streptokinase resulted in a 42% decrease in early (five-week) mortality.

A review of all antiplatelet studies was carried out by the Antiplatelet Trialists' Collaborative Group.[54] They calculated that aspirin treatment reduced vascular deaths by approximately 13% and resulted in a 31% decrease in non-fatal myocardial infarction. The latter observation was consistent with the Aspirin and Myocardial Infarction Study. The use of aspirin in unstable angina also reduces mortality and recurrent ischemic attacks.[12,13]

Studies examining the combination of aspirin and dipyridamole have failed to demonstrate any additional benefit.[55] Dipyridamole therapy alone also appears to have little or no role in the treatment of ischemic heart disease at the present time. Other antiplatelet agents have also been studied. Sulfinpyrazone was tested in post myocardial infarction patients and although clouded by confused analysis, did not appear to have a beneficial effect on mortality rate.[56] More recently, ticlopidine, another antiplatelet agent, has been under study.[57] At present, the development of monoclonal antibodies directed against surface active receptors on platelets is under investigation.[58]

The contrasting degrees of beneficial effect of aspirin in the hyperacute phase of ischemia compared to the late convalescent phase suggest that there are perhaps two different phases of coronary arterial occlusion. One, dominated by active thrombogenesis, comprises the hyperacute phase; the other, during the late convalescent phase, results from progressive narrowing of the vascular intima and subintimal layers. As observed with aspirin, other antiplatelet agents under development may be effective in this early phase of unstable angina and AMI.

Primary preventive therapy with low dose aspirin was examined in the Physicians' Health Study.[59] Over 20,000 physicians without previous heart disease were studied. No benefit in mortality was demonstrated, but a decrease in non-fatal infarction occurred in the aspirin-treated group. A similar but somewhat smaller study in

England failed to demonstrate any benefit for aspirin therapy and suggested that the incidence of stroke actually increased in the aspirin-treated patients.[60] Unfortunately, widespread publicity of the results of the Physicians' Health Study has led to a misplaced enthusiasm for the routine use of low dose aspirin in all males.

Angiotensin Converting Enzyme Inhibitors

Angiotensin converting enzyme inhibitors are the most recent entry into the post-infarction therapeutic regimen. Advocated initially for the treatment of patients with left ventricular dysfunction, they are currently under investigation for routine administration after an AMI. These agents have a number of unique effects, the most significant of which are their ability to decrease peripheral resistance and to modify the pattern of ventricular contractility. Studies by Sharp et al[61] and Pfeffer et al[62] have demonstrated that captopril led to improved left ventricular function after acute infarction, when compared to diuretics or placebo (Figure 6). In addition, angiotensin converting enzyme inhibitors have been used very effectively as adjunctive therapy in

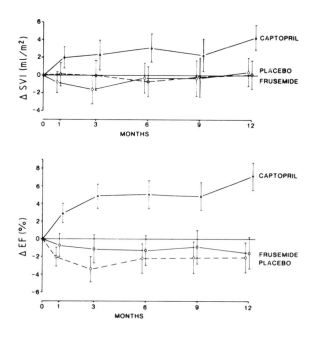

Figure 6. *Effect of captopril therapy on stroke volume index and ejection fraction in post-myocardial infarction patients. Values shown are least squares means with upper and lower least significant difference intervals (p < 0.05). From Sharpe et al,[61] with permission.*

patients with advanced left ventricular dysfunction associated with AMI.[63] When enalapril was combined with digitalis, diuretics and a coronary dilator, a substantial decrease in total mortality at six months and one year (Figure 7) was observed. Animal studies[64] and some clinical investigations[65] indicate that this class of drugs may have additional antifibrillatory and antiarrhythmic effects in acute ischemia and chronic heart failure.

Digitalis

Digitalis has also been used in post-infarction patients in the treatment of left ventricular dysfunction, although its use has been controversial. Studies by Moss et al[66] suggest that digitalis given in the first week of myocardial infarction is associated with an increased mortality rate, particularly in those patients with ventricular premature contractions. A retrospective study of the Beta Blocker Heart Attack Trial[67] and the Coronary Artery Surgical Study[68] failed to show any adverse effect in patients who were, by the design of those studies, started on digoxin therapy two to three weeks after their infarction. Analysis of these two studies failed to incriminate digoxin as a cause of post-myocardial infarction mortality.

SUMMARY

Beta-adrenergic blocking agents and aspirin appear to be the only well-studied agents with the ability to reduce both morbidity and mortality following a myocardial infarction. Calcium channel blockers may have some beneficial effects in selected patients in whom left ventricular function remains intact after a myocardial infarct. Although results with anticoagulants appear promising, further information is required. Angiotensin converting enzyme inhibitors also appear to hold promise, but again, more data will be necessary in order to evaluate the role of these agents.

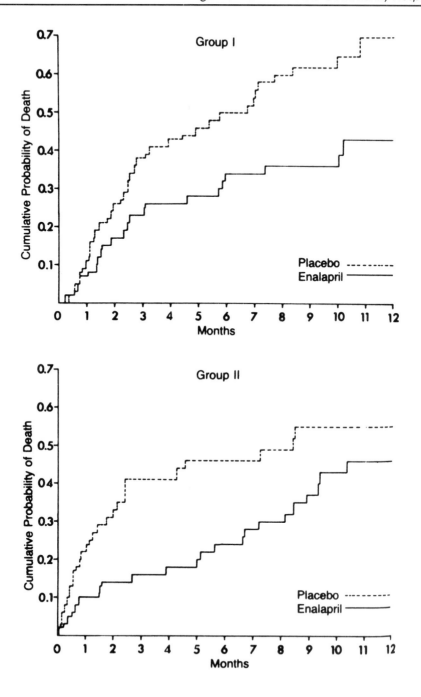

Figure 7. *Cumulative probability of death in patients not taking vasodilators (Group 1) and in patients taking vasodilators (Group 2) at the time of random assignment. From reference 63, with permission.*

REFERENCES

1. The Coronary Drug Project Research Group: The Coronary Drug Project: initial findings leading to modifications of its research protocol. JAMA 1970;214:1303-1306.

2. Beta Blocker Heart Attack Trial Research Group: A randomized trial of propranolol in patients with acute myocardial infarction. 1. Mortality results. JAMA 1982;247:1707-1714.

3. The Norwegian Multicenter Study Group: Timolol-induced reduction in mortality and reinfarction in patients surviving acute myocardial infarction. N Engl J Med 1981;304:801-807.

4. The Multicenter Postinfarction Research Group: Risk stratification and survival after myocardial infarction. N Engl J Med 1983;309:331-336.

5. Haywood LJ, for the BHAT Research Group: Coronary heart disease mortality/morbidity and risk in blacks. I. Clinical manifestation and diagnostic criteria: The experience of the Beta-Blocker Heart Attack Trial. Am Heart J 1984;108:787-793.

6. Ruberman W, Weinblatt E, Goldberg JD, et al: Ventricular premature beats and mortality after myocardial infarction. N Engl J Med 1977;297:750-757.

7. Davis HT, DeCamilla J, Bayer LW, et al: Survivorship patterns in the posthospital phase of myocardial infarction. Circulation 1979;60:1252-1258.

8. Schulze RA Jr, Strauss HW, Pitt B: Sudden death in the year following myocardial infarction: relation to ventricular premature contractions in the late hospital phase and left ventricular ejection fraction. Am J Med 1977;62:191-199.

9. Bigger JT Jr, Fleiss JL, Kleiger R, et al, for the Multicenter Post-Infarction Research Group: The relationships among ventricular arrhythmias, left ventricular dysfunction and mortality in the 2 years after myocardial infarction. Circulation 1984;69:250-258.

10. Goldstein S, Friedman L, Hutchinson R, et al, and the Aspirin Myocardial Infarction Study Research Group: Timing, mechanism and clinical setting of witnessed deaths in postmyocardial infarction patients. J Am Coll Cardiol 1984;3:1111-1117.

11. Kao W, Khaja F, Goldstein S, et al: Cardiac event rate after non-Q-wave acute myocardial infarction and the significance of its anterior location. Am J Cardiol 1989;64:1236-1242.

12. Lewis HD, Davis JW, Archibald DG, et al: Protective effects of aspirin against acute myocardial infarction and death in men with unstable angina. N Engl J Med 1983;309:396-403.

13. Cairns JA, Gent M, Singer J, et al: Aspirin, sulfinpyrazone, or both in unstable angina. N Engl J Med 1985;313:1369-1375.

14. Gibson RS, Boden WE, Therous P, et al: Diltiazem and reinfarction in patients with non Q wave MI. N Engl J Med 1986;315:423-429.

15. Wilhelmsson C, Vedin J, Wilhelmsen L: Reduction of sudden deaths after myocardial infarction by treatment with alprenolol: preliminary results. Lancet 1974;2:1157-1159.

16. ISIS-1 Collaborative Group: A randomized trial of intravenous atenolol among 16,027 cases of suspected acute myocardial infarction. Lancet 1986;2:57-66.

17. Gundersen T, Grottum P, Pederson T, et al: Effect of timolol on mortality and reinfarction after acute myocardial infarction: Prognostic importance of heart rate at rest. Am J Cardiol 1986;58:20-24.

18. Kloner RA, Fishbein MC, Braunwald E, et al: Effect of propranolol on mitochondrial morphology during acute myocardial ischemia. Am J Cardiol 1978;41:880-886.

19. ISIS-1 Collaborative Group: Mechanisms for the early mortality reduction produced by beta-blockade started early in acute myocardial infarction. Lancet 1988;2:921-923.

20. Peter T, Norris RM, Clarke ED, et al: Reduction of enzyme levels by propranolol after acute myocardial infarction. Circulation 1978;57:1091-1095.

21. Anderson JL, Roder HE, Green LS: Comparative effects of beta-adrenergic blocking drugs on experimental ventricular fibrillation threshold. Am J Cardiol 1983;51:1196-1202.

22. Friedman LM, Byington RP, Capone RJ, et al, for the Beta-Blocker Heart Attack Trial Research Group: Effect of propranolol in patients with myocardial infarction and ventricular arrhythmia. J Am Coll Cardiol 1986;7:1-8.

23. Ryden L, Ariniego R, Arnman K, et al: A double-blind trial of metoprolol in acute myocardial infarction: effects on ventricular tachyarrhythmias. N Engl J Med 1983;308:614-618.

24. Muller JE, Stone PH, Turi ZG, et al: Circadian variation in the frequency of onset of acute myocardial infarction. N Engl J Med 1985;313:1315-1322.

25. Peters RW, Muller JE, Goldstein S, et al, for the Beta-Blocker Heart Attack Trial Study Group: Propranolol and the morning increase in the frequency of sudden cardiac death (BHAT Study). Am J Cardiol 1989;63:1518-1520.

26. Tofler GH, Brezinski D, Schafer AI, et al: Concurrent morning increase in platelet aggregability and the risk of myocardial infarction and sudden cardiac death. N Engl J Med 1987;316:1514-1518.

27. Angleton P, Chandler WL, Schmer G: Diurnal variation of tissue-type plasminogen activator and its rapid inhibitor (PAI-1). Circulation 1988;79:101-106.

28. Weksler BB, Gillich M, Pink J: Effect of propranolol on platelet function. Blood 1977;49:185-196.

29. Green D, Rossi EC, Haring O: The Beta Blocker Heart Attack Trial: Studies of Platelets and Factor VIII. Thromb Res 1982;28:261-267.

30. Willich SN, Pohjola-Sintonen S, Bhatia SJS, et al: Suppression of silent ischemia by metoprolol without alteration of morning increase of platelet aggregability in patients with stable coronary artery disease. Circulation 1989;79:557-565.

31. Lichstein E, Morganroth J, Harrist R, et al, for the Beta Blocker Heart Attack Trial Study Group: Effect of propranolol on ventricular arrhythmia: The Beta-Blocker Heart Attack Trial Experience. Circulation 1983;67:I-5-I-10.

32. Gundersen T, Abrahamsen AM, Kjekshus J, et al, for the Norwegian Multicentre Study Group: Timolol-related reduction in mortality and reinfarction in patients ages 65-75 years surviving acute myocardial infarction. Circulation 1982;66:1179-1184.

33. Chadda K, Goldstein S, Byington R, et al: Effect of propranolol after acute myocardial infarction in patients with congestive heart failure. Circulation 1986;73:503-510.

34. Furberg CD, Hawkins CM, Lichstein E, for the Beta-Blocker Heart Attack Trial Study Group: Effect of propranolol in postinfarction patients with mechanical or electrical complications. Circulation 1984;69:761-765.

35. Baber NS, Lewis JA: Beta-adrenoceptor blockade and myocardial infarction: when should treatment start and for how long should it continue? Circulation 1983;67:I-71-I-75.

36. Hansteen V, Moinichen E, Lorentsen E, et al: One year's treatment with propranolol after myocardial infarction: preliminary report of Norwegian Multicenter Trial. Br Med J 1982;284:155-159.

37. Jafri SM, Tilley BC, Peters R, et al: Effects of cigarette smoking and propranolol in survivors of acute myocardial infarction. Am J Cardiol (in press).

38. The European Infarction Study Group: A secondary prevention study with slow release oxprenolol after myocardial infarction: morbidity and mortality. Eur Heart J 1984;5:189-202.

39. Australian and Swedish Pindolol Study Group: The effect of pindolol on the two years mortality after complicated myocardial infarction. Eur Heart J 1983;4:367-375.

40. The Holland Interuniversity Nifedipine/Metoprolol Trial (HINT) Research Group: Early treatment of unstable angina in the coronary care unit: A randomised, double-blind, placebo controlled comparison of recurrent ischaemia in patients treated with nifedipine or metoprolol or both. Br Heart J 1986;56:400-413.

41. Secondary Prevention Reinfarction Nifedipine Trial (SPRINT): A randomized intervention trial of nifedipine in patients with acute myocardial infarction. Eur Heart J 1988;9:354-364.

42. The Danish Study Group on Verapamil in Myocardial Infarction: Verapamil in acute myocardial infarction. Eur Heart J 1984;5:518-528.

43. The Danish Study Group on Verapamil in Myocardial Infarction: Effect of verapamil on mortality and major events after acute myocardial infarction (The Danish Verapamil Infarction Trial II - DAVIT II). Am J Cardiol 1990;66:779-785.

44. Multicenter Diltiazem Post-infarction Research Group: The effect of diltiazem on mortality and reinfarction after acute myocardial infarction. N Engl J Med 1988;319:385-392.

45. Wright IS, Marple CD, Beck DF: Report of the Committee for the Evaluation of Anticoagulants in the Treatment of Coronary Thrombosis with Myocardial Infarction (A Progress Report on the Statistical Analysis of the First 800 Cases Studied by this Committee). Am Heart J 1948;36:801-815.

46. Chalmers TC, Matta RJ, Smith H Jr, et al: Evidence favoring the use of anticoagulants in the hospital phase of acute myocardial infarction. N Engl J Med 1977;297:1091-1094.

47. Smith P, Arnesen H: Oral anticoagulants reduce mortality, reinfarction and cerebrovascular events after myocardial infarction — Waris Study. N Engl J Med 1990;323:147-151.

48. AIMS Trial Study Group: Effect of intravenous APSAC on mortality after acute myocardial infarction: preliminary report of a placebo-controlled clinical trial. Lancet 1988;1:545-549.

49. Jugdutt BI, Sivaram CA, Wortman C, et al: Prospective two-dimensional echocardiographic evaluation of left ventricular thrombus and embolism after acute myocardial infarction. J Am Coll Cardiol 1989;13:554-564.

50. Funke Kupper AJ, Verheugt FWA, Peels CH, et al: Left ventricular thrombus incidence and behavior studied by serial two-dimensional echocardiography in acute anterior myocardial infarction: left ventricular wall motion, systemic embolism and oral anticoagulation. J Am Coll Cardiol 1989;13:1514-1520.

51. The Coronary Drug Project Research Group: Aspirin in coronary heart disease. J Chronic Dis 1976;29:625-642.

52. Aspirin Myocardial Infarction Study Research Group: A randomized, controlled trial of aspirin in persons recovered from myocardial infarction. JAMA 1980;243:661-669.

53. ISIS-2 Collaborative Group: Randomized trial of IV streptokinase, oral aspirin, both, or neither among 17,187 cases of suspected acute myocardial infarction. Lancet 1988;2: 349-360.

54. Antiplatelet Trialists' Collaboration: Secondary prevention of vascular disease by prolonged antiplatelet treatment. Br Med J 1988;296:320-331.

55. Persantine-Aspirin Reinfarction Study Research Group: Persantine and aspirin in coronary heart disease. Circulation 1980;62:449-461.

56. Anturane Reinfarction Trial Research Group: Sulfinpyrazone in the prevention of sudden death after myocardial infarction. N Engl J Med 1980;302:250-256.

57. Berglund U, Lassvik C, Wallentin L: Effects of the platelet inhibitor ticlopidine on exercise tolerance in stable angina pectoris. Eur Heart J 1987;8:25-30.

58. Coller BS, Folts JD, Smith SR, et al: Abolition of in vivo platelet thrombus formation in primates with monoclonal antibodies to the platelet GPIIb/IIIa receptor. Circulation 1989;80:1766-1774.

59. Steering Committee of the Physicians' Health Study Research Group: Final report on the aspirin component of the ongoing Physicians' Health Study. N Engl J Med 1989;321:129-135.

60. Peto R, Gray R, Collins R, et al: Randomised trial of prophylactic daily aspirin in British male doctors. Br Med J 1988;296:13-16.

61. Sharpe N, Murphy J, Smith H, et al: Treatment of patients with symptomless left ventricular dysfunction after myocardial infarction. Lancet 1988;1:255-259.

62. Pfeffer MA, Lamas GA, Vaughn DE, et al: Effect of captopril on progressive ventricular dilatation after anterior myocardial infarction. N Engl J Med 1988;319:80-86.

63. The CONSENSUS Trial Study Group: Effects of enalapril on mortality in severe congestive heart failure. N Engl J Med 1987;316:1429-1435.

64. Linz W, Scholkens BA, Han YF: Beneficial effects of the converting enzyme inhibitor, ramipril, in ischemic rat hearts. J Cardiovasc Pharmacol 1986;8:S91-S99.

65. Cleland JGF, Dargie HJ, Hodsman GP, et al: Captopril in heart failure: a double blind controlled trial. Br Heart J 1984;52:530-535.

66. Moss AJ, Davis HT, Conard DL, et al: Digitalis-associated cardiac mortality after myocardial infarction. Circulation 1981;64:1150-1156.

67. Byington R, Goldstein S, for the BHAT Research Group: Association of digitalis therapy with mortality in survivors of acute myocardial infarction: observations in the Beta-Blocker Heart Attack Trial. J Am Coll Cardiol 1985;6:976-982.

68. Ryan TJ, Bailey KR, McCabe CH, et al: The effect of digitalis on survival in high-risk patients with coronary artery disease. The Coronary Artery Surgery Study. Circulation 1981;64(suppl IV):IV-83-IV-87.

Chapter 17

DIETARY AND LIFESTYLE INTERVENTIONS AFTER ACUTE MYOCARDIAL INFARCTION

Frank G. Yanowitz

"...if a physician is to deserve the exalted stature granted by society, he or she must have as a major concern, regardless of the degree of specialization or even subspecialization, the adoption by all of his or her patients of a lifestyle likely to minimize the development or progression, or both, of degenerative diseases that will lead to premature morbidity or mortality."

Henry D. McIntosh, M.D.[1]

INTRODUCTION

In an era of interventional cardiology which increasingly relies on such technologic feats as "crackers, breakers, stretchers, drillers, scrapers, shavers, burners, welders, and melters,"[2] there is a tendency to lose sight of the comprehensive rehabilitation needs of the post-myocardial infarction patient. To be sure, the "future treatment of atherosclerotic coronary artery disease"[2] will involve the use of these interventional devices to remove or remodel atherosclerotic plaque in an effort to restore myocardial blood flow. Nevertheless, the long-term prognosis in these patients will ultimately be determined by the success, if any, of those measures directed towards slowing, halting, or reversing the progression of coronary atherosclerosis.

This chapter addresses dietary and lifestyle interventions for patients recovering from acute myocardial infarction (AMI) or other coronary disease events. These interventions are directed towards achieving three long term therapeutic objectives: 1) restoration of function; 2) restoration of confidence; and 3) prevention of coronary disease recurrences.

Restoration of function and confidence are the usual end points of formal cardiac rehabilitation programs. Although there are many advantages of participating in hospital-based or free-standing cardiac rehabilitation programs, many patients do not have the opportunity to join such programs. The primary focus of this chapter, therefore, is on rehabilitation and prevention strategies applicable to practicing primary care physicians who often play pivotal roles in the long term management of coronary disease patients.

"Secondary prevention" is a term used in reference to programs designed to prevent recurrences of coronary disease complications in patients with known disease. In many respects these programs are a continuation of strategies found to be effective or useful in the primary prevention of coronary disease: namely interventions dealing with smoking cessation, hyperlipidemia, hypertension, exercise and stress management. Studies published in the last two decades have shown that the progression of coronary atherosclerosis as well as the subsequent morbidity and mortality from coronary disease are strongly determined by levels of established coronary risk factors.[3-6] Furthermore, interventions which favorably alter the coronary risk profile have been associated with a reduction of coronary morbidity and mortality and, in some instances, with a slowing, halting, or reversal of atherosclerotic lesions.[7-10] For these reasons it is imperative for physicians managing patients with coronary disease to emphasize dietary and lifestyle changes which are known to reduce risk, enhance function and improve quality of life.

Three general intervention programs are discussed in this chapter: 1) smoking cessation; 2) dietary intervention; and 3) exercise training. The emphasis is on clinical strategies that can be recommended or offered by primary care physicians in an office practice and subsequently carried out by patients at home or in an environment of their choice. Several recent reviews deal with more formal cardiac rehabilitation programs.[11-15]

SMOKING CESSATION

For the coronary disease patient who smokes, there is no greater secondary prevention priority than smoking cessation. Unfortunately, this is often the most difficult and least successful lifestyle change to implement. The continuation of cigarette smoking after myocardial infarction is often the single most important determinant of subsequent mortality.[16-18] Smoking may also precipitate ischemic episodes, both symptomatic and silent,[19,20] and attenuate the effects of antianginal medications.[21] Cessation of smoking after myocardial infarction, on the other hand, can be associated with up to 50% reductions in sudden death and fatal reinfarction.[22,23] Physicians caring for these patients, therefore, must be challenged to develop effective smoking cessation programs that can be administered in their office environment. The following discussion focuses on general strategies applicable to all smoking interventions and on those more intensive strategies often needed for the hard-core, nicotine-dependent smokers.

Office-based Smoking Cessation Strategies

Much has been written to encourage physicians to help their patients quit smoking.[24-27] In many respects post-myocardial infarction patients are an ideal group to work with since they are usually quite concerned about their own health status and motivated to consider appropriate lifestyle changes. Unfortunately many physicians are pessimistic about their ability to achieve long-term success in changing smoking behaviors.[28] This attitude often interferes with the ability to provide a comprehensive smoking cessation program; thus, a vicious circle of half-hearted efforts leading to more pessimism is likely to ensue.

In an attempt to overcome this pessimistic and often lethargic attitude among physicians, more structured smoking cessation programs have been developed, along with an intense effort by many national medical organizations to educate physicians in the use of these programs. Table 1 lists some general elements of effective smoking cessation programs. It is clear from a review of the literature that no one particular intervention strategy is any more effective than others, and what works for some smokers will not necessarily work for others. The most important component of successful interventions, however, is the combination of face-to-face advice by physicians and other clinic staff members with repeated follow-up visits over the longest possible duration of follow-up.[29]

Office and staff organization

Developing an office-based smoking intervention program requires several months of planning in order to organize the clinic environment optimally and enlist the support of the clinic staff.[26] The office should be a smoke-free environment in order to reinforce the antismoking message. Staff involvement will help facilitate changes that

Table 1. *Tactics of an effective smoking cessation program*

1. Involve office staff
2. Identify all smokers
3. Provide a strong smoking cessation message
4. Set a firm quit date
5. Provide self-help literature
6. Anticipate relapse
7. Provide for adequate follow-up
8. Provide list of smoking cessation resources

have to be made in record keeping and will ensure smooth day-to-day operation of the program once it gets underway.

Self-help patient education materials should be made available in the waiting room along with displays of appropriate antismoking posters. These materials may be obtained from a variety of local and national sources including the National Cancer Institute,[30] the American Academy of Family Physicians,[31] the American Cancer Society,[32] the American Lung Association,[33,34] and the American Heart Association and its affiliates. In addition a number of high-quality antismoking kits have been developed to help physicians implement their smoking cessation programs.[35-37]

Identification and classification of smokers

All smokers in an office practice should be identified and the "problem" placed on the problem list in the patient's chart. A smoking history includes the duration and amount of smoking (pack-years), the brand smoked, reasons for success or failure of previous attempts to quit, the longest period of abstinence, and withdrawal symptoms, if any. Other family members and significant others who smoke should also be identified and encouraged to participate in the smoking cessation program.

Because many heavy smokers become physically addicted to nicotine, intense withdrawal symptoms may occur within a day after quitting. These symptoms, which include irritability, anxiety, restlessness, difficulty concentrating, mouth sores, constipation, chest tightness and cough, present a serious obstacle to becoming a non-smoker. Table 2 illustrates a simple self-administered questionnaire developed by Fagerstrom[38] that helps identify patients who are nicotine-dependent. A score greater than 7 indicates "high nicotine dependence;" 4-7 indicates "medium dependence;" and 0-3 indicates "low dependence." Patients identified as nicotine-dependent can be prepared to anticipate their withdrawal symptoms and perhaps minimize them through the use of bronchodilators, high fiber diets, and counseling.[24]

A strong antismoking message

For many smokers a brief but strongly worded antismoking message from their personal physician describing the dangers of smoking and the benefits of quitting is sufficient to achieve long term abstinence. Six-month quit rates of up to 20% have been reported in trials of brief counseling carried out in the office setting.[24] Even more impressive, however, is the evidence that over 60% of smokers recovering from AMI will quit after receiving brief cessation advice and remain abstinent for one year or longer.[39] While delivering the antismoking message it is also important to emphasize other cardiac risk factor data since the continuation of smoking is likely to worsen the impact of these risk factors on the atherosclerotic process.

384

Table 2. *The Fagerstrom Nicotine Addiction Questionnaire*

Question	0 Points	1 Point	2 Points	Score
1. How soon after you wake up do you smoke your first cigarette?	After 30 min	Before 30 min	—	____
2. Do you find it difficult to refrain from smoking in places where it is forbidden?	No	Yes	—	____
3. Which cigarette smoked during the day is most satisfying?	Any other but the first one	The first one	—	____
4. How many cigarettes per day do you smoke?	1-15	16-25	> 25	____
5. Do you smoke more in the morning than the rest of the day?	No	Yes	—	____
6. Do you smoke when you are so ill that you are in bed most of day?	No	Yes	—	____
7. Does the brand smoked have low, medium, or high nicotine content?	Low	Medium	High	____
8. How often do you inhale smoke from cigarette?	Never	Sometimes	Often	____
			Total:	____

Score > 7 points: highly nicotine-dependent
Score = 4-7: medium dependence
Score = 0-3: low dependence
Adapted from Fagerstrom[38]

The exact wording of the antismoking message will vary from patient to patient depending on the particular psychosocial needs of the patient and on the doctor-patient relationship. There may be a tendency among some physicians not to insist strongly enough that their patients quit smoking because of previous unsuccessful attempts with other patients. Some physicians, on the other hand, feel so strongly about this issue that they will refuse to provide long-term care to their cardiac patients who continue to smoke.[1] This is likely to be a very effective strategy for patients who are emotionally attached to their personal physicians.

Setting a firm quit date

Once a patient has agreed to consider a smoking cessation intervention, it is important to set a reasonably firm quit date, preferably during a relatively stress-free time in the patient's life. This allows time for the patient and significant others to prepare for withdrawal symptoms and, perhaps, to arrange for distractions to help minimize these symptoms. As an example, sedentary smokers might choose this time to begin an exercise program which not only would provide distraction but would also prevent the weight gain that frequently accompanies cessation from smoking. A quit date also implies a commitment from the patient and indicates that he or she has assumed the responsibility for making a major behavioral change.

An additional useful strategy is the signing of a "contract" between the patient and the physician which explicitly commits the patient to quit smoking on a particular date. The reasons for stopping as well as the methods to achieve cessation may also be included in the contract. The physician, in turn, commits to following up with the patient by telephone and appropriately timed office visits to discuss progress made and to help the patient manage the withdrawal symptoms. Copies of the contract should be placed in the patient's medical record and also given to the patient along with pertinent self-help literature on smoking cessation.

Relapse prevention

For many smokers who are initially successful in quitting, the greatest recurrent problem is the high probability of relapse. Because this is a major obstacle to long-term abstinence, most comprehensive antismoking programs incorporate relapse prevention strategies along with methods to promote maintenance of the smoke free state. According to Greene et al,[25] three important behavioral techniques can be utilized to avert a relapse: 1) creation of a strong social support network; 2) acquisition of coping skills; and 3) cognitive restructuring.

A social support network is made up of family members, friends, neighbors, and co-workers. Ongoing support from these individuals in providing encouragement and positive feedback is an important adjunct to the antismoking intervention. Other smokers in the patient's sphere of influence should be urged to join the program for the mutual benefit of all.

Coping skills are necessary to help manage those special situations in which relapse is most likely to occur. Shiffman[40] has identified four particularly dangerous scenarios for the new ex-smoker to be aware of: 1) at home, following meals; 2) social drinking especially when other smokers are present; 3) stressful moments at work; and 4) alone at home during periods of anxiety or loneliness. Patients should be taught to anticipate these situations and either avoid them when possible or learn to substitute more healthful behaviors.

Cognitive restructuring is a valuable stress management technique for preventing relapse that focuses on changes in self-perception, knowledge, and attitudes. Although this is not always easy to achieve, physicians can help their patients by encouraging them to become more actively involved in the decision to quit smoking and to assume more responsibility for their actions. Often the change from being a passive recipient of medical services to an active participant in the health care process leads to a new self-image: one of being in control. This does much to facilitate the changes in knowledge and attitudes necessary to sustain the smoke-free state.

Intensive Strategies for Nicotine-dependent Smokers

There are, unfortunately, many smokers who will not respond to the brief intervention strategies just considered, which rely primarily on physician counseling. These are usually the nicotine-dependent smokers who, although motivated to quit, cannot manage their withdrawal symptoms. For them more intensive and often formal smoking cessation interventions are required. There are many options to consider when choosing a particular intervention strategy including office-based programs, community or hospital-based programs, pharmacologic adjuncts, and various nonpharmacologic techniques. Physicians should be familiar with the various options even though they may not be directly involved in administering them, since they are often asked by patients and their families for information regarding them.

If physicians are to become involved in more comprehensive office-based interventions, they should have previous experience and success with brief counseling techniques as well as a great deal of interest in smoking cessation.[24] The greater their involvement, the greater the success that can be achieved. Patients seem to prefer working with their personal physicians to joining more formal smoking cessation groups.

Pharmacologic adjuncts

Pharmacologic interventions, the most common of which is nicotine polacrilex (nicotine gum), can be a significant aid in smoking cessation, providing it is used as part of a comprehensive behavior modification program.[24,25] Studies suggest a doubling of the quit rate when nicotine gum is added to behavioral counseling in nicotine-dependent patients participating in formal smoking cessation programs.[41] It is unfortunate, however, that practicing physicians have been less successful using this product in their office-based practices.[24,42,43]

Success with nicotine polacrilex requires meticulous attention to detail when prescribing this product. Patients should be given written instructions such as those provided in the product insert or found in *The Physicians' Desk Reference* (PDR).[44] In a sense, the term "nicotine gum" is a misnomer since this product is not to be chewed like ordinary chewing gum. In fact, regular chewing causes the released nicotine to become mixed with saliva which, when swallowed, never reaches the circulation. At most, 10-15 slow chews should be sufficient to release the nicotine and create sufficient alkalinity in the mouth to insure absorption. After several slow chews a bitter and tingling sensation appears, at which time the flattened piece of gum should be moved with the tongue to the space between the upper molar teeth and the cheek. The gum should be left in place at least several minutes until the tingling sensation disappears and then chewed slowly to release more nicotine before moving it to a different location between the molar teeth and the cheek. This can be repeated several more times over a 30-minute period allowing absorption to occur from other areas of the mouth. It cannot be overemphasized that chewing and swallowing should be minimized. In addition, patients should avoid drinking liquids while the gum is in the mouth.

The purpose of nicotine polacrilex is to reduce the withdrawal symptoms that occur when nicotine-dependent smokers abruptly quit smoking. The nicotine in the gum, when absorbed through the mouth tissues, serves as a substitute for the nicotine in cigarettes. Unlike cigarettes, however, where inhaled nicotine reaches the circulation within seconds, the absorption of nicotine from the mouth is slower, taking 10-15 minutes to achieve adequate blood levels. The successful use of this product, therefore, requires a careful analysis of the patient's smoking behavior before the quit date.

Two types of smokers can be identified: 1) the situational smoker, and 2) the regimented smoker.[45] The situational smoker is one who smokes primarily during certain social or occupational situations rather than regularly throughout the day. In contrast, regimented smokers, who represent the majority of hard-core addicted smokers, smoke regularly in a structured pattern all day long. Once the patient's smoking pattern has been established through several weeks of monitoring, a dosing schedule for nicotine gum can be designed to ameliorate the withdrawal symptoms by providing an alternate source of nicotine during those periods of intense craving for cigarettes. It is recommended, however, that no more than 30 pieces of gum be used in any 24-hour period. It is further suggested that the patient learn to anticipate the nicotine craving and use the gum 10-15 minutes before in order to allow time for the slow absorption through the mouth.

After a successful replacement pattern has been established and used for several weeks, the patient should be given a schedule for gradually diminishing the daily dosage of drug until full withdrawal has been accomplished. The rate of withdrawal will vary according to the patient's particular needs. Physicians should maintain close contact with their patients during the active treatment phase to monitor progress, assess side effects, and reinforce behavioral strategies. *The Cooper/Clayton Method to Stop Smoking* is a detailed description of a well-designed and effective smoking cessation program using nicotine polacrilex to supplement behavior modification.[45]

Contraindications to the use of nicotine polacrilex include: 1) the immediate post-myocardial infarction period; 2) uncontrolled arrhythmias; 3) severe or worsening angina pectoris; 4) pregnancy and lactation; 5) active temporomandibular joint disease; 6) peripheral vasospastic diseases; and 7) oral and pharyngeal irritation. In general, nicotine polacrilex should only be used in those patients where the benefits of smoking cessation using this drug outweigh the risks. This is especially important in patients with hypertension, peptic ulcer disease, esophagitis, hyperthyroidism and Type I diabetes. Further warnings, precautions, and side effects can be found in the *Physicians' Desk Reference.*[44]

Clonidine is a non-nicotine pharmacologic agent under study in smoking cessation programs because it appears to reduce the craving for tobacco.[46] The use of this drug in both oral and transdermal forms is still considered investigational, since randomized controlled studies have shown both positive[47] and negative[48] results when clonidine was compared to placebo.

Nonpharmacologic methods

A variety of other methods has been suggested to decrease psychological dependency on nicotine.[25] Aversive methods such as rapid smoking, smoke holding, and smoking to satiation are rarely successful when used alone and are relatively contraindicated in patients with active coronary heart disease. Hypnosis and acupuncture are two promising approaches which have varying degrees of success depending on patient motivation, particular methodologies, length of treatment, and incorporation of other behavioral techniques.[27]

Summary

Cigarette smokers can quit providing they are given the tools and the enthusiastic support of their personal physicians. The methods considered above are ones that can be effectively carried out in an office-based medical practice. There are, however, two major requirements for a successful outcome: 1) a knowledgeable, interested physician who has the necessary clinical and counseling skills to match the most appropriate smoking cessation strategies to the particular needs of the patient, and 2) a motivated patient who has learned the necessary cognitive and coping skills to take responsibility for smoking cessation.

Office-based smoking cessation programs must also have documented cost/benefit adequacy.[26] This requires that the costs of implementing a program should be determined and built into the charges for physician counseling and patient education. Studies have already shown that the cost-effectiveness of physician counseling during routine office visits is substantial and at least as great as many other preventive medical practices.[49]

DIETARY INTERVENTION

Most patients recovering from AMI or other recent coronary events are motivated to consider dietary interventions that might reduce their likelihood of recurrent morbidity or mortality. Numerous studies have now shown that aggressive management of hyperlipidemia in patients with coronary disease can modify the progression of coronary atherosclerosis and improve outcome.[7-10,50,51] Although these studies focused primarily on lipid-lowering drugs, the implications for dietary intervention are no less significant, since dietary management is always the initial strategy in the treatment of hyperlipidemia.[52] Dietary intervention is also advantageous to the patient's family members who have yet to experience coronary disease but who share in the familial (genetic plus environmental) predisposition for the disease.

Nutritional information is usually offered to patients early in their hospital stay in the form of one-on-one conferences with a dietitian, small group classes organized by the cardiac rehabilitation or nursing staff, and self-help literature. The shortened hospital course, so characteristic of modern coronary care is, however, not sufficient to ensure the success of any recommended dietary intervention. As a result the focus on diet and nutrition must shift to the practicing physician in the office setting. This section considers several strategies for implementing appropriate dietary changes for controlling hyperlipidemia and other risk factors. Pharmacologic management of hyperlipidemia is discussed in several recent reviews.[52-55]

Rationale for Dietary Intervention

The relationship between a diet rich in cholesterol, saturated fat and total calories and coronary heart disease risk is unequivocal and supported by numerous clinical, epidemiologic, and animal research studies.[56] The "diet-heart hypothesis" is no longer a matter of loose speculation based on a few epidemiologic surveys but one that has achieved etiologic significance in the development of coronary heart disease. In other words, "rich" diet has emerged as a major causal factor in the twentieth century mass epidemic of coronary heart disease.[56] Most important, however, is the growing public and professional awareness that the treatment of hyperlipidemia with diet and drugs will significantly lower coronary disease morbidity and mortality.[52]

Several pathophysiologic mechanisms explain the diet-heart relationship. An atherogenic diet high in cholesterol (> 450 mg/day) and saturated fat (> 15% of calories) is a major determinant of elevated blood total cholesterol (TC) and low-density lipoprotein cholesterol (LDL-C).[57-59] Increased LDL-C, in turn, is a major factor in the process of atherogenesis.[60,61] In patients with established coronary artery disease, moreover, increased LDL-C may initiate plaque rupture and thrombus formation which are precursors of the three acute coronary heart disease syndromes: unstable angina, myocardial infarction, and sudden death.[62] Finally, increases in total calories and dietary sodium contribute to obesity and hypertension, both of which are known to accelerate the progression of atherosclerosis.[56]

Dietary Management of Hyperlipidemia

The first order of business in the dietary management of patients with established coronary heart disease is an assessment of the patient's lipid profile. This evaluation can begin as early as the day of admission for AMI, since it has been shown that total cholesterol (TC) measured within 24 hours of AMI accurately reflects the patient's baseline value.[63]

Total cholesterol levels greater than 200 mg/dL should be followed up during the patient's convalescence with a fasting lipoprotein analysis. This consists of measuring total cholesterol, high-density lipoprotein cholesterol (HDL-C), and triglycerides (TG) after an overnight fast. From these three measurements the low-density lipoprotein cholesterol (LDL-C) can be estimated by the formula: LDL-C = TC – (HDL-C + TG/5), providing triglycerides are below 400 mg/dL.[52] Values above this require direct measurement of LDL-C by ultracentrifugation in a specialized laboratory; fortunately this is an uncommon problem.

Treatment decisions are based on elevations of LDL-C, with a goal of achieving levels below 130 mg/dL.[52] Before considering specific therapies it is necessary to exclude secondary and possibly reversible causes of hyperlipidemia: hypothyroidism, nephrotic syndrome, diabetes mellitus, obstructive liver disease, and drugs (progestins, anabolic steroids and thiazide diuretics). Once these are excluded, the focus turns to dietary management.

The American Heart Association[64] and the National Heart, Lung, and Blood Institute's National Cholesterol Education Program[52] have recommended a two-step approach to the dietary management of hyperlipidemia, beginning with a Step-One Diet and followed, if necessary, with a more restrictive Step-Two Diet. The generic characteristics of these two diets are listed in Table 3. Physicians and their office staffs should feel comfortable in prescribing the Step-One Diet, since this diet is similar to the dietary modifications long recommended to the general public by the American Heart Association and other national organizations.

The usual approach to managing hypercholesterolemia is to begin with the Step-One Diet, recheck blood levels in four to six weeks and again at three months, and, if the target goal is not achieved, progress to the Step-Two Diet for three more months.[52] For most patients it is adequate and less costly to monitor nonfasting total cholesterol

Table 3. *Dietary management of elevated LDL-cholesterol*

Nutrient	Step-One Diet	Step-Two Diet
Total Fat	< 30% total calories	< 30% total calories
Saturated Fat	< 10% " "	< 7% " "
Polyunsaturated	< 10% " "	< 10% " "
Monounsaturated	10-15% " "	10-15% " "
Carbohydrates	50-60% " "	50-60% " "
Protein	10-20% " "	10-20% " "
Cholesterol	< 300 mg/day	< 200 mg/day
Calories	to achieve and maintain desirable body weight	

levels since total cholesterol levels of 200 and 240 mg/dL roughly correspond to LDL cholesterol levels of 130 and 160 mg/dL, respectively. If the TC goal of < 200 mg/dL is achieved after three months of the Step-One Diet, a fasting lipoprotein analysis should follow to confirm that the LDL-C goal of < 130 mg/dL has been met. Once the desired goal has been attained, the patient should be congratulated and long-term monitoring begun; TC levels should be checked four times during the first year and twice yearly thereafter.

The success of dietary therapy requires that physicians have the necessary knowledge, skills and attitudes to motivate their patients to change eating behaviors. Because changing behaviors takes valuable physician time, the physician may assign office personnel to work out the specific details of a diet after the patient has been presented with an overview of the dietary plan. In some situations, particularly with the more restrictive Step-Two Diet, referral to a registered dietitian may be necessary for more intensive education and behavior counseling. Self-help materials and suggestions for specific cook books[65-67] are important adjuncts in implementing a dietary change program. It is necessary for patients to realize, from the beginning, that these recommended dietary changes are to last a lifetime. Fortunately, with well-motivated patients, enthusiastic physicians and creative dietary counseling, the low-fat, low-cholesterol diets are generally well accepted.

For many patients with established coronary heart disease and especially for those with severe hypercholesterolemia (TC > 300 mg/dL, LDL-C > 200 mg/dL), it is not appropriate to continue diet therapy for six months before adding lipid-lowering drugs. Some of these patients have familial disorders that require more specialized laboratory evaluations and treatment programs. If possible patients with severe lipid disorders should be referred to specialists. Dietary considerations for the familial hyperlipidemias and recommendations for drug therapy have been carefully described in the Expert Panel's report of the National Cholesterol Education Program.[52]

In addition to reducing dietary cholesterol and saturated fat consumption, it is important to emphasize the need to reduce salt (especially in hypertensives), achieve and maintain desired body weight, and increase the intake of complex carbohydrates. In particular, recent evidence suggests that an increased intake of water-soluble fiber in the form of oat bran, barley, legumes, fresh fruits and vegetables significantly lowers total and LDL cholesterol by 5-15%.[68,69] Additionally, fish-oil supplements containing omega-3 fatty acids are being nationally advertised as effective cholesterol- and triglyceride-lowering products as well as having favorable antiplatelet activity.[70] However, considerable uncertainty exists in the medical community regarding the fish-oil supplements because of their potential side effects including adverse lipid changes, bleeding, and vitamin E deficiency.[70] However, the substitution of fish high in omega-3 fatty acids for other animal sources of protein is highly recommended in both the Step-One and Step-Two diets.[52,64]

EXERCISE TRAINING

The definite and possible benefits of exercise training in patients with established coronary heart disease are listed in Table 4. Possible benefits are those that may only be realized in a small subset of the coronary disease population. Although definite benefits occur in most patients, the range of improvement varies considerably and also depends on the quality of the training program.

Table 4. *Benefits of exercise training in patients with coronary heart disease*

Definite	Possible
1. Improved physical work capacity	1. Improved cardiac function and contractility
2. Reduction in ischemic manifestations	2. Improved myocardial perfusion
3. Reduction in coronary risk factors	3. Reversal or slowed progression of atherosclerosis
4. Psychologic benefits	4. Antiarrhythmic benefits
	5. Reduction in mortality and morbidity

The role of exercise training after myocardial infarction is still controversial in spite of the long tradition of cardiac rehabilitation services.[11-15] At the center of the controversy is the question of medical supervision. Do all patients recovering from acute coronary events require supervised, monitored exercise programs to restore function? This is unlikely to be the case, since studies have shown that most uncomplicated post-AMI patients recover functional capacity spontaneously by 11 weeks without formal exercise training.[71] While it is true that a supervised exercise program may result in a somewhat greater improvement in physical work capacity compared to spontaneous recovery, this increased function is not large enough to justify the expense of providing cardiac rehabilitation services for all patients.

Improved physical work capacity is the most clearly defined benefit of exercise training and occurs in practically all patients. In post-AMI patients, however, almost all of the functional improvement during the first 6-12 months is secondary to peripheral conditioning of skeletal muscles, with only minimal improvement in cardiac function or contractility.[72] In fact, a recent study suggests that ventricular function may deteriorate due to infarct expansion when exercise training is begun too soon after a large anterior wall infarction.[73] Parameters of ventricular function and contractility may eventually improve in some patients who continue to train for one year or longer.[72,74,75]

The second well defined benefit of exercise training is a reduction in anginal symptoms and other ischemic manifestations.[76] This is due to the physiologic adaptations that occur with training which lower myocardial oxygen demands during submaximal work. After training a given cardiac output can be delivered at a lower heart rate and greater stroke volume than before training. Since heart rate is a more important determinant of myocardial oxygen demand than stroke volume, the training effect improves the efficiency of cardiac work. Myocardial oxygen requirements are further reduced by peripheral adaptations to training including a lowering of systemic vascular resistance and improved oxygen extraction by skeletal muscles.[77] Reduction in ischemic symptoms may also reflect improved myocardial perfusion, although the evidence for this is not impressive.[75]

The reduction in coronary risk factors that occurs with exercise training is mostly indirect in the sense that the enhanced physical and psychological well-being often leads to other positive behavioral changes. It is easier for patients to give up bad habits after succeeding with a positive behavioral change. There are, however, several direct, albeit small, effects of exercise on cardiac risk factors.[14] Patients with hypertension may experience an improvement in their blood pressure due to the decrease in systemic vascular resistance with training. There is also a modest increase in HDL-cholesterol and decrease in triglycerides with training.

Exercise training is an effective strategy for dealing with the psychological and social disabilities associated with recovery from recent coronary events. Measures of depression and anxiety are significantly reduced in patients who train as compared with patients who do not exercise.[78] Return-to-work statistics are also improved after exercise training.[79] The restoration of confidence so frequently seen in patients who regain or even surpass their previous level of functioning should be regarded by both patients and physicians as an important prerequisite for returning to productive roles in society. These benefits, although difficult to measure and frequently overlooked, cannot be overemphasized.

The other benefits listed as "possible" in Table 4 are more speculative but certainly deserve consideration. The evidence that exercise training after myocardial infarction reduces morbidity and mortality is minimal. Oldridge et al[80] recently performed a meta-analysis of previously reported randomized controlled trials of cardiac rehabilitation and concluded that all-cause and cardiovascular mortality were significantly lower by 25% in the rehabilitation groups than in controls. The same analysis, however, showed no difference in nonfatal recurrent myocardial infarction. Reduction or slowed progression of atherosclerosis, although difficult to document, may actually occur in some patients who participate in exercise programs combined with intensive efforts to modify other risk factors.[81] Finally, antiarrhythmic benefits are purely speculative, although several theoretical reasons suggest that this may occur. As already discussed, training may reduce myocardial ischemia during submaximal work and, therefore, ischemic arrhythmias. The trained state is also associated with reduced sympathetic tone and lowered circulating catecholamines, thus reducing the arrhythmogenic potential.

Exercise Programs for Cardiac Patients

Given the evidence supporting the benefits of exercise for patients recovering from acute coronary events, how is this best accomplished? Ideally, although not always cost effective, patients should be encouraged to join comprehensive cardiac rehabilitation programs whenever possible. Such programs offer considerable assistance to physicians hoping to improve their patients' lifestyles and reduce their risk for recurrent disease complications. Unfortunately, because of the increasingly serious financial issues facing the various medical reimbursement plans, future cardiac rehabilitation programs are likely to be restricted to a subset of patients who are at increased risk of exercise-related complications.

In an effort to develop realistic guidelines for cardiac rehabilitation services, the Health and Public Policy Committee of the American College of Physicians (ACP) has published a set of recommendations[82] based on a comprehensive review of cardiac rehabilitation by Greenland and Chu.[14] Three categories of post-AMI patients were defined in these recommendations: 1) low-risk patients; 2) intermediate-risk patients; and 3) high-risk patients.

Low-risk patients are those recovering from uncomplicated myocardial infarctions who already have an adequate functional capacity — defined as 8 METS or

395

greater at 3 weeks post-AMI. One MET (metabolic equivalent) refers to a person's resting energy requirements and is defined as 3.5 ml O_2/kg/min. Eight METS, or 8 times the resting oxygen uptake, represents a level of functional capacity adequate for most occupational or recreational activities engaged in by sedentary individuals. In the exercise testing laboratory 8 METS is approximately the end of Stage 7 of the modified Naughton protocol[83] or the first minute of Stage III of the Bruce protocol.[84] The ACP position paper appropriately suggests that these patients do not need supervised exercise programs.[82]

Intermediate-risk patients are those who have an intermediate risk for recurrent cardiac events or who have functional capacities less than 8 METS. These are patients who may have had heart failure during hospitalization or ischemic ECG changes (less than 2 mm ST-segment depression) during post-AMI exercise testing. They may also be patients who cannot adequately monitor their own heart rates during exercise. The ACP position paper suggests that these patients may benefit from a shortened cardiac rehabilitation program in which the need for ECG monitoring is left to the supervising physician's discretion.[82] Patients should remain in the program long enough to develop self-monitoring skills and achieve an adequate functional capacity for return to normal activities.

High-risk patients generally require ECG monitored exercise programs because of their greatly increased risk of recurrent cardiac events and exercise related complications. Patients in this group usually have one or more of the following features:[82]

1. severely depressed left ventricular function with ejection fractions < 30%;
2. complex ventricular arrhythmias at rest;
3. ventricular arrhythmias increasing in severity with exercise;
4. systolic blood pressure fall of 15 mm Hg or more during exercise;
5. recent myocardial infarction complicated by serious ventricular arrhythmias;
6. severe ischemia (> 2 mm ST-segment depression) or angina during exercise testing;
7. survival of sudden cardiac arrest.

All patients being considered for exercise programs, whether home-based or supervised, should undergo a careful medical assessment including symptom-limited exercise testing at approximately 3 weeks after a recent cardiac event to classify risk category and determine a safe exercise prescription. Contraindications to exercise testing and training include unstable angina, medically refractory angina, severe hypertension at rest defined as systolic blood pressure > 200 mm Hg or diastolic > 100 mm Hg, severe aortic stenosis, active pericarditis or myocarditis, and other debilitating cardiac or noncardiac diseases which preclude exercise activities.[11] The prescription of exercise for patients participating in supervised cardiac rehabilitation programs is discussed in the cardiac rehabilitation literature and will not be covered in this chapter.[11,85]

Home exercise training

The exercise prescription for cardiac patients should be individualized to meet the occupational and recreational needs of each patient while, at the same time, remaining within the patient's functional capabilities. There are five major components to the exercise prescription:[85] 1) type of exercise; 2) intensity; 3) duration; 4) frequency; and 5) mode of progression. The specific details will depend on the patient's clinical status, the results of exercise testing, and the patient's particular needs and desires. To qualify for unsupervised home exercise training patients should not have any of the high-risk characteristics or contraindications previous discussed.

Type of exercise

Any exercise activity that uses large muscle groups in a repetitive rhythmic manner is acceptable for exercise training providing the remaining requirements in the exercise prescription are met. Examples of activities include walking, cycling, stair climbing, jogging, rowing, rope jumping, swimming, and many recreational games. At the beginning of an exercise program, however, competitive sports activities are not recommended because of the difficulty of staying within safe intensity guidelines. These more strenuous activities may be permitted once the patient's functional capacity has improved and their safety established in the exercise laboratory.

Intensity

The safety of exercise is assessed primarily by heart rate monitoring and perceived exertion. Prior to undergoing an exercise assessment patients should be encouraged to continue those activities begun in the hospital and at heart rates no greater than 20 beats/min above resting heart rate. After a symptom limited exercise test, performed approximately 3-6 weeks post-cardiac event, the intensity of exercise can be defined as a heart rate range representing 65-85% of either the maximal heart rate achieved or the heart rate at which ischemic manifestations such as angina, ST-segment depression, or arrhythmias occurred.

During the first several weeks of training the patient should remain at the lower end of this heart rate range in order to ensure comfort and minimize the risk of exercise complications. Later in the program patients may choose to increase the intensity towards the higher end of the training range. It must be emphasized, however, that low-intensity exercise training is all that is necessary to improve cardiovascular fitness when initiating an exercise program.[85] This is especially important for older patients as well as those with more compromised ventricular function.

The widespread use of β-blockers after myocardial infarction complicates the prescription of exercise intensity. One approach is to slowly taper and discontinue the β-blocker before exercise testing. Although controversial, some physicians discontinue β-blockers permanently if the exercise test shows good functional recovery and no ischemia. A second approach is to perform the exercise test with the patient on β-blockers and use the blunted heart rate response to calculate the training range as discussed previously. In some patients who are heavily beta-blocked, this may not be an adequate training range to improve functional capacity. Under these circumstances cautious increments in the exercise heart rate are reasonable, providing no ischemic manifestations occurred during exercise testing.

It is important that patients learn self-monitoring skills at the onset of an exercise program. One effective method is to use the time immediately after exercise testing to go over the test results and outline an exercise prescription. It is also helpful if the patient's spouse or partner is present during this session. After a training heart rate range is determined, patients should be observed taking their pulse over a 10-second interval. The exercise heart rate range can also be given in beats per 10 seconds. During the initial weeks of an exercise program the patient should monitor exercise heart rates frequently and increase or decrease the level of exertion whenever appropriate.

After several months of exercise training patients often learn to associate a particular perception of exertional symptoms with the training heart rate range. Substituting this level of perceived exertion in place of frequent pulse checks is permissible, providing that the patient's clinical condition is stable and that no significant ischemic manifestations appear on exercise testing.

Frequency and duration

These two components of an exercise prescription are straight forward. Initially after hospital discharge patients may exercise 10-15 minutes once or twice daily at heart rates < 20 beats/min above resting. After establishing the training heart rate range based on exercise test findings, patients should gradually increase the duration of exercise and decrease the frequency. The goal during the first three months is to achieve a duration of 45 minutes 3-5 days a week, avoiding more than two days between exercise sessions. The 45 minute sessions should include a 5-10 minute warm-up, 20-30 minutes of aerobic exercise within the training heart rate range, and a 5-10 minute cool-down period. Warm-up and cool-down activities consist of lower intensity aerobic activities as well as stretching, range-of-motion exercises, and light weights especially for the upper extremities.

Mode of progression

An exercise program can be conceptualized as involving three distinct phases: initial, improvement, and maintenance. The rate of progression through these phases depends upon the patient's age, functional capacity, overall health status, and particular needs or goals.

The initial phase for coronary patients should last at least three months. This is a most critical time for beginning exercisers, since a bad experience during this period is likely to result in noncompliance with further exercise recommendations. For these reasons, emphasis is placed on a slowly progressive and gentle program as previously discussed. A major behavioral goal during this phase is to develop the exercise habit. This involves not only learning the various exercise routines but also restructuring daily activities to include the exercise program.

After three months of training patients are usually anxious to assess their progress, and repeat exercise testing is often carried out at this time. In addition to documenting improved functional capacity, the exercise test offers an opportunity to revise the exercise prescription. Many patients who have regained confidence will push to a higher symptom-limited maximal heart rate which results in upgrading the training range.

The improvement phase is designed to increase the patient's functional capacity to a level compatible with long term occupational and recreational needs. This varies considerably from patient to patient. Again, the emphasis is on slow progression, making small increments in duration and/or intensity every few weeks. A reasonable goal for many patients is 30-60 minutes of aerobic exercise, 3-5 days a week at 70-85% of maximal achieved heart rate during exercise testing. During this period patients may substitute endurance sports for other aerobic activities in order to enhance enjoyment providing the clinical disease states are stable and compatible with these exercise activities.

The final phase is long-term maintenance and should continue as long as the patient remains stable. Changes in clinical status are common in patients with chronic coronary heart disease, and patients need to maintain close relationships with their personal physicians. New symptoms of chest discomfort, unusual dyspnea, palpitations, lightheadedness, extreme fatigue, and weight gain need to be quickly recognized, evaluated and treated appropriately. Periodic exercise testing every 6-12 months or whenever there is a questionable change in clinical status provides useful information for subsequent therapeutic decisions and revisions in the exercise prescription.

RETURN-TO-WORK GUIDELINES

Guidelines for returning cardiac patients to occupational activities have been published in the "20th Bethesda Conference: Insurability and Employability of the Patient with Ischemic Heart Disease."[86] The full report of this conference offers the practicing physician a wealth of information aimed at maximizing the return-to-work potential of cardiac patients. This issue continues to be a major challenge for the medical

Table 5. *Factors influencing return-to-work status*

1. Severity of disease: number of myocardial infarctions, extent of damage, severity of ischemia, functional status.

2. Age > 50 years: fewer patients return to work.

3. Social class/education: lower levels less likely to return to work.

4. Occupation: manual laborers less likely to return to work.

5. Perceived job stress: fewer patients return to unpleasant jobs.

6. Emotional disturbances: patients with anxiety, depression, pessimism, loss of self-efficacy are less likely to work.

7. Location of residence: patients in rural areas are less likely to return to work.

8. Labor market/unemployment/social benefits: varies with economics and social conditions in different areas of the country.

9. Employer misconceptions about ability of cardiac patients to work.

10. Attending physician's attitude: negative attitudes reduce likelihood of return to work.

11. Overprotection by the patient's family.

12. Inadequate or delayed return-to-work evaluation.

13. Lack of cardiac rehabilitation programs in the area.

profession, government agencies, and private industry since misconceptions abound regarding the employability and/or insurability of cardiac patients. Impediments to returning to work are listed in Table 5.

The determination of occupational working capacity requires a consideration of both the patient's clinical and functional status as well as the physical, environmental and psychological requirements of the particular job (Table 6). Important prognostic factors that might interfere with certain occupational activities include left ventricular dysfunction, ischemic manifestations, and electrophysiologic disturbances. These are usually assessed by exercise testing 3-5 weeks post-AMI. Maximal exercise ECG testing is adequate for most work evaluations unless resting ECG abnormalities preclude recognition of ischemic findings (diffuse ST-T changes, bundle branch block, digitalis effects, etc.). Exercise thallium testing and radionuclide ventriculography are often helpful in these situations. Cardiac imaging studies during exercise also provide important functional and anatomic information which can contribute to the occupational work assessment.

Table 6. *Return-to-work evaluation*

    I. Occupational Considerations
       A. Physical requirements
          1. Dynamic vs. static exercises
          2. Upper extremity work
          3. Work intensity and duration
       B. Environmental conditions
          1. Temperature
          2. Humidity
          3. Air pollution
          4. Altitude
       C. Psychological factors

    II. Patient Considerations
       A. Prognostic factors
          1. Left ventricular dysfunction
          2. Myocardial ischemia
          3. Electrophysiologic disturbances
       B. Exercise assessment
          1. Exercise capacity in METS
          2. Exercise induced abnormalities
             a. ST segment response
             b. Peak work load achieved
             c. Arrhythmias
             d. Blood pressure response

The patient's physical working capacity, reflected by the peak exercise test workload, is an important determinant of return to work potential. It is recommended that the maximal safe workload achieved during exercise testing be at least twice the average physical requirements at work.[87] This is generally not a problem for low risk patients who have an 8 MET or greater exercise capacity, since most jobs in today's high-tech society have limited physical requirements. For intermediate or high risk patients, however, there is a need for a more careful match of clinical status with the particular physical, environmental and psychological requirements of the job. Often a period of cardiac rehabilitation is recommended to improve the patient's working capacity and mental status (perception of self-efficacy) before returning to occupational activities.

The average energy requirements of many occupations have been published, but, at best, they are gross approximations.[87] Often it is necessary to perform ambulatory ECG or blood pressure monitoring during work if there is uncertainty about either the specific job demands or the patient's cardiovascular response to these activities.

CONCLUSION

Most physicians are more comfortable dealing with matters relating to the mechanistic aspects of health and disease (ie, body-as-a-machine concept) than they are with the psychosocial aspects (ie, mind-body and mind-environment interactions). Nevertheless, it is becoming increasingly apparent that mental phenomena and related lifestyle patterns play an important role in the pathogenesis and management of many chronic diseases including coronary heart disease.

As stated at the beginning of this chapter, the goals of comprehensive cardiac rehabilitation are restoration of function, restoration of confidence and prevention of recurrent coronary events. Achievement of these goals requires compliance with comprehensive treatment regimens that include medications, diet, exercise, and other lifestyle interventions such as smoking cessation. Compliance with these prescribed regimens, however, is often adversely affected by various emotional reactions experienced by patients recovering from acute coronary events.

For many patients the emotional distress associated with acute coronary events — anxiety, depression, anger — are self-limited and usually respond to supportive measures initiated in the hospital. For others the restoration of function achieved with medical management, exercise training, and other lifestyle modifications is sufficient to restore confidence and alleviate these emotional reactions. In some patients, however, psychological dysfunction persists long after hospital discharge and contributes to chronic illness behaviors characterized by multiple somatic complaints, depression, and loss of self-efficacy.[88] Although some of these patients may benefit from referral to mental-health professionals for short-term psychotherapy, many others can be managed successfully by primary care physicians who take the time to incorporate the psychological and social aspects of disease management along with the physical aspects.

REFERENCES

1. McIntosh HD: Office strategies to reduce the risk of coronary heart disease. J Am Coll Cardiol 1988;12:1095-1097.

2. Waller BF: "Crackers, breakers, stretchers, drillers, scrapers, shavers, burners, welders and melters" — the future treatment of atherosclerotic coronary artery disease? A clinical-morphologic assessment. J Am Coll Cardiol 1989;13:969-987.

3. Schlant RC, Forman S, Stamler J, et al: The natural history of coronary heart disease: Prognostic factors after recovery from myocardial infarction in 2789 men. Circulation 1982;66:401-409.

4. The Coronary Drug Project Research Group: The natural history of myocardial infarction in the Coronary Drug Project: Long-term prognostic implications of serum lipid levels. Am J Cardiol 1978;42:489-498.

5. The Coronary Drug Project Research Group: Cigarette smoking as a risk factor in men with a prior history of myocardial infarction. J Chronic Dis 1979;32:415-424.

6. Jenkins CD, Zyzanski SJ, Roseman RH: Risk of new myocardial infarction in middle-aged men with manifest coronary heart disease. Circulation 1976;53:342-347.

7. Blankenhorn DH, Nessim SA, Johnson RL, et al: Beneficial effects of combined colestipol-niacin therapy on coronary atherosclerosis and coronary venous bypass grafts. JAMA 1987;257:3233-3240.

8. Selvester R, Sanmarco M, Blessey R: Risk reduction and coronary progression and regression in humans, in Roskamm H (ed): *Myocardial Infarction At Young Age.* Berlin, Heidelberg, New York, Springer, 1981, pp 196-200.

9. Arntzenius AC, Kromhout D, Barth JD, et al: Diet, lipoproteins, and the progression of coronary atherosclerosis. The Leiden International Trial. N Engl J Med 1985;318:805-811.

10. Nash DT, Gensini G, Esente P: Effect of lipid-lowering therapy on the progression of coronary atherosclerosis assessed by scheduled repetitive coronary angiography. Int J Cardiol 1982;2:53-55.

11. Fardy PS, Yanowitz FG, Wilson PK: *Cardiac Rehabilitation, Adult Fitness, and Exercise Testing, ed. 2.* Philadelphia, Lea & Febiger, 1988, pp 1-402.

12. Wenger NK, Alpert JS: Rehabilitation of the coronary patient in 1989. Arch Intern Med 1989;149:1504-1506.

13. Wenger NK: Rehabilitation of the coronary patient: Status 1986. Prog Cardiovasc Dis 1986;29:181-204.

14. Greenland P, Chu JS: Efficacy of cardiac rehabilitation services with emphasis on patients after myocardial infarction. Ann Intern Med 1988;109:650-663.

15. Oldridge NB, Guyatt GH, Fisher ME, et al: Cardiac rehabilitation after myocardial infarction. Combined experience of randomized clinical trials. JAMA 1988;260:945-950.

16. Meinert CL, Forman S, Jacobs DR, et al: Cigarette smoking as a risk factor in men with a prior history of myocardial infarction. J Chron Dis 1979;32:415-423.

17. Mulcahy R, Hickey N, Graham I, et al: Factors influencing long term prognosis in male patients surviving a first coronary attack. Br Heart J 1975;37:158-63.

18. Sparrow D, Dawber TR, Colton T: The influence of cigarette smoking on prognosis after a first myocardial infarction. J Chron Dis 1978;31:426-433.

19. Barry J, Mead K, Nabel EG, et al: Effect of smoking on activity of ischemic heart disease. JAMA 1989;261:398-402.

20. Deanfield JE, Shea MJ, Wilson RA, et al: Direct effects of smoking on the heart: Silent ischemic disturbances of coronary flow. Am J Cardiol 1986;57:1005-1009.

21. Deanfield JE, Wright C, Krikler S, et al: Cigarette smoking and the treatment of angina with propranolol, atenolol, and nifedipine. N Engl J Med 1984;310:951-954.

22. Salonen J: Stopping smoking and long-term mortality after acute myocardial infarction. Br Heart J 1980;43:463-469.

23. Wilhelmsen L: Cessation of smoking after myocardial infarction: Effects on mortality after ten years. Br Heart J 1983;49:416-422.

24. Prochazka A, Boyko EJ: How physicians can help their patients quit smoking: A practical guide. West J Med 1988;149:188-194.

25. Greene HL, Goldberg RJ, Ockene JK: Cigarette smoking: the physician's role in cessation and maintenance. J Gen Intern Med 1988;3:75-87.

26. Kottke TE, Solberg LI, Brekke ML, et al: Smoking cessation strategies and evaluation. J Am Coll Cardiol 1988;12:1105-1110.

27. Health and Public Policy Committee, American College of Physicians: Methods for stopping cigarette smoking. Ann Intern Med 1986;105:281-291.

28. Wechsler H, Levine S, Idelson RK, et al: The physician's role in health promotion — a survey of primary-care practitioners. N Engl J Med 1983;308:97-100.

29. Kottke TE, Battista RN, DeFriese GH, et al: Attributes of successful smoking cessation interventions in medical practice: A meta-analysis of 39 controlled trials. JAMA 1988;259:2883-2889.

30. Quit For Good. Bethesda, Maryland: National Cancer Institute. DHHS National Institutes of Health Publication No. (PHS) 85-1824 and 85-2494.

31. AAFP stop smoking program. Patient stop smoking guide. Kansas City, Kansas: American Academy of Family Physicians, 1987.

32. I Quit Kit. American Cancer Society, 4 West 35th Street, New York, New York 10019.

33. Freedom From Smoking in 20 Days. American Lung Association, 1740 Broadway, New York, New York 10019.

34. A Lifetime of Freedom from Smoking. American Lung Association, 1740 Broadway, New York, New York 10019.

35. Davis RM: Uniting physicians against smoking: The need for a coordinated national strategy. JAMA 1988;259:2900-2901.

36. The Physician's Guide: How to Help Your Hypertensive Patients Stop Smoking. National Heart, Lung, and Blood Institute, Smoking Education Program, Building 31;4A-21, 9000 Rockville Pike, Bethesda, MD 20892. (NIH Publication 83-1271, 1983)

37. Clinical Opportunities For Smoking Intervention: A Guide for the Busy Physician. National Heart, Lung, and Blood Institute, Smoking Education Program, Building 31;4A-21, 9000 Rockville Pike, Bethesda, MD 20892 (NIH Publication 86-2178, 1986)

38. Fagerstrom KO: Measuring the degree of physical dependence to tobacco smoking with reference to individualization of treatment. Addict Behav 1978;3:235-241.

39. Bart A, Thornley P, Illingworth D: Stopping smoking after myocardial infarction. Lancet 1974;1:304-306.

40. Schiffman S: A cluster analytic classification of relapse episodes. Addict Behav 1986; 11:295-317.

41. Lam W, Sze PC, Sacks HS: Meta-analysis of randomized controlled trials of nicotine chewing gum. Lancet 1987;2:27-29.

42. Hughes JR, Gust SW, Keenan RM, et al: Nicotine vs. placebo gum in general medical practice. JAMA 1988;261:1300-1305.

43. Cummings SR, Hansen B, Richards RJ, et al: Internists and nicotine gum. JAMA 1988; 260:1565-1569.

44. *Physicians' Desk Reference.* Edward R. Barnhart (Publisher). Oradell, Medical Economics Company, 1990, p 1127.

45. Clayton RR, Cooper TM: *The Cooper-Clayton Method to Stop Smoking.* SBC/SBC Inc., 826 Glendover, Lexington, Ky 40502, 1989.

46. Ornish SA, Zisook S, McAdams LA: Effects of transdermal clonidine treatment on the withdrawal symptoms associated with smoking cessation: A randomized, controlled trial. Arch Intern Med 1988;148:2027-2031.

47. Glassman AH, Stetner F, Walsh BT, et al: Heavy smokers, smoking cessation, and clonidine. Results of a double-blind, randomized trial. JAMA 1988;259:2863-2866.

48. Franks P, Harp J, Bell B: Randomized, controlled trial of clonidine for smoking cessation in a primary care setting. JAMA 1989;262:3011-3013.

49. Cummings SR, Rubin SM, Oster G: The cost-effectiveness of counseling smokers to quit. JAMA 1989;261:75-79.

50. Canner PL, Berge KG, Wenger NK, et al: Fifteen year mortality in coronary drug project: Long-term benefit with niacin. J Am Coll Cardiol 1986;8:1245-1255.

51. Carlson LA, Rosenhamer G: Reduction of mortality in the Stockholm Ischemic Heart Disease Secondary Prevention Study by combined treatment with clofibrate and nicotinic acid. Acta Med Scand 1988;223:405-415.

52. National Cholesterol Education Program. Report of the expert panel on detection, evaluation, and treatment of high blood cholesterol in adults. Arch Intern Med 1988;148:36-69.

53. Lavie CJ, Gau GT, Spuires RW, et al: Management of lipids in primary and secondary prevention of cardiovascular diseases. Mayo Clin Proc 1988;605-621.

54. Hoeg JM, Gregg RE, Brewer B: An approach to the management of hyperlipoproteinemia. JAMA 1986;255:512-521.

55. Tobert TA: New developments in lipid-lowering therapy: The role of inhibitors of hydroxymethylglutaryl-coenzyme A reductase. Circulation 1987;76:534-538.

56. Stamler J: Epidemiology, established major risk factors, and the primary prevention of coronary heart disease, in Parmley WW, Chatterjee K (eds), *Cardiology*, Volume 2. Philadelphia, JB Lippincott Co 1989, pp 1-41.

57. Mattson FH, Erickson BA, Kligman AM: Effect of dietary cholesterol on serum cholesterol in man. Am J Clin Nutr 1972;25:589-594.

58. Shekelle RB, Shyrock AM, Lepper PO, et al: Diet, serum cholesterol and death from coronary heart disease: The Western Electric Study. N Engl J Med 1981;304:65-70.

59. Schonfeld G, Patsch W, Rudel LL, et al: Effects of dietary cholesterol and fatty acids on plasma lipoproteins. J Clin Invest 1982;69:1072-1080.

60. Goldstein JL, Brown MS: The low-density lipoprotein pathway and its relation to athero-sclerosis. Ann Rev Biochem 1977;46:897-930.

61. Carew TE: Role of biologically modified low-density lipoprotein in atherosclerosis. Am J Cardiol 1989: 64:18G-22G.

62. Stein B, Israel DH, Cohen M, et al: Pathogenesis of coronary occlusion. Hosp Pract 1988; April 15:65.

63. Gore JM, Goldberg RJ, Matsumoto AS, et al: Validity of serum total cholesterol level obtained within 24 hours of acute myocardial infarction. AM J Cardiol 1984;54:722-725.

64. AHA Special Report: Recommendations of treatment of hyperlipidemia in adults. Circu-lation 1984: 69:1065A-1090A.

65. Connor SL, Connor WE: *The New American Diet.* New York, Simon & Schuster, Inc, 1986.

66. Gaunt L: Recipes to Lower Your Fat Thermostat. Vitality House International Inc, Provo, 1984.

67. *Low Fat, Low Cholesterol Cookbook*, Scott Grundy (ed). New York, Times Books, 1989.

68. Council on Scientific Affairs (AMA): Dietary fiber and health. JAMA 1989;262:542-546.

69. Anderson JW: Dietary fiber, lipids and atherosclerosis. Am J Cardiol 1987;60:17G-22G.

70. Yetiv JZ: Clinical applications of fish oils. JAMA 1988;260:665-670.

71. DeBusk RF, Houston N, Haskell W, et al: Exercise training soon after myocardial infarc-tion. Am J Cardiol 1979;44:1223-1229.

72. Paterson DH, Shephard RJ, Cunningham D, et al: Effects of physical training on cardio-vascular function following myocardial infarction. J Appl Physiol 1979;47:482-489.

73. Jugdutt BI, Michorowski BL, Kappagoda CT: Exercise training after anterior Q-wave myocardial infarction: Importance of regional left ventricular function and topography. J Am Coll Cardiol 1988;12:362-372.

74. Ehsani AA, Martin WH III, Heath GW, et al: Cardiac effects of prolonged and intense exercise training in patients with coronary artery disease. Am J Cardiol 1982;50:246-256.

75. Froelicher V, Jensen D, Genter F, et al: A randomized trial of exercise training in patients with coronary heart disease. JAMA 1984;252:1291-1297.

76. Redwood DR, Rosing DR, Epstein SE: Circulatory and symptomatic effects of physical training in patients with coronary artery disease and angina pectoris. N Engl J Med 1972;286:959-965.

77. Clausen JP: Circulatory adjustments to dynamic exercise and effect of physical training in normal subjects and in patients with coronary artery disease. Prog Cardiovasc Dis 1976;18:459-495.

78. Taylor CB, Houston-Miller N, Ahn DK, et al: The effects of exercise training programs on psychosocial improvement in uncomplicated postmyocardial infarction patients. J Psychosom Res 1986;30:581-587.

79. Krasemann EO, Jungmann H: Return to work after myocardial infarction. Cardiol 1979; 30:581-587.

80. Oldridge NB, Guyatt GH, Fisher ME, et al: Cardiac rehabilitation after myocardial in-farction. Combined experience of randomized clinical trials. JAMA 1988;260:945-950.

81. Kallio V, Hamalainen H, Hakkila J, et al: Reduction of sudden death by a multifactorial intervention program after acute myocardial infarction. Lancet 1979;2:1091-1094.

82. Health and Public Policy Committee, American College of Physicians: Cardiac rehabilitation services. Ann Intern Med 1988;109:671-673.

83. Starling MR, Crawford MH, Kennedy GT, et al: Exercise testing soon after myocardial infarction: Predictive value for subsequent unstable angina and death. Am J Cardiol 1980;46:909-917.

84. Bruce RA, Kusumi F, Hosner D: Maximal oxygen intake and normographic assessment of functional capacity. Am Heart J 1973;85:346-351.

85. *American College of Sports Medicine: Guidelines for Exercise Testing and Prescription, Third Edition.* Lea & Febiger, Philadelphia 1986, pp 1-179.

86. 20th Bethesda Conference: Insurability and Employability of the Patient with Ischemic Heart Disease. J Am Coll Cardiol 1989;14:1003-1044.

87. Haskell WL, Brachfeld N, Bruce RA, et al: Task force II: Determination of occupational working capacity in patients with ischemic heart disease. J Am Coll Cardiol 1989;14:1025-1034.

88. Blumenthal JA, Bradley W, Dimsdale JE: Task force III: Assessment of psychosocial status in patients with ischemic heart disease. J Am Coll Cardiol 1989;14:1034-1042.

Chapter 18

CURRENT AND FUTURE CARDIAC IMAGING TECHNIQUES IN ACUTE MYOCARDIAL INFARCTION

Brian D. Williamson
Andrew J. Buda

INTRODUCTION

With rapid evolution in the management of acute myocardial infarction (AMI) has come the need for progressively more sophisticated cardiac imaging modalities to better evaluate the outcome of therapy. It is now possible to measure noninvasively not only cardiac structure but also regional contractility, myocardial perfusion, and even metabolism on a clinical basis. Each of the diagnostic cardiac studies to be discussed in this chapter has inherent advantages and disadvantages, and the choice of study needs to be tailored to the individual clinical setting. Often, more than one imaging study will be necessary to obtain complementary information.

There are a wide variety of clinical situations in which cardiac imaging provides information vital to the management of the infarct patient. The assessment of ventricular function and residual ischemia, recognition of mechanical complications, development of clinical algorithms, and the identification of ischemic but viable myocardium represent a few such examples.

Ventricular function has been identified as an important predictor of survival post-infarction. Furthermore, a jeopardized blood supply to remaining myocardium places the infarct patient at high risk for future adverse cardiac events and requires a more aggressive approach. Several noninvasive measures of function and inducible ischemia are now available to evaluate these important clinical parameters.

The improved survival of patients since the introduction of coronary care units (CCUs) has changed the demographics of those who die early following an infarction. With successful therapy for ventricular dysrhythmias, mechanical complications such as myocardial rupture are now the second most common cause of early death, after cardiogenic shock due to massive myocardial necrosis. Early diagnosis of mechanical complications is readily made using cardiac imaging techniques, and prompt surgical intervention offers a favorable prognosis in otherwise fatal conditions.

The widespread use of thrombolytic therapy has decreased the mortality from infarction and has preserved myocardial function in survivors. Clinical algorithms remain to be developed to recognize those who fail thrombolytic therapy and to identify those who require additional interventional strategies. The diagnostic studies discussed in this chapter offer the capability of providing this information.

Perhaps the most exciting new prospect in the area of cardiac imaging is the potential to identify ischemic but viable myocardium and differentiate it from irreversibly infarcted tissue. This would allow identification of those in whom revascularization could salvage myocardium with limited existing perfusion, and improve functional recovery.

New technologies loom on the horizon, as well as new applications of established ones, which may add to the considerable armamentarium currently available to analyze myocardial structure, function and metabolism. The clinician must have a sound understanding of these diagnostic studies in order to maximize their application to clinical decision-making in the management of the patient with myocardial infarction.

ECHOCARDIOGRAPHY

Echocardiography remains an excellent imaging modality in the setting of AMI. It offers the advantages of widespread availability in most institutions, absence of radiation exposure to the patient or staff, low cost compared with other imaging techniques, and the potential for portable use in the CCU setting. Several studies have confirmed the utility of echocardiography in demonstrating and localizing regional left ventricular asynergy seen in myocardial infarction.[1,2] In addition to left ventricular myocardial infarction, echocardiography can also demonstrate right ventricular wall motion abnormalities suggesting right ventricular infarction. Furthermore, improvement in function following successful reperfusion may be detected by echocardiography. Echocardiography can also be used to detect mechanical complications of infarction, such as myocardial rupture or thrombus formation. Future use of echocardiographic techniques may be expanded to include ultrasonic characterization of tissue properties. These applications of echocardiography will be discussed individually and are summarized in Table 1.

Echocardiographic Assessment of Ventricular Function

In-hospital and long-term prognosis in patients with AMI correlates with location and extent of the infarct. Echocardiography can provide this information. Interruption of

Table 1. *Clinical uses of echocardiography in acute myocardial infarction*

Systolic function and regional wall motion abnormalities

Infarct extension (new necrosis)

Infarct expansion (dilation)

Aneurysm/Pseudoaneurysm

Myocardial rupture

Ventricular thrombus

Tissue characterization (experimental)

coronary flow promptly results in systolic wall motion abnormalities which can be easily imaged by two-dimensional echocardiography. One may see a failure of normal systolic wall thickening or actual thinning and paradoxical systolic bulging of the infarcted segment. Such wall motion abnormalities may be detected by echocardiography with up to 90% sensitivity.[1,2]

In 66 patients with their first Q wave myocardial infarction, Visser et al[3] found 62 had similar infarct localization by echocardiography and electrocardiography. They also found a good correlation (r = 0.87) between asynergic area and infarct size estimated by creatine kinase value (in the absence of reperfusion). Echocardiography may provide particularly useful information on infarct size and location in patients in whom limited information is available from the electrocardiogram, such as those with left bundle branch block or a permanent pacemaker. In addition, asynergy of the right ventricular wall may be detected, suggesting the diagnosis of right ventricular infarction. Right ventricular wall motion abnormalities have been seen in the setting of normal right-sided hemodynamics, suggesting that in some cases echocardiography may be more sensitive than hemodynamic measures in the diagnosis of right ventricular infarction.[4]

Although a relatively good correlation exists between wall motion abnormalities and infarct size, the functional abnormality imaged by two-dimensional echocardiography modestly overestimates the extent of necrosis because of a lateral tethering effect of the ischemic segments on the adjacent normal myocardium.[5-7] On the other hand, the actual area of necrotic myocardium would be no greater than the zone of dysfunction estimated by echocardiography.

While the diagnosis of AMI or the decision to admit to the CCU is usually made on the basis of clinical parameters other than echocardiography, two-dimensional echocardiography can nevertheless provide important prognostic information early in the hospital course. Horwitz et al[8] examined 80 patients with acute chest pain syndrome and found two-dimensional echocardiography to be a useful technique to stratify patients according to their subsequent clinical outcome. Thirty-one of 33 patients (94%) who proved to have an AMI had regional wall motion abnormalities on their initial echocardiogram. All the patients with normal two-dimensional echoes had an uneventful hospital course, while 10 of 36 patients with initial wall motion abnormalities had a complicated hospital stay. Other studies have confirmed that patients with significant myocardial dysfunction identified by echocardiography early following infarction are at several times higher risk for in-hospital complications than those with little or no functional impairment.[9,10] Thus, two-dimensional echocardiography may be useful in early identification of those patients at high risk of in-hospital morbidity or mortality who may benefit from more aggressive management.

Serial studies following infarction using echocardiography and nuclear techniques have shown that, in the absence of reperfusion, patients with significant initial functional abnormalities have only minor improvement in these abnormalities over time.[11] On the other hand, successful early reperfusion may result in demonstrable improvement in regional function. A number of studies have shown that successful reperfusion by thrombolysis, angioplasty, or a combination of the two can result in improved wall motion index scores.[12,13] However, while echocardiography may be useful to document improved regional function following successful reperfusion, it does not have sufficient specificity and sensitivity to accurately predict a patent infarct-related vessel. Other cardiac imaging techniques discussed later in this chapter may offer this capability.

Patients who experience extension of their myocardial infarction (new areas of myocardial necrosis, as opposed to infarct expansion, which involves thinning and dilation of the infarct zone without new necrosis) appear to have a worse prognosis than those without this complication. Traditionally, this diagnosis is made by a new rise in creatine kinase values and ECG changes. It is often difficult to identify those episodes of acute ischemia which represent infarct extension. Serial echocardiograms can identify infarct extension by new areas of wall motion abnormality, and echocardiography may be superior to electrocardiography in distinguishing acute ischemia from infarct extension.[14] As expected, those patients with worsening regional asynergy, with infarct extension following initial presentation, have a worse prognosis.

Infarct expansion, seen as thinning and dilation of the region of infarcted myocardium, is a mechanical complication of myocardial infarction associated with impaired hemodynamics, ventricular aneurysm formation, ventricular rupture and increased mortality.[15-17] It may result from stretching or slippage of adjacent myofibrils.[18]

Myocardial infarct expansion can be readily detected by two-dimensional echocardiography. Eaton et al[19] reported that in 28 patients with transmural myocardial infarction, 8 demonstrated transmural thinning and dilation of the infarcted region. In this study, patients with expansion had a significantly higher eight-week mortality (4 of 8 versus 0 of 20 patients without expansion). Recognition of this phenomenon is important, since early therapy to decrease heart load using nitroglycerin or angiotensin converting enzyme inhibitors may limit the extent of infarct expansion.[20,21]

True ventricular aneurysms are localized areas of ventricular wall dilation and bulging. They may result in impaired stroke volume leading to congestive heart failure, increased wall tension with increased oxygen demand, and refractory angina; they may also cause malignant ventricular dysrhythmias. Echocardiography can readily detect the presence of ventricular aneurysms following infarction[22] and can also predict aneurysm resectability.[23] Echocardiography can also differentiate true aneurysms from pseudoaneurysms.[24] Pseudoaneurysms are characterized by a narrow opening in the ventricular wall that communicates with a contained area in the pericardial space and represents in essence a limited myocardial rupture. Unlike true aneurysms, however, pseudoaneurysms are at high risk of free rupture into the pericardial space, leading to sudden death. Hence, early recognition of pseudoaneurysms and subsequent surgical repair is essential.

Echocardiographic Evaluation of Myocardial Rupture

Myocardial rupture now represents the second most common cause of early death in myocardial infarction, after cardiogenic shock. This diagnosis has usually been made at postmortem, and it continues to carry an extremely high mortality. The clinical challenge is to recognize myocardial rupture early enough to allow surgical intervention for an otherwise fatal complication.

Reddy and Roberts[25] examined the incidence of myocardial rupture in necropsy patients at the Pathology Branch of the National Heart, Lung, and Blood Institute following the introduction of CCUs in 1968. In 648 patients who died of fatal myocardial infarction (MI), 204 patients, or 31%, had cardiac rupture. The site of rupture was the left ventricular free wall in 137 patients (67%), the ventricular septum in 55 patients (27%), and both the left ventricular free wall and ventricular septum in 7 patients (4%). The left ventricular free wall and papillary muscle were involved in five patients (2%). The MILIS Study Group recently reported that of 849 patients enrolled in their database, documented rupture occurred in only 14 cases (1.7%).[26] Nevertheless, rupture accounted for 14% of the in-hospital deaths, which translates into an estimated 25,000 deaths per year in the United States.

Left Ventricular Free Wall Rupture

The most common time for myocardial rupture to occur is early in the course of infarction. In the MILIS study, 7 of 14 deaths from myocardial rupture occurred in the first two days following infarction, and a total of 10 occurred within the first four days following infarction. This complication may present with recurrent chest pain and

413

hemopericardium leading to cardiac tamponade with hemodynamic decompensation, electromechanical dissociation, and sudden death. However, patients may also have a subacute presentation with hypotension and cardiac tamponade. These patients may survive long enough to undergo echocardiography, which demonstrates a pericardial effusion with the characteristic echocardiographic features of tamponade, including right atrial and right ventricular collapse.[27,28] Unfortunately, only a minority of patients with free wall rupture present with subacute symptoms which allow time for surgical intervention. In the MILIS study, only one patient with free wall rupture had a subacute course which allowed diagnosis and successful surgical repair; nevertheless, this patient was in good health at two-year follow-up.

Ventricular Septal Rupture

Ventricular septal rupture tends to be better tolerated hemodynamically than free wall rupture. Although septal rupture is less common than free wall rupture, it nevertheless accounts for approximately 5% of the early in-hospital deaths from myocardial infarction, which translates into a yearly mortality of over 8,000 patients.[29]

Most often, ventricular septal rupture occurs as a complication of anteroseptal myocardial infarction. Early recognition is essential, because these patients may live long enough to undergo surgery if the diagnosis is made promptly. Without surgical intervention the mortality is 25% within 24 hours and 65% within two weeks.[30]

Clinically, patients suddenly develop a pansystolic murmur, which must be distinguished from acute mitral regurgitation due to papillary muscle injury. Fortunately, two-dimensional echocardiography provides a readily available, noninvasive means of diagnosis in the majority of cases, allowing direct visualization of the defect in the muscular septum. Several views may be utilized to visualize the septal defect, while angulation off-axis in each standard view may further improve detection.[31] The presence of necrotic and fibrotic tissue adjacent to the septal defect may enhance the contrast between the myocardial tissue and the defect, improving the detection capability.

Perforations in the septum may, however, take complex forms which are hard to detect by two-dimensional echocardiography. These appearances may include jagged linear lacerations, serpiginous tunnels between chambers, openings into the two ventricles at different planes, or multiple holes.[32] In this setting, the peripheral administration of a saline bolus provides echocardiographic contrast to demonstrate the presence of an interventricular shunt. With this procedure, a negative contrast effect in the right ventricle (displacement of bubbles in the right ventricle from the left to right shunt), and/or a positive contrast effect in the left ventricle (the presence of bubbles in the left ventricle) may be visualized, confirming the diagnosis. Drobac et al[33] reported the usefulness of contrast in demonstrating ventricular septal defects; of 13 patients with ventricular septal defects, 6 were imaged with two-dimensional echocardiography

414

alone. The administration of contrast yielded an additional 6 patients in whom a ventricular septal defect was found.

The addition of Doppler echocardiography may further improve sensitivity. Doppler sampling along the ventricular septum is performed in multiple views, as well as in the right ventricular chamber and outflow tract to demonstrate the abnormal left to right blood flow. Miyatake et al[34] documented septal rupture in 2 of 6 patients by two-dimensional echocardiography. An additional patient was diagnosed by contrast injection, whereas the remaining 3 patients required Doppler echocardiography to make the diagnosis. Several other studies have confirmed the utility of Doppler echocardiography in septal rupture.[35-40]

The development of color flow Doppler has provided an additional technique to aid in the diagnosis of acute ventricular septal defect complicating myocardial infarction. The addition of color allows immediate visualization of shunted blood and aids the echocardiographer in directing the Doppler sample volume to the proper location to characterize the flow pattern occurring from the interventricular shunt, as shown in Figure 1. A recent study has demonstrated the potential utility of color flow Doppler in the diagnosis of septal rupture.[40]

Papillary Muscle Rupture

Papillary muscle rupture can lead to acute mitral regurgitation and severe pulmonary edema. While it is less common than either free wall or ventricular septal rupture, it may still cause up to 5% of the acute mortality from myocardial infarction.[41] Untreated, papillary muscle rupture is associated with an 80-90% mortality rate. The majority of these patients develop an apical systolic murmur, which is classically loud, holosystolic, constant, and radiates to the axilla and back. The most common time of occurrence is 2-5 days post-myocardial infarction (with a mean of 4 days). Rupture occurs primarily in first-time infarctions, like other types of rupture. The entire trunk of the papillary muscle may rupture, with loss of support for half of the chordae tendineae to both mitral leaflets, resulting in severe mitral regurgitation and cardiogenic shock. Fortunately, it is more common for just one of the muscle heads to rupture, affecting fewer chordae, which is generally better hemodynamically tolerated but may still lead to significant pulmonary edema.

While the presence of a systolic murmur may suggest the possibility of papillary muscle rupture, a murmur may not be audible due to high left atrial pressures causing a fall in the transmitral pressure gradient.[42] In addition, the systolic murmur associated with papillary muscle rupture must be distinguished from that of a ventricular septal defect. Papillary muscle rupture may be recognized directly by echocardiography as diastolic fluttering of the flail leaflet, or the ruptured portion of the papillary muscle may be seen as a mass attached to the chordae, prolapsing into the left atrium during systole.[30,43,44]

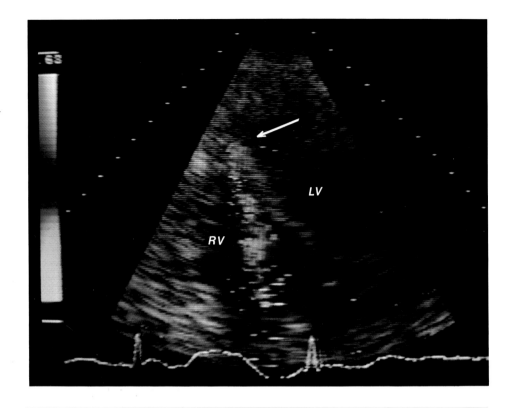

Figure 1. *Color-flow Doppler echocardiographic image in an off-axis longitudinal view showing the left to right shunt (in blue) due to a ventricular septal defect complicating an acute myocardial infarction. The septal defect is located near the apex in this patient. RV = right ventricle, LV = left ventricle, arrow denotes the septal defect.*

Doppler techniques complement two-dimensional echocardiography in evaluating the severe mitral regurgitation that accompanies papillary muscle rupture. Doppler sampling in the left atrium in the parasternal apical view can readily demonstrate the holosystolic regurgitation into the left atrium. In addition, in the unlikely occurrence of a concomitant ventricular septal defect and papillary muscle rupture, Doppler techniques can help distinguish the resultant jets of blood.[45] Early detection and prompt surgical intervention for ruptured papillary muscle following AMI is essential in order to reduce the high mortality when this complication is untreated.

Echocardiography and Left Ventricular Thrombus

The development of left ventricular thrombus is a relatively common event following AMI, particularly anterior Q wave infarcts.[46] Two-dimensional echocardiography allows direct visualization of regional asynergy and intramural thrombus with a 95% sensitivity and 86% specificity for ventricular thrombus.[47] The diagnosis is normally made when an echo-dense mass distinct from the endocardium is visualized in more than one view throughout the cardiac cycle, as shown in Figure 2. The incidence of thrombus formation is limited to Q wave infarction, particularly involving the anterior wall.[48] Jugdutt and Sivaram recently reported observations in 541 patients prospectively studied following their first myocardial infarction, with no evidence of thrombus formation at the first study.[49] None of these patients received thrombolytic therapy

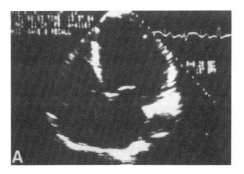

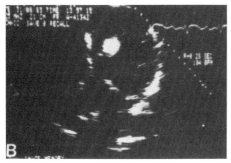 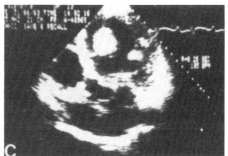

Figure 2. *A large pedunculated thrombus. This thrombus was not seen in the apical four chamber view (A), but was clearly visible after rotating the transducer (B and C). This thrombus was highly mobile and was associated with fatal embolism.*
Reproduced with permission from Jugdutt BI, Sivaram CA, Wortman C, Trudell C: Prospective two-dimensional echocardiographic evaluation of left ventricular thrombus and embolism after acute myocardial infarction. J Am Coll Cardiol 1989;13: 554-564.

during the study period. With serial studies, they found echocardiographic evidence of subsequent left ventricular thrombus in 21% of patients. The echocardiographic features associated with an increased risk of embolization were thrombus mobility, hyperkinesia of the adjacent myocardial wall (which contributes to thrombus mobility), and thrombus protrusion into the chamber in more than one view.[50,51] The incidence of embolism was greatest in the first month following infarction. In the Jugdutt study, the incidence of early embolism was 23% in patients with thrombus who were not adequately anticoagulated, whereas no embolism occurred in patients who were adequately anticoagulated. One might expect that thrombolytic therapy would further reduce the incidence of thrombus formation, either by improvement of ventricular function or by direct lytic activity. However, in one randomized trial, thrombolytic therapy did not reduce the incidence of thrombus formation below that seen in anticoagulated patients.[52]

Thus, two-dimensional echocardiography appears to be useful, not only in detecting ventricular thrombi, but also in identifying those at risk for systemic embolization. Since anticoagulation appears to prevent embolization of ventricular thrombus, echocardiography may prove to be a useful guide in identifying those patients requiring anticoagulation. Furthermore, serial echocardiograms allow the opportunity to follow the resolution of thrombus while on anticoagulation and may provide a guide for length of therapy. Nevertheless, the debate over the indications for anticoagulation continues; in a recent study of 53 patients with anterior myocardial infarctions treated with antiplatelet agents and subcutaneous heparin, 40 percent developed left ventricular thrombus, yet none of the patients developed systemic embolism, and in fact, the patients with mural thrombus had a lower morbidity and mortality than those without thrombus.[53] Based on these findings the authors argue for "masterly inactivity" in treating patients with ventricular thrombus. Additional prospective trials are needed to resolve the issue of the indications for and the duration of anticoagulation.

Tissue Characterization by Echocardiography

In addition to quantifying ventricular structure and function, echocardiography may also be used to provide ultrasonic characterization of cardiac muscle tissue properties which may provide further insight into physical changes after infarction and clinical implications for prognosis. Infarction results in pathological changes in myocardial physical properties which are reflected in ultrasonic indices of integrated back scatter.[54-56] These changes in ultrasonic properties appear to be directly related to the duration of ischemia and may be attenuated by reperfusion. A recent study in humans found depressed cyclic variation of integrated back-scatter following infarction, which recovered in reperfused infarct regions prior to any observed recovery of wall motion.[57] These findings suggest that such ultrasound indices may, in the future, have significant implications in the evaluation of therapeutic interventions.

418

Thus, a considerable amount of experience has been accumulated with echocardiographic imaging following AMI. Despite the many newer imaging modalities which have been developed, echocardiography continues to have widespread clinical applications.

PYROPHOSPHATE AND INFARCT SCINTIGRAPHY

Pyrophosphate Scintigraphy

As previously discussed, the size and location of the myocardial infarction have important prognostic and therapeutic implications.[58,59] Radiopharmaceuticals which localize to infarcted myocardium have provided valuable diagnostic tools for certain clinical settings. The most commonly used infarct-avid imaging modality is technetium-labeled pyrophosphate. Following intravenous injection, pyrophosphate binds to albumin and circulates to infarcted myocardium where it binds to calcium and deposits in infarcted myocardial cells.

Pyrophosphate imaging was first performed using planar techniques. However, problems with overlapping activity from other structures (such as sternum, chest wall, and breast) limited application to large transmural anterior myocardial infarctions. The development of tomographic imaging using single photon emission computed tomography (SPECT) has largely resolved this problem, allowing cross-sectional imaging of myocardium with the ability to localize areas of infarction distinct from overlapping structures. The amount of pyrophosphate uptake correlates well with the amount of actual tissue necrosis (Figure 3) and has a direct relationship to prognosis.[60,61] Pyrophosphate scintigraphy during the 2 to 3 days post-infarction has been shown to have up to a 95% sensitivity for transmural infarction and a 70-80% sensitivity in nontransmural infarction.[62] Depending on the threshold used for a positive test, the specificity ranges from 60-80%.

Pyrophosphate imaging can be useful in diagnosing myocardial infarction in several clinical situations. In patients who present with infarction after the peak release of creatine kinase, pyrophosphate scanning can confirm a diagnosis of recent infarction and indicate the severity of muscle necrosis. It may also be helpful in localizing the region of infarction in patients with an abnormal baseline ECG, such as a paced rhythm or left bundle branch block. In addition, it is a sensitive method to detect and localize perioperative infarction associated with coronary bypass.[63] The diagnosis of infarction in the perioperative period can be difficult to make: ST changes are nonspecific, and Q waves are often insensitive, while CK-MB levels may be nonspecifically elevated from surgical trauma or diffuse intraoperative myocardial ischemia.[64,65] On the other hand, while pyrophosphate scintigraphy detects infarcts which would not otherwise have been detected, routine use in uncomplicated bypass patients is not indicated, as the few additional infarcts diagnosed are small enough that their discovery would not affect therapy or prognosis.

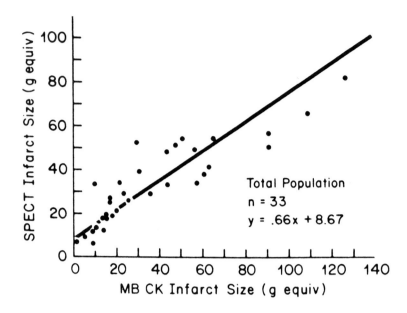

Figure 3. *Comparison of size of infarction determined by single photon-emission computed tomography (SPECT) using technetium-99 pyrophosphate and that by MB-CK analysis in patients with transmural myocardial infarctions.*
Reproduced with permission from Jansen DE, Corbett JR, Wolfe CL, et al: Quantification of myocardial infarction: A comparison of single photon-emission computed tomography with pyrophosphate to serial plasma MB-creatine kinase measurements. Circulation 1985;72:327-333.

A recent application of pyrophosphate scintigraphy is in the assessment of reperfusion following thrombolytic therapy.[66,67] It appears that strongly positive early scans correlate with a patent infarct-related vessel. Kondo et al[66] studied 29 patients who received thrombolytic therapy and found that a strongly positive early pyrophosphate scan had a 73% sensitivity and a 100% specificity for successful recanalization, with a positive predictive accuracy for reperfusion of 90%.

In addition to size, the pattern of pyrophosphate uptake may have prognostic significance. Rude et al[68] found that patients in whom pyrophosphate uptake resembled a doughnut (with intense peripheral uptake and decreased central uptake) had a much higher risk of left ventricular failure. Likewise, a persistently positive technetium pyrophosphate scintigram during a follow-up period of 11.6 months was found to correlate with a higher incidence of cardiac death, non-fatal recurrent myocardial infarction, unstable angina pectoris, or the development of congestive heart failure.[69]

Antimyosin Imaging

Monoclonal antibodies directed against myosin (antimyosin antibodies or AMA) have been radiolabeled with a number of radioisotopes for imaging infarcted myocardium. Potential advantages of this modality over pyrophosphate scanning include the absence of rib and sternal uptake and a more homogenous background activity, allowing for more dependable background subtraction. In addition, animal studies have shown that anti-myosin antibody imaging is less likely to overestimate infarct size compared with pyrophosphate.[70] Several groups have reported using indium-111 radiolabeled commercially available murine antimyosin antibody in patients with acute infarction. In one study of 57 patients, its clinical utility was compared with electrocardiogram, echocardiogram, technetium-99m pyrophosphate, and cardiac catheterization.[71] No patient had an adverse reaction from injection of antimyosin antibodies, and AMA infarct localization showed a good correlation with the other techniques. The sensitivity and specificity for infarction were 98% and 85%, respectively, and no uptake occurred in old infarctions. Another recent study used tomographic techniques (SPECT) to measure myocardial infarct size following injection of indium-111 anti-myosin antibody in 27 patients.[72] The indium-111 antimyosin infarct size correlated well with the thallium-201 perfusion defect, suggesting that AMA imaging may be useful in estimating the extent of myocardial damage.

One disadvantage of this technique is the potential for allergic reaction to the murine-derived monoclonal antibody. This has not proven to be a problem so far, although patients selected for clinical trials did not have a history of previous allergic reactions. Additional clinical trials are necessary to define the role of this modality, but it may become an extremely useful method for myocardial infarct detection, localization, and prognostication.

RADIONUCLIDE ANGIOGRAPHY

Radionuclide angiography allows noninvasive measurement of ventricular volumes, ejection fraction, and the quantification of global and regional wall motion. The availability of portable gamma cameras permits early imaging of infarct patients while still in the CCU. Numerous studies have established the prognostic significance of the left ventricular ejection fraction determined in the first 24 hours following myocardial infarction. Becker et al[73] found that infarct patients with an initial left ventricular ejection fraction of 35% or less had a six-month mortality of 60%, whereas patients with an ejection fraction greater than 35% had a six-month mortality of 11%. The multicenter post-infarction research group reported that in 866 patients studied from 1979 to 1980, the only risk factors which were independent predictors of mortality were ejection fraction below 40%, 10 or more premature ventricular depolarizations per hour, advanced New York Heart Association functional class prior to infarction, and evidence of rales (Figure 4).[74] Several other studies have confirmed the relationship between early ejection fraction and survival.

Serial measurements of left ventricular ejection fraction following discharge can help identify patients who are at risk for early morbidity and mortality. Patients with an initially low or falling ejection fraction over time are at higher risk for mortality than patients with a normal ejection fraction or those whose ejection fraction improves to normal over time.[75] Thus, resting radionuclide angiography may be used to identify those patients at increased risk of mortality who require closer follow-up, as well as those who are likely to do well and may increase their functional activities relatively quickly.

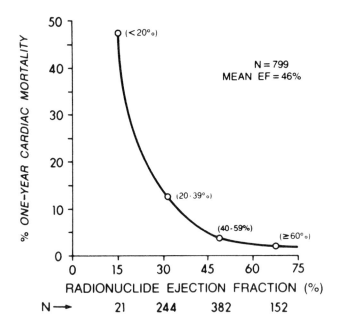

Figure 4. *Cardiac mortality rate in four categories of radionuclide ejection fraction (EF) determined before discharge. N denotes the number of patients in the total population and in each category. Of 811 patients in whom the ejection fraction was recorded, 12 were lost to follow-up during the first year after hospitalization.*
Reproduced with permission from The Multicenter Postinfarction Research Group: Risk stratification and survival after myocardial infarction. N Engl J Med 1983;309: 331-336.

First-pass radionuclide ventriculography may suggest right ventricular infarction by demonstrating right ventricular dilation, impaired ejection fraction, or abnormal wall motion. Patients with inferior or posterior myocardial infarction often have concomitant involvement of the right ventricle. Right ventricular infarction may be associated with clinically significant hypotension, particularly in the setting of hypovolemia or nitrate therapy. However this suspicion is best confirmed with hemodynamic correlates from right heart catheterization.[76,77]

While a resting radionuclide ventriculogram reflects the extent of previous myocardial injury and remaining functional myocardium, an exercise radionuclide ventriculogram can indicate viable myocardium with insufficient coronary flow reserve. Corbett et al[78] performed submaximal exercise radionuclide ventriculograms in 117 patients within two to three weeks after AMI. No complications resulted from the submaximal exercise testing. Using multivariate analysis of scintigraphic variables, they found that change in left ventricular ejection fraction and end systolic volume were the most important in predicting future cardiac events (death, recurrent myocardial infarction, unstable angina or heart failure). The accuracy in predicting cardiac events from an abnormal change with exercise in left ventricular ejection fraction or end systolic volume was 93% and 91%, respectively.[78] Exercise testing post-infarction will be discussed further in the section on myocardial perfusion imaging.

Radionuclide ventriculography can indicate the presence of left ventricular aneurysms. It is most reliable for detecting apical and anterior aneurysms, where most aneurysms occur. It is less sensitive for detecting less common posterobasal aneurysms.[79] Radionuclide angiography may also suggest the presence of a left ventricular pseudoaneurysm. As previously mentioned, the pseudoaneurysm occurs as a consequence of rupture of the myocardium into the pericardial sac. The extent of the rupture is limited, preventing the development of tamponade. The pseudoaneurysm has a narrow neck which opens into a larger cavity, the wall of which is composed of fibrous and necrotic tissue. A first pass study, in which a bolus of radiopharmaceutical is given and images are rapidly acquired within a few seconds as the bolus travels through the pulmonary circulation and then the left heart, is the primary scintigraphic method for detecting a pseudoaneurysm, since filling of the left ventricle proper precedes the filling of the pseudoaneurysm. By contrast, a true aneurysm fills at the same time as the remaining left ventricle during a first pass study.

Quantitative radionuclide angiography also is useful for determining the ratio of pulmonary to systemic blood flow. This calculation allows the determination of left to right shunts. In the setting of AMI, a left to right shunt suggests an acute ventricular septal defect.[80] Echocardiography, however, is more useful in demonstrating the precise location of the septal defect, especially when used in conjunction with contrast, Doppler, or color flow techniques, as previously discussed.

MYOCARDIAL PERFUSION IMAGING
Thallium-201

Another radionuclide technique which has demonstrated considerable cardiac application is myocardial perfusion imaging. The radiopharmaceutical best known for this use is thallium-201. Thallium, a metallic element in the III A group in the periodic table, shares many properties with potassium in biological systems, such as uptake by Na-K ATPase. While the uptake of radiolabeled thallium parallels that of radiolabeled potassium, imaging quality is better with thallium. Animal studies have shown that thallium is quickly taken up from the bloodstream into myocardial tissue, allowing imaging within a few minutes of injection. The uptake of thallium is proportional to regional perfusion in situations of normal or decreased flow. In the setting of reactive hyperemia, the uptake of thallium is augmented, although at extremes this relationship is no longer linear.[81]

Thallium-201 scintigraphy is a sensitive technique for diagnosing and localizing acute infarction. Wackers et al[82] reported in 1976 that in a series of 96 patients with AMI imaged during the first 24 hours, 90 were positive. Earlier in the course of infarction the sensitivity of thallium was even greater; in 44 patients who had thallium scans within the first six hours after the onset of symptoms, all were positive. The extent of the thallium defect diminishes over time, either because of subsequent reperfusion or other mechanisms which improve regional perfusion. Postmortem studies have shown thallium to be more accurate than the ECG in determining infarct location.[83]

In the past, the two-dimensional nature of planar thallium scintigraphy posed a limitation due to tissue overlap in different planes. The development of tomographic imaging of thallium uptake has improved the utility of this technique. Single photon emission computed tomography (SPECT) provides a three-dimensional view of the myocardium, with better resolution of perfusion defects. Fintel et al[84] recently reported that in 112 patients in whom both planar and SPECT imaging were performed, SPECT was more accurate over a range of decision thresholds in the detection and localization of perfusion defects. Computerized quantitative techniques which have the potential to define more precisely the location and size of infarction are under development. Such quantitative definition of perfusion defects will probably become routine in the future. Although visual analysis of thallium images by trained interpreters will remain important, quantitative measures of perfusion defects will limit inter- and intra-observer variability and provide a more precise measure of treatment interventions both clinically and experimentally.[85-87]

Thallium imaging may provide quantitative information concerning the extent of myocardial injury. A recent study compared infarct size determined by SPECT thallium imaging with that estimated by plasma creatine kinase-MB activity in 30 patients.[88] None of these patients had received therapy to restore infarct vessel patency (since reperfusion affects the enzyme levels measured). A good correlation was found between scintigraphic and enzymatic estimate of infarct size (Figure 5), which was stronger in anterior than inferior infarctions (r = 0.91 versus 0.50). The lesser correlation in inferior infarctions was attributed to the contribution of creatine kinase from right ventricular necrosis, which often accompanies inferior infarctions.

Thallium imaging may also be useful in evaluating the success of thrombolytic therapy. Several studies have demonstrated that following successful thrombolysis, regional myocardial thallium-201 uptake improves.[89-91] However, care must be taken in the interpretation of thallium findings in the setting of reperfusion. Myocardial blood flow is dynamic, with well recognized post-ischemic hyperemia following reperfusion. This may result in transient thallium overestimation of blood flow, despite the presence of myocardial necrosis, if thallium is given at the time of reperfusion. On the other hand, residual critical coronary stenoses may limit post-perfusion flow, and thallium washout may vary considerably during early reperfusion. Thus,

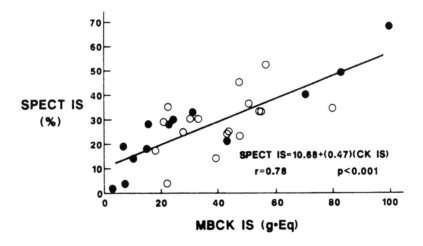

Figure 5. *Linear regression analysis comparing SPECT thallium and enzymatic estimates of infarct size for all patients. IS = infarct size; filled circles = anterior infarction; empty circles = inferior infarction*
Reproduced with permission from Mahmarian JJ, Pratt CM, Borges-Neto S, et al: Quantification of infarct size by thallium-201 single-photon emission computed tomography during acute myocardial infarction in humans: Comparison with enzymatic estimates. Circulation 1988;78:831-839.

thallium activity may be highly dependent on the timing of the administration of thallium in relation to reflow.[92]

Another potential limitation to the use of thallium for determining successful thrombolysis is the "no-reflow" phenomenon. In this situation, prolonged ischemia may result in myocardial cell or microvascular injury, which impairs reperfusion on a local tissue level despite a patent epicardial vessel and normal contrast runoff at angiography.[93] In addition, because thallium redistributes over time, a pretreatment imaging study should be performed immediately before thrombolytic therapy is given. Since this would delay therapy, in practice, pretreatment studies are often omitted. Thus, thallium imaging has several limitations for use in evaluating the efficacy of thrombolytic therapy, which has prompted investigations into other imaging agents.

Technetium-99m Isonitrile

An exciting new type of perfusion radiopharmaceutical, technetium-99m isonitrile, has several advantages over thallium imaging. Technetium-99m methoxy isobutyl isonitrile (MIBI) is one agent in this class. MIBI has low uptake in lung and liver, which improves image resolution, and unlike thallium, it does not redistribute after transient ischemia. Once the agent is given, imaging can be delayed if necessary, without resulting in a change in image with time. To evaluate flow at a different time, another injection can be given once radioactivity has worn off, a different radioisotope may be used, or computer subtraction techniques may be used. In addition to better image resolution and shorter imaging times, the more intense emission allows concomitant wall motion analysis by electrocardiogram (ECG)-gated imaging acquisition.

Because no redistribution occurs with these agents, the tracer can be given prior to thrombolytic therapy, and imaging may be delayed until a more convenient time without interfering with the administration of thrombolytic therapy. This initial pretreatment study can then be compared with subsequent post-therapy studies to assess the success of thrombolytic therapy. Wackers et al[94] examined the ability of planar technetium-99 isonitrile imaging to assess the success of thrombolytic therapy. Patients with acute infarction were treated with recombinant tissue-plasminogen activator (rt-PA) and injected with technetium-99 isonitrile at or shortly before the administration of thrombolytic therapy. Because technetium-99 MIBI does not redistribute, images which were obtained several hours later still represented the area of myocardium at risk pre-therapy. Technetium-99 isonitrile injection and imaging were repeated at 18-48 hours and 6-24 days later to define the final area of infarction. Patients successfully reperfused had, on average, a 50% decline in technetium-99 isonitrile defect size. All patients successfully reperfused had at least a 30% reduction in defect (Figure 6). There was also an inverse relationship between the pre-discharge ejection fraction and the size of the initial technetium-99 isonitrile defect.

THROMBOLYSIS

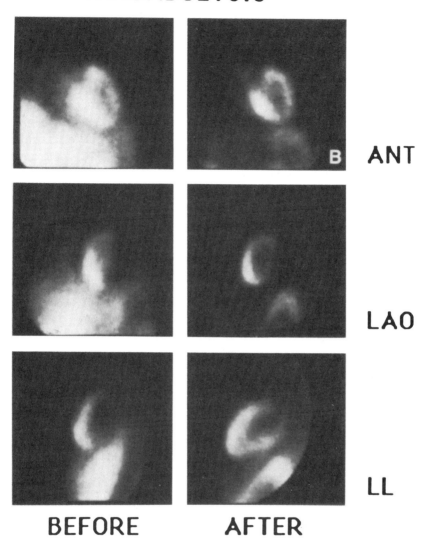

Figure 6. *Serial technetium-99m isonitrile imaging during thrombolysis in the anterior (ANT), left anterior oblique (LAO), and left lateral (LL) views. These views are from a patient with acute inferolateral myocardial infarction and successful reperfusion of the infarct-related artery. The total three view defect size integral was 49 before thrombolytic treatment and 28 after thrombolysis, yielding a 42% change in defect size.*
Reproduced with permission from Wackers FJT, Gibbons RJ, Verani MS, et al: Serial quantitative planar technetium-99 isonitrile imaging in acute myocardial infarction: Efficacy for noninvasive assessment of thrombolytic therapy. J Am Coll Cardiol 1989;14:861-873.

In addition to the considerable research potential which this agent appears to have for interventional trials, it may also have significant clinical applications. Patients with acute infarctions could receive technetium-99 isonitrile at the time of presentation and then be scanned within the next few hours after receiving thrombolytic therapy. Those patients found to have small initial defects would be at low risk and could be treated conservatively. Patients with large initial defects would be at a high risk and would have repeat post-treatment imaging to assess the efficacy of thrombolysis. Those patients with large initial defects which did not decrease significantly would be assumed to have failed reperfusion and could be considered for triage to invasive techniques for "rescue." Clearly data to address these issues are scant, and more research will need to be done in this area.

Pre-Discharge Stress Testing

Exercise testing following myocardial infarction can provide important prognostic information. Patients with AMI are at increased risk of further cardiac events, which most commonly occur within several weeks of infarction. The utility and safety of predischarge exercise testing to identify those at higher risk of cardiac events has been established.[95-97] Evidence of post-infarction ischemia such as exercise induced ST depression, angina, or poor exercise tolerance on pre-discharge submaximal exercise stress tests has been associated with an increased risk of future cardiac events.[95] The addition of thallium imaging to exercise testing improves the sensitivity. Thallium images predictive of a low risk of future cardiac events are characterized by a single region thallium defect without redistribution or increased lung uptake. Thallium findings associated with high risk include thallium defects in more than one region, evidence of delayed redistribution, and increased lung uptake. Gibson et al[96] performed thallium scintigraphy and coronary angiography in 140 consecutive patients and found a low risk thallium scan was more predictive of a good prognosis than either ST depression or angiography. Also, thallium scintigraphy was more sensitive in detecting patients at increased risk than either exercise ECG changes or coronary angiography, as shown in Figure 7.

After successful thrombolysis, a significant residual coronary stenosis is often present which may be at risk of reocclusion. These lesions may be detected by thallium scintigraphy by demonstrating an exercise-induced defect with redistribution at rest. A recent study reported that an exercise thallium study can be safely performed as early as the third hospital day following reperfusion therapy in uncomplicated patients and is predictive of subsequent in-hospital complications.[97] In 40 patients with a negative exercise thallium, none had an in-hospital complication, while 4 of 14 patients with a positive stress thallium went on to extend their infarction or develop post-infarction angina or ventricular tachycardia. Thus, exercise thallium can be used

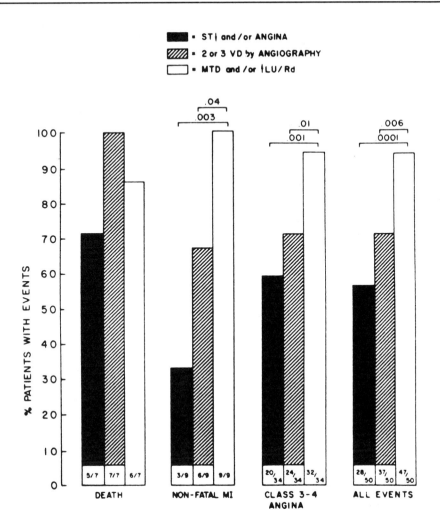

Figure 7. *Sensitivity of exercise test, angiographic, and thallium-201 scintigraphic findings for identifying postinfarction patients who died, experienced reinfarction, or developed NYHA class III or IV angina pectoris. VD = vessel disease; MTD = thallium defects involving multiple vascular regions; LU = lung uptake of thallium-201; Rd = redistribution. See text for further explanation.*

Reproduced with permission from Gibson RS, Watson DD, Craddock GB, et al: Prediction of cardiac events after uncomplicated myocardial infarction: a prospective study comparing predischarge exercise thallium-201 scintigraphy and coronary angiography. Circulation 1983;68:321-336.

safely following infarction to distinguish those at low risk, who may advance their activity and be discharged early, from those with residual ischemia, who are at high risk of further cardiac events and may require more aggressive management. In patients who are unable to exercise, dipyridamole thallium imaging offers another method to identify those at risk for future events.[98,99] Although some patients may experience angina, this study is generally tolerated without serious complications. A recent report compared the prognostic utility of predischarge dipyridamole thallium imaging to submaximal exercise electrocardiography (without thallium imaging) in 40 patients who had not previously received thrombolytic therapy or coronary bypass surgery.[100] Redistribution was commonly seen in the region of infarction and was not predictive of subsequent cardiac events. However, redistribution *outside* the region of infarction was as sensitive for cardiac events (63%), and had improved specificity (75%) over using *any* redistribution as a criterion for a positive test. The negative predictive values for further cardiac events of dipyridamole thallium and submaximal exercise electrocardiography were both 88 percent. Thus a dipyridamole thallium showing redistribution in regions outside the infarct zone is a relatively sensitive and specific indication of a significant risk for further cardiac events post-infarction. It is a useful test for patients who are unable to exercise, and it can identify those who are at high risk who should undergo coronary angiography and consideration for revascularization.

POSITRON EMISSION TOMOGRAPHY

Positron emission tomography currently holds the unique distinction of being the only imaging modality which allows correlation of regional blood flow with myocardial metabolism. Positron-emitting radionuclides such as ^{11}C, ^{13}N, ^{15}O, and ^{18}F are cyclotron-generated and incorporated into biologically active molecules. These radionuclides decay by emitting pairs of photons, 180 degrees apart, which are simultaneously counted by paired scintillation detectors. Radioactivity emitted is proportional to radionuclide uptake into tissue and is measured tomographically. Computerized tomography allows generation of transverse sections of the local emission profile in the organ of interest. Considerable experience has been accumulated with various tracers measuring blood flow and metabolism, as shown in Table 2.[101] Regional blood flow has been measured using ^{15}O, ^{82}Rb, and ^{13}N ammonia. More importantly, concomitant substrate utilization can also be measured. ^{18}F-2-fluoro-2-deoxyglucose (FDG) can serve as a useful measure of glucose utilization. In moderate ischemia, with a relative absence of sufficient oxygen, lactate production is accelerated, resulting in acceleration of glucose uptake and more intense FDG imaging. ^{11}C-labeled palmitate can be used as a measure of fatty acid metabolism, while ^{11}C acetate serves to quantify activity of the tricarboxylic acid (Krebs) cycle. In contrast to moderate ischemia, there

Table 2. *Tracers used in cardiac positron emission tomography*

BLOOD FLOW

^{13}N ammonia

^{15}O water

^{82}Rb

SUBSTRATE UTILIZATION

Glucose:
^{18}F 2-deoxyglucose

Fatty acids:
^{11}C palmitate

Krebs cycle: (oxygen consumption)
^{11}C acetate

Adapted from Schelbert[101]

is a matched absence of both blood flow and metabolic activity in irreversibly infarcted tissue.

PET and Infarct Localization

Initial clinical studies using PET demonstrated reliability in localizing and quantifying infarctions by diminished regional perfusion and metabolic activity as measured by uptake of ^{11}C palmitate substrate.[102] In fact, PET scanning may have some advantage over thallium or technetium imaging in demonstrating small infarcts in patients in whom ECG changes or cardiac enzymes are nondiagnostic. Geltman et al[103] reported that in 22 patients with Q wave myocardial infarctions, all had homogeneously depressed accumulation of ^{11}C palmitate in a region of their transmural infarction. In patients with non-Q wave myocardial infarctions, while only 61 percent had abnormal thallium scintigrams, 96 percent had abnormalities in the uptake of ^{11}C palmitate. In those patients with non-Q wave infarctions, the uptake of palmitate was frequently manifested as thinning in the zone of infarction.

PET and Tissue Viability

The application of PET scanning in acute infarction which offers the most exciting potential is in distinguishing irreversibly infarcted myocardium from potentially viable myocardium. Marshall et al[104] studied 15 patients with recent myocardial infarction using ^{18}F 2-deoxyglucose (FDG) as a measure of glucose metabolism and ^{13}N ammonia as a measure of myocardial perfusion in 19 areas of documented infarction. Fourteen had concordant diminished glucose uptake and tissue perfusion; however, in another 11 regions glucose utilization was relatively increased in the setting of decreased perfusion, consistent with anaerobic metabolism. These regions were defined as having a mismatch between blood flow and metabolism, suggesting areas which were ischemic but viable. These findings corresponded with clinical evidence of ischemia by electrocardiogram, post-infarction angina, and reversible regional wall motion abnormalities. In a subsequent study to evaluate the clinical significance of the mismatch between anaerobic metabolism and regional blood flow, Tillisch et al[105] studied 17 patients before and after coronary artery bypass surgery. They found that regions with abnormal wall motion and PET images showing on-going glucose metabolism had improvement in wall motion after revascularization, whereas regions with wall motion abnormalities and impaired glucose uptake had no improvement in wall motion after revascularization. They were able to correctly predict reversible wall motion abnormalities with 85% accuracy and those which were irreversible with 92% accuracy.

Thus, positron emission tomography has the potential to determine whether areas with poor or absent blood flow may be salvaged with revascularization. The traditional measurement of tissue viability has been thallium imaging, based on the premise that reversible thallium defects on delayed imaging indicate ischemic but viable tissue, while fixed defects on 3 to 4 hour delayed images indicate non-viable tissue. However, it has been shown that despite persistent defects on exercise and rest thallium imaging, tissue function may return once revascularized by either PTCA or CABG.[106,107] Preservation of glucose metabolism was demonstrated by PET in 47% of fixed thallium defects and in 65% of partially reversible thallium defects.[108] These findings suggest that persistent thallium defects may overestimate irreversibly infarcted tissue and that positron emission tomography may be a better measure of potentially viable tissue.

As further evidence of the potential of PET in evaluating tissue viability, Schwaiger et al[109] studied 13 patients with AMI within three days of the onset of symptoms using ^{18}F deoxyglucose and ^{13}N ammonia to measure glucose metabolism and regional blood flow, respectively. Regional blood flow measured by ammonia uptake was depressed in 32 myocardial segments; 16 of these segments demonstrated a matched decrease in glucose metabolism. In these matched segments, regional function did not improve when re-examined an average of six weeks later. However, the remaining 16 segments with depressed ammonia uptake had continued ^{18}F deoxyglucose uptake, suggesting remaining viable tissue. These patients had a variable outcome; 8 demonstrated improvement of wall motion, 6 had no change in wall motion over time, and in 2, wall motion worsened over time. Thus, the findings in this study suggest that patients with a matched defect in blood flow and metabolism have irreversible myocardial injury, while patients with mismatched glucose metabolism in the absence of perfusion may benefit from aggressive measures to salvage remaining viable tissue post-infarction (Figure 8).

Although the development of, or lack of Q waves following infarction does not necessarily correspond to pathologic transmural or nontransmural infarctions, the absence of Q wave development following infarction suggests a smaller amount of

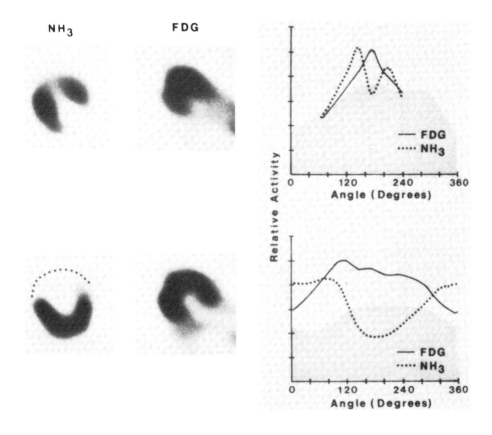

Figure 8. *Cross-sectional images after administration of ^{13}N ammonia (NH_3) and ^{18}F deoxyglucose (FDG) 40 hours after the onset of symptoms. The two consecutive planes through the left ventricle are displayed. There is decreased ^{13}N ammonia uptake in the anterior segments of the left ventricle and the ^{18}F deoxyglucose images reveal increased glucose utilization in these segments with decreased flow. The respective circumferential profiles of relative ^{13}N and ^{18}F activity distribution show a clear mismatch of tracer uptake from 80 to 280 degrees ("PET viability"). The shaded areas represent values more than two standard deviations below the normal mean.*
Reproduced with permission from Schwaiger M, Brunken R, Grover-McKay M, et al: Regional myocardial metabolism in patients with acute myocardial infarction assessed by positron emission tomography. J Am Coll Cardiol 1986;8:800-808.

injury. Nevertheless, it is widely felt that patients with non-Q wave infarctions are at risk for additional tissue infarction. This is demonstrated by the more frequent appearance of segmental ^{18}F deoxyglucose uptake in infarcted regions in patients with non-Q wave infarctions, consistent with residual viable myocardium.[110]

In the future, PET scanning may be used commonly following myocardial infarction to identify those patients in whom a large area of ischemic but potentially viable tissue remains, who may be candidates for revascularization.

PET Evaluation of Reperfusion Therapy

To evaluate the ability of PET scanning to evaluate the success of reperfusion therapy, Sobel et al[111] performed positron emission tomography with ^{11}C palmitate in 19 patients immediately on presentation of the first transmural infarction and again within 48 to 72 hours after thrombolytic therapy. There was no change in PET scans over a three day period in 8 patients who failed thrombolysis. In each of the 11 patients in whom thrombolysis was successful, the myocardial accumulation of ^{11}C palmitate improved on average 29 percent from the early to the late study. Thus, PET demonstrated that successful thrombolysis was associated with improved regional myocardial metabolism. Future PET studies of patients following thrombolytic therapy will undoubtedly provide additional insights into appropriate clinical management algorithms. For the interested reader, excellent comprehensive reviews of the clinical applications of PET in myocardial ischemia have recently been published.[101,112]

COMPUTED TOMOGRAPHIC SCANNING

Experimental studies have reported that x-ray computed tomography can distinguish infarcted myocardium from normal tissue without requiring contrast infusion, due to radiodensity changes related to edema. However, this distinction has been made infrequently in human studies, except when calcification occurs in the region of infarction. This may be due to resolution limitations as a consequence of cardiac motion. A negative filling defect in the region of infarction is commonly seen within a few minutes after contrast infusion. Once contrast enhancement of normal tissue has washed out, late enhancement of the infarct region sometimes occurs. This was first reported in animal studies, which found the ratio of iodine in infarcted myocardium was 8.5 times that of normal tissue at three hours after contrast infusion.[113] However, human studies have less frequently demonstrated late contrast enhancement of infarcted tissue. This may be due to the much higher concentration of contrast used in animal studies, or alternatively, to the greater collaterals present in dogs, which were used as the animal model.[114]

Computed tomography can also detect post-infarction ventricular wall thinning, which is postulated to occur due to wall stretch or loss of necrotic tissue that occurs with the healing process. Due to the slice angle of the CT exam, thinning is best visualized in anterior or apical wall infarctions. Although a number of simpler techniques can be used as previously discussed, ventricular aneurysms can also be readily imaged by CT (with or without contrast infusion). In a study by Masuda et al, 39 of 103 infarct patients were found to have anterior or apical ventricular aneurysms.[114] Contrast-enhanced CT may be better than echocardiography for detecting left ventricular mural thrombi, which are recognized as filling defects in the ventricular chamber. In the study by Masuda et al, 20 patients were found to have left ventricular thrombi by CT, yet only 13 had definite echocardiographic criteria for left ventricular thrombus.[114] Of the remaining 7, 2 had a suggestion of thrombus by echocardiography, while in the remaining 5, no thrombi could be demonstrated by echocardiography. Pericardial effusions and pericardial calcifications have also been detected easily by conventional non-enhanced CT. Figure 9 illustrates typical CT findings following myocardial infarction.

Improvements in cine computed tomography now allow imaging of 8mm sections at 17 frames per second (51 msec per image). Animal studies have shown that cine computed tomography is capable of precise measurements of right and left ventricular volumes and stroke volumes which correlate well with invasive measures of cardiac output.[115] Cine computed tomography has also been used for quantitative assessment of left ventricular wall thickening in response to various drug interventions.[116] With more rapid acquisition capabilities, more precise evaluation of wall motion abnormalities by cine CT will be possible, although further studies will be necessary to define its role in clinical practice. However, cine CT may prove helpful in cases where other imaging modalities are inadequate — for example, in obese patients or those on mechanical ventilators in whom echocardiography is inadequate.

Nuclear Magnetic Resonance Imaging

Recently, considerable attention has focused on magnetic resonance imaging (MRI) of cardiac structures, due to the absence of either ionizing radiation or the need for contrast media. In addition to the ability of MRI to image gross structural and functional features of the myocardium with high resolution, it may also be capable of characterizing tissue properties.

Magnetic resonance imaging of the thorax and heart produces varying signal intensities from different tissues. Bone, calcified structures, flowing blood and air produce little or no signal intensity and appear as dark structures. Subcutaneous and epicardial fat produce high signal intensity, and vascular and myocardial tissues produce an intermediate signal intensity. The high contrast that results between myocar-

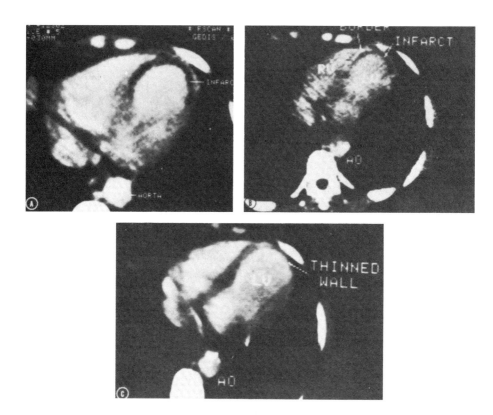

Figure 9. *(A) Contrast-enhanced computed transmission tomography (CTT) obtained 5 days after infarction, at the completion of contrast infusion, showing a transmural crescent of unenhanced myocardium involving the septal, anterior, and lateral walls of the left ventricle and extending into the free wall of the right ventricle. (B) CTT image obtained 20 minutes after the image in A, showing a smaller area of abnormal myocardium and the appearance of a bright halo at the infarct border. (C) Image obtained 3 months after infarction in the same patient, showing disappearance of contrast-poor myocardium and thinning of the infarcted wall.*
Reproduced with permission from Kramer PH, Goldstein JA, Herkins RJ, Lipton MJ, Brundage BH: Imaging of acute myocardial infarction in man with contrast-enhanced computed transmission tomography. Am Heart J 1984;108:1514-1523.

dium and the blood filled cavity, and the myocardium and epicardial fat and surrounding lungs, leads to precise definition of endocardial and epicardial borders (Figure 10). Thus, left ventricular wall thickness and thickening dynamics can be measured.

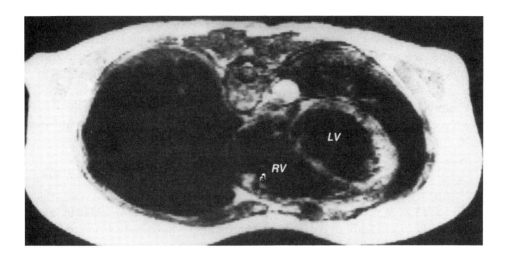

Figure 10. *Noncontrast end-diastolic gated magnetic resonance image taken in transverse section through the heart demonstrating the high contrast between moving blood and myocardium and the surrounding lung parenchyma in a patient with coronary artery disease and normal ventricular function.*
Reproduced with permission from Dilworth LR, Aisen AM, Mancini GBJ, et al: Determination of left ventricular volumes and ejection fraction by nuclear magnetic resonance imaging. Am Heart J 1987;113:24-32.

Magnetic Resonance Imaging in AMI

Magnetic resonance imaging can demonstrate segmental wall motion abnormalities following myocardial infarction, which correlate well with those demonstrated by echocardiographic and ventriculographic studies.[117-119] A recent study confirmed that abnormalities of regional systolic wall thickening in experimental animals and in humans correlate well with wall motion abnormalities assessed by ventriculography.[120] Furthermore, MR determination of ejection fraction also correlates well with systolic function by echocardiography or left ventriculography.[121]

Magnetic resonance imaging may also prove to be useful in the assessment of tissue properties of the infarcted region and potential changes following reperfusion. MRI can uniquely assess tissue characterization by the proton relaxation parameters T1 (spin-lattice relaxation time) and T2 (spin-spin relaxation time). These relaxation parameters vary with the type of tissue and its biophysical and biochemical milieu. During ischemia and reperfusion, changes in tissue lipid and, particularly, tissue water produce increases in T1 and T2. These alterations in T1 and T2 alter image intensity in a complex manner. Animal studies suggest that proton MRI distinguishes hypoperfused and infarcted myocardium from normal myocardium but overestimates the actual infarct size.[122] The area of infarction appears as increased signal intensity on the MRI images and most likely reflects regional edema associated with tissue necrosis. Experimental studies using paramagnetic contrast agents suggest that these agents may be useful in detecting acute regional myocardial perfusion abnormalities.[123]

A number of recent studies have demonstrated that proton MRI imaging can detect myocardial ischemia and infarction in man.[124-126] However, until recently, the greater expense of magnetic resonance imaging, prolonged acquisition times, and interference by the magnetic field with the function of certain electronic devices such as pacemakers, mechanical ventilators, and infusion pumps have limited the application of MRI for the routine assessment of wall motion abnormalities or ventricular volumes. One recent study examined the feasibility of obtaining MRIs within the first 24 hours of chest pain while in the CCU.[127] Monitoring facilities were arranged in the MR imaging suite to allow the same level of safety as would be available in the standard CCU. Complete studies were obtained within 30 minutes, and no patient developed complications while in the imaging suite; 16 of 18 patients had technically adequate MRI images, and 13 demonstrated increased signal intensity in the infarcted region. Wall motion abnormalities also corresponded well with two-dimensional echocardiography and contrast angiography. Using analysis of signal intensity and wall thickness, the sensitivity, specificity, and accuracy for diagnosing the region of the infarction were 93, 80, and 87% respectively. Of interest, no significant change in the relative intensity of infarcted myocardium occurred between 4 and 12 days post-infarction, suggesting that regional myocardial edema following myocardial infarction persists throughout the initial in-hospital period.[128]

Magnetic resonance imaging may also prove useful in demonstrating myocardial reperfusion. Infarct signal intensity in the T-2 images increases following successful reperfusion. Therefore changes in magnetic resonance relaxation parameters may help determine the success of reperfusion therapy in a noninvasive fashion. Further clinical studies will be necessary to examine this clinical problem.

Phosphorus magnetic resonance spectroscopy

Another area in which magnetic resonance techniques may have considerable application in the future is in the measurement of high energy phosphates by P-31 NMR spectroscopy. This technique allows measurement of myocardial pH, phosphocreatine, adenosine triphosphate, and inorganic phosphate levels in a variety of conditions. P-31 MRI can show a significant reduction in high-energy phosphate stores following myocardial ischemia and infarction.[129] The ability to measure phosphate stores has potential application in measuring the extent of injury from infarction as well as the response to intervention. Recent animal studies have suggested that P-31

MRI can distinguish normal from reperfused infarcted as well as reperfused but viable myocardium based upon their phosphorus-31 spectroscopy (Figure 11).[123,130] Phosphorus spectroscopy has been largely limited to animal models thus far because of technical considerations. However, initial studies in man demonstrate the feasibility of this technique.[131] With further technological improvements, phosphorus spectroscopy will likely expand the evaluation of myocardial tissue properties into previously unexamined areas.

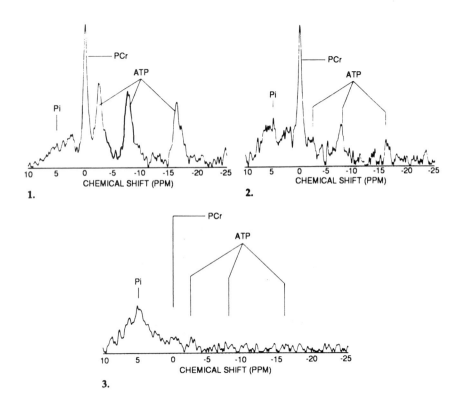

Figure 11. *P-31 MR spectra of risk-zone myocardium. (1) Before coronary occlusion. (2) Reperfused-viable group, after reperfusion. (3) Reperfused-infarcted group, after reperfusion. The spectra are displayed with identical scaling. PCr = creatine phosphate; Pi = inorganic phosphate; ATP = adenosine triphosphate; PPM = parts per million*
Reproduced with permission from Rehr RB, Tatum JL, Hirsch JI, et al: Reperfused-viable and reperfused-infarcted myocardium: Differentiation with in vivo P-31 MR spectroscopy. Radiology 1989;172:53-58.

CONCLUSION

Many advances have occurred in noninvasive cardiac imaging which offer the potential for increasingly sophisticated evaluation of myocardial structures, function, and metabolism. Table 3 attempts to summarize the current applications of the common modalities to various clinical questions. As emphasized at the beginning of this chapter, the use of a given study should be individualized to the clinical setting, and some patients may require several studies for proper management. More clinical experience with the newer imaging modalities is necessary for a clearer understanding of their role in routine evaluation. Future advances in cardiac imaging promise to have an impact on not only clinical management, but also on the basic understanding of acute ischemic heart disease.

Table 3. Comparison of imaging techniques in acute myocardial infarction

	Echo-cardiography	RNA	Technetium	Thallium	CT	PET	NMR
Diagnosis	Good	Good	Excellent	Excellent	Good	Good	Good
Infarct Size	Fair	Fair	Good	Good	Fair	Good	Fair
Prognosis	Good	Excellent	Good	Excellent	—	Fair	—
RV Infarction	Good	Good	Good	—	Good	—	Good
Ventricular function	Good	Excellent	—	—	Good	—	Good
Exercise-induced ischemia	Fair	Good	—	Excellent	—	—	—
Successful reperfusion	Suggestive	—	Possibly	Fair	—	Good	Possibly
Viable myocardium	—	—	—	Fair	—	Excellent	Possibly
Aneurysm	Excellent	Good	—	—	Excellent	—	Excellent
LV thrombus	Excellent	Suggestive	—	—	Excellent	—	Fair
Septal rupture	Excellent	Indirect	—	—	Good	—	Possibly
Papillary rupture	Excellent	—	—	—	Good	—	Possibly
Pericardial disease	Good	Suggestive	—	—	Excellent	—	Good

Abbreviations: Echo= echocardiography; RNA= radionuclide angiography; Technetium = technetium-99m pyrophosphate imaging; Thallium = thallium-201 imaging; CT = computed tomography; PET = positron emission tomography; NMR = nuclear magnetic resonance imaging; Possibly = of potential but unproven value; (—) = of no demonstrated value

REFERENCES

1. Heger JJ, Weyman AE, Wann LS, et al: Cross-sectional echocardiography in acute myocardial infarction: Detection and localization of regional left ventricular asynergy. Circulation 1979;60:531-538.

2. Gibson RS, Bishop HL, Stamm RB, Crampton RS, Beller GA, Martin RP: Value of early two-dimensional echocardiography in patients with acute myocardial infarction. Am J Cardiol 1982;49:1110-1119.

3. Visser CA, Lie KI, Kan G, et al: Detection and quantification of acute, isolated myocardial infarction by two dimensional echocardiography. Am J Cardiol 1981;47:1020-1025.

4. Lopez-Sendon J, Garcia-Fernandez MA, Coma-Canella I, et al: Segmental right ventricular function after acute myocardial infarction: Two-dimensional echocardiographic study in 63 patients. Am J Cardiol 1983;51:390-396.

5. Lieberman AN, Weiss JL, Jugdutt BI, et al: Two-dimensional echocardiography and infarct size: relationship of regional wall motion and thickening to the extent of infarction in the dog. Circulation 1981;63:739-746.

6. Buda AJ, Zotz RJ, Gallagher KP: Characterization of the functional border zone around regionally ischemic myocardium using circumferential regionally ischemic myocardium using circumferential regional flow-function maps. J Am Coll Cardiol 1986;8:150-158.

7. Force T, Kemper A, Perkins L, et al: Overestimation of infarct size by quantitative two-dimensional echocardiography: the role of tethering and of analytic procedures. Circulation 1986;73:1360-1368.

8. Horwitz RRS, Morganroth J, Parrotto C, et al: Immediate diagnosis of acute myocardial infarction by two-dimensional echocardiography. Circulation 1982;65:323-329.

9. Nishimura RA, Tajik AJ, Shub C, et al: Role of two-dimension echocardiography in the prediction of in-hospital complications after acute myocardial infarction. J Am Coll Cardiol 1984;4:1080-1087.

10. Heger JJ, Weyman AE, Wann S, et al: Cross-sectional echocardiographic analysis of extent of left ventricular asynergy in acute myocardial infarction. Circulation 1980;61:1113-1124.

11. Van Reet RE, Quinones MA, Poliner LR, et al: Comparison of two-dimensional echocardiography with gated radionuclide ventriculography in the evaluation of global and regional left ventricular function in acute myocardial infarction. J Am Coll Cardiol 1984;4:243-252.

12. Presti CF, Gentile R, Armstrong WF, et al: Improvement in regional wall motion after percutaneous transluminal coronary angioplasty during acute myocardial infarction: utility of two-dimensional echocardiography. Am Heart J 1988;115:1149-1155.

13. Bourdillon PD, Broderick TM, Williams ES, et al: Early recovery of regional left ventricular function after reperfusion in acute myocardial infarction assessed by serial two-dimensional echocardiography. Am J Cardiol 1989;63:641-646.

14. Isaacsohn JL, Earle MG, Kemmper AJ, et al: Postmyocardial infarction pain and infarct extension in the coronary care unit: role of two-dimensional echocardiography. J Am Coll Cardiol 1988;11:246-251.

15. Merzlish JL, Berger HJ, Plankey M, et al: Functional left ventricular aneurysm formation after acute anterior transmural myocardial infarction: incidence, natural history, and prognostic implications. N Engl J Med 1984;311:1001-1006.

16. Erlebacher JA, Weiss JL, Kallman C, et al: Late effects of acute infarct dilation of heart size: a two-dimensional echocardiographic study. Am J Cardiol 1982;49:1120-1126.

17. Schuster EH, Bulkley BH: Expansion of transmural myocardial infarction: a pathophysiologic factor in cardiac rupture: Circulation 1979;60:1532-1538.

18. Weisman H, Bush D, Kallman C, et al: Cellular mechanism of infarct expansion: stretch vs slippage. Circulation 1983;68(suppl III):III-253, (abstract).

19. Eaton LW, Weiss JL, Bulkley BH, et al: Regional cardiac dilation after acute myocardial infarction: Recognition by two-dimensional echocardiography. N Engl J Med. 1979;300:57-62.

20. Jugdutt BI, Warnica JW: Intravenous nitroglycerin therapy to limit myocardial infarct size, expansion, and complications: Effect of timing, dosage, and infarct location. Circulation 1988;78:906-919.

21. Pfeffer MA, Lamas GA, Vaughan DE, et al: Effect of captopril on progressive ventricular dilation after anterior myocardial infarction. 1988;319:80-86.

22. Baur HR, Daniel JA, Nelson RR: Detection of left ventricular aneurysm on two dimensional echocardiography. Am J Cardiol. 1982;50:191-196.

23. Visser CA, Kan G, Meltzer RS, et al: Assessment of left ventricular aneurysm resectability by two-dimension echocardiography. Am J Cardiol 1985;56:857-860.

24. Gatewood RP, Nanda NC: Differentiation of left ventricular pseudoaneurysm from true aneurysm with two dimensional echocardiography. Am J Cardiol 1980;46:869-878.

25. Reddy SG, Roberts WC: Frequency of rupture of the left ventricular free wall or ventricular septum among necropsy cases. A fatal acute myocardial infarction since introduction of coronary care units. Am J Cardiol 1989;63:906-911.

26. Pohjola-Sintonen S, Muller JE, Stone PH, et al: Ventricular septal and free wall rupture complicating acute myocardial infarction: Experience in the Multicenter Investigation of Limitation of Infarct Size. Am Heart J 1989;117:809-816.

27. Singh S, Wann LS, Schuchard GH, et al: Right ventricular and right atrial collapse in patients with cardiac tamponade — a combined echocardiographic and hemodynamic study. Circulation 1984;70:966-971.

28. Gillam LD, Guyer DE, Gibson TC, et al: Hydrodynamic compression of the right atrium: a new echocardiographic sign of cardiac tamponade. Circulation 1983;68:294-301.

29. Radford MJ, Johnson RA, Dagget WM, et al: Ventricular septal rupture: a review of clinical and physiologic features and an analysis of survival. Circulation 1981;64:545-553.

30. Sanders RJ, Kern WH, Blount SG Jr: Perforation of the inter-ventricular septum complicating myocardial infarction. Am Heart J 1956;51:736-748.

31. Mintz GS, Victor MF, Kotler MN, Parry WR, Segal BL: Two-dimensional echocardiographic identification of surgically correctable complications of acute myocardial infarction. Circulation 1981;64:91-96.

443

32. Edwards BS, Edwards WD, Edwards JE: Ventricular septal rupture complicating acute myocardial infarction: identification of simple and complex types in 53 autopsied hearts. Am J Cardiol 1984;54:1201-1205.

33. Drobac M, Gilbert B, Howard R, et al: Ventricular septal defect after myocardial infarction: diagnosis by two-dimensional contrast echocardiography. Circulation 1983;67: 335-341.

34. Miyatake K, Okamoto M, Kinoshita N, et al: Doppler echocardiographic features of ventricular septal rupture in myocardial infarction. J Am Coll Cardiol 1985; 5:182-187.

35. Recusani F, Raisaro A, Sgalambro AL, et al: Ventricular septal rupture after acute myocardial infarction: diagnosis by two-dimensional and pulsed Doppler echocardiography. Am J Cardiol 1984;54:277-281.

36. Karen G, Sherez J, Roth A, et al: Diagnosis of ventricular septal rupture from acute myocardial infarction by combined two-dimensional and pulsed Doppler echocardiography. Am J Cardiol 1984;53:1202-1203.

37. Panidis IP, Mintz GS, Goel I, et al: Acquired ventricular septal defect after myocardial infarction: detection by combined two-dimensional and Doppler echocardiography. Am Heart J 1986;111:427-429.

38. MacLeod D, Fananapazir L, DeBono D, et al: Ventricular septal defect after myocardial infarction: assessment by cross-sectional echocardiography with pulsed wave Dopplers. Br Heart J 1987;58:214-217.

39. Bhatia SJS, Plappert T, Theard MA, et al: Transseptal Doppler flow velocity profile in acquired ventricular septal defect in acute myocardial infarction. Am J Cardiol 1987; 60:372-373.

40. Harrison MR, Halamart EA, Gurley JC, et al: Evaluation of ventricular septal defect complicating acute myocardial infarction: identification, localization and differentiation from mitral regurgitation by color flow imaging. J Am Coll Cardiol 1989;13(2):209A.

41. Wei JY, Hutchins GM, Bulkley BH: Papillary muscle rupture in fatal acute myocardial infarction: A potentially treatable form of cardiogenic shock. Ann Int Med 1979;90:149-153.

42. Nishimura RA, Schaff HV, Shado C, et al: Papillary muscle rupture complicating acute myocardial infarction: analysis of 17 patients. Am J Cardiol 1983;51:373-377.

43. Mintz GS, Victor MF, Kotler MN, et al: Two-dimensional echocardiographic identification of surgically correctable complications of acute myocardial infarction. Circulation 1981;64:91-96.

44. Come PC, Riley MF, Weintraub R, et al: Echocardiographic detection of complete and partial papillary muscle rupture during acute myocardial infarction. Am J Cardiol 1985; 56:787-789.

45. Eisenberg BR, Barzilai B, Perez JE: Non-invasive detection by Doppler echocardiography of combined ventricular septal rupture and mitral regurgitation in acute myocardial infarction. J Am Coll Cardiol 1984;4:617-620.

46. Asinger RW, Mickell, FL, Elsberger J, et al: Incidence of left ventricular thrombus after acute transmural myocardial infarction: serial evaluation by two-dimensional echocardiography. N Engl J Med 1981;305:297-302.

47. Stratton, Lightly GW, Pearlman AS, Ritchie JL: Detection of left ventricular thrombus by two-dimensional echocardiography: sensitivity, specificity, and causes of uncertainty. Circulation 1982;66:156-166.

48. Friedman MJ, Carlson K, Marcus, FI, Woolfenden JM: Clinical correlations in patients with acute myocardial infarction and left ventricular thrombus detected by two-dimensional echocardiography. Am J Med 1982;72:894-898.

49. Jugdutt BI, Sivaram CA. Prospective two-dimensional echocardiographic evaluation of left ventricular thrombus and embolism after acute myocardial infarction. J Am Coll Cardiol 1989;13:554-64.

50. Stratton, Lightly GW, Pearlman AS, Ritchie JL: Detection of left ventricular thrombus by two-dimensional echocardiography: sensitivity, specificity, and causes of uncertainty. Circulation 1982;66:156-166.

51. Visser CA, Can G, Meltzer RS, Dunning AJ, Roelandt J: Embolic potential of left ventricular thrombus after myocardial infarction: a two-dimensional echocardiographic study of 119 patients. J Am Coll Cardiol 1985;5:1276-1280.

52. Stratton JR, Speck SM, Caldwell JH, et al: Late effects of intracoronary streptokinase on regional wall motion, ventricular aneurysm and left ventricular thrombus in myocardial infarction: Results from the Western Washington Randomized Trial. J Am Coll Cardiol 1985;5:1023-1028.

53. Nihoyannopoulos P, Smith GC, Maseri A, et al: The natural history of left ventricular thrombus in myocardial infarction: A rationale in support of masterly inactivity. J Am Coll Cardiol 1989;14:903-911.

54. Parisi AF, Nieminen M, O'Boyle JE, et al: Enhanced detection of the evolution of tissue changes after acute myocardial infarction using color-encoded two-dimensional echocardiography. Circulation 1982;66:764-772.

55. Pandian NG, Nichols J, Koyanhei SS, et al: Detection of acute myocardial infarction in closed chest dogs by analysis of regional two-dimensional echocardiographic gray level distributions. Circ Res 1983;52:36-44.

56. Barzilai B, Madaras EI, Sobel BE, et al: Effects of myocardial contraction on ultrasonic back scatter before and after ischemia. Am J Physiol 1984;247:H417-H483.

57. Milunski MR, Mohr GA, Perez JE, et al: Ultrasonic tissue characterization with integrated back scatter: acute myocardial ischemia, reperfusion, and stunned myocardium in patients. Circulation 1989;80:491-503.

58. Page DL, Caulfield GB, Kastor JA, et al: Myocardial changes associated with cardiogenic shock. N Engl J Med 1971;285:133-137.

59. Alonso DR, Scheidt W, Post M, et al: Pathophysiology of cardiogenic shock. Quantification of myocardial necrosis: clinical, pathologic, and electrocardiographic correlations. Circulation 1973;40:588-596.

60. Holman BL, Goldhader SZ, Kirsch CM, et al: Measurement of infarct size using single photon emission computed tomography and technetium 95-pyrophosphate: a description of the method and comparison with patient prognosis. Am J Cardiol 1982;50:503-511.

61. Lewis SE, Devous MD, Corbett JR, et al: Measurement of infarct size in acute canine myocardial infarction by single-photon computed emission tomography with technetium-99M pyrophosphate. Am J Cardiol 1984;54:193-199.

62. Poliner LR, Buja LM, Parkey RW, et al: Clinical pathological findings in 52 patients studied by technetium-99-stannous pyrophosphate myocardial scintigraphy. Circulation 1979;59:257-267.

63. Burns RJ, Gladstone PJ, Tremblay PC, et al: Myocardial infarction determined by technetium-99 pyrophosphate single-photon tomography complicating elective coronary artery bypass grafting for angina pectoris. Am J Cardiol 1989;63:1429-1434.

64. Val PG, Pelletier LC, Hernandez MG, et al: Diagnostic criteria and prognosis of perioperative myocardial infarction following coronary bypass. J Thorac Cardiovasc Surg l983;86:878-886.

65. Gardiner MJ, Johnstone DE, Lalonde L, et al: Perioperative myocardial infarction with coronary artery surgery: diagnosis, incidence, and consequences. Can J Cardiol l987;3:336-341.

66. Kondo M, Takahashi M, Matsuda T, et al: Clinical significance of early myocardial 99M TC-pyrophosphate uptake in patients with acute myocardial infarction. Am Heart J 1987;113:250-256.

67. Wheeland K, Wolfe C, Corbett J, et al: Early positive technetium-99M stannous pyrophosphate images as a marker for reperfusion after thrombolytic therapy for acute myocardial infarction. Am J Cardiol 1985;56:252-256.

68. Rude RE, Parkey RW, Bonte FJ, et al: Clinical implications of the technetium-99m stannous pyrophosphate myocardial scintigraphic "Doughnut" pattern in patients with acute myocardial infarcts. Circulation 1979;59:721-730.

69. Olson HG, Lyons KP, Aronow WS. Prognostic value of a persistently positive technetium-99M stannous pyrophosphate myocardial scintigram after myocardial infarction. Am J Cardiol 1979;43:889-898.

70. Khaw BA, Strauss HW, Moore R, et al: Myocardial damage delineated by indium-111 antimyosin Fab and technetium-99m pyrophosphate. J Nucl Med 1987;28:76-82.

71. Volpini M, Giubbini R, Gei P, et al: Diagnosis of acute myocardial infarction by indium-111 antimyosin antibodies and correlation with the traditional techniques for the evaluation of extent and localization. Am J Cardiol 1989;63:7-13.

72. Antunes ML, Seldin DW, Wall RM, et al: Measurement of acute Q-wave myocardial infarct size with single photon emission computed tomography imaging of indium-111 antimyosin. Am J Cardiol 1989;63:777-783.

73. Becker RC, Silverman KJ, Bulkley BH, et al: Comparison of early thallium-201 scintigraphy and gated blood pool imaging for predicting mortality in patients with acute myocardial infarction. Circulation l983;67:1272-1282.

74. The Multi-Center Post Infarct Research Group. Risk stratification and survival after myocardial infarction. New Engl J Med 1983;309:331-336.

75. Schelbert HR, Henning H, Ashburn WL, et al: Serial measurements of left ventricular ejection fraction by radionuclide angiography early and late after myocardial infarction. Am J Cardiol 1976;38:407-415.

76. Sharpe DM, Votvinick EH, Shames DM, et al: Noninvasive diagnosis of right ventricular infarction. Circulation 1978;57:483-490.

77. Shah PK, Maddahi J, Berman DS, et al: Scintographically detected predominant right heart dysfunction in acute myocardial infarction: Clinical and hemodynamic correlates and implications for therapy and prognosis. J Am Coll Cardiol 1985;6:1264-1272.

78. Corbett JR, Nicod P, Lewis SE, et al: Prognostic value of submaximal radionuclide ventriculography after myocardial infarction. Am J Cardiol 1983;52:82A-91A.

79. Friedman ML, Canter RE: Reliability of gated heart scintigrams for detection of left-ventricular aneurysm: concise communication. J Nucl Med 1979;20:720-723.

80. Askenazi J, Ahnberg DS, Korngold E, et al: Quantitative radionuclide angiocardiography: detection and quantitation of left to right shunts. Am J Cardiol 1976;37:382-387.

81. Strauss HW, Harrison K, Langan JK, et al: Thallium-201 for myocardial imaging: Relation of thallium-201 to regional myocardial perfusion. Circulation 1975;51:641-645.

82. Wackers FJT, Sokole EB, Samson G, et al: Value and limitations of Thallium-201 scintigraphy in the acute phase of myocardial infarction. N Engl J Med 1976;295:1-5.

83. Wackers FJT, Becker A, Samson G, et al: Location and size of acute transmural myocardial infarction estimated from thallium-201 scintiscans: A clinicopathological study. Circulation 1977;56:72-78.

84. Fintel DJ, Links JM, Brinker JA, et al: Improved diagnostic performance of exercise thallium-201 single photon emission computed tomography over planar imaging in the diagnosis of coronary artery disease: a receiver operating characteristic analysis. J Am Coll Cardiol 1989;13:600-612.

85. Prigent F, Maddahi J, Gercia EV, et al: Quantification of myocardial infarct size by thallium-201 single-photon emission computed tomography: experimental validation in the dog. Circulation 1986;74:852-861.

86. Prigent F, Maddahi J, Gercia EV, et al: Comparative methods for quantifying myocardial infarct size by thallium-201 SPECT. J Nucl Med 1987;28:325-333.

87. Maublant JC, Peycelon P, Cardot JC, et al: Value of myocardial defect size measured by thallium-201 SPECT: results of a multicenter trial comparing heparin and a new fibrinolytic agent. J Nucl Med 1988;29:1486-1491.

88. Mahmarian JJ, Pratt CM, Borges-Neto S, et al: Quantification of infarct size by 201Tl single-photon emission computed tomography during acute myocardial infarction in humans. Comparison with enzymatic estimates: Circulation 1988;78:831-839.

89. De Coster PM, Melin JA, Detry JR, Vrassuer LA, Beckers C, Col J: Coronary artery reperfusion in acute myocardial infarction: Assessment by pre- and post-intervention thallium-201 myocardial perfusion imaging. Am J Cardiol 1985;55:889-895.

90. Markis JE, Malagold M, Parker JA, et al: Myocardial salvage after intracoronary thrombolysis with streptokinase in acute myocardial infarction. N Engl J Med 1981;305:777-782.

91. Schwarz F, Schuler G, Katus H, et al: Intracoronary thrombolysis in acute myocardial infarction: Correlations among serum enzymes, scintigraphic and hemodynamic findings. Am J Cardiol 1982;50:32-38.

92. Granato JE, Watson DD, Flanagan TL, et al: Myocardial thallium-201 kinetics during coronary occlusion and reperfusion: influence of methods of reflow and timing of thallium-201 administration. Circulation 1986;73:150-160.

93. Schofer G, Montz R, Mathey DG: Scintigraphic evidence of the "no-reflow" phenomenon in human beings after coronary thrombolysis. J Am Coll Cardiol 1985;5:593-598.

94. Wackers FJTH, Gibbons RJ, Verani MS, et al: Serial quantitative planar technetium-99m-isonitrile imaging in acute myocardial infarction: efficacy for noninvasive assessment of thrombolytic therapy. J Am Coll Cardiol 1989:14;861-873.

95. Theroux P, Waters DD, Halphen C, et al: Prognostic value of exercise testing soon after myocardial infarction. N Engl J Med 1979;301:341-345.

447

96. Gibson RS, Watson DD, Craddock GB, et al: Prediction of cardiac events after uncomplicated myocardial infarction: a prospective study comparing predischarge exercise thallium-201 scintigraphy and coronary angiography: Circulation 1983;68:321-336.

97. Topol EJ, Juni JE, O'Neill WW, et al: Exercise testing three days after onset of acute myocardial infarction: Am J Cardiol 1987;60:958-962.

98. Leppo JA, O'Brien J, Rothendler JA, et al: Dipyridamole thallium-201 scintigraphy in the prediction of future cardiac events after acute myocardial infarction. N Engl J Med 1984;310:1014-1018.

99. Younis LT, Byers S, Shaw L, et al: Prognostic value of intravenous dipyridamole thallium scintigraphy after an acute myocardial ischemic event. Am J Cardiol 1989;64:161-166.

100. Gimple LW, Hutter AM, Guiney TE, et al: Prognostic utility of predischarge submaximal exercise electrocardiography and maximal exercise thallium imaging after uncomplicated acute myocardial infarction. Am J Cardiol 1989;64:1243-1248.

101. Schelbert HR. Myocardial ischemia and clinical applications of positron emission tomography. Am J Cardiol 1989;64:46E-53E.

102. Sobel BE, Weiss ES, Welch MJ, et al: Detection of remote myocardial infarctions with position emission transaxial tomography and intravenous 11C-palmitate. Circulation 1977;55:853-857.

103. Geltman EM, Biello D, Welch MJ, et al: Characterization of nontransmural myocardial infarction by positron-emission tomography. Circulation 1982;65:747-755.

104. Marshall RC, Tillisch JH, Phelps ME, et al: Identification and differentiation of resting myocardial ischemia and infarction in man with positron computed tomography, 18F-labelled fluorodeoxyglucose and N-13 ammonia. Circulation 1983;67:766-778.

105. Tillisch J, Brunken R, Marshall R, et al: Reversibility of cardiac wall-motion abnormalities predicted by positron tomography. N Engl J Med 1986;314:884-888.

106. Liu P, Kiess MC, Okada RD, et al: The persistent defect on exercise thallium imaging and its fate after myocardial revascularization: does it represent scar or ischemia? Am Heart J 1985;110:996-1001.

107. Gibson RS, Watson DD, Taylor GJ, et al: Perspective assessment of regional myocardial perfusion before and after coronary revascularization surgery by quantitative thallium-201 scintigraphy. J Am Coll Cardiol 1983;1:804-815.

108. Brunken R, Kotton S, Nienaber C, et al: PET detection of viable tissue in myocardial segments with persistent defects at T1-201 SPECT. Radiology 1989;172:65-73.

109. Schwaiger M, Brunken R, Grover-McKay M, et al: Regional myocardial metabolism in patient with acute myocardial infarction assessed by positron emission tomography. J Am Coll Cardiol 1986;8:800-808.

110. Hashimoto TH, Kambara H, Fudo T, et al: Non-Q wave versus Q wave myocardial infarction: Regional myocardial metabolism and blood flow assessed by positron emission tomography. J Am Coll Cardiol 1988;12:88-93.

111. Sobel BE, Geltman EM, Tiefenbrunn AJ, et al: Improvement of regional myocardial metabolism after coronary thrombolysis induced with tissue-type plasminogen activator or streptokinase. Circulation 1984;69:983-990.

112. Schelbert HR, Buxton D. Insights into coronary artery disease gained from metabolic imaging. Circulation 1988;78:496-505.

113. Higging CB, Sovak M, Schmidt W, et al: Differential accumulation of radiouptake contrast material in acute myocardial infarction. Am J Cardiol 1979;43:47-51.

114. Masuda J, Yoshida H, Morooka N, et al: The usefulness of x-ray computed tomography for the diagnosis of acute myocardial infarction. Circulation 1984;70:217-225.

115. Reiter SJ, Rumberger JA, Feiring AJ, et al: Precision of measurements of right and left ventricular volume by cine computed tomography. Circulation 1986;74:890-900.

116. Lanzer P, Garrett J, Lipton MJ, et al: Quantitation of regional myocardial function by cine computed tomography: pharmacologic changes in wall thickness. J Am Coll Cardiol 1986;8:682-692.

117. Sechtem U, Sommerhoff BA, Markiewicz W, et al: Regional left ventricular wall thickening by magnetic resonance imaging: evaluation in normal persons and patients with global and regional dysfunction. Am J Cardiol 1986;59:145-51.

118. Adkins EW, Hill JA, Sievers KW, Conti CR. Assessment of left ventricular wall thickness in the healed myocardial infarction by magnetic resonance imaging. Am J Cardiol 1987;59:23-28.

119. White RD, Cassidy MM, Cheitlin ND, et al: Segmental evaluation of left ventricular wall motion after myocardial infarction: magnetic resonance imaging vs echocardiography. Am Heart J 1988;115:166-175.

120. Peshock RM, Rokey R, Malloy CM, et al: Assessment of myocardial systolic wall thickening using nuclear magnetic resonance imaging. J Am Coll Cardiol 1989;14:653-659.

121. White RD, Holt WW, Cheitlin NDK, et al: Estimation of the functional and anatomic extent of myocardial infarction using magnetic resonance imaging. Am Heart J 1988;115:740-747.

122. Buda AJ, Aisen AN, Juni JE, et al: Detection and sizing of myocardial ischemia in infarction by nuclear magnetic resonance imaging in the canine heart. Am Heart J 1985;110:1284-1290.

123. Wolfe CL, Mosely ME, Wikstrom MG, et al: Assessment of myocardial salvage after ischemia and reperfusion using magnetic resonance imaging and spectroscopy. Circulation 1989;80:969-982.

124. Wesbey G, Higgins CB, Lanzer P, et al: Imaging and characterization of acute myocardial infarction in vivo by gated nuclear magnetic resonance. Circulation 1984;69:125-130.

125. McNamara MT, Higgins CB, Schechtmann N, et al: Detection and characterization of acute myocardial infarction in man with use of gated magnetic resonance. Circulation 1985;71:717-724.

126. Johnston DL, Thompson RC, Liu P, et al: Magnetic resonance imaging during acute myocardial infarction. Am J Cardiol 1986;57:1059-1065.

127. Johnston DJ, Mulbagh SR, Cashion RW, et al: Nuclear magnetic resonance imaging of acute myocardial infarction within 24 hours of chest pain onset. Am J Cardiol 1989;64:172-179.

128. Dilworth LR, Aisen AM, Mancini GBJ, et al: Serial nuclear magnetic resonance imaging in myocardial infarction in man. Am J Cardiol 1987;59:1203-1205.

129. Bottomlay PA, Herfkens RJ, Smith LS, et al: Altered phosphate metabolism in myocardial infarction: P-31 MR spectroscopy. Radiology 1987;165:703-707.

130. Rehr RB, Tatum JL, Hirsch JI, et al: Reperfused-viable and reperfused-infarcted myocardium: differentiation with in vivo P-31 MR spectroscopy. Radiology 1989;172:53-58.

131. Schaefer S, Gober J, Valenza M, et al: Nuclear magnetic resonance imaging-guided phosphorus-31 spectroscopy of the human heart. J Am Coll Cardiol 1988;12:1449-1455.

FUTURE DIRECTIONS IN MANAGEMENT OF MYOCARDIAL INFARCTION AND THE ISCHEMIC SYNDROME

Section VI

Chapter 19

OUT-OF-HOSPITAL ASSESSMENT OF THE ACUTE MYOCARDIAL INFARCTION PATIENT AND INITIATION OF THROMBOLYTIC THERAPY

W. Douglas Weaver

for the MITI Project Investigators

RATIONALE

Investigations into the feasibility and effectiveness of prehospital initiation of thrombolytic therapy have been precipitated by observations from several placebo-controlled trials of thrombolytic therapy. There is general consensus that the earlier thrombolytic therapy is initiated, the better the result.[1-8] One trial showed a 47% reduction in mortality in patients treated within the first hour after onset of symptoms.[4] In a substantial number of patients the only possible way to treat within this time frame is to initiate thrombolytic therapy in the prehospital setting.

In an effort to reduce delay from hospital admission to initiation of treatment, the decision for thrombolytic therapy and the location where treatment is initiated have changed from the cardiologist in the coronary care unit to the physician in the emergency department. Because of the importance of time, delays associated with consultation with the patient's physician or a cardiologist prior to treatment must be minimized or obviated by a previously devised plan. The hospital emergency department and cardiology staff must develop protocols aimed at rapid triage and selection of appropriate patients for initiation of thrombolytic therapy or emergent catheterization followed by mechanical or pharmacologic methods of coronary reperfusion.

Because prehospital evaluation, stabilization, and transport of the patient combined with further hospital assessment and initiation of treatment in the emergency department consume 1-2 hours, a better way to routinely minimize the time to treatment would be to initiate thrombolytic therapy to appropriate patients in the prehospital setting.

The initial description of prehospital administration of thrombolytic therapy from Israel showed that resulting left ventricular ejection fraction was substantially higher (56% ± 15 vs. 47% ± 14) and infarct size (measured by QRS scoring methods) was substantially smaller when intravenous streptokinase was begun within 90 minutes from onset of chest pain compared to later treatment.[9] In this small study, most patients treated had thrombolytic therapy begun in their homes by emergency ambulance physicians.

Prehospital emergency care in the U.S. is provided by either nurses or paramedics. Until recently these paramedical personnel have had limited training in making the diagnosis of acute myocardial infarction (AMI). Prehospital assessment in the past has simply included a short medical history and physical examination aimed primarily at rapidly triaging patients with presumed cardiac pain due to any suspected acute coronary syndrome for further hospital evaluation and treatment. In the prehospital setting, physician control and supervision are provided by a medical director who establishes protocols and policies and emergency department staff who provide remote consultation and prescription of therapy. The benefit of paramedic management of patients with cardiac arrest and other serious medical and surgical emergencies has been enormous. Survival of patients with out-of-hospital cardiac arrest has improved from 5% to 25% with the advent of prehospital treatment in many cities.[10-15]

The major factor preventing immediate widespread implementation of prehospital initiation of thrombolytic therapy is the relative lack of evidence to demonstrate that paramedics working alone or with a remotely located physician can effectively select appropriate patients for treatment. Second, it has not yet been shown that the time savings achieved by this strategy will result in less myocardial necrosis and lower hospital morbidity and mortality than traditional in-hospital treatment. Several studies, however, are in progress, and early results show that this approach is both feasible and safe.[16-20]

OBSTACLES TO PREHOSPITAL INITIATION OF THROMBOLYTIC THERAPY

Perhaps the greatest impediment to prehospital initiation of thrombolytic treatment is the same as that which applies in the hospital setting. Most patients with chest pain evaluated in the prehospital setting are not appropriate candidates for systemic thrombolytic therapy, at least using the currently accepted indications. In the Seattle metropolitan area registry of patients with AMI established in the Myocardial Infarction, Triage and Intervention (MITI) Project in 1988, only 22% of all patients admitted with chest pain and who developed evidence of AMI were treated with systemic thrombolytic therapy (Figure 1). The remainder either had non-diagnostic electrocardiographic changes or relative contraindications (advanced age, hypertension, other co-morbidity) to systemic thrombolysis. The present indications for treatment emphasize selection of

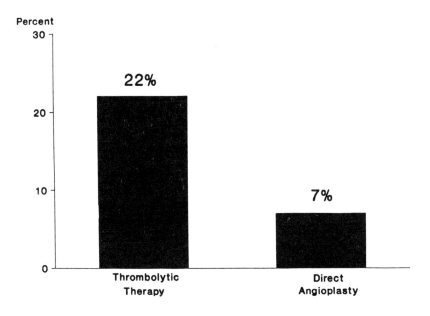

Figure 1. *Use of thrombolytic therapy and direct angioplasty in 2,043 patients with acute myocardial infarction treated in 19 Seattle metropolitan area hospitals in 1988. The strict criteria used to select suitable candidates for thrombolytic therapy and the yet unproven role of direct angioplasty have resulted in the selection of relatively few patients for these emergent reperfusion strategies.*

the young, those with symptoms of short duration, and those with a small potential risk of serious bleeding problems. This practice excludes the majority of patients presenting with suspected myocardial infarction.

A second obstacle to prehospital care of most patients with acute coronary thrombosis is prolonged patient delays prior to seeking medical care. Despite the fact that paramedic services and a central 911 emergency telephone number have become widely available in the past 20 years, even in Seattle only half of all patients with symptoms of AMI call 911. Instead, many seek medical attention by "walking in," often relatively late, at a time when thrombolytic therapy is less effective. Even fewer patients may seek prompt attention in other cities with more recently established or less well organized emergency systems. The patient's decision of when and how to seek care can and will be modified, as patient and public educational programs are developed to influence behavior following the onset of symptoms.[21,22]

Another requirement for the earlier treatment of patients with AMI is the enhancement of both diagnostic and treatment abilities of all prehospital cardiac care providers. Simple triage of cardiac chest pain patients to hospitals is no longer good enough. Instead, consistent screening protocols and 12-lead electrocardiography, which permit the prehospital diagnosis of acute infarction, need to become standard practice.

Prehospital Selection of Appropriate Patients

The MITI Project is a multiphase evaluation of feasibility, safety and benefit of prehospital initiation of thrombolytic therapy.[16] Seattle and suburban King county have a population of 1.4 million people and 19 hospitals with coronary care units. The emergency medical system is tiered; first emergency responders (firefighters) provide first-aid level care, and 13 strategically located emergency medical units are staffed by paramedics trained to triage and treat most medical emergencies. During an 8 1/2 month feasibility phase aimed primarily at developing accurate and safe patient selection criteria to identify prehospital patients with suspected acute coronary thrombosis, almost 2,500 patients with chest pain of presumed cardiac origin were evaluated by paramedics using a clinical checklist designed to screen patients with chest pain and select those who would be appropriate candidates for thrombolytic therapy (Figure 2). This represented approximately 12% of all medical emergencies attended by paramedics during this time.[18] The checklist provided a straight-forward and uniform means to quickly assess patients and did not require additional time to complete. The in-field evaluation and treatment time was 26 ± 9.3 minutes compared to 24 ± 12 minutes in the previous year when it did not exist. The checklist also permitted paramedics to obtain a great deal more patient information.

The importance and meaning of each of the selection criteria and the operation of the specialized cellular telephone transmitted electrocardiogram were taught (Figure 3). This instruction and practice required 3-4 hours spread over a two-day period in order to maximize the amount of knowledge retained. Operation of the cellular electrocardiograph continues to be practiced by paramedics each morning in order to test the device and retain the technical skills required of the operator.

Following the checklist assessment, the subset of patients with presumed acute coronary thrombosis and with no potential contraindications to thrombolytic therapy had prehospital 12-lead electrocardiograms. The electrocardiogram itself required approximately seven minutes, most of which was used in skin preparation and electrode placement. The actual electrocardiogram acquisition, digital storage and cellular telephone transmission time was 30 seconds or less. In order to minimize any further delay caused by this additional diagnostic testing, acquisition of the electrocardiogram was integrated into overall patient assessment and treatment; thus, the total

456

HEART PAIN CHECKLIST (For Paramedic Use)

YES (☑ = meets criteria)		NO
☐	ORIENTED, CAN COOPERATE	—
☐	HEART PAIN	—
☐	PAIN FOR MORE THAN 15 MINUTES AND LESS THAN 6 HOURS	—
☐	AGE (35-74)	—
	BP RIGHT ARM ______/______	
	BP LEFT ARM ______/______	
☐	SYSTOLIC IS MORE THAN 80 AND LESS THAN 180	—
☐	SYSTOLIC RIGHT ARM VERSUS LEFT ARM IS LESS THAN 20	—
☐	DIASTOLIC IS LESS THAN 120	—
—	STROKE, SEIZURES, BRAIN SURGERY	☐
—	CENTRAL LINES OR TRAUMA	☐
—	TAKES WARFARIN, COUMADIN	☐
—	KNOWN BLEEDING PROBLEMS	☐
—	GI BLEED IN LAST 12 MONTHS	☐
—	SURGERY IN LAST 2 MONTHS	☐
—	CANCER, TERMINAL	☐
—	KIDNEY, LIVER PROBLEMS, DIABETES	☐
—	COLITIS, CROHN'S ENTERITIS	☐
	IF ABOVE BOXES ARE CHECKED, PROCEED WITH ECG	
☐	ECG DONE	—
☐	ECG RECEIVED BY DOCTOR	—
☐	MEETS CRITERIA FOR PRE-HOSP t-PA	—
☐	PATIENT INFORMED	—
	KIT ID #__________	
☐	t-PA GIVEN, AMT INCL BOLUS _____	—
☐	ASA (5gr) GIVEN	—

TIMES

PAIN BEGAN	____:____
DECISION TIME	____:____
t-PA BOLUS	____:____
BEGIN TRANSPORT	____:____
HOSPITAL ARRIVAL	____:____

Figure 2. *The prehospital medical record was modified to include this checklist of criteria to select from all patients with chest pain those who are suitable candidates for electrocardiography and treatment. The protocol approach did not require any additional time over an undirected history and exam, and it consistently provided more information to the receiving hospital staff.*

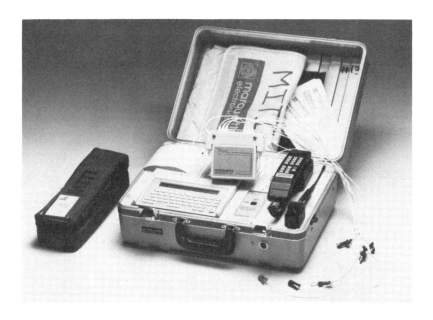

Figure 3. *The cellular electrocardiograph consists of a battery powered computer interpretive electrocardiograph coupled with a cellular telephone which transmits a duplicate record of the electrocardiogram to the emergency department. Electrocardiogram transmission required 30 seconds and was possible in 92% of patients in which it was attempted. The remainder were lost due to deficiencies in the cellular telephone transmission system.*

in-field and transport time was the same for patients in whom electrocardiograms were obtained compared to those patients with chest pain in whom they were not (45 ± 11 vs. 45 ± 10 minutes, respectively). The electrocardiograms were computer interpreted (12 SL interpretive program, versions 6.0-8.0, Marquette Electronics, Inc., Milwaukee, Wisconsin) and overread by remote emergency department physicians who made the diagnosis and prepared to treat the patient, even before the patient arrived.

This technology combined with the clinical checklist permits a prehospital diagnosis in patients with suspected acute coronary thrombosis. The prehospital diagnosis allows more rapid patient triage and shortens the time to treatment after the patient is admitted. In 522 patients evaluated with prehospital electrocardiograms in the feasibility phase of the MITI Project, 24% were candidates for thrombolytic therapy and were treated in the hospital 57 ± 50 minutes after hospital arrival. During the same period, 75 other patients also transported by paramedics but without prehospital electrocardiography were treated. The average time to treatment was 75 ± 67 minutes, sig-

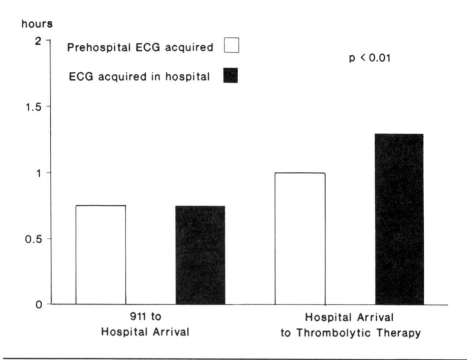

Figure 4. *The prehospital electrocardiogram did not add to the time required for prehospital assessment, stabilization and transport. On the other hand, the prehospital diagnosis of acute myocardial infarction made possible by the cellular transmitted electrocardiogram reduced the hospital delay from admission until initiation of treatment in patients receiving this assessment.*

nificantly longer than in those in whom a prehospital diagnosis had been made (p < 0.01) (Figure 4). The benefit of prehospital electrocardiography and diagnosis has also been noted in other cities; in Salt Lake City the delay from hospital admission to initiation of treatment was reduced from 68 ± 29 minutes to 48 ± 12 minutes following initiation of a prehospital diagnosis program.[23] No matter what the outcome of prehospital trials of thrombolytic therapy, it is already apparent that this new diagnostic technology improves emergency cardiac care and should be part of the standard equipment used by all prehospital providers.

A study in Göteborg, Sweden underscored the additional importance of prehospital electrocardiography.[24] In that city, patients with suspected AMI were evaluated using the history alone, and a subset with appropriate symptoms was selected for thrombolytic treatment by paramedics and nurses in the prehospital setting. Electrocardiograms were not obtained in the prehospital setting. Only those patients who were later determined to have ST-segment elevation derived benefit from early thrombolysis treatment, and patients with other electrocardiographic findings had the same infarct size as placebo-treated controls. Thus, electrocardiography enabled the selection of a group of patients who could benefit from very early treatment.

Several alternatives are available for obtaining prehospital electrocardiograms, but each has advantages and disadvantages. Single-lead electrocardiogram radio telemetry has been used for years. However, this technique requires considerable time to acquire and transmit all 10 leads, and the possibility of non-standardization between leads and lack of simultaneous lead acquisition make this approach unacceptable. Ten-lead simultaneous acquisition is associated with the fewest problems and pitfalls and represents the method of choice at present.

Battery powered electrocardiographs have recently been coupled to both landline and cellular telephones.[25] Using cellular telephone technology, electrocardiograms can be acquired and transmitted from the location where the patient is initially assessed, to the hospital, even if no landline telephone is available. This approach minimizes the time to diagnosis. The electrocardiogram can be acquired and transmitted during the prehospital evaluation of the patient and does not consume additional time for patient assessment. Cellular telephone technology is expanding rapidly, becoming more reliable, and will soon be used for many types of data transmission. This type of transmission will likely become even more widespread and less expensive as future technologic developments occur.

Prehospital electrocardiographs can also be coupled to a minicomputer to provide an immediate and continuously available "expert" interpretation. In 460 prehospital acquired electrocardiograms, the diagnostic accuracy of a computer algorithm (Marquette 12 SL/ versions 6.0-8.0) was in some ways superior to that of an emergency physician and an electrocardiographer reading the record "blind."[26] In making the diagnosis of acute injury (ST elevation consistent with acute thrombosis), the computer interpretation had a sensitivity of 71% and a specificity of 99.4%. The sensitivity was similar to that of the emergency physician readings. More importantly, the specificity (correct exclusion of patients without AMI) was superior (essentially 100%) to that of both the electrocardiographer (94%) and the emergency physician (88%) (p < 0.01). In the absence of an electrocardiographer, the computer interpretation provided the safest and best means for immediate selection of appropriate patients for treatment with systemic thrombolytic therapy. With further algorithm development, computer interpretations can likely be made even more highly sensitive and specific.

On the other hand, the myriad of computer generated statements used to describe the various electrocardiographic diagnoses associated with suspected coronary thrombosis, ischemia and prior infarction can, in fact, be confusing to the non-electrocardiographer. In order to simplify appropriate selection in the MITI project, a simple statement — a "flag" — was added to discriminate all electrocardiographic diagnoses consistent with findings of acute coronary thrombosis. This "flag" improved the diagnostic accuracy of the emergency physician selecting patients for possible treatment (Figure 5). If the computer interpretation is used to make treatment decisions, this simplification provides an ideal way to minimize errors on the part of the user. It is also clear that before other interpretative algorithms are used in this manner, clinical studies of their accuracy are mandatory. Few manufacturers have published evaluations of the accuracy of their interpretations when compared to actual clinical findings, a necessary requirement of safe and appropriate patient selection. For example, the MITI study found that the diagnostic accuracy of the most recent Marquette 12SL (versions 6.0 and later) algorithm was significantly better than earlier versions from the same manufacturer. This illustrates the value of rigorous testing of any computer interpretation software to be used to select appropriate patients. The potential benefit of computerized electrocardiography in this setting is enormous.

Time Savings With Prehospital Initiated Treatment

Three major components contribute to treatment delays: 1) the time from symptom onset until the patient seeks emergency care; 2) hospital transport time; and 3) the delay from hospital arrival until initiation of treatment. The findings from at least nine

Table 1. *Potential time savings due to prehospital initiation of thrombolytic therapy*

Reference	Symptom onset to prehospital diagnosis or treatment initiated (hr:min)	Hospital initiated treatment (hr:min)
MITI Project (Phase I)		
- Seattle[18]	1:11	2:24
EMIP[19]	2:00	4:00
Castaigne et al[20]	2:11	3:00
Weiss et al[27]	1:03	1:54
Villemant et al[28]	2:35	3:39
Bippus et al[29]	1:24	2:04
Oemrawsingh et al[30]	1:10	2:05
Roth et al[31]	1:33	2:17
Bossaert et al[32]	1:31	2:17

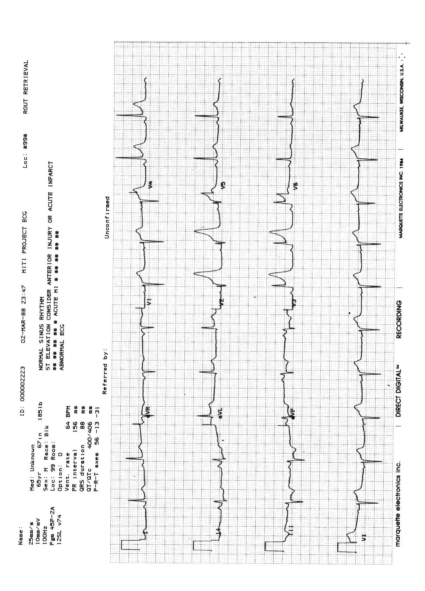

Figure 5. *The standard available computer interpretative statements were modified to permit a simple report which "flagged" all records with evidence of ST segment elevation consistent with acute coronary thrombosis. This approach was important in maximizing specificity of the emergency department physician and excluding any inappropriate patients for consideration of treatment with thrombolytic therapy. This method was superior to physician interpretation alone and provides an instant "expert" reading available 24 hours a day.*

studies suggest that prehospital initiation of thrombolytic therapy could save up to an hour or more from symptom onset to initiation of treatment (Table 1).[18-20,27-32]

The factors affecting patient decision time are only partially understood. In the MILIS study, patients who were older, had a prior history of cardiac disease, diabetes, or hypertension, or who were prescribed nitroglycerine or β-blocker treatment delayed longer than patients without such histories.[33] Other studies have shown that women, patients who are older, and those with symptoms during waking hours delay longer than their counterparts.[34-36] Patients who are alone at the time of onset of symptoms have longer decision times than those who are with someone else at the time of symptom onset.[37] It is discouraging that the patients who should know the most about cardiac disease delay longer than others; these findings suggest that it may be quite difficult to modify this behavior. Two recent pilot studies carried out in Seattle and Milwaukee were aimed at mass media education of the community about the importance of early emergency medical care following onset of chest pain.[22,*] Both the Milwaukee study, sponsored by the local AHA affiliate and Genentech, Inc., and a similar study in Seattle failed to substantially reduce the time from chest pain onset to patient action. In Seattle, the median delay was reduced from 2.6 hours to 2.3 hours after the campaign (an insignificant reduction in time), although it was clear from random telephone surveys of the public that the message had been seen and remembered.[22] In a year-long effort in Göteborg, Sweden, an intensive mass media educational effort reduced the time delay from 2.6 to only 2.2 hours.[21] More effective and cost efficient approaches for reducing these times are vitally needed.

Transport time to the hospital represents a moderate delay in most urban communities, averaging 30 minutes or less, although, admittedly it can be considerably longer in highly congested or rural areas.

Surprisingly, hospital-related delays are among the most significant obstacles to early treatment. Data from several Western Washington trials of thrombolytic therapy provide insight into the magnitude of these delays (Table 2).[16,38,39] The MITI registry of patients with AMI surveyed hospital delay times in 19 hospitals in the Seattle metropolitan area. The average delay in 1988 from hospital admission to initiation of treatment of patients with acute infarction was still 1 hour and 8 minutes. This time may reflect the general lack of efficient hospital protocols for rapidly selecting patients and initiating treatment after hospital arrival. Patient registration, redundant assessments by nursing and emergency and consultant physician staff plus the preliminary use of unnecessary laboratory testing and inadequate pharmacy support may all contribute to this delay. In a recent study, these delays averaged 90 minutes after hospital arrival. Treatment in the emergency department rather than the coronary care unit reduced the time by half.[40]

* Personal communication, Samuel Teischman, MD, Genentech, Inc., South San Francisco, CA

Table 2. *Average times from hospital admission to initiation of thrombolytic therapy in Western Washington Thrombolytic Studies*

Study/Site	No. of patients	Entry criteria	Mean time from patient arrival to treatment (hr:min)
Intravenous Alteplase/ Emergency Department*[16]	160	< 6 hours (< 1 hour after hospital arrival)	0:46
Intracoronary Streptokinase/ Catheterization Laboratory[38]	250	< 12 hours	2:23
Intravenous Streptokinase/ Coronary Care Unit[39]	368	< 6 hours	1:41
MITI Project - 1988/ All Area-Wide Hospitals	450	none	1:08

* Entry requirement that treatment be initiated within one hour of hospital admission

Projecting the Magnitude of Benefit of Prehospital Treatment

Phase I of the MITI study examined the feasibility and safety of prehospital initiation of thrombolytic therapy. Of 400 patients who developed evidence of AMI, 24% would have been candidates for prehospital initiation of treatment.[18] The clinical criteria chosen were conservative, since the objective was to select a subset with a very low likelihood of complications and the greatest potential benefit from treatment. If less strict age, duration of symptoms, blood pressure, and electrocardiographic criteria are utilized, perhaps 35-40% of patients with acute infarction would be suitable candidates for initiation of thrombolytic therapy (Table 3). After the diagnosis was made in the prehospital setting, it took 20 ± 8 minutes to prepare and transport the patient to hospital where therapy was initiated 57 ± 50 minutes after hospital arrival. Thus, in this preliminary evaluation of the feasibility and benefit of prehospital initiated treatment, one hour or more could be saved by initiating treatment in the field.

Unresolved Issues

It is unclear at present whether a thrombolytic agent which requires a continuous infusion because of a short half-life has greater disadvantages associated with its use

464

Table 3. Cross-tabulation of the percent of eligible AMI patients meeting various combinations of prehospital inclusion/exclusion criteria MITI AMI database — phase 1

	Age 35-74	CP >15m & <6 hrs	Not Hypotens	Not Hypertens	Diff. in arm BPs <20	No Hx of Stroke	No Recent GI Bleed	No Recent Surgery	No Bleeding Problems	No Cancer/Terminal	No Other Misc. Problems	No Previous MI	ST Elevation on ECG	ST Elv. or Depres.
Age 35-74		67%	69%	62%	68%	71%	73%	73%	72%	74%	63%	52%	43%	57%
CP >15m & <6 hrs			83%	71%	82%	83%	86%	87%	86%	88%	77%	60%	51%	70%
Not Hypotensive				77%	88%	89%	92%	92%	91%	94%	82%	64%	51%	73%
Not Hypertensive					75%	76%	78%	78%	78%	80%	71%	54%	46%	61%
Diff. in arm BPs <20						87%	89%	90%	89%	91%	80%	60%	52%	71%
No Hx of Stroke							92%	92%	91%	93%	80%	65%	52%	72%
No Recent GI Bleed								95%	95%	97%	83%	66%	54%	76%
No Recent Surgery									95%	97%	84%	66%	54%	75%
No Bleeding Porblems										96%	84%	65%	54%	75%
No Cancer/Terminal											85%	67%	56%	77%
No Other Misc. Cond.												58%	50%	67%
No Previous MI													41%	52%
ST Elevation on ECG														56%
ST Elev. or Depression														

Influence of various clinical and electrocardiographic criteria on suitability of patients for prehospital administration of thrombolytic therapy. The crosstabulation provides a way of evaluating the relationship of one characteristic with another (eg, the electrocardiographic findings in patients with no prior history of stroke).

than others which have longer half-lives and also disrupt coagulation for several hours. Continuous infusion does not preclude prehospital use, although admittedly bolus injection is inherently easier to deliver. When clear differences in drug efficacy exist, the drug used in the prehospital setting will probably be determined primarily by its efficacy and not by its ease of administration. Patency rates in patients receiving prehospital therapy may be much higher than prior reports because treatment can be initiated within the first hour of symptom onset for most patients.

The widespread use of prehospital electrocardiography may shorten hospital delays associated with initiating treatment to the extent that no advantage will be gained by starting therapy in the out-of-hospital setting, provided, of course, that transport times are short. The results from studies in the United States as well as those from the EMIP Trial in Europe will help clarify the value of this treatment strategy.[19,20] There is no doubt, however, that prehospital treatment is the only way to initiate treatment within the first hour of symptom onset to any meaningful proportion of patients with AMI.

The use of prehospital protocols and electrocardiography may also permit triage of selected patients, particularly those with hemodynamic compromise, to tertiary cardiac care facilities, so that further diagnostic testing, reperfusion treatments and surgery are immediately available if needed. The benefits associated with such a policy could be analogous to those seen with the triage and treatment of the severe trauma or burn patient. Perhaps the greatest advantage of prehospital initiated treatment is the potential delivery of therapy to the majority of patients within the first hour after the onset of chest pain.

In summary, prehospital selection of appropriate patients for initiation of thrombolytic therapy is feasible, safe, and saves time. The ultimate role of out-of-hospital initiated treatment awaits the results of ongoing studies.

REFERENCES

1. ISIS-2 (Second International Study of Infarct Survival) Collaborative Group: Randomised trial of intravenous streptokinase, oral aspirin, both, or neither among 17 187 cases of suspected acute myocardial infarction: ISIS-2. Lancet 1988;2:349-360.

2. ISAM Study Group: A prospective trial of intravenous streptokinase in acute myocardial infarction (ISAM). N Engl J Med 1986;314:1465-1471.

3. Ritchie JL, Cerqueira M, Maynard C, et al: Ventricular Function and infarct size: The western Washington intravenous streptokinase in myocardial infarction trial. J Am Coll Cardiol 1988;11:689-697.

4. Gruppo italiano per lo studio della streptochinasi nell'infarto miocardioco (GISSI): Effectiveness of intravenous thrombolytic treatment in acute myocardial infarction. Lancet 1986;8478:397-422.

5. Maynard C, Althouse R, Olsufka M, et al: Early versus late hospital arrival for acute myocardial infarction in the western Washington thrombolytic therapy trials. Am J Cardiol 1989;63:1296-1300.

6. Van de Werf F, Arnold AER: Intravenous tissue plasminogen activator and size of infarct, left ventricular function, and survival in acute myocardial infarction. Brit Med J 1988; 297:1374-1379.

7. Verheugt FWA, Kupper AJF, Sterkman LGW, et al: Emergency room infusion of intravenous streptokinase in acute myocardial infarction: Feasibility, safety, and hemodynamic consequences. Am Heart J 1989;117:1018-1022.

8. Topol EJ, Bates ER, Walton JA, et al: Community hospital administration of intravenous tissue plasminogen activator in acute myocardial infarction: Improved timing, thrombolytic efficacy and ventricular function. J Am Coll Cardiol 1978;10:1173-1177.

9. Koren G, Weiss AT, Hasin Y, et al: Prevention of myocardial damage in acute myocardial ischemia by early treatment with intravenous streptokinase. N Engl J Med 1985;313: 1384-1389.

10. Stults KR, Brown DD, Schug VL, et al: Prehospital defibrillation performed by emergency medical technicians in rural communities. N Engl J Med 1984;310:219-223.

11. Cobb LA, Werner JA, Trobaugh BG: Sudden cardiac death. 1: A decade's experience with out-of-hospital resuscitation. Mod Concepts Cardiovasc Dis 1980;49:31-36.

12. Eisenberg MS, Bergner L, Hallstrom A: Out-of-hospital cardiac arrest: Improved survival with paramedic services. Lancet 1980;i;812-815.

13. Lewis RP, Stang JM, Fulkerson PK, et al: Effectiveness of advanced paramedics in a mobil coronary care system. JAMA 1979;214;1902-1904.

14. Roth R, Stewart RD, Rogers K, et al: Out-of-hospital cardiac arrest: Factors associated with survival. Ann Emerg Med 1984;13:237-243.

15. Eisenberg MS, Hallstrom AP, Copass MK, et al: Treatment of ventricular fibrillation. Emergency medical technician defibrillation and paramedic services. JAMA 1984;251:1723-1728.

16. Kennedy JW, Weaver WD: Potential use of thrombolytic therapy before hospitalization. Am J Cardiol 1989;64:8A-11A.

17. Castaigne AD, Duval AM, Dubois-Rande JL, et al: Prehospital administration of anisoylated plasminogen streptokinase activator complex in acute myocardial infarction. Drugs 1987;33(suppl 3):231-234.

18. Weaver WD, Eisenberg MS, Martin JS, et al: Myocardial infarction, triage and intervention project — Phase I: patient characteristics and feasibility of prehospital initiation of thrombolytic therapy. J Am Coll Cardiol 1990;15(5):925-931.

19. Report of the European Myocardial Infarction Project (EMIP) Sub-Committee: Potential time savings with pre-hospital intervention in acute myocardial infarction. Eur Heart J 1988;9:118-124.

20. Castaigne AD, Herve C, Duval-Moulin A, et al: Prehospital use of APSAC: Results of a placebo-controlled study. Am J Cardiol 1989;64:30A-33A.

21. Herlitz J, Hartford M, Blohm M, et al: Effect of a media campaign on delay times and ambulance use in suspected acute myocardial infarction. Am J Cardiol 1989;64:90-93.

22. Ho MT, Eisenberg MS, Litwin PE, et al: Delay between onset of chest pain and seeking medical care: The effect of public education. Ann Emerg Med 1989;18:727-731.

23. Karagounis L, Ipsen SK, Jessop MR, et al: Impact of field-transmitted electrocardiography on time to in-hospital thrombolytic therapy in acute myocardial infarction. Circulation 1989;80(suppl IV):1406 (abstract).

24. Holmberg S, Hartford M, Herlitz J, et al: Very early thrombolysis with rt-PA in acute myocardial infarction. Circulation 1988;78(4):1101.

25. Grim P, Feldman T, Martin M, et al: Cellular telephone transmission of 12-lead electrocardiograms from ambulance to hospital. Am J Cardiol 1987;60:715-720.

26. Kudenchuk PJ, Ho MT, Litwin PE, et al: Accuracy of Cardiologist vs computerized ECG analysis in selecting patients for out-of-hospital thrombolytic therapy. Circulation 1988;78(suppl IV):957 (abstract).

27. Weiss AT, Fine DG, Applebaum D, et al: Prehospital coronary thrombolysis. A new strategy in acute myocardial infarction. Chest 1987;92:124-128.

28. Villemant D, Barriot P, Biou B, et al: Achievement of thrombolysis at home in cases of acute myocardial infarction. Lancet 1987;8526:228-229.

29. Bippus PH, Storch WH, Andresen D, et al: Thrombolysis started at home in acute myocardial infarction: Feasibility and time-gain. Circulation 1987;76(suppl IV):122 (abstract).

30. Oemrawsingh PV, Bosker HA, Vander Laarse A, et al: Early reperfusion by initiation of intravenous streptokinase infusion prior to ambulance transport. Circulation 1988;78(suppl II):110 (abstract).

31. Roth A, Barbash GI, Hod H, et al: Should rt-PA be administered by the mobile intensive care unit teams? Circulation 1988;78(suppl II):187 (abstract).

32. Bossaert LL, Demey HE, Colemont LJ, et al: Prehospital thrombolytic treatment of acute myocardial infarction with anisoylated plasminogen streptokinase activator complex. Crit Care Med 1988;16:823-830.

33. Turi ZG, Stone PH, Muller JE, et al: Implications for acute intervention related to time of hospital arrival in acute myocardial infarction. Am J Cardiol 1986;58:203-209.

34. Tjoe SL, Luria MH: Delays in reaching the cardiac care unit: an analysis. Chest 1972;61:617-621.

35. Moss AJ, Wynar B, Goldstein S: Delay in hospitalization during the acute coronary period. Am J Cardiol 1969;24:659-665.

36. Hackett TP, Cassem NH: Factors contributing to delay in responding to the signs and symptoms of acute myocardial infarction. Am J Cardiol 1969;24;651-658.

37. Alonzo AA: The impact of the family and lay others on care-seeking during life-threatening episodes of suspected coronary artery disease. Soc Sci Med 1986;22:1297-1311.

38. Kennedy JW, Ritchie JL, Davis KB, et al: Western Washington randomized trial of intracoronary streptokinase in acute myocardial infarction. N Engl J Med 1983;309: 1477-1482.

39. Kennedy JW, Martin GV, David KB, et al: The western Washington intravenous streptokinase in acute myocardial infarction randomized trial. Circulation 1988;77(2):345-352.

40. Sharkey SW, Bruneete DD, Ruiz E, et al: An analysis of time delays preceding thrombolysis for acute myocardial infarction. JAMA 1989;262:3171-3174.

Chapter 20

NEW DEVICE THERAPY IN THE MANAGEMENT OF CORONARY ARTERY DISEASE AND ACUTE ISCHEMIC SYNDROME

Michael H. Sketch, Jr.
Richard S. Stack

INTRODUCTION

The preservation and protection of myocardial tissue through cardiac revascularization is the principle behind the management of coronary artery disease and the treatment of acute myocardial infarction. A new era in revascularization was ushered in with the introduction of percutaneous transluminal coronary angioplasty (PTCA) by Gruentzing et al in 1979.[1] The subsequent huge popularity of this technique was reflected in a four-fold increase in the numbers performed in the USA between 1983 and 1986. It is estimated that 184,000 PTCA procedures were performed in the United States in 1987.[2] Despite recent advances in balloon catheter technology allowing access to most lesions within the coronary vasculature, acute vessel occlusion and late restenosis persist as unpredictable complications of this technique in a significant number of cases.[3] New interventional techniques are increasingly being pursued in an effort to develop safer and more efficacious alternatives to PTCA and to extend the horizons of percutaneous revascularization to include patients currently considered unsuitable, such as those with diffuse coronary disease or left mainstem stenosis. These newer approaches to coronary revascularization include autoperfusion balloon angioplasty, atherectomy, intracoronary stents, and intra-arterial laser therapy.

This chapter will discuss autoperfusion balloon angioplasty, atherectomy, and intracoronary stents. Intra-arterial laser therapy is discussed in Chapter 21.

PTCA: THE "GOLD STANDARD"

Since PTCA is the "gold standard" for the interventional treatment of coronary athero-sclerosis, an understanding of PTCA is fundamental to the quest for new techniques that might replace or complement it. The major mechanism by which balloon an-gioplasty appears to increase intravascular diameter involves atherosclerotic plaque breaking, cracking, fracturing or splitting.[4]

There are at least three postulated elements behind the success of this disruptive process. First, the plaque fractures or cracks produced by balloon dilatation improve vessel patency by creating additional channels or avenues for coronary blood flow. Second, intimal fractures with localized tears or dissections of the underlying media may result in improvement in luminal cross-sectional area. An absence of medial involvement may result in subsequent restenosis. A third mechanism of coronary artery dilatation appears to be the stretching of plaque-free wall segments of eccentric atherosclerotic lesions. Inflation of angioplasty balloons across eccentric lesions may distend or stretch the normal wall segment and produce minimal, if any, damage to the plaque on the remaining portions of the arterial wall. This initial improvement in luminal diameter may be lost within hours, days or weeks after the dilatation, as the stretched segment relaxes toward the pre-dilatation state.[4,5]

Successful angioplasty may necessitate this disruptive process; however, the biological response to this injury may result in acute occlusive dissection and resteno-sis. Plaque fracture with stretching of the intima and media may unpredictably result in acute occlusive dissection in 2-12% of patients undergoing balloon dilation.[6] Fur-thermore, secondary sequelae of this disruptive process, such as thrombosis, elastic recoil and neointimal hyperplasia, may contribute to the 30-40% incidence of reocclu-sion or restenosis within six months of an apparently successful dilatation.[7] These limitations of PTCA have been the impetus behind the development of new inter-ventional technologies.

AUTOPERFUSION BALLOON ANGIOPLASTY

The maximum duration of balloon inflation during conventional PTCA is usually short (30-60 seconds), limited by patient intolerance to chest pain and hemodynamic or electrical instability. Numerous pharmacologic and mechanical techniques have been used to effect longer balloon catheter inflation times. These techniques have included pretreatment with β-blockers, calcium channel blockers, or nitrates and at-tempts at perfusion using fluorocarbons, retrograde perfusion via the coronary sinus or perfusion pump systems.[8,9] However, the majority of these techniques have re-sulted in only modest increases in balloon inflation times and have occasionally been associated with significant ventricular arrhythmias. A subsequent solution was the development of an autoperfusion balloon catheter which would allow continuous myocardial perfusion through a central lumen in the inflated balloon, thus maintaining distal coronary blood flow and allowing more gradual and prolonged balloon catheter inflation.

Theoretically, prolonged and gradual expansion of the balloon may result in less trauma to the vessel and less risk of a large dissection and acute occlusion. Prolonged balloon dilatation may desiccate the plaque and compromise nutrient flow to the media through compression of the vasa vasorum, thus possibly reducing proliferation of smooth muscle cells which can lead to restenosis. Thus, autoperfusion angioplasty may reduce the two major limitations of conventional angioplasty: acute occlusive dissection and restenosis.

Several different varieties of autoperfusion balloon catheters (PBC) have been used to perform coronary angioplasty in the animal model and in humans.[10-13] The PBC used by the authors is a 4.5 French double lumen polyethylene catheter with the central lumen open to linear sideholes (Stack Perfusion Catheter,™ Advanced Cardiovascular Systems, Inc., Santa Clara, CA). It has 10 proximal side holes and 4 distal side holes with a radiopaque marker at the distal end and in the middle of the 20 mm balloon (Figures 1 and 2), and is available in 2.5, 3.0, and 3.5 mm balloons with profiles of 0.064, 0.065, and 0.067 inches.

Our current method for using this catheter is as follows. The autoperfusion catheter with a balloon-to-artery ratio of 1.1 to 1.0 is prepared and advanced across the lesion over a 0.018-inch high torque floppy guidewire. If the target lesion is too tight to permit initial passage of the autoperfusion catheter, an initial dilatation with a 2 mm balloon will be performed. After placement of the PBC, the guide catheter is with-

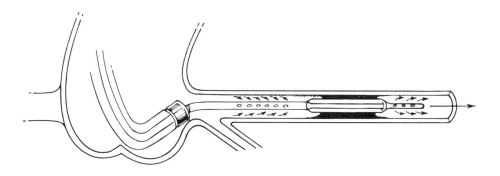

Figure 1. *Diagrammatic representation of an autoperfusion balloon catheter. Multiple side holes are present proximal and distal to the balloon segment. From Stack RS, et al: Interventional cardiac catheterization at Duke University Medical Center. Am J Cardiol 1988;62:3F-24F, with permission.*

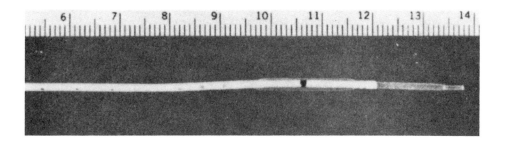

Figure 2. *Photograph of the distal portion of the Stack Perfusion Catheter™ (Advanced Cardiovascular Systems, Inc., Santa Clara, CA). From Stack RS, et al: Perfusion balloon catheter. Am J Cardiol 1988;61:77G-80G, with permission.*

drawn slightly to facilitate entry of blood into the proximal side holes. The balloon is gradually expanded at a rate of 1 atmosphere every 30 seconds to a maximum of 6 atmospheres with a target inflation period of 15 minutes. Once the balloon is inflated, the guidewire is pulled back to the guide catheter to allow maximum flow through the central balloon lumen. The central lumen is flushed with 1,000 units of heparin every 3 minutes. Following deflation of the PBC, the guidewire is reinserted taking care not to pass the wire out the side holes, and the PBC is removed from the system.

Due to the design of the catheter, not all lesions are suitable for PTCA using the PBC. The profile of the PBC is larger than standard balloon catheters, and it may thus be more difficult to place especially across distal lesions. In lesions close to major side branches, inflation of the balloon may occlude these branches and produce ischemia. Also, there is the possibility of damage to the vessel from the portion of the catheter beyond the balloon, and therefore angled or tandem lesions are not suitable. Adequate systemic heparinization and frequent flushing of the catheter, as noted above, is necessary to prevent thrombosis within the central lumen. Finally, an adequate blood pressure must be maintained to ensure perfusion through the catheter and into the myocardium. Thus, an intraaortic balloon pump should be inserted prior to treating a patient in cardiogenic shock with the PBC.

In the initial human studies on the safety of the PBC, 50 consecutive patients undergoing elective angioplasty with this catheter were examined for evidence of myocardial damage or hemolysis.[14] Myocardial damage was assessed with serial electrocardiograms and cardiac enzymes in all 50 patients and with pre- and post-procedure ventriculography in a subgroup of 15 patients. Hemolysis was assessed with plasma free hemoglobin, serum haptoglobin and lactate dehydrogenase in the first 25 consecutive patients. Mean inflation time was 15 minutes, and antegrade flow during inflation was at least TIMI 2 in all patients. Cardiac enzyme assays and electrocardiograms were negative for evidence of myocardial damage in all patients. No statistically significant change in left ventricular function was apparent. Evidence of hemolysis was absent. The authors concluded that prolonged perfusion balloon angioplasty can be performed without evidence of myocardial damage or hemolysis.

Potential Applications of the PBC

There are four potential applications for the use of autoperfusion balloon catheters: to perform routine PTCA, to perform high-risk PTCA, to salvage failed PTCA and to maintain perfusion prior to emergency bypass surgery.

Use of the PBC for Routine PTCA

To assess the efficacy of the PBC as a primary device, the results in the first 122 consecutive patients undergoing elective coronary angioplasty with the PBC at Duke University Medical Center and The Christ Hospital were analyzed.[15] The lesion location was the left anterior descending (50%), right coronary (44%) and left circumflex in 6% of the patients. Coronary angioplasty with the PBC was successful in 120 of the 122 patients (98%) with a reduction in mean diameter stenosis from 85 to 17%. Emergency coronary bypass surgery was necessary in only one patient, and one patient had a late in-hospital coronary occlusion. The mean PBC inflation duration was 13.8 minutes to a maximum inflation pressure of 6.5 ± 0.7 atmospheres. In this series, 63 of the 67 patients eligible for six-month angiographic follow-up were restudied and had an angiographic restenosis rate of 30% (19/63 patients). These preliminary results suggest that the PBC is associated with a high acute success rate and low in-hospital complication rate. Further studies are necessary to compare restenosis rates six months after either PBC or conventional PTCA.

At present, a large multicenter prospective, randomized clinical trial is underway to test the hypothesis that primary PTCA with prolonged inflations will provide better in-hospital anatomic and clinical success and reduce long-term restenosis. Patients not having an acute myocardial infarction and with lesions suitable for the PBC are randomized to short versus long inflations. The short arm consists of two, one minute inflations, while the prolonged inflations are for 15 minutes. Patients are followed for six months with clinical follow-up, exercise treadmill test and second look cardiac catheterization.

Use of the PBC for High-Risk PTCA

Gradual and prolonged inflations of stenoses in proximal large dominant coronary arteries with conventional balloon catheters are usually poorly tolerated due to chest pain or hemodynamic or electrical instability. These high-risk lesions with a large mass of myocardium at risk have been successfully dilated using the PBC.

Use of the PBC to Salvage Failed PTCA

In a recent study, 28 consecutive patients were treated with the PBC for persistent total or subtotal occlusive dissection after failed elective PTCA despite repeated, long inflations using conventional balloon catheters.[16] The mean inflation time with the PBC was 21.4 minutes. Success ($\leq 50\%$ residual stenosis) was achieved in 16 of the 28 patients (57%). Ten of the 12 unsuccessful patients underwent emergency surgery. In conclusion, the PBC can salvage vessel patency in approximately half of the patients who fail conventional balloon angioplasty.

Use of the PBC to Maintain Perfusion Prior to Emergency Bypass Surgery

In cases where coronary patency cannot be achieved after PTCA, the PBC has been used to maintain adequate coronary perfusion and thus maintain hemodynamic and electrical stability en route to surgical revascularization.

Summary

In summary, the PBC can reduce ischemia during PTCA allowing gradual and pro-longed inflations without myocardial damage, even in high risk patients. The PBC appears to be associated with a low incidence of coronary dissection and a high primary success rate. Although the preliminary coronary restenosis rate at 6 month follow-up after either PBC or conventional angioplasty appears to be similar, this will be further defined by the ongoing multicenter trial. However, even if autoperfusion angioplasty proves not to offer significant restenosis-reduction benefits, it may make angioplasty safer, more effective and less uncomfortable for the patient, especially if abrupt vessel closure occurs during the procedure.

ATHERECTOMY

One of the new mechanical approaches designed to overcome many of the limitations of current balloon angioplasty is atherectomy. As the name implies, atherectomy is the mechanical excision and removal of atheromatous plaque. The concept of atherec-tomy centers around the hypothesis that by excising and removing plaque a better local rheological environment may be achieved in the treated vessel segment with less trauma to the vessel wall, thereby reducing the potential for acute occlusion and restenosis to occur. In contrast to surgical endarterectomy, the percutaneous atherec-tomy procedure is intended to remove a portion of the atherosclerotic plaque to create a smooth surface and large lumen without injuring the normal segment of the vessel.

476

At present, three atherectomy devices are undergoing clinical evaluation in human coronary arteries. These devices include Atherocath™ (Devices for Vascular Interventional Inc., Redwood City, CA), Transluminal Extraction-Endarterectomy Catheter – TEC™ (Interventional Technologies Inc., San Diego, CA) and Rotablator™ (Squibb, Inc., Princeton, NJ).

Atherocath™

The Atherocath was developed by Dr. John B. Simpson, the pioneer in this field, and was the first atherectomy catheter tested in humans. This device was initially tested in the peripheral vessels for the treatment of obstructive disease,[17] and clinical investigation of this device in coronary artery disease began in October, 1986.[18]

The Atherocath is shown in Figure 3. This catheter combines a "cutting and retrieval" housing unit and a small balloon attached to the housing. The housing is a cylindric tube with a longitudinal opening on one side through which an enclosed cup-shaped cutter can gain access to atheromatous plaque. The support balloon attaches to the back of the housing opposite the longitudinal opening. The balloon is inflated to less than 20 psi and is designed to hold the housing against the vessel wall. The catheter shaft is a double-lumen structure with sufficient torsional control to direct the housing opening toward the diseased area of the vessel. A hand-held battery-powered motor drive unit is attached to the proximal end of the catheter and drives a cable which rotates the cutter at 2,000 rpm. The catheter is operated over an 0.014-inch guidewire. The coronary catheter sizes are 5, 6, and 7 French.

The procedure is diagrammatically depicted in Figure 4. After intubation of the coronary ostium with the 11 French guiding catheter, the cutter and guidewire assembly are directed through the lesion under fluoroscopic control. The atherectomy catheter is positioned so that the longitudinal opening is directed toward the thickest portion of the atheroma. The support balloon is inflated to stabilize the housing unit and the opening against the atheroma. The motor drive unit is activated, and the tissue within the window is excised and trapped within the nose cone of the catheter. The balloon is deflated, and the window is rotated to another portion of the plaque to remove additional atheromatous material. Several passes with the cutter are possible before the nose cone of the housing unit is full.

In a recent abstract, preliminary results of the coronary Atherocath in the treatment of 260 consecutive patients with 308 lesions were reported.[19] The primary lesion angiographic success rate was 91%. Success was defined as 50% or less residual diameter stenosis and greater than 20% reduction of stenosis. The mean diameter stenosis was reduced from $76 \pm 14\%$ to $13 \pm 22\%$. Complications included 3.5% coronary bypass surgery (9/260 patients), 1.5% Q wave infarction (4/260 patients), 1.2% perforation (3/260 patients) and 0.7% abrupt vessel closure (2/260 patients).

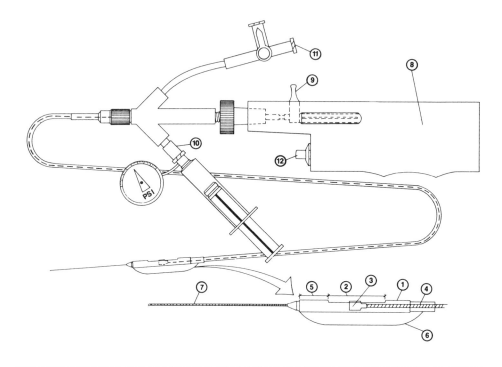

Figure 3. *Peripheral Atherocath™ system. The coronary catheter is similar except for a coaxial over-the-wire design and an overall system miniaturization. The catheter components include: 1) cylindrical housing; 2) longitudinal opening; 3) cutter; 4) cutter drive cable to motor; 5) specimen collection site; 6) balloon support mechanism; 7) fixed guide wire; 8) motor; 9) cutter-advance lever; 10) balloon inflation port; 11) flush port; and 12) on/off switch for motor. From Simpson JB, et al: Transluminal athrectomy for occlusive peripheral vascular disease. Am J Cardiol 1988;61:96G-101G, with permission.*

A recent study evaluated restenosis in native coronary arteries following a successful atherectomy procedure with the Atherocath.[20] Of the 91 patients eligible for follow-up, 75 (82.4%) with 91 lesions had angiographic follow-up. Restenosis was defined as greater than 50% luminal narrowing as measured by electronic calipers. The overall restenosis rate was 40% (37/91 lesions). A proximal lesion location and a vessel size $\geq$ 3.25 mm were associated with lower restenosis rates of 26 and 23%, respectively.

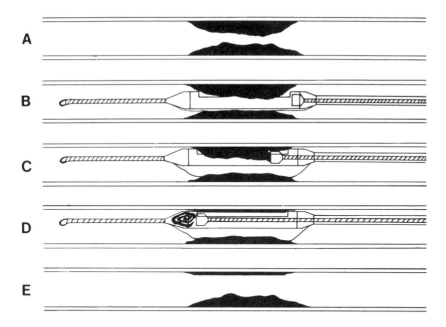

Figure 4. *Diagrammatic representation of an atherectomy procedure with the Atherocath.™*
A: lesion prior to procedure
B: catheter in position across the lesion
C: balloon support inflated
D: cutter advanced and specimen trapped in housing
E: balloon deflated and catheter removed
From Simpson JB, et al: Transluminal athrectomy for occlusive peripheral vascular disease. Am J Cardiol 1988;61:96G-101G, with permission.

Transluminal Extraction-Endarterectomy Catheter

A second atherectomy device is the transluminal extraction-endarterectomy catheter (TEC), which was invented by InterVentional Technologies Inc. and developed in conjunction with Dr. Richard S. Stack at Duke University Medical Center. Early experiments with the TEC involved in vitro and in vivo safety and efficacy studies performed in both normal and atherosclerotic arteries.[21] In December 1987, clinical atherectomy with the TEC was begun in the peripheral arteries, and coronary atherectomy was begun in July, 1988.

The TEC is a wire-based, motor-driven, rotating flexible torque tube designed to excise and extract atherosclerotic plaque. As diagrammatically depicted in Figure 5, the TEC is slowly advanced across the atherosclerotic plaque by tracking over a steerable 0.014-inch guide wire. Plaque is excised by 2 rotating stainless steel blades at the conical head of the catheter. The excised fragments are extracted through the central lumen by continuous vacuum suction. Figure 6 shows a close-up of the conical head of the catheter. Attached to the proximal end of the TEC is the hand-held control piece (Figure 7) which houses the motor and trigger with sites for attachment of a remote battery power source and a vacuum bottle for retrieval of excised material. The trigger activates both the cutting blade rotation and the vacuum system. On the side of the control piece is a lever which controls the relative position, advanced or retracted, of the cutting blades to the lesion. The coronary catheter sizes are 5.5, 6.0, 6.5, 7.0, and 7.5 French.

The procedure is performed via a percutaneous transfemoral technique similar to PTCA. After positioning the 10 French guide catheter in the coronary orifice, a 0.014-inch guide wire is advanced through the guide catheter and across the stenosis to the distal portion of the vessel. The torque tube cutter is then advanced over the guide wire to the origin of the lesion. Intracoronary nitroglycerin (0.1-0.3 mg) is administered before activation of the cutter. A lactated Ringer's solution is infused through the guide catheter during periods of cutter activation. One, two or three excursions are made initially with the smallest catheter across the lesion, each cut lasting 10-15 seconds. Repeat arteriography is performed after each series of cuts to assess the result with progression to successively larger cutter sizes as necessary,

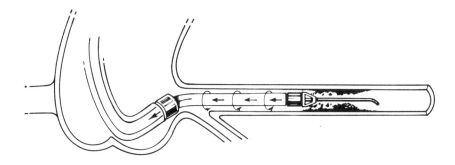

Figure 5. *Diagrammatic depiction of the transluminal extraction-endarterectomy catheter being advanced across an atherosclerotic plaque by tracking over a steerable 0.014-inch guide wire. The excised fragments are extracted through the central lumen by continous vacuum suction. From Stack RS, et al: Interventional cardiac catheterization at Duke University Medical Center. Am J Cardiol 1988; 62:3F-24F, with permission.*

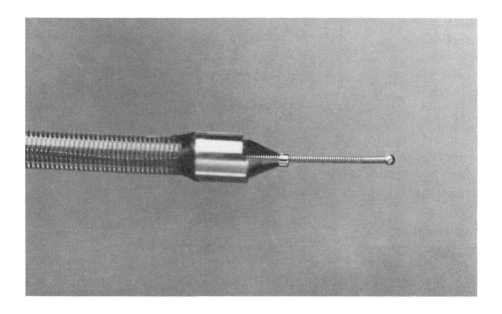

Figure 6. *A close-up of the torque tube and cutter head of the TEC™ over a 0.014-inch guide wire.*

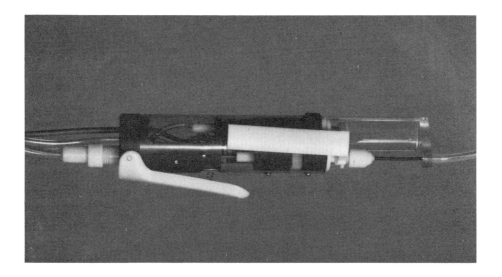

Figure 7. *The hand-held control piece of the TEC™ which houses the motor and trigger with sites for attachment of a remote battery power source and vacuum bottle for retrieval of the excised material.*

depending on the normal internal vessel diameter. If the result remains visually unsatisfactory due to persistent residual stenosis, particularly in patients with large coronary vessels, adjunctive PTCA is performed to optimize the angiographic appearance.

In 1990 we reported the preliminary results of a multicenter study of coronary atherectomy using the TEC.[22] This study included 66 patients at four medical centers. The lesion location was 42% LAD, 42% RCA, 9% circumflex, 5% saphenous vein graft and 2% protected left main stem. The TEC alone was used in 45 patients, and TEC with PTCA was used in 21 patients. The primary angiographic success rate was 92% (61/66 patients, with success being defined as 50% or less residual diameter stenosis). The 5 patients who were not successfully treated with the TEC underwent successful immediate bypass surgery. In all cases, there was no evidence of distal embolization.

A preliminary study on restenosis following a successful TEC procedure was presented at the American Heart Association Scientific Sessions in November 1989.[23] At that time, only 18 patients treated with the TEC alone were eligible for follow-up and all had angiographic follow-up. Restenosis occurred in 6 of the 18 patients (33%). In these patients, if the post-procedural residual stenosis was $\leq 30\%$, the restenosis rate was 14% (1/7 patients).

Rotablator™

The third atherectomy device is the Rotablator which was designed to pulverize plaque material without retrieval. This catheter was developed by Dr. David C. Auth. The Rotablator consists of a high-speed rotary, oblong metal burr in sizes ranging from 1.0 to 2.0 mm in diameter (Figure 8). The distal half of the burr is embedded with

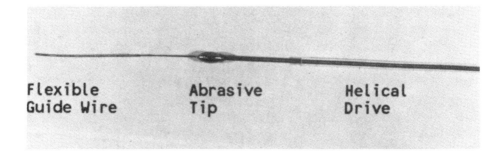

Flexible   Abrasive   Helical
Guide Wire   Tip   Drive

Figure 8. *Photograph of the distal portion of the Rotablator™ with a 1.25 mm diameter, rotation abrasive tip. From Hansen DD, et al: Rotation endarterectomy in normal canine coronary arteries: preliminary report. J Am Coll Cardiol 1988;11(5): 1073-1077. Reprinted with permission.*

fine diamond abrasive particles (30-40 µm) and rotates at approximately 180,000 rpm. The flexible drive shaft is housed in a 4 French Teflon sheath and connected to a turbine which is powered by compressed air. The rotational speed is controlled by the air pressure. The burr and drive shaft track over a central coaxial 0.009-inch guide wire. The steerable guide wire does not rotate with the burr during the atherectomy procedure.[24,25]

The percutaneous intravascular delivery technique used with this atherectomy device is similar to balloon angioplasty. After positioning the 9 French guide catheter in the coronary ostium, the guide wire is advanced across the lesion to the distal portion of the vessel, and the burr is advanced to the origin of the lesion. The burr is rotated at a speed of approximately 180,000 rpm while advancing slowly over the guidewire through the lesion. After 6-8 passes through the lesion, the rotation is stopped, and the burr is withdrawn into the guide catheter. As the majority of particles are less than 5 to 10 µm in size, they can travel downstream through the capillary system to be trapped in the reticuloendothelial activating system.[24,25]

In a recent study, 30 patients underwent percutaneous coronary rotational atherectomy with the Rotablator.[26] The treated vessel was the RCA in 8 patients, LAD in 12 patients, circumflex in 7 patients, posterior descending in 1 patient, and a saphenous vein graft in 2 patients. The angiographic success rate was 97% (29/30 patients). Success was defined as 50% or less residual diameter stenosis. Elevated cardiac enzymes were documented in 5 patients. A no-reflow phenomenon occurred in 6 patients; however, flow was restored in 5 of the patients after administration of intracoronary nitroglycerin and sublingual nifedipine. Angiographic follow-up was obtained in 18 of the patients, and restenosis was documented in 8 of the 18 patients (44%).

Summary

This new and rapidly evolving nonsurgical approach for selectively excising or pulverizing arterial stenoses has demonstrated a high initial success rate and low complication rate. With limited follow-up data, final conclusions about atherectomy restenosis rates cannot be made, although rates appear to be similar to those reported for PTCA.

As each atherectomy device is in the early stages of clinical testing in the coronary arteries, the exact advantages and limitations of each device are unknown. If these devices are found to be safe and effective, they may play a complementary role in the treatment of coronary artery disease. An example of such a synergistic relationship might be the use of the Atherocath for large vessels or eccentric lesions, the use of the TEC for lesions in coronary vessels less than 3 mm (particularly tight lesions or long diffuse lesions) and the use of the Rotablator for smaller vessels, especially short discrete lesions in distal vessels.

The advantages and disadvantages of these atherectomy procedures compared to angioplasty or other newer modalities remain to be determined in prospective controlled trials.

INTRACORONARY STENTS

Another evolving coronary technology is the coronary stent prosthesis. Interest in stenting dates back to 1969 when Dotter placed a tubular coiled wire stent into canine femoral arteries to prevent restenosis after angioplasty.[27] Due to the development of significant narrowing over time, these stents were not used in a clinical setting. Subsequently, interest in stents was rekindled by other investigators who designed and developed a variety of metallic stents which differed in the type of metal used, the arrangement of the metallic components, the amount of metallic surface exposed to the vascular lumen and the deployment technique.[28-31]

The hypothesis behind the insertion of an intracoronary stent at the site of PTCA is two-fold. First, the risk of acute vessel closure would be reduced by both the "tacking up" of intimal flaps and the circumferential application of homogenous radial stress to the vessel wall. This homogenous radial stress would provide a smoother surface and a more concentric dimension to the intraluminal aspect of the vessel after PTCA. Second, the incidence of restenosis would be reduced by the increased blood flow and the decreased blood turbulence resulting in a more favorable rheologic environment.

Certain characteristics are requisite in the creation of an ideal stent. An ideal stent would be: 1) flexible and easily deployable; 2) biocompatible with both the artery into which it is placed and the blood components that traverse it; 3) durable or degradable; and 4) radiopaque.[32]

At present, there are at least four stents under investigation for use in human coronary arteries. These include the Medinvent stent, the nitinol coil stent, the Palmaz-Schatz stent (Johnson & Johnson, Inc., New Brunswick, NJ), and the Gianturco-Roubin stent (Cook Inc., Bloomington, IN).

The Medinvent Stent

The first human intracoronary stent was the Medinvent stent developed by Dr. Ulrich Sigwart.[33] This stent is composed of a stainless steel alloy and has a self-expanding mesh design (Figures 9a,9b,9c). The mesh design incorporates 16 filaments with a standard diameter of 0.09 mm and ranges in length from 15 to 23 mm. Prior to implantation, a doubled-over membrane maintains the stent constrained and elongated on the end of a 1.6 mm diameter delivery catheter.

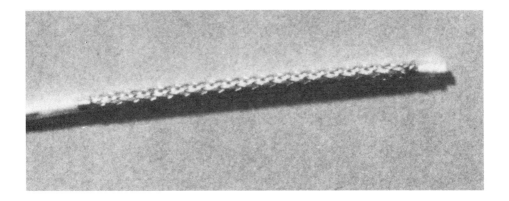

Figure 9a. *The Medinvent stent constrained and elongated on the end of a delivery catheter.*

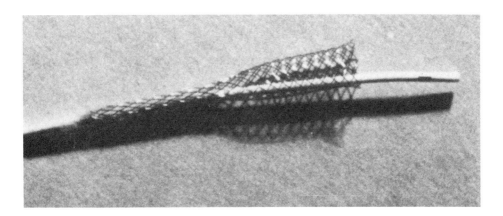

Figure 9b. *Deployment of the stent by withdrawal of a doubled-over membrane. The stent expands with distal to proximal release.*

Prior to stent implantation, the stenosis is dilated in the usual fashion. Subsequently, the balloon catheter is exchanged for the stent-bearing delivery catheter over a 0.014-inch guide wire. After positioning the delivery catheter, the membrane is withdrawn, and the stent expands with distal to proximal release. Once the stent has been deployed, it cannot be retrieved. The size of the selected stent is based on a fully expanded diameter approximately 15% larger than the estimated normal lumen of the recipient artery so that it will be stable once positioned and exert a residual radial pressure on the vessel wall.

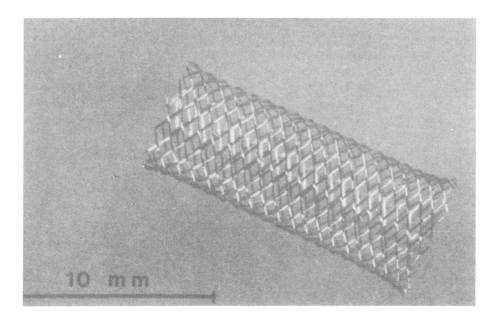

Figure 9c. *A fully expanded Medinvent stent. From Sigwart U, et al: Intravascular stents to prevent occlusion and restenosis after transluminal angioplasty. N Engl J Med 1987;316:701-706. Reprinted with permission.*

The Nitinol Coil Stent

Nitinol is a nickel-titanium alloy with a unique thermal recovery property. If a nitinol wire is annealed at greater than 500° C while being constrained to a desired shape, it will memorize that shape. After cooling, the wire can be straightened and introduced into the body via a catheter. At or near body temperature, the wire will assume its original annealed shape (Figure 10).[34,35] Thus, this unique property would allow nitinol coils to be straightened and passed into the body through relatively small catheters without destroying the coil shape, as would occur with stainless steel wire. At present, no clinical studies have been reported on the use of this stent.

The Palmaz-Schatz Stent

This stent consists of 0.08 mm stainless steel filaments arrayed in a slotted configuration, which when expanded deploy as a meshwork of adjacent parallelograms (Figure 11). An articulation point is present in the center of this 15 mm-long stent to optimize the fit into tortuous arterial segments. In contrast to the self-expanding stent design, the Palmaz-Schatz stent is balloon-expandable. As pioneered by Dr. J.C. Palmaz, this

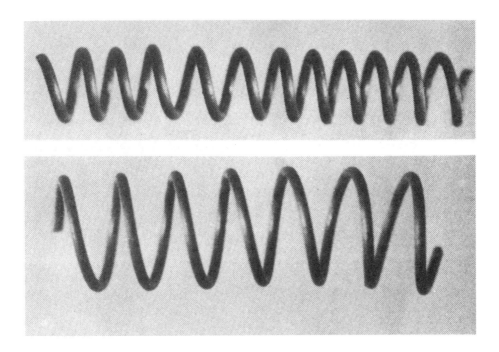

Figure 10. *A nitinol coil stent seen in the compacted configuration (above) and in the original annealed configuration (below). From Dotter C, et al: Transluminal expandable nitinol coil stent grafting: preliminary report. Radiology 1983;147:259-260, with permission.*

design relies on the concept of plastic deformation, whereby a metal will not change shape once it is stretched beyond a certain limit.[32,36]

After placing the stent-balloon apparatus at the site of the pre-dilated stenosis, the stent is deployed by inflating the balloon to 8-10 atmospheres for 15 seconds. The balloon is then deflated and withdrawn. To obtain an optimal stent-to artery ratio of 1.0-1.1, additional inflations with a larger balloon may be needed.[37]

The Gianturco-Roubin Stent

This balloon-expandable stent was developed at Emory University by Drs. C. Gianturco and G.S. Roubin. The stent is made of mono-filamentous stainless steel (0.08 mm in diameter) and is formed into an interdigitating coil structure (Figure 12). The stent is

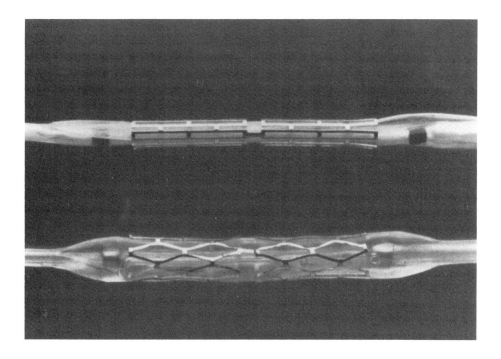

Figure 11. *The Palmaz-Schatz stent shown before and after expansion over a standard balloon angioplasty catheter. From Ellis SE: The Palmza-Schatz stent: potential coronary applications in Topol EJ (ed): Textbook of Interventional Cardiology. Philadelphia, W.B. Saunders Company, 1990, pp 623-632, with permission.*

wrapped firmly around a standard, deflated balloon catheter, thus providing a relatively flexible, low-profile device. The length of the stent is 20 mm. This stent tends to undergo slight elastic recoil; thus a stent intended for a 3 mm diameter vessel is mounted on a 3.5 mm balloon catheter. The deployment of this stent is similar to the Palmaz-Schatz stent.[38]

All four stent designs have advantages and disadvantages. The thickness of the 0.08 mm filaments of the Medinvent stent, in contrast to the 0.015 mm filaments of the Palmaz-Schatz and Gianturco-Roubin stents, may play a role in the reported increased frequency of thrombosis.[37,39] Nitinol coil stents may expand prematurely in the guiding catheter and inhibit deployment.[35] Both the Palmaz-Schatz stent and Gianturco-Roubin stent have the potential for dislodgement from the balloon catheter during delivery to the placement site. Also, all of these stents except the Nitinol coil stent are radiolucent. In essence, the ideal stent has not yet been created.

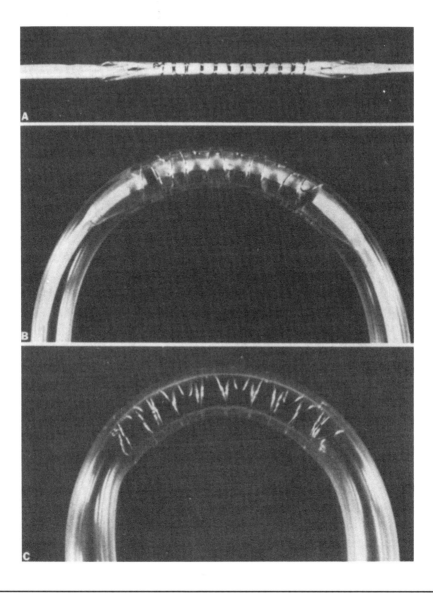

Figure 12. *The Gianturco-Roubin stent:*
A. the stent wrapped around a standard deflated balloon catheter;
B. the stent expanded in transparent flexible tubing after inflation of the balloon catheter;
C. the stent expanded after removal of the deflated balloon catheter.
From Roubin GS, et al: Early and late results of intracoronary arterial stenting after coronary angioplasty in dogs. Circulation 1987;76:891-897. Reprinted with permission.

Summary

Because intracoronary stents are in their infancy, their utility in obviating the need for bypass surgery after an acute occlusion or preventing restenosis remains to be determined. However, preliminary studies support the use of stents as an alternative to emergency bypass surgery after acute vessel occlusion in selected patients.[40,41] Their ability to lower the restenosis rate remains to be determined in long-term follow-up.

In an attempt to develop an ideal stent, future designers may coat stents with heparin and various antiplatelet agents, seed endothelial cells onto stents, and create bioabsorbable stents.

CONCLUSION

Interventional cardiology is an exciting and rapidly expanding field. The technologic explosion that has occurred since the introduction of PTCA by Andreas Gruentzig in 1979 has resulted in a multitude of new devices. After completion of their developmental phases, these devices must undergo prospective randomized trials in comparison with the current state-of-the-art techniques: balloon angioplasty and coronary artery bypass surgery. Finally, all these new devices must be directly compared with each other to determine the best use of each new technology.

REFERENCES

1. Gruentzig AR, Senning A, Siegenthaler WE: Nonoperative dilatation of coronary-artery stenosis: percutaneous transluminal coronary angioplasty. N Engl J Med 1979;301:61-68.

2. Kozak LJ: Hospital inpatient surgery: United States 1983-1987. Advanced data from vital and health statistics, no. 169. DHHS publication no. (PHS) 89-1250. Public Health Service, Hyattsville, Maryland.

3. Cowley MJ, Dorros G, Kelsey SF, Van Roden K, Detre KM: Acute coronary events associated with percutaneous transluminal coronary angioplasty. Am J Cardiol 1984;53:12C-16C.

4. Waller BF: "Crackers, breakers, stretchers. drillers, scrapers, shavers, burners, welders and melters" — the future treatment of atherosclerotic coronary artery disease? A clinical-morphologic assessment. J Am Coll Cardiol 1989;13:969-987.

5. Block PC: Mechanism of transluminal angioplasty. Am J Cardiol 1984;53:69C-71C.

6. Simpfendorfer C, Belardi J, Bellamy G, Galan K, Franco I, Hollman J: Frequency, management and follow-up of patients with acute coronary occlusion after percutaneous transluminal angioplasty. Am J Cardiol 1987;59:267-269.

7. Blackshear JL, O'Callaghan WG, Califf RM: Medical approaches to prevention of restenosis after coronary angioplasty. J Am Coll Cardiol 1987;9:834-48.

8. Lasala JM, Cleman NW: Myocardial protection during percutaneous transluminal coronary angioplasty. Cardiology Clinics 1988;6(3):329-343.

9. Zalewski A, Goldberg S: Protection of the ischemic myocardium during coronary angioplasty. Cardiovasc Clin 1988;19:79-98.

10. Stack RS, Quigley PJ, Collins G, Phillips HR: Perfusion balloon catheter. Am J Cardiol 1988;61:77G-80G.

11. Erbel R, Clas W, Busch V, Von Seelan W, Brennecke R, Blomer H, Meyer J: New balloon catheter for prolonged percutaneous transluminal coronary angioplasty and bypass flow in occluded vessels. Cathet Cardiovasc Diagn 1986;12:116-123.

12. Turi ZG, Campbell CA, Gottimukkala M, Loner R: Preservation of distal coronary perfusion during prolonged balloon inflation with an autoperfusion angioplasty catheter. Circulation 1987;75:1273-1280.

13. White CJ, Ramee SR, Banks AK, Ross TC, Graeber GM, Berman M, Sogard D, Slaughter J, Price HL: A new passive perfusion PTCA catheter. Circulation 1988;78(suppl II):II-104.

14. Muhlestein JB, Quigley PJ, Phillips HR, Smith JE, Enos SM, Navetta FI, Tcheng JE, Stack RS: Does myocardial damage or hemolysis occur during prolonged perfusion balloon angioplasty? J Am Coll Cardiol 1990;15:250A.

15. Quigley PJ, Kereiakes DJ, Abbottsmith CW, Bauman RP, Tcheng JE, Muhlestein JB, Phillips HR, Stack RS: Prolonged autoperfusion angioplasty: immediate clinical outcome and angiographic follow-up. J Am Coll Cardiol 1989;13:155A.

16. Smith JE, Quigley PJ, Tcheng JE, Bauman RP, Thomas J, Stack RS: Can prolonged perfusion balloon inflations salvage vessel patency after failed angioplasty? Circulation 1989;80(suppl II):II-373.

17. Simpson JB, Johnson DE, Thapliyal HV, Marks DS, Braden LJ: Transluminal atherectomy: a new approach to the treatment of atherosclerotic vascular disease. Circulation 1985;72(suppl II):III-146.

18. Simpson JB, Robertson GC, Selmon MR: Percutaneous coronary atherectomy. Circulation 1988;78(suppl II):II-82.

19. Simpson J, Rowe M, Robertson G, Selmon M, Vetter J, Braden L, Hinohara T: Directional coronary atherectomy: success and complication rates and outcome predictors. J Am Coll Cardiol 1990;15:196A.

20. Hinohara T, Rowe M, Sipperly ME, Johnson D, Robertson G, Selmon M, Leggestt J, Simpson J: Restenosis following directional coronary atherectomy of native coronary arteries. J Am Coll Cardiol 1990;15:196A.

21. Perez JA, Hinohara T, Quigley PJ, Lee MM, Hoffman PU, Mikat EM, Phillips HR, Stack RS: In-vitro and in-vivo experimental results using a new wire-guided concentric atherectomy device. J Am Coll Cardiol 1988;11:109A.

22. Stack RS, Phillips HR, Quigley PJ, Tcheng JE, Bauman RP, Ohman EM, O'Neill WW, Galichia JT, Walker C: Multicenter registry of coronary atherectomy using the transluminal extraction-endarterectomy catheter. J Am Coll Cardiol 1990;15:196A.

23. Sketch MH, Quigley PJ, Tcheng JE, Bauman RP, Phillips HR, Stack RS: Restenosis following coronary transluminal extraction-endarterectomy. Circulation 1989;80(suppl II):II-583.

24. Hansen DD, Auth DC, Hall M, Ritchie JL: Rotational endarterectomy in normal canine coronary arteries: preliminary report. J Am Coll Cardiol 1988;11:1073-1077.

25. Ahn SS, Auth D, Marcus DR, Wesley SM: Removal of focal atheromatous lesions by angioscopically guided high-speed rotary atherectomy. J Vasc Surg 1988;7:292-300.

26. O'Neill WW, Friedman HZ, Cragg D, Strzelecki MR, Gangadharan V, Levine AB, Ramos RG: Initial clinical experience and early follow-up of patients undergoing mechanical rotary endarterectomy. Circulation 1989;80(suppl II):II-584.

27. Dotter CT: Transluminally-placed coilspring endarterial tube grafts: long-term patency in canine popliteal artery. Invest Radiol 1969;4:392-332.

28. Cragg A, Lund G, Rysavy J, Castaneda F, Castaneda-Zuniga WR, Amplatz K: Non-surgical placement of arterial endoprosthesis: a new technique using nitinol wire. Radiology 1983;147:261-263.

29. Maas D, Zollikofer CL, Largiader F, Senning A: Radiological follow-up of transluminally inserted vascular endoprosthesis: an experimental study using expendable spirals. Radiology 1984;152:659-663.

30. Palmaz JC, Sibbitt RR, Reuter SR, Tio FO, Rice WJ: Expandable intraluminal graft: a preliminary study. Radiology 1985;156:73-77.

31. Wright KC, Wallace S, Charnsangavej C, Carrasco CH, Gianturco C: Percutaneous endovascular stents: an experimental evaluation. Radiology 1985;156:69-72.

32. Ellis E, Topol EJ: Intracoronary stents: will they fulfill their promise as an adjunct to angioplasty? J Am Coll Cardiol 1989;13:1425-1430.

33. Sigwart U, Poel J, Mirkovitch V, Joffie F, Kappenberger L: Intravascular stents to prevent occlusion and restenosis after transluminal angioplasty. N Engl J Med 1987;316:701-706.

34. Dotter CT, Bushmann RW, McKinney MK, Rosch J: Transluminal expandable nitinol coil stent grafting: preliminary report. Radiology 1983;147:259-260.

35. Cragg A, Lund G, Rysavy J, Castaneda F, Castaneda-Zuniga WR, Amplatz K: Non-surgical placement of arterial endoprosthesis: a new technique using nitinol wire. Radiology 1983;147:261-263.

36. Schatz RA: A view of vascular stents. Circulation 1989;79:445-457.

37. Ellis SE: The Palmaz-Schatz stent: potential coronary applications, in Topol EJ (ed): *Textbook of Interventional Cardiology.* Philadelphia, WB Saunders Co, 1990, pp 623-632.

38. Roubin GS, Robinson KA, King SB, Gianturco C, Black AJ, Brown JE, Siegel RJ, Douglas JS: Early and late results or intracoronary arterial stenting after coronary angioplasty in dogs. Circulation 1987;76:891-897.

39. Sigwart U, Urban P, Sadeghi H, Kappenberger L: Implantation of 100 coronary artery stents: learning curve for the incidence of acute early complications. J Am Coll Cardiol 1989;13:107A.

40. Sigwart U, Urban P, Golf S, Kaufmann U, Imbert C, Fischer A, Kappenberger L: Emergency stenting for acute occlusion after coronary balloon angioplasty. Circulation 1988; 78:1121-1127.

41. Roubin GS, Douglas JS, Lembo NJ, Black AJ, King SB: Intracoronary stenting for acute closure following PTCA. Circulation 1988;78(suppl II):II-407.

Chapter 21

FUTURE APPLICATIONS OF LASER THERAPY IN CORONARY ARTERY DISEASE

G. Michael Vincent

INTRODUCTION

The application of laser energy to the cardiovascular system is relatively new and holds considerable promise for the future. The excitement surrounding laser applications stems in part from the "star wars" appeal of laser light, but more importantly from the unique characteristics of the laser. LASER, an acronym for **L**ight **A**mplification by **S**timulated **E**mission of **R**adiation, describes a process whereby a light of one color (monochromatic) is propagated in a single direction (spatial coherence) with all waves oscillating together in time (temporal coherence). When coupled with high levels of energy, these characteristics give the laser its remarkable poser. With respect to cardiovascular applications, this power is both an asset and a drawback. The laser can heat tissue causing coagulation of proteins, vaporize tissue by thermal mechanisms, remove tissue by photochemical and electromechanical means, and can cut a sharply demarcated line or remove a desired volume of tissue. The light can be delivered to a very small or a large area, by direct illumination from the laser or by transmission via optical fibers, giving enormous flexibility and precise control to the laser application. However, harnessing this tremendous power has proven to be a difficult task, especially in the area of angioplasty, where confinement of the laser effect to the atherosclerotic plaque and prevention of injury to adjacent or underlying vascular tissue have been significant challenges.

Laser applications to the cardiovascular system have been investigated since the late 1970s, with particular interest directed at laser angioplasty of atherosclerotic vessels.[1-3] Early results demonstrated the ability of argon, CO_2 and Nd:YAG lasers to effectively remove plaque.[4-7] These lasers, however, when used in the continuous wave (cw) mode [the continuous application of laser energy, as opposed to pulsed application, the delivery of the energy over microsecond to millisecond intervals] all caused significant thermal damage to the area surrounding the treatment site. This was manifested by charring of the surface of the irradiated area and vacuolization of the surrounding tissue from the explosive effects of vaporization. Also, these lasers were found to be non-selective with respect to the injury produced, with the arterial wall as susceptible as the plaque. Subsequent studies reported a high incidence of perforation and damage to the vessel wall when forward surface illumination from a bare optical fiber was used.[8-10] It became apparent that harnessing laser power was a substantial challenge, and efforts since that time have focussed largely on safer delivery systems.

A fundamental initial question was whether laser vaporization of plaque produced particulate matter which would embolize to distal vascular beds, or if noxious gases or other compounds would be produced. The principal byproducts are nontoxic gases such as CO_2, nitrogen, and hydrocarbons, and particulate materials of a few microns in diameter, with little evidence of embolic material,[11-14] but larger particulate debris of several hundred or more microns has been identified as well.[15] Embolic events have been uncommon in clinical trials.

LASER ANGIOPLASTY

At present, no systems are approved for routine use in coronary artery disease. The two peripheral angioplasty systems include innovations which attempt to prevent the wall damage and perforation previously seen with bare optical fiber irradiation noted above.

Metal Capped Laser Fibers

Early work on metal capped fibers demonstrated more uniform effect on the vessel wall than direct beam angioplasty and a decreased incidence of perforation.[16-18] This system, also referred to as the "Laserprobe," "thermal angioplasty," and "Hot Tip angioplasty," incorporates a metal cap at the end of the optical fiber, which is heated by the laser energy to a temperature of 150° to 400° C. Usually the laser probe is used in conjunction with balloon angioplasty in which case it is referred to as "laser assisted balloon angioplasty." Two probe designs are available. A solid tip with a blunt-nosed bullet shaped configuration is used for complete occlusions and is advanced while heated with modest pressure until the lesion is recanalized. The other probe has an eccentric guidewire channel. This probe is used for laser therapy of stenotic lesions. After a guide wire is passed through the narrowed segment, the probe is passed "over the wire" through the lesion. This guidance system significantly reduces the risk of extraluminal passage of the probe and consequent vessel perforation. The commonly used laser probes have a diameter of 1.0 to 2.5 mm and can easily be passed through a percutaneously placed 8 Fr sheath. The channel created by the laser probe is generally somewhat smaller than the tip diameter.[19,20] Balloon dilatation is therefore used to produce greater luminal enlargement.

Figures 1a and 1b show an example of Laserprobe angioplasty. A 4 cm severely stenotic segment is seen in Figure 1a, and Figure 1b shows the vessel after passage of a 2.5 mm probe. The result was improved further after balloon angioplasty with a 5 mm balloon. In addition to the solid metal tips, a new version of the Laserprobe called the Spectraprobe has an opening at the tip of the metal cap allowing a percentage of the laser energy (about 20%) to be emitted from the tip of the fiber, with the majority of the laser energy still used to heat the metallic cap. The actual mechanism of recanalization of vessels with these probes is somewhat uncertain. Early experimental studies[16-20] suggested that vaporization of the plaque material was the principal mechanism.

An example of metal tip angioplasty showing plaque ablation is shown in Figures 2a and 2b. A severely diseased tibial vessel in an amputated limb was subjected to laser angioplasty using a 2.0 mm probe. Figure 2a shows the severely stenotic tibial vessel before laser application. Figure 2b shows the vessel after passage of the metal capped fiber. In this example, it appears that atherosclerotic material has been vaporized by the laser probe. However, subsequent studies have suggested that vaporization

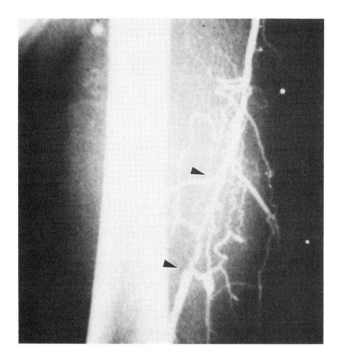

Figure 1a. *Distal superficial femoral artery of a 76-year-old woman with claudication and a resting ABI (ankle-brachial index) of 0.34. A severely stenotic 4 cm long segment is seen between the arrows.*

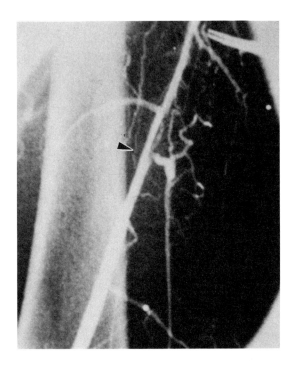

Figure 1b. *Angiograms following passage of a 2.5 mm Trimedyne Laser Probe over a guidewire passed through the lesion, but prior to balloon angioplasty. The hemostat tip indicates the proximal side of the severely stenotic segment seen in panel A, and the arrow the distal extent. Following laser/balloon angioplasty, the ABI was 0.81.*

of plaque may not be the major mechanism of successful recanalization, and that alternative mechanisms are likely.[21-24] Based on extensive experience and angiographic findings, Diethrich et al[22] suggested that the probe is usually extraluminal during recanalization of a totally obstructed vessel, and therefore would not vaporize the plaque but might open a channel in the media or subintimal layers by either thermal or mechanical means. White et al[21] demonstrated both plaque vaporization and extraluminal recanalization and concluded that the laser probe takes the path of least resistance, which is often subintimal or in a plane in the media or medial-adventitial boundary, passing back into the lumen of the vessel at a distal location in successful cases. In unsuccessful cases the probe does not return to the lumen or exits out the adventitia causing a perforation. Calcification appears to be a common cause of difficulty, deflecting the hot tip away from the lumen and into the medial layers.[19,21,22]

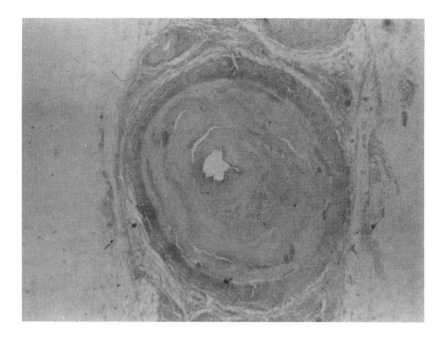

Figure 2a. *Photomicrography of an H & E stained section of an atherosclerotic human tibial vessel x 40. Note the severe luminal narrowing and extensive athero-sclerosis.*

Even in stenotic lesions the effect may not be vaporization primarily, but a combination of some vaporization, thermal remodeling, and mechanical dilatation by the probe.[23,24]

The results of hot tip angioplasty in patients are still preliminary, since the device has been available for only a relatively short time. Several large clinical studies have reported the short-term effects, however.[19,22,25,26] Diethrich et al[25] reported on 206 consecutive, unselected patients with lower extremity peripheral vascular disease in whom 358 laser/balloon procedures were performed.[25] In this series, both percutaneous entry (52%) and open surgical entry (48%) were used. Complications were noted in 11.1%. Perforation occurred in 15 (4.2%), thrombosis in 16 (4.5%), spasm in 5 (1.4%), and a false aneurysm at the femoral puncture site in 7 (2.0%). Success, as defined by relief of symptoms and an increase in the ankle-brachial index of > 0.15, occurred in 65%. Success was most likely in short occlusions, stenotic lesions, and in

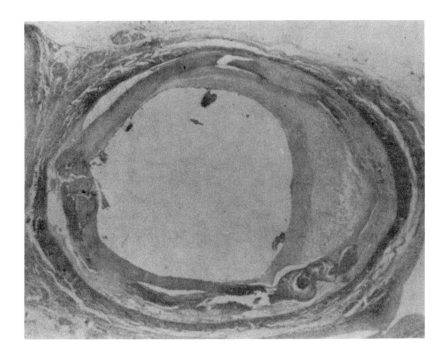

Figure 2b. *Photomicrograph of the same tibial vessel after passage of a 2.0 mm laser probe using 10 watts argon power and a 10 second exposure as the probe was passed through the lesion x 2. The probe would not pass through the lesion "cold."*

larger, proximal vessels. Failure was associated with calcification, inadequate distal runoff circulation, and inability to control/prevent reocclusion and restenosis.

Sanborn et al[20,26] and Cumberland et al[19] have reported an initial success rate of 75-85% in selected patients. In 129 patients, one-year follow-up of the 99 initial successes showed an overall clinical patency of 77%.[26] Patency was highest for stenoses (95%) and 1-3 cm occlusions (93%), lower for the 4-7 cm occlusions at 76%, and significantly lower (58%) for occlusions greater than 7 cm.

As noted earlier, a newer probe design from Trimedyne called the Spectraprobe PLR has become available. It is a hybrid probe, with 20% of the laser energy delivered as a direct beam from the tip of the fiber and 80% heating the metal tip. A preliminary clinical study in 9 iliac and 23 femoral occlusions showed successful recanalization in 78%, 25/32.[27] No follow-up was reported to assess the patency rate. There were two perforations, without sequelae. Other preliminary reports in high-risk patients[28] and in those with extensive vascular disease requiring simultaneous surgical intervention[29] showed only modest success. Several investigators have used the Laserprobe to recanalize occluded femoral popliteal grafts with an approximately 70% success rate.[25,30,31]

"Hot tip" devices heated by energy sources other than laser are also being studied. A radiofrequency heated metal tip, 2.3 mm diameter, has been used in 12 patients with 13 total occlusion or stenotic lesions in the superficial femoral artery and popliteal system.[32] Recanalization, followed by balloon dilation was possible in 9 patients, 75%, with improvement in symptoms and ankle-brachial index. No complications were reported. This device may be a less expensive alternative to the laser heated systems.

Direct Argon Laser Angioplasty

The other device currently approved for peripheral laser angioplasty is the LASTAC system.[33] This system uses an 18 Watt argon laser which effectively vaporizes plaque by a thermal mechanism, with thermal charring and vacuolization around the irradiated area. The laser energy is transmitted through an optical fiber which is passed through a catheter placed in the targeted vessel. The perforation problem associated with bare optical fibers has been addressed by placing a balloon at the end of the guiding catheter. The balloon acts as a centering mechanism and interrupts blood flow. Heparinized saline or Ringers solution is used to flush blood from the treatment area to prevent damage to the fiber tip and allow unobstructed delivery of laser energy to the plaque. In addition, the flush solution may cool the surrounding tissue and minimize the thermal injury to adjacent vessel wall. A potential advantage of the direct laser angioplasty system is the possibility that more tissue is vaporized than with the hot tip method, and presumably, this could lead to an improved outcome and reduced restenosis.

In one study,[34] 24 patients were treated, 13 with total occlusions (3-12 cm) of the superficial femoral artery, 6 with stenosis of the superficial femoral artery, 3 with stenosis of the popliteal artery, and 2 with stenoses of a peroneal or posterior tibial artery. Success was obtained in 16/24 (67%), and over 18 months of follow-up 3 patients have shown some decline in clinical findings. In another study, 33 arteries, 29 superficial and 4 iliac, were irradiated.[35] Primary success rate was reported at 91%, with mean ABI increasing from 0.6 to 0.81. At five months the patency rate was 72%. Complications included 2 intimal dissections which caused failure of the angioplasty, 1 perforation without sequelae, and 1 embolus. An updated report by these investigators on 53 peripheral and 5 coronary cases showed initial success in 92%. Total occlusions of mean length of 9 cm in the femoral artery showed success in 30/33, and there was 100% success in 11 stenoses. Total occlusion of the iliac was successfully treated in 8/9. Six-month follow-up revealed a 71% patency rate. Of 12 arteries which closed, 5 occurred within 24 hours of the procedure. Complications included 3 perforations, without consequence, and 2 emboli. These initial results with the direct argon LASTAC system appear to be comparable to or better than the metal capped laser probe results, but it is not possible to determine if comparable patients were selected. There is still a significant restenosis/reocclusion rate, however, which needs further study.

EXPERIMENTAL ANGIOPLASTY SYSTEMS IN CLINICAL TRIALS

Clinical Trials of Coronary Angioplasty Using the Laserprobe and LASTAC Lasers

The coronary trials of the LASTAC system are very preliminary. Foschi et al[36] reported on 36 patients (31 men) in whom 37 total occlusion lesions were treated. Success, defined as recanalization with a 20% increment in luminal diameter and a residual luminal stenosis of 2%, was achieved in 31/37 (84%). There were 2 arterial dissections related to the laser delivery, 1 of which required emergency bypass surgery, a 2.7% (1/37) rate, similar to that occurring with conventional balloon angioplasty. Other complications included reversible arrhythmias (type and frequency not reported) and femoral puncture site hematomas. During a follow-up of 0 to 7.3 months on 30 patients there were 8 reclosures (27%).

Coronary interventions with the metallic capped Laserprobe are also preliminary. Cumberland et al[37] reported initial results with four patients. There was 1 dissection, thought to be mechanical in origin, but recanalization was apparently successful in all 4. However, two patients with left anterior descending angioplasty had an anterior myocardial infarction within 4-12 hours after angioplasty, a 50% serious complication rate. A second study by Crea et al[38] described three patients treated at the time of coronary artery bypass surgery, presumably with somewhat greater control of the probe than with the percutaneous application. Even in these circumstances, 1/3 had perforation and unsuccessful recanalization, while in 2 there was recanalization. There was no follow-up reported on these patients, so the patency rate and subsequent complications are not known. Sanborn et al[39] reported on seven patients receiving percutaneous coronary Laserprobe angioplasty. Recanalization was successful in 4, and no significant complications were encountered. One of the patients in whom recanalization occurred required bypass surgery during the short follow-up reported.

Spectroscopic Guidance of Laser Angioplasty

Fluorescence spectroscopy may be useful for identifying plaque in preparation for laser angioplasty. A low-powered laser is used to induce tissue fluorescence, and the fluorescent signals from plaque have been reported to be different from those from normal wall,[40-43] allowing differentiation of plaque from normal wall. In addition, the fluorescence patterns may identify plaque composition.[44] It has also been suggested that plaque removal is accompanied by a return of the fluorescence signal to a normal pattern, thus providing an endpoint for the angioplasty procedure.[45,46] This technique has been coupled with a 480 nm laser[47,48] into a system called the "Smart Laser."

Geschwind et al[49] described the results in 19 patients with total occlusions of the superficial femoral artery 4-25 cm in length. The patients included some with calcified vessels. The report indicated successful recanalization in all patients, allowing subsequent balloon dilatation to be performed. A potential disadvantage of this promising system is the cost, currently about $250,000. A similar system using a krypton-fluorine excimer laser at 248 nm for both diagnostic fluorescence induction and plaque treatment is also being investigated.[50]

Spears Laser Balloon Angioplasty

Balloon angioplasty of the coronary arteries is complicated by an acute closure rate of 4-6%[51,52] and a restenosis rate of 25% or more.[53,54] Hiehle et al[55] proposed that heat sealing of the vascular wall during balloon inflation would avoid some of these complications, and subsequently laser balloon angioplasty (LBA) was developed. The Spears Laser Balloon incorporates a laser fiber wrapped in a helical fashion around the balloon enclosed portion of the balloon catheter. An Nd:YAG laser is used to provide laser energy during balloon inflation. The balloon displaces blood from vascular lumen, and since the balloon itself is transparent to the laser, laser energy, and therefore heat, is applied to the vessel wall. The fractured segments and dissections of the vessel wall and separations of plaque from vessel wall which result from the balloon inflation are fused and 'heat sealed.'

Studies in iliac arteries of the atherosclerotic rabbit compared the effect of laser balloon angioplasty (LBA) with that of balloon angioplasty alone.[56] LBA at a laser energy level of 176 joules produced a statistically larger lumen both initially and at one month follow-up than conventional balloon angioplasty. However, LBA using higher laser power, 300 J, caused coagulation necrosis of the vessel wall, intimal proliferation, and extravascular fibrosis, and loss of the initial increase in luminal diameter at one-month follow-up. No perforation or thrombosis occurred. In clinical studies the laser balloon treatment has been associated with a restenosis rate of 30-50%, thus limiting its usefulness.[57,58]

Excimer Laser Angioplasty

The excimer lasers, with wavelengths in the ultraviolet range of the electromagnetic spectrum, have different effects on tissue than the previously mentioned continuous wave lasers. Histologic examination reveals very precise removal of tissue with sharp margins and minimal evidence of adjacent thermal damage.[59,60]

Clinical trials with peripheral and coronary vessels have shown promising results. Wollenek et al[61] successfully recanalized a 7 cm total occlusion of the superficial femoral artery with a 308 nm laser transmitted through a 1 mm diameter fiber. The channel created in the 6-7 mm vessel was approximately 1 mm, the same size as the fiber, and the procedure was completed by balloon angioplasty. No complications occurred. Litvak et al[62] reported on 23 patients with peripheral vascular disease treated with the 308 nm laser. Sixteen patients with total occlusions (< 5 to > 20 cm length) and 7 patients with stenoses were treated. Recanalization was possible in 81% of occlusions, with 2 of the failures occurring in occlusions greater than 20 cm in length. No mention was made of balloon dilatation. After a mean follow-up of four months, 12/13 vessels were patent, for a reocclusion rate of 8% and a short-term overall success rate of 75%. The success in stenoses was disappointing. Initial success was described in 5/7, but there were 3 restenoses (60%), for an overall success rate of only 29%. Recent reports of coronary excimer laser angioplasty indicate good initial results, complication rates similar to balloon angioplasty, but restenosis rates of 32 to 56%.[63,64] Thus, like other interventional procedures in the coronary arteries, restenosis continues to be the "Achilles heel" of laser angioplasty. One disadvantage of the excimer laser is the cost, currently ranging from about $120,000 to $200,000.

Selective Ablation of Plaque

All of the laser techniques described so far cause damage to the plaque and arterial wall in a non-selective fashion. A laser system which selectively removes the plaque while leaving the normal wall intact would therefore be a significant improvement. It has been proposed that selective absorption of laser energy by endogenous pigments[47,48] or by exogenously administered pigments which accumulate in plaque[65] may provide this selectivity. Prince et al[47] demonstrated that yellow-fatty plaque had a different absorption spectrum than normal arterial wall in the wavelength range of 420-530 nm. Application of laser energy in this "window" of wavelengths seemed to allow preferential ablation of plaque. Concern has been expressed that atherosclerotic plaque is a heterogeneous and complex material and that not all plaques are the yellow, fatty variety, and therefore all may not preferentially absorb laser energy at these wavelengths. A preliminary report by Orme et al[48] has demonstrated a large disparity of absorption spectra in a set of heterogeneous plaques, including fatty, fibrous, mixed, calcified, and hemorrhagic specimens. It is not certain whether any consistent natural chromophore exists in plaque which will preferentially absorb a given wavelength.

Spears et al[65] reported preferential accumulation of hematoporphyrin derivative in plaque, an observation confirmed by several other investigators,[66-68] and preferential accumulation of dihematoporphyrin ether and tetraphenyl porphine sulfonate, with a 2 to 3 times greater concentration of the pigments in plaque than in non-plaqued arterial wall.[68] Selective ablation of porphyrin photosensitized plaque using 630 nm laser has been demonstrated both in vitro[69] and in vivo.[70] Tetracycline may also be retained preferentially in plaque compared to the arterial wall.[71,72]

Angioscopic Guidance

Angioscopic guidance also holds promise for a safer and more directed laser angioplasty process. An example of angioscopy in a rabbit aorta is shown in Figure 3. Several studies using new ultrathin angioscopes have demonstrated the technical feasibility of angioscopy, including coronary angioscopy, and have suggested the angioscope as a tool for guidance of laser energy.[73-76] Human angioscopic studies have provided important information regarding the pathoanatomy of coronary lesions, helping to define the important role of complex anatomy and thrombus in unstable angina.[77] To be an effective adjunct to laser angioplasty, the angioscope must have enough tip articulation so

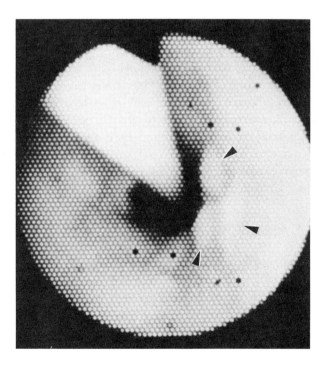

Figure 3. *Angioscopic image of a rabbit aorta. The raised areas around the wall are atherosclerotic fatty deposits, showing mild irregularity of the lumen. In the upper left quadrant is a 400 micron laser fiber passing through the aorta.*

that the geometry of the plaque and its relationship to the diseased vessel lumen can be identified and the laser beam precisely directed at the target. At present, angioscopes small enough to be used in diseased coronary arteries do not have this degree of tip control.

Ultrasound Guidance

Perhaps more interesting is the use of ultrasound imaging to assess the geometry and distribution of atherosclerotic lesions and the composition of plaque. Preliminary studies suggest that both three-dimensional geometry and plaque composition can be accurately determined by intravascular imaging with small ultrasound catheters.[78,79] This could be of enormous benefit for any of the laser systems described, as well as for a number of non-laser atherectomy devices and stents that are under current investigation. A further possibility is the use of ultrasound for plaque ablation.[80] The ultrasound catheter could then be used both for the diagnosis (detection, localization, composition) and for the angioplasty. Other possible techniques include acoustic and plasma-guided systems.[81]

LASER ABLATION OF THROMBUS

A possible laser application may be vaporization of intravascular thrombus as well as atherosclerotic plaque. Laser energy might be an alternative to the combination of thrombolytic therapy followed by PTCA in acute coronary syndromes. The thrombus initiating the ischemic event could be vaporized, followed by definitive laser therapy of the underlying lesion. Preliminary data suggest that highly selective laser ablation of a thrombus is possible, at least in vitro.[82] These interesting findings require additional study, but may be applicable in venous thrombosis and pulmonary embolism in the coronary arteries in patients with unstable angina and acute myocardial infarction.

ARRHYTHMIA ABLATION

Operative intervention for intractable life-threatening ventricular arrhythmias has been performed for more than a decade, with relatively good success in this particularly high risk patient population. Procedures have included endocardial excision,[83] encircling ventriculotomy[84] and cryotherapy.[85] Endocardial mapping has significantly enhanced the success of such interventions.[86] Cryotherapy has become the preferred technique, but the rather large cryoprobe and the nature of the freezing process dictate that the injury is difficult to confine to a precise region, and the cryoprobe cannot easily be applied in some locations in the ventricle. These limitations have led to the use of laser energy as an alternative mechanism for destruction of arrhythmogenic myocardium. Preliminary studies have shown that laser energy can produce either

506

vaporization of myocardium or coagulation necrosis with subsequent scarring, and that the degree of injury is highly predictable based on the amount of laser energy delivered.[87-91]

The application of the laser is performed using a flexible fiber, with a spot size of 2-3 mm up to 2 cm depending upon the distance of the fiber tip from the tissue. This system allows the energy to be directed very precisely to the target myocardium. The area treated can be carefully controlled by movement of the laser beam, and the depth of injury controlled by the amount of energy applied. In animal studies, one-half to full-thickness coagulation necrosis injury was produced without vaporization of myocardium, perforation or aneurysm formation.[92]

Laser therapy for intractable ventricular arrhythmias in humans is in the investigational stage. Initial reports, however, have been quite favorable.[93,94] At the time of open heart surgery, ventricular tachycardia is induced by programmed electrical stimulation. The electrical activity of the epicardium and endocardium is then mapped to identify the apparent source(s) of the ventricular tachycardia. Following source identification, the area is treated with the laser beam.

Svenson et al[95] found that the surface area of endocardium which needs to be treated in order to ablate the arrhythmia source is 12.6 ± 1.9 cm^2. In a subgroup in which more precise electrophysiologic mapping was possible, irradiation of 6.7 ± 1.1 cm^2 of tissue was required for termination of the arrhythmias.[95] Their protocol uses the Nd:YAG laser and photocoagulation of the myocardium as the treatment methodology. In 17 patients with 55 ventricular tachycardia morphologies, success was obtained with 52/55 morphologies. Surgical mortality was 11.7%, compared to a range of 9-36% which they found on a review of the literature. Saksena et al[94] reported on 5 patients with 7 ventricular tachycardia morphologies. An Argon laser was employed, and the endocardium was vaporized rather than photocoagulated. The endocardial vaporization technique is anatomically similar to surgical endocardial excision by scalpel, whereas photocoagulation produces coagulation necrosis with subsequent scarring, which is similar to the injury produced by cryotherapy. In spite of the differences in technique, the results were similar. Saksena et al eliminated the 7 morphologies in their 5 patients. Thus, both series, while small and preliminary, reported a very high degree of success. Saksena et al[94] also studied the effect of laser surgery on left ventricular ejection fraction, cardiac index and pulmonary artery wedge pressure, and found no change from preoperative values. Svenson et al[93] found no change in ejection fraction in their patients.

While the addition of laser during open-heart surgery has been valuable, the operative mortality, morbidity, and cost are significant. Laser application to the endocardium by cardiac catheterization has therefore been suggested as an alternative delivery technique.[96-99]

REFERENCES

1. Abela GS, Normann SJ, Cohen DM, et al: Laser recanalization of occluded atherosclerotic arteries in vivo and in vitro. Circulation 1985;71:403-411.

2. Choy DSJ, Stertzer S, Myler RK, et al: Human coronary laser recanalization. Clin Cardiol 1984;7:377-381.

3. Ginzburg R, Kim OS, Gunthaner D, et al: Salvage of an ischemic limb by laser angioplasty:description of a new technique. Clin Cardiol 1984;7:54-58.

4. Lee G, Ikeda RM, Kozina J, et al: Laser-dissolution of coronary atherosclerotic obstruction. Am Heart J l981;102:1074-1075.

5. Abela GS, Normann S, Cohen D, et al: Effects of carbon dioxide, Nd:YAG and argon laser radiation on coronary atheromatous plaques. Am J Cardiol 1982;50:1199-1204.

6. Eldar M, Battler A, Neufeld HN, et al: Transluminal carbon dioxide-laser catheter angioplasty for dissolution of atherosclerotic plaques. J Am Coll Cardiol 1984;3:135-137.

7. Livesay JJ, Cooley DA. Laser coronary endarterectomy: proposed treatment for diffuse coronary atherosclerosis. Tex Heart Inst J 1984;11:276-279.

8. Lee G, Ikeda RM, Theis JH, et al: Acute and chronic complications of laser angioplasty:Vascular wall damage and formation of aneurysms in the atherosclerotic rabbit. Am J Cardiol 1984;53:290-293.

9. Crea F, Fenech A, Smith W, et al: Laser recanalization of acutely thrombosed coronary arteries in live dogs: Early results. J Am Coll Cardiol 1985;6:1052-1056.

10. Isner JM, Donaldson RF, Funai JT, et al: Factors contributing to perforations resulting from laser coronary angioplasty: Observations in an intact human postmortem preparation of intraoperative laser coronary angioplasty. Circulation 1985;72(suppl II):191-199.

11. Choy DSJ, Stertzer S, Loubeau JM, et al: Embolization and vessel wall perforation in argon laser recanalization. Lasers Surg Med 1985;5:297-308.

12. Abela GS, Crea F, Smith W, et al: In vitro effects of argon laser radiation on blood. Quantitative and morphologic analysis. J Am Coll Cardiol 1985;5:231-237.

13. Isner JM, Clarke RH, Donaldson RF, et al: Identification of photo-products liberated by in vitro argon irradiation of atherosclerotic plaque, calcified cardiac valves, and myocardium. Am J Cardiol 1985;55:1192-1196.

14. Case RB, Choy DSJ, Dwyer EM, et al: Absence of distal emboli during in vivo laser recanalization. Lasers Surg Med 1985;5:281-289.

15. Grewe DD, Castaneda-Zuniga WR, Nordstrom LA, et al: Debris analysis after laser photorecanalization of atherosclerotic plaque. Semin Inter Radiol 1986;3:53-60.

16. Lee G, Ikeda RM, Chan MC, et al: Dissolution of human atherosclerotic disease by fiber optic laser heated metallic tip. Am Heart J 1984;107:777-778.

17. Abela GS, Fenech A, Crea F, et al: "Hot Tip": Another method of laser vascular recanalization. Lasers Surg Med 1985;5:327-335.

18. Sanborn TA, Faxon DP, Haudenschild CC, et al: Experimental Angioplasty: Circumferential distribution of laser thermal energy with a laser probe. J Am Coll Cardiol 1985; 5:934-938.

19. Cumberland DC, Sanborn TA, Tayler DI, et al: Percutaneous laser thermal angioplasty: Initial clinical results with a laser probe in total peripheral artery occlusions. Lancet 1986;i:1457-1459.

20. Sanborn TA, Greenfield AJ, Guben JK, et al: Human percutaneous and intraoperative laser thermal angioplasty: Initial clinical results as an adjunct to balloon angioplasty. J Vasc Surg 1987;5:83-90.

21. White RA, White GH, Vlasak J, et al: Histopathology of human laser thermal angioplasty recanalization. Lasers Surg Med 1988;8:469-476.

22. Diethrich EB, Timbadia Ej, Bahadir I, et al: Argon laser-assisted peripheral angioplasty. Vasc Surg 1988;22:77-87.

23. Tobis JM, Smolin M, Mallery J, et al: Laser assisted thermal angioplasty in human peripheral occlusions: mechanism of recanalization. J Am Coll Cardiol 1989;13:1547-1554.

24. Vincent GM, Johnson M, Fox J, et al: Thermal laser contact probe angioplasty. Influence of constant tip temperature. Circulation 1988;78:II-504.

25. Diethrich EB, Timbadia E, Bahadir I. Applications and limitations of laser-assisted angioplasty. Eur J Vasc Surg 1989;3:61-70.

26. Sanborn TA, Cumberland DC, Greenfield AJ, et al: Percutaneous laser thermal angioplasty: Initial results and 1-year follow-up in 129 femoropopliteal lesions. Radiology 1988;168:121-125.

27. Cumberland DC, Belli AM, Myler RK, et al: Combined laser/thermal recanalization of peripheral artery occlusions. J Am Coll Cardiol 1989;13:13A.

28. Seeger JM, Abela GS: Laser recanalization in high risk patients. Lasers Surg Med 1989(suppl 1);1:8.

29. Dixon SH, Harding GS: The "Laserprobe" and peripheral vascular surgery. Lasers Surg Med 1988;8:151.

30. Labs JD, White RI, Anderson JH, et al: Laser thrombectomy and arterial prosthetic graft recanalization. Surg Forum 1987;38:326-328.

31. Seeger JM, Abela GS, Klingman N: Laser radiation in the treatment of prosthetic graft stenosis. J Vasc Surg 1987;6:221-225.

32. Grundfest W, Litvack F, Hickey A, et al: Radiofrequency thermal angioplasty for the treatment of peripheral vascular occlusive disease: Preliminary results of a clinical trial. J Am Coll Cardiol 1989;13:14A.

33. Nordstrom LA, Castaneda-Zuniga, Grewe DD, et al: Laser-enhanced transluminal angioplasty: The role of coaxial fiber placement. Semin Int Radiol 1986;3:47-52.

34. Richter EI: Laser Angioplasty: Clinical results from Germany. Lastext 1989;1:7-8.

35. Nordstrom LA: Laser-enhanced angioplasty: The use of direct argon exposure as an alternative to contact probe plaque ablation. Lasers Surg Med 1988;8:151.

36. Foschi AE, Myers GE, Flamm D: Laser-enhanced coronary angioplasty via direct argon laser exposures: Early clinical results in totally occluded native arteries. Circulation 1989;80:II-478.

37. Cumberland DC, Starkey IR, Oakley GDG, et al: Percutaneous laser assisted coronary angioplasty. Lancet 1986;ii:214.

38. Crea F, Davies G, McKenna W, et al: Percutaneous laser recanalization of coronary arteries. Lancet 1986;ii:214-215.

39. Sanborn TA, Faxon DP, Kellett MA, et al: Percutaneous coronary laser thermal angioplasty. J Am Coll Cardiol 1986;8:1437-1440.

40. Kittrell C, Willett RL, de los Santos-Pacheo DLK, et al: Diagnosis of fibrous arterial atherosclerosis using fluorescence. Appl Optics 1985;24:2280-2281.

41. Deckelbaum LI, Lam JK, Cabin HS, et al: Discrimination of normal and atherosclerotic aorta by laser-induced fluorescence. Lasers Surg Med 1987;7:330-335.

42. Gmitro AF, Cutruzzola FW, Stetz ML, et al: Measurement depth of laser-induced tissue fluorescence with application to laser angioplasty. Appl Optics 1988;27:1844-1849.

43. Deckelbaum LI, Sarembok IJ, Stetz ML, et al: In-vivo fluorescence spectroscopy of normal and atherosclerotic arteries. Optical Fibers Med III 1988;906:314-319.

44. Gaffney EJ, Clarke RH, Lucas AR, et al: Correlation of fluorescence emission with the plaque content and intimal thickness of atherosclerotic coronary arteries. Lasers Surg Med 1989;9:215-228.

45. Cutruzzola FW, Stetz ML, O'Brien KM, et al: Change in laser-induced arterial fluorescence during ablation of atherosclerotic plaque. Lasers Surg Med 1989;9:109-116.

46. Deckelbaum LI, Stetz ML, O'Brien KM, et al: Fluorescence spectroscopy guidance of laser ablation of atherosclerotic plaque. Lasers Surg Med 1989;9:205-214.

47. Prince MR, Deutsch TF, Mathews-Roth MM, et al: Preferential light absorption in atheromas in vitro. J Clin Invest 1986;78:295-302.

48. Orme EC, McClane RW, Straight RC: Absorption coefficient analysis of in vitro human normal and atherosclerotic arteries. Lasers Surg Med 1989(suppl 1);9:12.

49. Geschwind HJ, Dubois-Rande JL, Shafton E, et al: Percutaneous pulsed laser-assisted balloon angioplasty guided by spectroscopy. Am Heart J 1989;117:1147-1152.

50. Laufer G, Wollenek G, Hohla K, et al: Excimer laser-induced simultaneous ablation and spectral identification of normal and atherosclerotic arterial tissue layers. Circulation 1988;78:1031-1039.

51. Cowley MJ, Dorros G, Kelsey SF, et al: Acute coronary events associated with percutaneous coronary angioplasty. Am J Cardiol 1984;53(suppl):12C-16C.

52. Detre K, Holubkov R, Kelsey S, et al: Percutaneous transluminal coronary angioplasty in 1985-1986 and 1977-1981. N Engl J Med 1988;318:265-270.

53. Holmes DR, Vlietstra RE, Smith HC, et al: Restenosis after percutaneous transluminal coronary angioplasty (PTCA): A report from the PTCA registry of the National Heart, Lung, and Blood Institute. Am J Cardiol 1984;53(suppl):77C-81C.

54. Serruys PW, Luitjen HE, Beatt KJ, et al: Incidence of restenosis after successful coronary angioplasty: A time-related phenomenon. A quantitative angiographic study in 342 consecutive patients at one, two, three, and four months. Circulation 1988;77:361-371.

55. Hiehle JF, Bourgelais BD, Shapshay S, et al: Nd:YAG fusion of human atheromatous plaque-arterial wall separations in vitro. Am J Cardiol 1985;56:953-957.

56. Jenkins RD, Sinclair IN, Leonard BM, et al: Laser balloon angioplasty versus balloon angioplasty in normal rabbit iliac arteries. Lasers Surg Med 1989;9:237-247.

57. Mast G, Plokker T, Bal E, et al: Laser balloon angioplasty does not reduce restenosis rate in type A and type B coronary lesions. Circulation 1990;82:III-312.

58. Reis GJ, Pomerantz RM, Jenkins RD, et al: Laser balloon angioplasty: clinical, angiographic and histologic results. Circulation 1990;82:III-672.

59. Grundfest WS, Litvack F, Forrester JS, et al: Laser ablation of human atherosclerotic plaque without adjacent tissue injury. J Am Coll Cardiol 1985;5:929-933.

60. Isner JM, Donaldson RF, Deckelbaum LI, et al: The excimer laser: Gross, light microscopic and ultrastructural analysis of potential advantages for use in laser therapy of cardiovascular disease. J Am Coll Cardiol 1985;6:1102-1109.

61. Wollenek G, Laufer G, Grabenwoger F: Percutaneous transluminal excimer laser angioplasty in total peripheral artery occlusion in man. Lasers Surg Med 1988;8:464-468.

62. Litvack F, Grundfest W, Adler L, et al: Percutaneous excimer laser angioplasty in humans. Circulation 1988;78:II-295.

63. Reeder GS, Bresnahan JF, Bresnahan DR: Excimer laser coronary angioplasty (ELCA) in patients with restenosis after prior balloon angioplasty (BA). Circulation 1990;82:III-672 (abstract).

64. Haase KK, Mauser M, Baumbach A, et al: Restenosis after excimer laser coronary atherectomy. Circulation 1990;82:III-672 (abstract).

65. Spears JR, Serur J, Shropshire D, et al: Fluorescence of experimental atheromatous plaques with hematoporphyrin derivative. J Clin Invest 1983;71:395-399.

66. Litvack F, Grundfest W, Forrester JS, et al: Effects of hematoporphyrin derivative and photodynamic therapy on atherosclerotic rabbits. J Am Coll Cardiol 1985;6:667-671.

67. Kessel D, Sykes E: Porphyrin accumulation by atheromatous plaques of the aorta. Photochem Photobiol 1984;40:59-61.

68. Vincent GM, Fox J, Scuderi L, et al: Laser photodynamic therapy and quantitative hematoporphyrin levels in swine atherosclerotic plaque. Circulation 1985;72:III-303.

69. Johnson M, Fox JB, Hammond EM, et al: In vitro removal of photosensitized rabbit atherosclerotic plaque by dye laser irradiation. Laser Institute of America ICALEO '87. Laser Res Med 1987;60:13-17.

70. Vincent GM, Mackie RW, Orme E, et al: In vivo photosensitizer enhanced laser angioplasty in atherosclerotic yucatan miniswine. J Am Coll Cardiol 1989;13:43A.

71. Murphy-Chutorian D, Kosek J, Mok W, et al: Selective absorption of ultraviolet laser energy by human atherosclerotic plaque treated with tetracycline. Am J Cardiol 1985; 55:1293-1297.

72. Lafont A, Avrillier S, Fabiani JN, et al: Is tetracycline able to guide excimer laser angioplasty by laser-induced fluorescence? Circulation 1990;82:III-104.

73. Spears JR, Marais HJ, Serur J, et al: In vivo coronary angioscopy. J Am Coll Cardiol 1983; 115:1311-1314.

74. Vincent GM, Fox J: Cardiovascular endoscopy. Cardiovascular Reviews and Reports 1985;6:1227-1234.

75. Litvack F, Grundfest WS, Lee ME, et al: Angioscopic visualization of blood vessel interior in animals and humans. Clin Cardiol 1985;8:65-70.

76. Abela GS, Seeger JM, Barbieri E, et al: Laser angioplasty with angioscopic guidance in humans. J Am Coll Cardiol 1986;8:184-192.

77. Sherman CT, Litvack F, Grundfest W, et al: Coronary angioscopy in patients with unstable angina pectoris. N Engl J Med 1986;315:913-919.

78. Pandian N, Dreis A, O'Donnell T, et al: Intraluminal two-dimensional ultrasound angioscopic quantitation of arterial stenosis: Comparisons with external high-frequency ultrasound imaging and anatomy. J Am Coll Cardiol 1989;13:5A.

79. Chandraratna PAN, Jones JP, Rahimtoola SH, et al: Evaluation of mixed atherosclerotic plaques by quantitative ultrasonic methods. J Am Coll Cardiol 1989;13:5A

80. Siegel RJ, Fishbein MC, Forrester J, et al: Ultrasonic plaque ablation. A new method for recanalization of partially or totally occluded arteries. Circulation 1988;78:1443-1448.

81. Bhatta KM, Rosen DI, Dretler SP: Acoustic and plasma-guided laser angioplasty. Lasers Surg Med 1989;9:117-123.

82. LaMuraglia GM, Anderson R, Parrish JA, et al: Selective laser ablation of venous thrombus: Implications for a new approach in the treatment of pulmonary embolus. Laser Surg Med 1988;8:486-493.

83. Josephson M, Harken AH, Horowitz LN: Endocardial excision, a new surgical technique for treatment of recurrent ventricular tachycardia. Circulation 1979;60:1430-1439.

84. Holman W, Ikeshita M, Douglas J, et al: Ventricular cryosurgery: short-term effects on intramural electrophysiology. Ann Thorac Surg 1983;35:386-393.

85. Camm J, Ward D, Cory-Pearce R, et al: The successful cryosurgical treatment of paroxysmal ventricular tachycardia. Chest 1979;75:621-624.

86. Gallagher J, Kassell J, Cox J, et al: Techniques of intraoperative electrophysiologic mapping. Am J Cardiol 1982;49:221-240.

87. Lee G, Ikeda RM, Theis J, et al: Effects of laser irradiation delivered by flexible fiber-optic system on the left ventricular internal myocardium. Am Heart J 1983;106: 587-590.

88. Isner JM, Michlowitz H, Clarke RH, et al: Laser photoablation of pathological endocardium: In vitro findings suggesting a new approach to the surgical treatment of refractory arrhythmias and restrictive cardiomyopathy. Ann Thorac Surg 1985;39:201-206.

89. Vincent GM, Knowlton K, Lee RG, et al: Effects of Nd:YAG laser on myocardial and valvular tissue. Dosimetry and gross and microscopic anatomy. J Am Coll Cardiol 1984; 3:536.

90. Saksena S, Ciccone JM, Chandran P, et al: Laser ablation of normal and diseased human ventricle. Am Heart J 1986;112:52-60.

91. Downar E, Butany J, Jares A, et al: Endocardial photoablation by excimer laser. J Am Coll Cardiol 1986;7:546-550.

92. Vincent GM, Fox J, Knowlton K, et al: Catheter-directed neodymium:YAG laser injury of the left ventricle for arrhythmia ablation: Dosimetry and hemodynamic, hematologic, and electrophysiologic effects. Lasers Surg Med 1989;9:446-453.

93. Svenson RH, Gallagher JJ, Selle JG, et al: Neodymium:YAG laser photocoagulation: A successful new map-guided technique for the intraoperative ablation of ventricular tachycardia. Circulation 1987;76:1319-1328.

94. Saksena S, Hussain M, Gielchinsky I, et al: Intraoperative mapping-guided argon laser ablation of malignant ventricular tachycardia. Am J Cardiol 1987;59:78-83.

95. Svenson RH, Gallagher JJ, Zimmern S, et al: Intraoperative Nd:YAG laser photocoagulative ablation of ventricular tachycardia: Observations relevant to transcatheter ablation techniques. J Am Coll Cardiol 1987;9:249A.

96. Vincent GM, Fox J, Benedick BA, et al: Laser catheter ablation of simulated ventricular tachycardia. Laser Surg Med 1987;7:421-425.

97. Lee BI, Gottdiener JS, Fletcher RD, et al: Trans-catheter ablation: Comparison between laser photoablation and electrode shock ablation in the dog. Circulation 1985;71:579-583.

98. Lee BI, Rodriquez ER, Notargiacoma A, et al: Thermal effects of laser and electrical discharge on cardiovascular tissue: Implications for coronary artery recanalization and endocardial ablation. J Am Coll Cardiol 1986;8:192-200.

99. Saksena S, Lim F, Prasher S, et al: Feasibility of trans-catheter argon laser ablation for ventricular tachycardia. Circulation 1987;76:IV-278.

INDEX

ABOUT THE EDITOR

Jeffrey L. Anderson is Professor of Internal Medicine (Cardiology) at the University of Utah Medical School, and Chief of the Division of Cardiology at LDS Hospital, Salt Lake City, Utah. The author or coauthor of over 260 journal articles, book chapters, and abstracts, and the editor of two books, he is a Fellow of the American College of Cardiology, American College of Physicians, Council on Clinical Cardiology of the American Heart Association, and American College of Chest Physicians, and a member of the American Society for Clinical Investigation, American Medical Association, and American Heart Association, among others. Dr. Anderson received the B.A. degree (1968) in chemistry from the University of Utah, Salt Lake City, and the M.D. degree (1972) from the Harvard Medical School, Boston, Massachusetts.